Roitt's Essential Immunology

Ivan M. Roitt

MA, DSc(Oxon), FRDPath, Hon FRCP(Lond), FRS
Emeritus Professor, Department of Immunology and Molecular Pathology,
University College London,
London W1T 4JF

Peter J. Delves

PhD
Department of Immunology and Molecular Pathology,
University College London,
London W1T 4JF

Blackwell
Science

© 1971, 1974, 1977, 1980, 1984, 1988, 1991, 1994, 1997, 2001 by Blackwell Science Ltd
a Blackwell Publishing company
Blackwell Science, Inc., 350 Main Street, Malden, Massachusetts 02148-5018, USA
Blackwell Science Ltd, 9600 Garsington Road, Oxford OX4 2DQ, UK
Blackwell Science Asia Pty Ltd, 550 Swanston Street, Carlton, Victoria 3053, Australia

The right of the Authors to be identified as the Authors of this Work has been asserted in accordance with the Copyright, Designs and Patents Act 1988.

First published 1971
Reprinted 1972 (twice), 1973 (twice)
Second edition 1974, Reprinted 1975
Third edition 1977, Reprinted 1978, 1979
Fourth edition 1980, Reprinted 1982, 1983
Fifth edition 1984
Sixth edition 1988, Reprinted 1988, 1989
Seventh edition 1991
Eighth edition 1994, Reprinted 1996
Ninth edition 1997, Reprinted 1999
Tenth edition 2001, Reprinted 2003

Spanish editions 1972, 1975, 1978, 1982, 1988, 1989, 1993
Italian editions 1973, 1975, 1979, 1986, 1988, 1990, 1993, 1995

Portuguese editions 1973, 1979, 1983
French editions 1975, 1979, 1990
Dutch editions 1975, 1978, 1982
Japanese editions 1976, 1978, 1982, 1986, 1988
German editions 1977, 1984, 1988, 1993
Polish edition 1977
Greek editions 1978, 1989, 1992
Turkish edition 1979
Slovak edition 1981
Indonesian editions 1985, 1991
Russian edition 1988
Korean edition 1991
ELBS editions 1977, 1982, 1988, Reprinted 1991
Chinese (Taiwan) editions 1991, 1994

Library of Congress Cataloging-in-Publication Data

Roitt, Ivan M. (Ivan Maurice)
   Roitt's essential immunology / Ivan M. Roitt, Peter J. Delves. — 10th ed.
       p.; cm.
   Includes bibliographical references and index.
   ISBN 0-632-05902-8 (pbk.)
     1. Immunology.
     I. Title: Essential immunology. II. Delves, Peter J. III. Title.
   [DNLM: 1. Immune System.
   2. Immunity.
   QW 504 R719e 2001]
   QR181 .R57   2001
   616.07′9 — dc21

                                                    2001025562

ISBN 0-632-05902-8

A catalogue record for this title is available from the British Library

Set by SNP Best-set Typesetter Ltd., Hong Kong
Printed and bound in India by Replika Press Pvt. Ltd, Kundli 131028

For further information on Blackwell Science, visit our website:
www.blackwellpublishing.com

Contents

Acknowledgements

The input of the editorial team of Nick Morgan, Meg Barton and Fiona Goodgame at Blackwell Science, the illustrator Graeme Chambers and the indefatigable secretarial assistance of Christine Griffin is warmly acknowledged. Wise counsel was provided by Kirsten Fischer Lindahl, Jurg Tschopp and Helen Turner concerning aspects of MHC gene organization, apoptosis and IgE receptor signaling respectively. We are much indebted to the co-editors of *Immunology*, J. Brostoff and D. Male, together with the publishers, Harcourt Health Sciences, and the following individuals for permission to utilize or modify their figures: J. Brostoff and A. Hall for figures 1.15 and 16.10; J. Horton for figure 12.20; G. Rook for figures 13.5 and 13.12; and J. Taverne for figure 13.21 and table 13.1.

Every effort has been made by the authors and the publisher to contact all the copyright holders to obtain their permission to reproduce copyright material. However, if any have been inadvertently overlooked, the publisher will be pleased to make the necessary arrangements at the first opportunity.

A number of scientists very generously provided illustrations for inclusion in this edition, and we have acknowledged our gratitude to them in the relevant figure legends.

Preface

It is now 30 years since the 1st Edition of *Essential Immunology* appeared, and it seemed that the time was now appropriate for the task of producing the 10th Edition to be shared. The new co-author, Peter Delves, has been a close colleague of Professor Roitt for many years and is a highly experienced teacher.

A wide range of subjects have been extensively revised, restructured or updated, and advanced material is included in the figure legends to avoid disruption of the basic text. These subjects include:

- dendritic cells
- intraepithelial lymphocytes
- NK-T and γδ T-cells
- NK receptors
- receptor editing relating to receptor diversity
- non-classical MHC and the presentation of non-peptidic antigens
- the role of chaperone proteins in antigen processing
- T-cell recognition of peptide–MHC reflecting the latest crystallographic studies
- arrays for analysis of gene expression
- tetramer evaluation of antigen-specific T-cells
- experimental genetic manipulation using conditional 'knockouts' employing the Lox/Cre system and 'knockins' to replace endogenous genes
- B- and T-cell signaling pathways and the role of adaptor proteins
- cytokine physiology
- chemokines and their receptors
- memory cells
- intimate links of innate and adaptive immunity
- the role of complement in modulating the adaptive immune response
- regulatory T-cells
- activation-induced cell death
- neuroendocrine influences on the immune system
- critical role of *Pax 5* in B-cell differentiation
- molecular basis of thymic development
- signaling through pattern recognition systems
- prions

- viral hijacking of host processes as evasion mechanisms
- DNA vaccines
- mucosal adjuvants
- 'shot gun' approach to identification of vaccine candidates
- primary immunodeficiency including IL-7 receptor mutation, and deficiency of *VDJ* recombination in severe combined immunodeficiency
- CCR5 co-receptor for HIV infection of cells
- the importance of highly active anti-retroviral drug therapy and of healthy CD8 response dependent on robust CD4 Th1 effectors in control of HIV infection
- pivotal role of IgE antibodies in pathogenesis of asthma and atopic dermatitis, and remarkable therapeutic benefit of monoclonal anti-IgE
- the excessive hygiene hypothesis related to the development of allergy
- the role of Fcγ receptors in the pathogenesis of type II and III hypersensitivities
- suppression of graft rejection by synergy between fungal metabolites and other drugs and by induction of antigen-specific tolerance with high-dose bone marrow transplantation combined with co-stimulatory blockade by anti-CD40L and CTLA-4-Ig
- engineering grafts from recipient cells
- the role of hsp70 and 90 in natural and induced tumor immunity
- peptide priming of dendritic cells to provoke anti-cancer cytotoxic responses
- the avoidance of graft vs. host disease in allogeneic bone marrow transplantation for leukemias
- inhibition of B-cell lymphomas and tumor angiogenesis by radiolabeled monoclonals
- thymic expression of some organ-specific antigens
- role of autoimmunity to hsp65 in atherosclerosis
- autologous stem cell transplantation after cytotoxic ablative therapy for some cases of SLE, scleroderma and juvenile rheumatoid arthritis.

All in all, quite a mouthful!

Abbreviations

Ab	antibody
ACh-R	acetylcholine receptor
ACTH	adrenocorticotropic hormone
ADA	adenosine deaminase
ADCC	antibody-dependent cellular cytotoxicity
Ag	antigen
AIDS	acquired immunodeficiency syndrome
ANCA	antineutrophil cytoplasmic antibodies
APC	antigen-presenting cell
ARRE-1	antigen receptor response element-1
ARRE-2	antigen receptor response element-2
AZT	zidovudine (3′-azido-3′-deoxythymidine)
B-cell	lymphocyte which matures in bone marrow
BCG	bacille Calmette–Guérin attenuated form of tuberculosis
BCR	B-cell receptor
BM	bone marrow
BSA	bovine serum albumin
BUDR	bromodeoxyuridine
C	complement
$C\alpha(\beta/\gamma/\delta)$	constant part of TCR $\alpha(\beta/\gamma/\delta)$ chain
CALLA	common acute lymphoblastic leukemia antigen
cAMP	cyclic adenosine monophosphate
CCP	complement control protein repeat
CD	cluster of differentiation
CDR	complementarity determining regions of Ig or TCR variable portion
CEA	carcinoembryonic antigen
CFA	complete Freund's adjuvant
cGMP	cyclic guanosine monophosphate
$C_{H(L)}$	constant part of Ig heavy (light) chain
CMI	cell-mediated immunity
CML	cell-mediated lympholysis
CMV	cytomegalovirus
Cn	complement component 'n'
Cñ	activated complement component 'n'
iCn	inactivated complement component 'n'
Cna	small peptide derived by proteolytic activation of Cn
CpG	guanosine–cytosine
CR(n)	complement receptor 'n'
CRP	C-reactive protein
CsA	cyclosporin A
CSF	cerebrospinal fluid
D gene	diversity minigene joining V and J segments to form variable region
DAF	decay accelerating factor
DAG	diacylglycerol
DC	dendritic cells
DNP	dinitrophenyl
DTP	diphtheria, tetanus, pertussis triple vaccine
EAE	experimental allergic encephalomyelitis
EBV	Epstein–Barr virus
ELISA	enzyme-linked immunosorbent assay
EM	electron microscope
Eϕ	eosinophil
ER	endoplasmic reticulum
ES	embryonic stem (cell)
F(B)	factor (B, etc.)
Fab	monovalent Ig antigen-binding fragment after papain digestion
F(ab′)$_2$	divalent antigen-binding fragment after pepsin digestion
FACS	fluorescence-activated cell sorter
Fc	Ig crystallisable-fragment originally; now non-Fab part of Ig
FcγR	receptor for IgG Fc fragment
FDC	follicular dendritic cells
(sc)Fv	(single chain) V_H–V_L antigen binding fragment
G	granulocyte
g.b.m.	glomerular basement membrane
GM-CSF	granulocyte–macrophage colony-stimulating factor
gp*n*	*n*kDa glycoprotein
g.v.h.	graft versus host
H-2	the mouse major histocompatibility complex
H-2D/K/L	main loci for classical class I (class II)
(A/E)	murine MHC molecules
HAMA	human antimouse antibodies
HBsAg	hepatitis B surface antigen
hCG	human chorionic gonadotropin
HEV	high walled endothelium of post capillary venule
Hi	high
HIV-1(2)	human immunodeficiency virus-1 (2)
HLA	the human major histocompatibility complex
HLA-A/B/C	main loci for classical class I (class II)
(DP/DQ/DR)	human MHC molecules
HRF	homologous restriction factor
HSA	heat-stable antigen
hsp	heat-shock protein
5HT	5-hydroxytryptamine
HTLV	human T-cell leukemia virus
H-Y	male transplantation antigen

ICAM-1	intercellular adhesion molecule-1	NADP	nicotinamide adenine dinucleotide phosphate
Id (αId)	idiotype (anti-idiotype)	NAP	neutrophil activating peptide
IDC	interdigitating dendritic cells	NBT	nitro blue tetrazolium
IDDM	insulin-dependent diabetes mellitus	NCF	neutrophil chemotactic factor
IFNα	α-interferon (also IFNβ, IFNγ)	NFAT	nuclear factor of activated T-cells
Ig	immunoglobulin	NFκB	nuclear transcription factor
IgG	immunoglobulin G (also IgM, IgA, IgD, IgE)	NK	natural killer cell
sIg	surface immunoglobulin	NO·	nitric oxide
IgM-α/Ig-β	membrane peptide chains associated with sIgM B-cell receptor	NOD	Nonobese diabetic mouse
		NZB	New Zealand Black mouse
IgSF	immunoglobulin superfamily	NZB × W	New Zealand Black mouse × NZ White F1 hybrid
IL-1	interleukin-1 (also IL-2, IL-3, etc.)	$\cdot O_2^-$	superoxide anion
iNOS	inducible nitric oxide synthase	OD	optical density
IP_3	inositol triphosphate	ORF	open reading frame
ISCOM	immunostimulating complex	OS	obese strain chicken
ITAM	immunoreceptor tyrosine-based activation motif	Ova	ovalbumin
ITIM	immunoreceptor tyrosine-based inhibitory motif	PAF(-R)	platelet activating factor (-receptor)
		PCA	passive cutaneous anaphylaxis
ITP	idiopathic thrombocytopenic purpura	PCR	polymerase chain reaction
JAK	Janus kinases	PG(E)	prostaglandin (E etc.)
J chain	peptide chain in IgA dimer and IgM	PHA	phytohemagglutinin
J gene	joining gene linking V or D segment to constant region	phox	phagocyte oxidase
		PIP_2	phosphatidylinositol diphosphate
Ka(d)	association (dissociation) affinity constant (usually Ag–Ab reactions)	PKC	protein kinase C
		PLC	phospholipase C
kDa	units of molecular mass in kilo Daltons	PMN	polymorphonuclear neutrophil
KLH	keyhole limpet hemocyanin	PMT	photomultiplier tube
LAK	lymphocyte activated killer cell	PNH	paroxysmal nocturnal hemoglobinuria
LATS	long-acting thyroid stimulator	PPD	purified protein derivative from *Mycobacterium tuberculosis*
LBP	LPS binding protein		
LCM	lymphocytic choriomeningitis virus	PTK	protein tyrosine kinase
Le$^{a/b/x}$	Lewis$^{a/b/x}$ blood group antigens	PWM	pokeweed mitogen
LFA-1	lymphocyte functional antigen-1	RA	rheumatoid arthritis
LGL	large granular lymphocyte	RANTES	*r*egulated upon *a*ctivation *n*ormal *T*-cell *e*xpressed and *s*ecreted chemokine
LHRH	luteinizing hormone releasing hormone		
LIF	leukemia inhibiting factor	RAST	radioallergosorbent test
Lo	low	RF	rheumatoid factor
LT(B)	leukotriene (B etc.)	Rh(D)	rhesus blood group (D)
LPS	lipopolysaccharide (endotoxin)	ROI	reactive oxygen intermediates
Mφ	macrophage	SAP	serum amyloid P
mAb	monoclonal antibody	SC	Ig secretory component
MAC	membrane attack complex	SCF	stem cell factor
MAdCAM	mucosal addressin cell adhesion molecule	scFv	single chain variable region antibody fragment ($V_H + V_L$ joined by a flexible linker)
MALT	mucosal-associated lymphoid tissue		
MAP kinase	mitogen-activated protein kinase	SCG	sodium cromoglycate
MBP	basic protein of eosinophils (also myelin basic protein)	SCID	severe combined immunodeficiency
		SDS-PAGE	sodium dodecylsulfate–polyacrylamide gel electrophoresis
MC	mast cell		
MCP	membrane cofactor protein (C′ regulation)	SEA(B etc.)	*Staphylococcus aureus* enterotoxin A (B etc.)
MCP-1	monocyte chemotactic protein-1	SIV	Simian immunodeficiency virus
M-CSF	macrophage colony-stimulating factor	SLE	systemic lupus erythematosus
MDP	muramyl dipeptide	SRID	single radial immunodiffusion
MHC	major histocompatibility complex	STAT	signal transducer and activator of transcription
MIF	macrophage migration inhibitory factor	TAP	transporter for antigen processing
MLA	monophosphoryl lipid A	T-ALL	T-acute lymphoblastic leukemia
MLR	mixed lymphocyte reaction	TB	tubercle bacillus
MMTV	mouse mammary tumor virus	Tc	cytotoxic T-cell
MS	multiple sclerosis	T-cell	thymus-derived lymphocyte
MSH	melanocyte stimulating hormone	TCR1(2)	T-cell receptor with γ/δ chains (with α/β chains)
MuLV	murine leukemia virus		

TdT	terminal deoxynucleotidyl transferase	tum–	strongly immunogenic mutant tumors
TG-A-L	polylysine with polyalanyl side-chains randomly tipped with tyrosine and glutamic acid	$V\alpha(\beta/\gamma/\delta)$	variable part of TCR $\alpha(\beta/\gamma/\delta)$ chain
TGFβ	transforming growth factor-β	*V* gene	variable region gene for immunoglobulin or T-cell receptor
Th(1/2)	T-helper cell (subset 1 or 2)	V_H	variable part of Ig heavy chain
Thp	T-helper precursor	VIP	vasoactive intestinal peptide
TLI	total lymphoid irradiation	V_L	variable part of light chain
TM	transmembrane	$V_{\kappa/\lambda}$	variable part of $\kappa(\lambda)$ light chain
TNF	tumor necrosis factor	VCAM	vascular cell adhesion molecule
TNP	trinitrophenol	VLA	very late antigens
Ts	suppressor T-cell	VNTR	variable number of tandem repeats
TSAb	thyroid stimulating antibodies	VP1	virus-specific peptide 1
TSH(R)	thyroid stimulating hormone (receptor)	XL	X-linked

User Guide

Throughout the illustrations standard forms have been used for commonly-occurring cells and pathways. A key to these is given in the figure below.

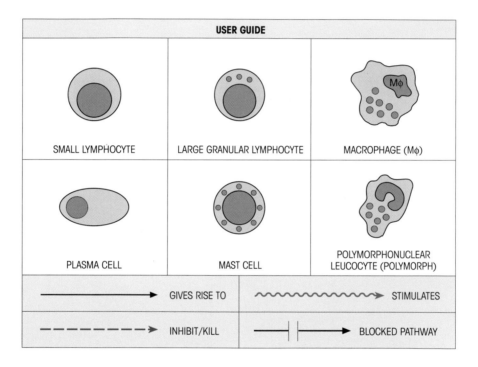

Innate immunity

INTRODUCTION

We live in a potentially hostile world filled with a bewildering array of infectious agents (figure 1.1) of diverse shape, size, composition and subversive character which would very happily use us as rich sanctuaries for propagating their 'selfish genes' had we not also developed a series of defense mechanisms at least their equal in effectiveness and ingenuity (except in the case of many parasitic infections where the situation is best described as an uneasy and often unsatisfactory truce). It is these defense mechanisms which can establish a state of immunity against infection (Latin *immunitas*, freedom from) and whose operation provides the basis for the delightful subject called 'Immunology'.

Aside from ill-understood constitutional factors which make one species innately susceptible and another resistant to certain infections, a number of relatively nonspecific antimicrobial systems (e.g. phagocytosis) have been recognized which are **innate** in the sense that they are not intrinsically affected by prior contact with the infectious agent. We shall discuss these systems and examine how, in the state of **specific acquired immunity**, their effectiveness can be greatly increased.

EXTERNAL BARRIERS AGAINST INFECTION

The simplest way to avoid infection is to prevent the microorganisms from gaining access to the body (figure 1.2). The major line of defense is of course the skin which, when intact, is impermeable to most infectious agents; when there is skin loss, as for example in burns, infection becomes a major problem. Additionally, most bacteria fail to survive for long on the skin because of the direct inhibitory effects of lactic acid and fatty acids in sweat and sebaceous secretions and the low pH which they generate. An exception is *Staphylococcus aureus* which often infects the relatively vulnerable hair follicles and glands.

Mucus, secreted by the membranes lining the inner surfaces of the body, acts as a protective barrier to block the adherence of bacteria to epithelial cells. Microbial and other foreign particles trapped within the adhesive mucus are removed by mechanical stratagems such as ciliary movement, coughing and sneezing. Among other mechanical factors which help protect the epithelial surfaces, one should also include the washing action of tears, saliva and urine. Many of the secreted body fluids contain bactericidal components, such as acid in gastric juice, spermine and zinc in semen, lactoperoxidase in milk and lysozyme in tears, nasal secretions and saliva.

A totally different mechanism is that of microbial

Figure 1.1. **The formidable range of infectious agents which confronts the immune system.** Although not normally classified as such because of their lack of a cell wall, the mycoplasmas are included under bacteria for convenience. Fungi adopt many forms and approximate values for some of the smallest forms are given.]►, range of sizes observed for the organism(s) indicated by the arrow; ◄[, the organisms listed have the size denoted by the arrow.

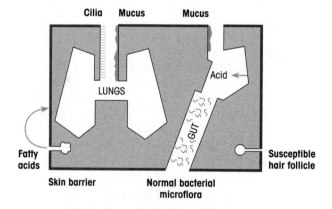

Figure 1.2. **The first lines of defense against infection:** protection at the external body surfaces.

antagonism associated with the normal bacterial flora of the body. This suppresses the growth of many potentially pathogenic bacteria and fungi at superficial sites by competition for essential nutrients or by production of inhibitory substances. To give one example, pathogen invasion is limited by lactic acid produced by particular species of commensal bacteria which metabolize glycogen secreted by the vaginal epithelium. When protective commensals are disturbed by antibiotics, susceptibility to opportunistic infections by *Candida* and *Clostridium difficile* is increased. Gut commensals may also produce colicins, a class of bactericidins which bind to the negatively charged surface of susceptible bacteria and insert a hydrophobic helical hairpin into the membrane; the molecule then

undergoes a 'Jekyll and Hyde' transformation to become completely hydrophobic and forms a voltage-dependent channel in the membrane which kills by destroying the cell's energy potential. Even at this level, survival is a tough game.

If microorganisms do penetrate the body, two main defensive operations come into play, the destructive effect of soluble chemical factors such as bactericidal enzymes and the mechanism of **phagocytosis**—literally 'eating' by the cell (Milestone 1.1).

PHAGOCYTIC CELLS KILL MICROORGANISMS

Neutrophils and macrophages are dedicated 'professional' phagocytes

The engulfment and digestion of microorganisms are assigned to two major cell types recognized by Metchnikoff at the turn of the last century as microphages and macrophages.

The polymorphonuclear neutrophil

This cell, the smaller of the two, shares a common hematopoietic stem cell precursor with the other formed elements of the blood and is the dominant white cell in the bloodstream. It is a nondividing short-lived cell with a multilobed nucleus and an array of granules which are virtually unstained by histologic dyes such as hematoxylin and eosin, unlike those

Milestone 1.1—Phagocytosis

The perceptive Russian zoologist, Elie Metchnikoff (1845–1916), recognized that certain specialized cells mediate defense against microbial infections, so fathering the whole concept of cellular immunity. He was intrigued by the motile cells of transparent starfish larvae and made the critical observation that, a few hours after the introduction of a rose thorn into these larvae, they became surrounded by these motile cells. A year later, in 1883, he observed that fungal spores can be attacked by the blood cells of *Daphnia*, a tiny metazoan which, also being transparent, can be studied directly under the microscope. He went on to extend his investigations to mammalian leukocytes, showing their ability to engulf microorganisms, a process which he termed **phagocytosis**.

Because he found this process to be even more effective in animals recovering from infection, he came to a somewhat polarized view that phagocytosis provided the main, if not the only, defense against infection. He went on to define the existence of two types of circulating phagocytes: the polymorphonuclear leukocyte, which he termed a 'microphage', and the larger 'macrophage'.

Figure M1.1.1. Caricature of Professor Metchnikoff from *Chanteclair*, 1908, No. 4, p. 7. (Reproduction kindly provided by The Wellcome Institute Library, London.)

Figure M1.1.2. Reproductions of some of the illustrations in Metchnikoff's book, *Comparative Pathology of Inflammation* (1893). (a) Four leukocytes from the frog, enclosing anthrax bacilli; some are alive and unstained, others which have been killed have taken up the vesuvine dye and have been colored; (b) drawing of an anthrax bacillus, stained by vesuvine, in a leukocyte of the frog; the two figures represent two phases of movement of the same frog leukocyte which contains stained anthrax bacilli within its phagocytic vacuole; (c and d) a foreign body (colored) in a starfish larva surrounded by phagocytes which have fused to form a multinucleate plasmodium shown at higher power in (d); (e) this gives a feel for the dynamic attraction of the mobile mesenchymal phagocytes to a foreign intruder within a starfish larva.

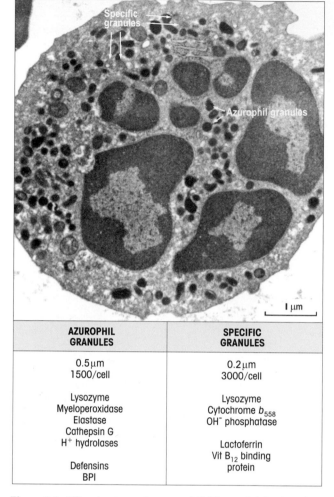

AZUROPHIL GRANULES	SPECIFIC GRANULES
0.5 μm 1500/cell	0.2 μm 3000/cell
Lysozyme Myeloperoxidase Elastase Cathepsin G H^+ hydrolases	Lysozyme Cytochrome b_{558} OH^- phosphatase
Defensins BPI	Lactoferrin Vit B_{12} binding protein

Figure 1.3. Ultrastructure of neutrophil. The multilobed nucleus and two main types of cytoplasmic granules are well displayed. (Courtesy of Dr D. McLaren.)

structures in the closely related eosinophil and basophil (figures 1.3 and 1.4). These neutrophil granules are of two main types: (i) the **primary azurophil granule** which develops early (figure 1.4e), has the typical lysosomal morphology and contains myeloperoxidase together with most of the nonoxidative antimicrobial effectors including defensins, bactericidal permeability increasing (BPI) protein and cathepsin G (figure 1.3), and (ii) the peroxidase-negative **secondary specific granules** containing lactoferrin, much of the lysozyme, alkaline phosphatase (figure 1.4d) and membrane-bound cytochrome b_{558} (figure 1.3). The abundant glycogen stores can be utilized by glycolysis enabling the cells to function under anerobic conditions.

The macrophage

These cells derive from bone marrow promonocytes which, after differentiation to blood monocytes, finally settle in the tissues as mature macrophages where they

constitute the **mononuclear phagocyte system** (figure 1.5). They are present throughout the connective tissue and around the basement membrane of small blood vessels and are particularly concentrated in the lung (figure 1.4h; alveolar macrophages), liver (Kupffer cells) and lining of spleen sinusoids and lymph node medullary sinuses where they are strategically placed to filter off foreign material. Other examples are mesangial cells in the kidney glomerulus, brain microglia and osteoclasts in bone. Unlike the polymorphs, they are long-lived cells with significant rough-surfaced endoplasmic reticulum and mitochondria (figure 1.8b) and, whereas the polymorphs provide the major defense against pyogenic (pus-forming) bacteria, as a rough generalization it may be said that macrophages are at their best in combating those bacteria (figure 1.4g), viruses and protozoa which are capable of living within the cells of the host.

Pattern recognition receptors (PRRs) on phagocytic cells recognize and are activated by pathogen-associated molecular patterns (PAMPs)

It hardly needs to be said but the body provides a very complicated internal environment and the phagocytes continuously encounter an extraordinary variety of different cells and soluble molecules. They must have mechanisms to enable them to distinguish these friendly self components from unfriendly and potentially dangerous microbial agents—as Charlie Janeway so aptly put it, they should be able to discriminate between 'noninfectious self and infectious nonself'. Not only must the infection be recognized, but it must also generate a signal which betokens 'danger' (Polly Matzinger).

In the interests of survival, phagocytic cells have evolved a system of receptors capable of recognizing molecular patterns expressed on the surface of the pathogens (PAMPs) which are conserved (i.e. unlikely to mutate), shared by a large group of infectious agents (sparing the need for too many receptors) and clearly distinguishable from self patterns. By and large these pattern recognition receptors (PRRs) are lectin-like and bind multivalently with considerable specificity to exposed microbial surface sugars with their characteristic rigid three-dimensional configurations (PAMPs). They do not bind appreciably to the galatose or sialic acid groups which are commonly the penultimate and ultimate sugars of mammalian surface polysaccharides. PAMPs linked to extracellular infections include Gram-negative lipopolysaccharide (LPS), Gram-positive lipoteichoic acid, yeast cell wall mannans (cf. figure 1.8) and mycobacterial glycolipids. Unmethy-

Figure 1.4. Cells involved in innate immunity. (a) Monocyte, showing 'horseshoe-shaped' nucleus and moderately abundant pale cytoplasm. Note the three multilobed polymorphonuclear neutrophils and the small lymphocyte (bottom left). Romanowsky stain. (b) Two monocytes stained for nonspecific esterase with α-naphthyl acetate. Note the vacuolated cytoplasm. The small cell with focal staining at the top is a T-lymphocyte. (c) Four polymorphonuclear leukocytes (neutrophils) and one eosinophil. The multilobed nuclei and the cytoplasmic granules are clearly shown, those of the eosinophil being heavily stained. (d) Polymorphonuclear neutrophil showing cytoplasmic granules stained for alkaline phosphatase. (e) Early neutrophils in bone marrow. The primary azurophilic granules (PG), originally clustered near the nucleus, move towards the periphery where the neutrophil-specific granules are generated by the Golgi apparatus as the cell matures. The nucleus gradually becomes lobular (LN). Giemsa. (f) Inflammatory cells from the site of a brain hemorrhage showing the large active macrophage in the center with phagocytosed red cells and promi-

nent vacuoles. To the right is a monocyte with horseshoe-shaped nucleus and cytoplasmic bilirubin crystals (hematoidin). Several multilobed neutrophils are clearly delineated. Giemsa. (g) Macrophages in monolayer cultures after phagocytosis of mycobacteria (stained red). Carbol-Fuchsin counterstained with Malachite Green. (h) Numerous plump alveolar macrophages within air spaces in the lung. (i) Basophil with heavily staining granules compared with a neutrophil (below). (j) Mast cell from bone marrow. Round central nucleus surrounded by large darkly staining granules. Two small red cell precursors are shown at the bottom. Romanowsky stain. (k) Tissue mast cells in skin stained with Toluidine Blue. The intracellular granules are metachromatic and stain reddish purple. Note the clustering in relation to dermal capillaries. (The slides from which illustrations (a), (b), (d), (e), (f), (i) and (j) were reproduced were very kindly provided by Mr M. Watts of the Department of Haematology, Middlesex Hospital Medical School; (c) was kindly supplied by Professor J.J. Owen; (g) by Professors P. Lydyard and G. Rook; (h) by Dr Meryl Griffiths; and (k) by Professor N. Woolf.)

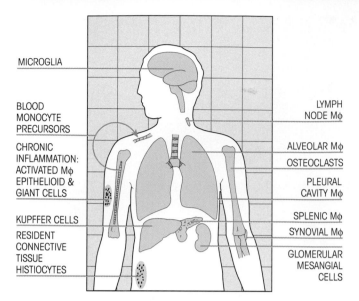

Figure 1.5. The mononuclear phagocyte system. Promonocyte precursors in the bone marrow develop into circulating blood monocytes which eventually become distributed throughout the body as mature macrophages (Mφ) as shown. The other major phagocytic cell, the polymorphonuclear neutrophil, is largely confined to the bloodstream except when recruited into sites of acute inflammation.

lated CpG (guanosine–cytosine) sequences in bacterial DNA and the double-stranded RNA from RNA viruses are examples of PAMPs linked to intracellular infections.

Engagement of the pattern recognition receptor generates a signal through an NFκB transcription factor pathway which alerts the cell to danger and initiates the phagocytic process. It may be worthwhile looking more closely at the handling of Gram-negative LPS (endotoxin) since failure to do so can result in septic shock. The biologically reactive lipid A moiety of LPS is recognized by a plasma LPS-binding protein and the complex captured by the CD14 scavenger molecule on the phagocytic cell. This then activates a Toll-like receptor which in turn unleashes a series of events culminating in the release of NFκB from its inhibitor; the free NFκB translocates to the nucleus and triggers phagocytosis with the release of proinflammatory mediators (figure 1.6).

Programed cell death (apoptosis; see below) is an essential component of embryonic development and the maintenance of the normal physiologic state. The dead cells need to be removed by phagocytosis but since they do not herald any 'danger' this must be done silently without setting off the alarm bells. Accordingly, recognition of apoptotic cells by macrophages directly through the CD14 receptor and indirectly through the binding of C1q to surface nucleosome blebs (see p. 425) proceeds without provoking the re-

lease of proinflammatory mediators. In sharp contrast, cells which are injured by infection and become necrotic release endogenous heat-shock protein 60 which acts as a danger signal to the phagocytic cells and establishes a protective inflammatory response.

Microbes are engulfed by activated phagocytic cells

After adherence of the microbe to the surface of the neutrophil or macrophage through recognition of a PAMP (figure 1.7.2), the resulting signal (figure 1.7.3) initiates the ingestion phase by activating an actin–myosin contractile system which extends pseudopods around the particle (figures 1.7.4 and 1.8); as adjacent receptors sequentially attach to the surface of the microbe, the plasma membrane is pulled around the particle just like a 'zipper' until it is completely enclosed in a vacuole (phagosome; figures 1.7.5 and 1.9). Events are now moving smartly and, within 1 minute, the cytoplasmic granules fuse with the phagosome and discharge their contents around the imprisoned microorganism (figure 1.7.7 and 1.9) which is subject to a formidable battery of microbicidal mechanisms.

There is an array of killing mechanisms

Killing by reactive oxygen intermediates

Trouble starts for the invader from the moment phagocytosis is initiated. There is a dramatic increase in activity of the hexose monophosphate shunt generating reduced nicotinamide-adenine-dinucleotide phosphate (NADPH). Electrons pass from the NADPH to a flavine adenine dinucleotide (FAD)-containing membrane flavoprotein and thence to a unique plasma membrane **cytochrome (cyt b_{558})**. This has the very low midpoint redox potential of $-245\,\text{mV}$ which allows it to reduce molecular oxygen directly to superoxide anion (figure 1.10a). Thus the key reaction catalysed by this NADPH oxidase, which initiates the formation of reactive oxygen intermediates (ROI), is:

$$\text{NADPH} + \text{O}_2 \xrightarrow{\text{oxidase}} \text{NADP}^+ + \cdot\text{O}_2^- \quad \text{(superoxide anion)}$$

The superoxide anion undergoes conversion to hydrogen peroxide under the influence of superoxide dismutase, and subsequently to hydroxyl radicals ($\cdot$OH). Each of these products has remarkable chemical reactivity with a wide range of molecular targets, making them formidable microbicidal agents; $\cdot$OH in particular is one of the most reactive free radicals known. Furthermore, the combination of peroxide, myeloper-

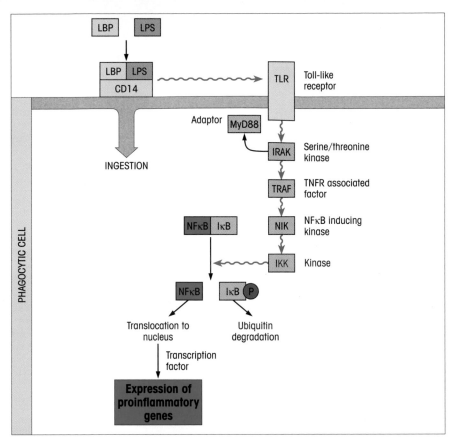

Figure 1.6. Activation of a phagocytic cell by a Gram-negative LPS (endotoxin) danger signal. Circulating LPS is complexed by LPS-binding protein (LBP) and captured by the CD14 (see p. 147 for CD definitions) surface scavenging receptor. This signals internalization of the complex and activates the Toll-like receptor (TLR), which then initiates a phosphorylation cascade mediated by different kinase enzymes, as a result of which the transcription factor NFκB is released from its inhibitor IκB and translocates to the nucleus, where it upregulates genes encoding defensive factors such as tumor necrosis factor (TNF), antibiotic peptides and the NADPH oxidase which generates reactive oxygen intermediates (see below). The Toll-like receptor is a leucine-rich molecule homologous with the Toll component which signals early embryonic differentiation events in *Drosophila*. The TLR is not itself a PRR and does not provide a signal for internalization, as shown by the ability of a double mutant of the MyD88 adaptor to internalize microorganisms attached to a PRR without producing inflammatory mediators such as TNF. The TLR appears to control the type of defensive response to different microbes. Thus TLR4 engineers the response to Gram-negative bacteria and LPS while TLR2 plays a key role in yeast and Gram-positive infections.

oxidase and halide ions constitutes a potent halogenating system capable of killing both bacteria and viruses (figure 1.10a). Although H_2O_2 and the halogenated compounds are not as active as the free radicals, they are more stable and therefore diffuse further, making them toxic to microorganisms in the extracellular vicinity.

Killing by reactive nitrogen intermediates

Nitric oxide surfaced prominently as a physiologic mediator when it was shown to be identical with endothelium-derived relaxing factor. This has proved to be just one of its many roles (including the mediation of penile erection, would you believe it!), but of major interest in the present context is its formation by an inducible NO· synthase (iNOS) within most cells, but particularly macrophages and human neutrophils, thereby generating a powerful antimicrobial system (figure 1.10b). Whereas the NADPH oxidase is dedicated to the killing of extracellular organisms taken up by phagocytosis and cornered within the phagocytic vacuole, the NO· mechanism can operate against microbes which invade the cytosol; so, it is not surprising that the majority of nonphagocytic cells which may be infected by viruses and other parasites are endowed with an iNOS capability. The mechanism of action may be through degradation of the Fe–S prosthetic groups of certain electron transport enzymes, depletion of iron and production of toxic ·ONOO radicals. The *N-ramp* gene linked with resistance to microbes such as bacille Calmette–Guérin (BCG), *Salmonella* and *Leishmania*, which can live within an intracellular habitat, is now known to express a protein forming a

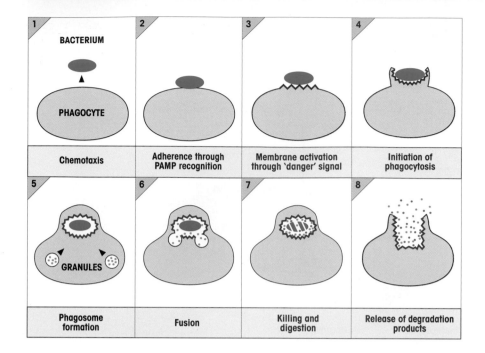

Figure 1.7. Phagocytosis and killing of a bacterium. Stage 3/4, respiratory burst and activation of NADPH oxidase; stage 5, damage by reactive oxygen intermediates; stage 6/7, damage by peroxidase, cationic proteins, antibiotic peptide defensins, lysozyme and lactoferrin.

Figure 1.8. Adherence and phagocytosis. (a) Phagocytosis of *Candida albicans* by a polymorphonuclear leukocyte (neutrophil). Adherence to the yeast wall surface mannan initiates enclosure of the fungal particle within arms of cytoplasm. Lysosomal granules are abundant but mitochondria are rare (×15 000). (b) Phagocytosis of *C. albicans* by a monocyte showing near completion of phagosome formation (arrowed) around one organism and complete ingestion of two others (×5000). (Courtesy of Dr H. Valdimarsson.)

Figure 1.9. Phagolysosome formation. (a) Neutrophil 30 minutes after ingestion of *C. albicans*. The cytoplasm is already partly degranulated and two lysosomal granules (arrowed) are fusing with the phagocytic vacuole. Two lobes of the nucleus are evident (×5000). (b) Higher magnification of (a) showing fusing granules discharging their contents into the phagocytic vacuole (arrowed) (×33 000). (Courtesy of Dr H. Valdimarsson.)

transmembrane channel which may be involved in transporting NO· across lysosome membranes.

Killing by preformed antimicrobials (figure 1.10c)

These molecules, contained within the neutrophil granules, contact the ingested microorganism when fusion with the phagosome occurs. The dismutation of superoxide consumes hydrogen ions and raises the pH of the vacuole gently, so allowing the family of cationic proteins and peptides to function optimally. The latter, known as **α-defensins**, are approximately 3.5–4 kDa and invariably rich in arginine, and reach incredibly high concentrations within the phagosome, of the order of 20–100 mg/ml. Like the bacterial colicins described above, they have an amphipathic structure which allows them to insert into microbial membranes to form destabilizing voltage-regulated ion channels (who copied whom?). These antibiotic peptides, at concentrations of 10–100 µg/ml, act as disinfectants against a wide spectrum of Gram-positive and -negative bacteria, many fungi and a number of enveloped viruses. Many exhibit remarkable selectivity for prokaryotic and eukaryotic microbes relative to host cells, partly dependent upon differential membrane lipid composition. One must be impressed by the ability of this surprisingly simple tool to discriminate large classes of nonself cells, i.e. microbes from self.

As if this was not enough, further damage is inflicted on the bacterial membranes both by neutral proteinase (cathepsin G) action and by direct transfer to the micro-bial surface of BPI, which increases bacterial permeability. Low pH, lysozyme and lactoferrin constitute bactericidal or bacteriostatic factors which are oxygen independent and can function under anaerobic circumstances. Finally, the killed organisms are digested by hydrolytic enzymes and the degradation products released to the exterior (figure 1.7.8).

By now, the reader may be excused a little smugness as she or he shelters behind the impressive antimicrobial potential of the phagocytic cells. But there are snags to consider; our formidable array of weaponry is useless unless the phagocyte can: (i) 'home onto' the microorganism, (ii) adhere to it, and (iii) respond by the membrane activation which initiates engulfment.

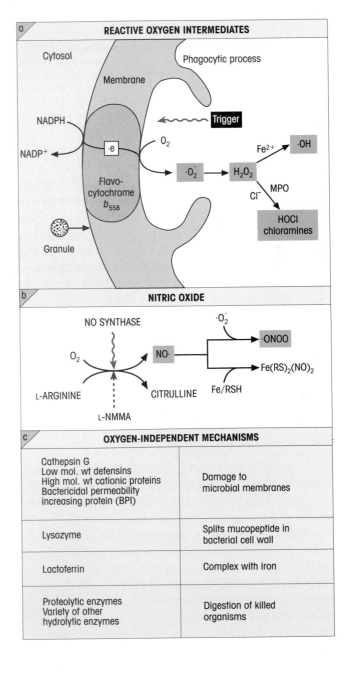

Figure 1.10. Microbicidal mechanisms of phagocytic cells. (a) Production of reactive oxygen intermediates. Electrons from NADPH are transferred by the flavocytochrome oxidase enzyme to molecular oxygen to form the microbicidal molecular species shown in the boxes. (*For the more studious*—The phagocytosis triggering agent binds to a classic G-protein-linked seven transmembrane domain receptor which activates an intracellular guanosine triphosphate (GTP)-binding protein. This in turn activates an array of enzymes: phosphoinositol-3 kinase concerned in the cytoskeletal reorganization underlying chemotactic responses (p. 10), phospholipase-Cγ2 mediating events leading to lysosome degranulation and phosphorylation of p47 phox through activation of protein kinase C, and the MEK and MAP kinase systems (cf. figure 9.6) which oversee the assembly of the NADPH oxidase. This is composed of the membrane cytochrome b_{558}, consisting of a p21 heme protein linked to gp91 with binding sites for NADPH and FAD on its intracellular aspect, to which phosphorylated p47 and p67 translocate from the cytosol on activation of the oxidase.) (b) Generation of nitric oxide. The enzyme, which structurally resembles the NADPH oxidase, can be inhibited by the arginine analog *N*-monomethyl-L-arginine (L-NMMA). The combination of NO· with superoxide anion yields the highly toxic peroxynitrite radical ·ONOO which cleaves on protonation to form reactive ·OH and NO_2 molecules. NO· can form mononuclear iron dithioldinitroso complexes leading to iron depletion and inhibition of several enzymes. (c) The basis of oxygen-independent antimicrobial systems.

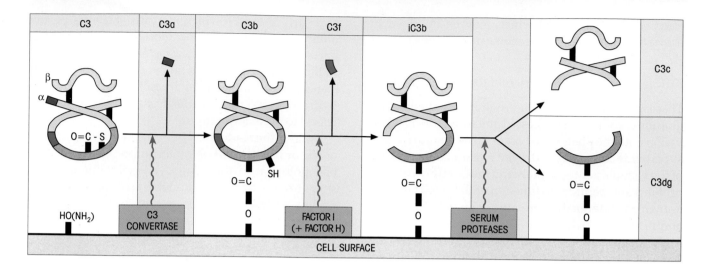

Figure 1.11. Structural basis for the cleavage of C3 by C3 convertase and its covalent binding to ·OH or ·NH$_2$ groups at the cell surface through exposure of the internal thiolester bonds. Further cleavage leaves the progressively smaller fragments, C3dg and C3d, attached to the membrane. (Based essentially on Law S.H.A. & Reid K.B.M. (1988) *Complement*, figure 2.4. IRL Press, Oxford.)

Some bacteria do produce chemical substances, such as the peptide formyl.Met.Leu.Phe, which directionally attract leukocytes, a process known as **chemotaxis**; many organisms do adhere to the phagocyte surface and many do spontaneously provide the appropriate membrane initiation signal. However, our teeming microbial adversaries are continually mutating to produce new species which may outwit the defenses by doing none of these. What then? The body has solved these problems with the effortless ease that comes with a few million years of evolution by developing the **complement** system.

COMPLEMENT FACILITATES PHAGOCYTOSIS

Complement and its activation

Complement is the name given to a complex series of some 20 proteins which, along with blood clotting, fibrinolysis and kinin formation, forms one of the triggered enzyme systems found in plasma. These systems characteristically produce a rapid, highly amplified response to a trigger stimulus mediated by a cascade phenomenon where the product of one reaction is the enzymic catalyst of the next.

Some of the complement components are designated by the letter 'C' followed by a number which is related more to the chronology of its discovery than to its position in the reaction sequence. The most abundant

and the most pivotal component is C3 which has a molecular weight of 195 kDa and is present in plasma at a concentration of around 1.2 mg/ml.

C3 undergoes slow spontaneous cleavage

Under normal circumstances, an internal thiolester bond in C3 (figure 1.11) becomes activated spontaneously at a very slow rate, either through reaction with water or with trace amounts of a plasma proteolytic enzyme, to form a reactive intermediate, either the split product C3b, or a functionally similar molecule designated C3i or C3(H$_2$O). In the presence of Mg^{2+} this can complex with another complement component, factor B, which then undergoes cleavage by a normal plasma enzyme (factor D) to generate C3b$\overline{\text{Bb}}$. Note that, conventionally, a bar over a complex denotes enzymic activity and that, on cleavage of a complement component, the larger product is generally given the suffix 'b' and the smaller 'a'.

C3b$\overline{\text{Bb}}$ has an important new enzymic activity: it is a **C3 convertase** which can split C3 to give C3a and C3b. We will shortly discuss the important biologic consequences of C3 cleavage in relation to microbial defenses, but under normal conditions there must be some mechanism to restrain this process to a 'tick-over' level since it can also give rise to more C3b$\overline{\text{Bb}}$, that is, we are dealing with a potentially runaway **positive-feedback loop** (figure 1.12). As with all potentially explosive triggered cascades, there are powerful regulatory mechanisms.

C3b levels are normally tightly controlled

In solution, the C3b$\overline{\text{Bb}}$ convertase is unstable and factor B is readily displaced by another component, factor

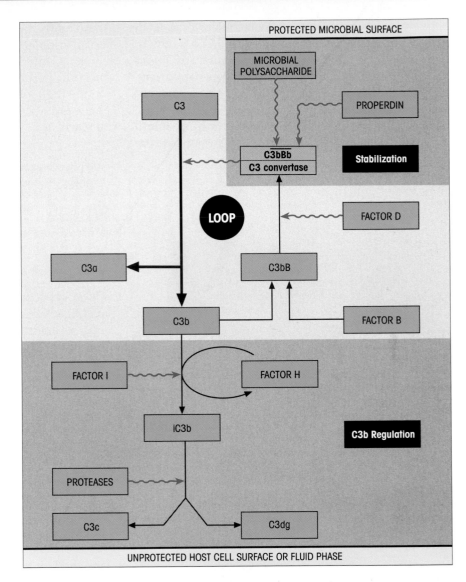

Figure 1.12. Microbial activation of the alternative complement pathway by stabilization of the C3 convertase (C3bBb), and its control by factors H and I. When bound to the surface of a host cell or in the fluid phase, the C3b in the convertase is said to be 'unprotected' in that its affinity for factor H is much greater than for factor B and is therefore susceptible to breakdown by factors H and I. On a microbial surface, C3b binds factor B more strongly than factor H and is therefore 'protected' from or 'stabilized' against cleavage—even more so when subsequently bound by properdin. Although in phylogenetic terms this is the oldest complement pathway, it was discovered after a separate pathway to be discussed in the next chapter, and so has the confusing designation 'alternative'. ⟿ represents an activation process. The horizontal bar above a component designates its activation.

H, to form C3bH which is susceptible to attack by the C3b inactivator, factor I (figure 1.12; further discussed on p. 307). The inactivated iC3b is biologically inactive and undergoes further degradation by proteases in the body fluids. Other regulatory mechanisms are discussed at a later stage (see p. 307).

C3 convertase is stabilized on microbial surfaces

A number of microorganisms can activate the C3bBb convertase to generate large amounts of C3 cleavage products by stabilizing the enzyme on their (carbohydrate) surfaces, thereby protecting the C3b from factor H. Another protein, properdin, acts subsequently on this bound convertase to stabilize it even further. As C3 is split by the surface membrane-bound enzyme to nascent C3b, it undergoes conformational change and its potentially reactive internal thiolester bond becomes exposed. Since the half-life of nascent C3b is less than $100\,\mu sec$, it can only diffuse a short distance before reacting covalently with local hydroxyl or amino groups available at the microbial cell surface (figure 1.11). Each catalytic site thereby leads to the clustering of large numbers of C3b molecules on the microorganism. This series of reactions leading to C3 breakdown provoked directly by microbes has been called **the alternative pathway** of complement activation (figure 1.12).

The post-C3 pathway generates a membrane attack complex

Recruitment of a further C3b molecule into the C3bBb enzymic complex generates a C5 convertase which activates C5 by proteolytic cleavage releasing a small polypeptide, C5a, and leaving the large C5b fragment loosely bound to C3b. Sequential attachment of C6 and C7 to C5b forms a complex with a transient membrane-binding site and an affinity for the β-peptide chain of C8. The C8α chain sits in the membrane and directs the conformational changes in C9 which transform it into an amphipathic molecule capable of insertion into the lipid bilayer (cf. the colicins, p. 2) and polymerization to an annular **membrane attack complex** (MAC; figures 1.13 and 2.4). This forms a transmembrane channel fully permeable to electrolytes and water, and due to the high internal colloid osmotic pressure of cells, there is a net influx of Na$^+$ and water frequently leading to lysis.

Complement has a range of defensive biological functions

These can be grouped conveniently under three headings.

1 C3b adheres to complement receptors

Phagocytic cells have receptors for C3b (CR1) and iC3b (CR3) which facilitate the adherence of C3b-coated microorganisms to the cell surface (discussed more fully on p. 258).

2 Biologically active fragments are released

C3a and C5a, the small peptides split from the parent molecules during complement activation, have several important actions. Both act directly on phagocytes, especially neutrophils, to stimulate the respiratory burst associated with the production of reactive oxygen intermediates and to enhance the expression of surface receptors for C3b and iC3b. Also, both are **anaphylatoxins** in that they are capable of triggering mediator release from mast cells (figures 1.4k and 1.14) and their circulating counterpart, the basophil (figure 1.4i), a phenomenon of such relevance to our present discussion that we have presented details of the mediators and their actions in figure 1.15; note in particular the chemotactic properties of these mediators and their effects on blood vessels. In its own right, C3a is a chemoattractant for eosinophils whilst C5a is a potent neutrophil chemotactic agent and also has a striking ability to act directly on the capillary endothelium to produce vasodilatation and increased permeability, an effect which seems to be prolonged by leukotriene B$_4$ released from activated mast cells, neutrophils and macrophages.

(a)

(b)

Figure 1.13. Post-C3 pathway generating C5a and the C5b–9 membrane attack complex (MAC). (a) Cartoon of molecular assembly. The conformational change in C9 protein structure which converts it from a hydrophilic to an amphipathic molecule (bearing both hydrophobic and hydrophilic regions) can be interrupted by an antibody raised against linear peptides derived from C9; since the antibody does not react with the soluble or membrane-bound forms of the molecule, it must be detecting an intermediate structure transiently revealed in a deep-seated structural rearrangement. (b) Electron micrograph of a membrane C5b–9 complex incorporated into liposomal membranes clearly showing the annular structure. The cylindrical complex is seen from the side inserted into the membrane of the liposome on the left, and end-on in that on the right. Although in itself a rather splendid structure, formation of the annular C9 cylinder is probably not essential for cytotoxic perturbation of the target cell membrane, since this can be achieved by insertion of amphipathic C9 molecules in numbers too few to form a clearly defined MAC. (Courtesy of Professor J. Tranum-Jensen and Dr S. Bhakdi.)

3 The terminal complex can induce membrane lesions

As described above, the insertion of the membrane attack complex into a membrane may bring about cell lysis. Providentially, complement is relatively inefficient at lysing the cell membranes of the autologous host due to the presence of control proteins (cf. p. 307).

Figure 1.14. The mast cell. (a) A resting cell with many membrane-bound granules containing preformed mediators. (b) A triggered mast cell. Note that the granules have released their contents and are morphologically altered, being larger and less electron dense. Although most of the altered granules remain within the circumference of the cell, they are open to the extracellular space. (Electron micrographs ×5400.) (Courtesy of Drs D. Lawson, C. Fewtrell, B. Gomperts and M.C. Raff from (1975) *Journal of Experimental Medicine* **142**, 391.)

COMPLEMENT CAN MEDIATE AN ACUTE INFLAMMATORY REACTION

We can now put together an effectively orchestrated defensive scenario initiated by activation of the alternative complement pathway (see figure 1.16).

In the first act, C3bBb is stabilized on the surface of the microbe and cleaves large amounts of C3. The C3a fragment is released but C3b molecules bind copiously to the microbe. These activate the next step in the sequence to generate C5a and the membrane attack com-

plex (although many organisms will be resistant to its action).

The mast cell plays a central role

The next act sees C3a and C5a, together with the mediators they trigger from the mast cell, acting to recruit polymorphonuclear phagocytes and further plasma complement components to the site of microbial invasion. The relaxation induced in arteriolar walls causes increased blood flow and dilatation of the small vessels, while contraction of capillary endothelial cells allows exudation of plasma proteins. Under the influence of the chemotaxins, neutrophils slow down and the surface adhesion molecules they are stimulated to express cause them to marginate to the walls of the capillaries where they pass through gaps between the endothelial cells (diapedesis) and move up the concentration gradient of chemotactic factors until they come face to face with the C3b-coated microbe. Adherence to the neutrophil C3b receptors then takes place, C3a and C5a at relatively high concentrations in the chemotactic gradient activate the respiratory burst and, hey presto, the slaughter of the last act can begin!

The processes of capillary dilatation (redness), exudation of plasma proteins and also of fluid (edema) due to hydrostatic and osmotic pressure changes, and accumulation of neutrophils are collectively termed the **acute inflammatory response**.

Macrophages can also do it

Although not yet established with the same confidence that surrounds the role of the mast cell in acute inflammation, the concept seems to be emerging that the tissue macrophage may mediate a parallel series of events with the same final end result. Nonspecific phagocytic events and certain bacterial toxins such as the lipopolysaccharides (LPSs) can activate macrophages, but the phagocytosis of C3b-opsonized microbes and the direct action of C5a generated through complement activation are guaranteed to goad the cell into copious secretion of soluble mediators of the acute inflammatory response (figure 1.17).

These upregulate the expression of adhesion molecules for neutrophils on the surface of endothelial cells, increase capillary permeability and promote the chemotaxis and activation of the polymorphonuclear neutrophils themselves. Thus, under the stimulus of complement activation, the macrophage provides a pattern of cellular events which reinforces the

PRE-FORMED	EFFECT
HISTAMINE	Vasodilatation, incr. capillary permeability chemokinesis, bronchoconstriction
PROTEOGLYCAN	Binds granule proteases
NEUTRAL PROTEASES β-GLUCOSAMINIDASE	Activates C3 Splits off glucosamine
ECF NCF	Eosinophil chemotaxis Neutrophil chemotaxis
PLATELET ACTIVATING FACTOR	Mediator release
INTERLEUKINS 3, 4, 5 & 6 GM-CSF, TNF	Multiple, including macrophage activation, trigger acute phase proteins, etc. (cf. Chapter 10)

NEWLY SYNTHESIZED	EFFECT
LEUKOTRIENES C_4, D_4 (SRS-A), B_4	Vasoactive, bronchoconstriction, chemotaxis
PROSTAGLANDINS THROMBOXANES	Affect bronchial muscle, platelet aggregation and vasodilatation

Figure 1.15. Mast cell triggering leading to release of mediators by two major pathways: (i) release of preformed mediators present in the granules, and (ii) the metabolism of arachidonic acid produced through activation of a phospholipase. Intracellular Ca^{2+} and cyclic AMP are central to the initiation of these events but details are still unclear. Mast cell triggering may occur through C3a, C5a and even by some microorganisms which can act directly on cell surface receptors. Mast cell heterogeneity is discussed on p. 323. ECF, eosinophil chemotactic factor; GM-CSF, granulocyte–macrophage colony-stimulating factor; NCF, neutrophil chemotactic factor. Chemotaxis refers to directed migration of granulocytes up the pathway concentration gradient of the mediator.

mast cell-mediated pathway leading to acute inflammation—yet another of the body's fail-safe redundancy systems (often known as the 'belt and braces' principle).

HUMORAL MECHANISMS PROVIDE A SECOND DEFENSIVE STRATEGY

Microbicidal factors in secretions

Turning now to those defense systems which are mediated entirely by soluble factors, we recollect that many microbes activate the complement system and may be

lysed by the insertion of the membrane attack complex. The spread of infection may be limited by enzymes released through tissue injury which activate the clotting system. Of the soluble bactericidal substances elaborated by the body, perhaps the most abundant and widespread is the enzyme lysozyme, a muramidase which splits the exposed peptidoglycan wall of susceptible bacteria (cf. figure 13.5).

Like the α-defensins of the neutrophil granules, the human β-defensins are peptides derived by proteolytic cleavage from larger precursors; they have β-sheet structures, 29–40 amino acids and three intramolecular disulfide bonds, although they differ from

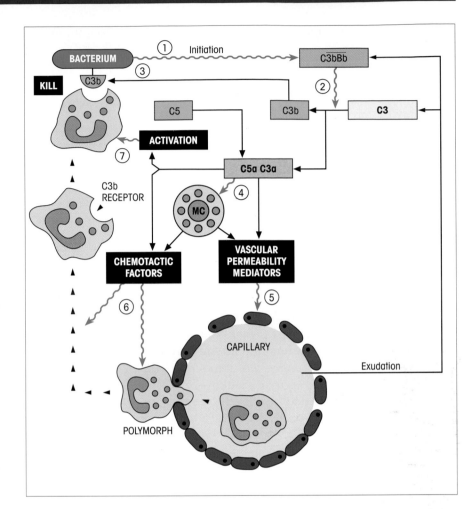

Figure 1.16. The defensive strategy of the acute inflammatory reaction initiated by bacterial activation of the alternative C pathway. Directions: ① start with the activation of the C3bBb C3 convertase by the bacterium, ② notice the generation of C3b (③ which binds to the bacterium), C3a and C5a, ④ which recruit mast cell mediators; ⑤ follow their effect on capillary dilatation and exudation of plasma proteins and ⑥ their chemotactic attraction of neutrophils to the C3b-coated bacterium and triumph in ⑦ the adherence and final activation of neutrophils for the kill.

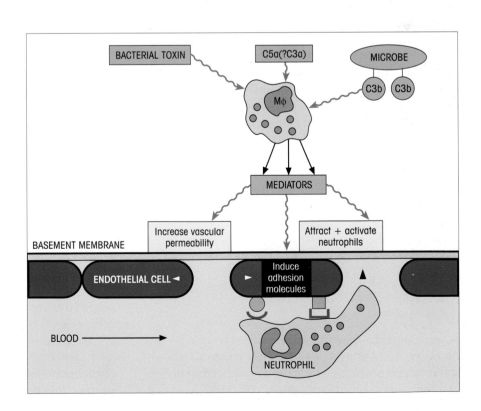

Figure 1.17. Stimulation by complement components and bacterial toxins such as LPS induces macrophage secretion of mediators of an acute inflammatory response. Blood neutrophils stick to the adhesion molecules on the endothelial cell and use this to provide traction as they force their way between the cells, through the basement membrane (with the help of secreted elastase) and up the chemotactic gradient.

the α-defensins in the placement of their six cysteines. The main human β-defensin, hDB-1, is produced abundantly in the kidney, the female reproductive tract, the oral gingiva and especially the lung airways. Since the word has it that we are all infected every day by tens of thousands of airborne bacteria, this must be an important defense mechanism. This being so, inhibition of hDB-1 and of a second pulmonary defensin, hDB-2, by high ionic strength could account for the susceptibility of cystic fibrosis patients to infection since they have an ion channel mutation which results in an elevated chloride concentration in airway surface fluids. Another airway antimicrobial active against Gram-negative and -positive bacteria is LL-37, a 37-residue α-helical peptide released by proteolysis of a cathelicidin (cathepsin L-inhibitor) precursor.

This theme surfaces again in the stomach where a peptide split from lactoferrin by pepsin could provide the gastric and intestinal secretions with some antimicrobial policing. A rather longer two-domain peptide with 108 residues, termed secretory leukoprotease inhibitor (SLPI), is found in many human secretions. The C-terminal domain is anti-protease but the N-terminal domain is distinctly unpleasant to metabolically active fungal cells and to various skin-associated microorganisms, which makes its production by human keratinocytes particularly appropriate. In passing, it is worth pointing out that many D-amino acid analogs of peptide antibiotics form left-handed helices which retain the ability to induce membrane ion channels and hence their antimicrobial powers and, given their resistance to catabolism within the body, should be attractive candidates for a new breed of synthetic antibiotics. Lastly, we may mention the two lung surfactant proteins SP-A and SP-D which, in conjunction with various lipids, lower the surface tension of the epithelial lining cells of the lung to keep the airways patent. They belong to a totally different structural group of molecules termed collectins (see below) which contribute to innate immunity through binding of their lectin-like domains to carbohydrates on microbes, and their collagenous stem to cognate receptors on phagocytic cells—thereby facilitating the ingestion and killing of the infectious agents.

Acute phase proteins increase in response to infection

A number of plasma proteins collectively termed acute phase proteins show a dramatic increase in concentration in response to early 'alarm' mediators such as macrophage-derived interleukin-1 (IL-1) released as a

Table 1.1. Acute phase proteins.

Acute phase reactant	Role
Dramatic increases in concentration:	
C-reactive protein	Fixes complement, opsonizes
Mannose binding protein	Fixes complement, opsonizes
α_1-acid glycoprotein	Transport protein
Serum amyloid P component	Amyloid component precursor
Moderate increases in concentration:	
α_1-proteinase inhibitors	Inhibit bacterial proteases
α_1-antichymotrypsin	Inhibit bacterial proteases
C3, C9, factor B	Increase complement function
Ceruloplasmin	$\cdot O_2^-$ scavenger
Fibrinogen	Coagulation
Angiotensin	Blood pressure
Haptoglobin	Bind hemoglobin
Fibronectin	Cell attachment

result of infection or tissue injury. These include C-reactive protein (CRP), mannose-binding protein (MBP) and serum amyloid P component (table 1.1). Other acute phase proteins showing a more modest rise in concentration include α_1-antichymotrypsin, fibrinogen, ceruloplasmin, C9 and factor B. Overall, it seems likely that the acute phase response achieves a beneficial effect through enhancing host resistance, minimizing tissue injury and promoting the resolution and repair of the inflammatory lesion.

To take an example, during an infection, microbial products such as endotoxins stimulate the release of IL-1, which is an endogenous pyrogen (incidentally capable of improving our general defenses by raising the body temperature), and IL-6. These in turn act on the liver to increase the synthesis and secretion of CRP to such an extent that its plasma concentration may rise 1000-fold.

Human CRP is composed of five identical polypeptide units noncovalently arranged as a cyclic pentamer around a Ca-binding cavity. These protein **pentraxins** have been around in the animal kingdom for some time, since a closely related homolog, limulin, is present in the hemolymph of the horseshoe crab, not exactly a close relative of *Homo sapiens*. A major property of CRP is its ability to bind in a Ca-dependent fashion, as a pattern recognition molecule, to a number of microorganisms which contain phosphorylcholine in their membranes, the complex having the useful property of activating complement (by the classical and not the alternative pathway with which we are at present familiar). This results in the deposition of C3b on the surface of the microbe which thus becomes **opsonized** (i.e. 'made ready for the table') for adherence to phagocytes.

Yet another member of this pentameric family is the serum amyloid P (SAP) component. This protein can complex with chondroitin sulfate, a cell matrix glycosaminoglycan, and subsequently bind lysosomal enzymes such as cathepsin B released within a focus of inflammation. The degraded SAP becomes a component of the amyloid fibrillar deposits which accompany chronic infections—it might even be a key initiator of amyloid deposition (cf. p. 385).

A most important acute phase opsonin is the Ca-dependent **mannose-binding protein (MBP)** which can react not only with mannose but several other sugars, so enabling it to bind with an exceptionally wide variety of Gram-negative and -positive bacteria, yeasts, viruses and parasites; its subsequent ability to trigger the classical C3 convertase through two novel associated serine proteases (MASP-1 and MASP-2) qualifies it as an opsonin. (Please relax, we unravel the secrets of the classical pathway in the next chapter.) MBP is a multiple of trimeric complexes, each unit of which contains a collagen-like region joined to a globular lectin-binding domain. This structure places it in the family of **collectins** (**col**lagen + **lectin**) which have the ability to recognize 'foreign' carbohydrate patterns differing from 'self' surface polysaccharides normally decorated by terminal galactose and sialic acid groups, whilst the collagen region can bind to and activate phagocytic cells through complementary receptors on their surface. The collectins, especially MBP and the alveolar surfactant molecules SP-A and SP-D mentioned earlier, have many attributes that qualify them for a first-line role in innate immunity. These include the ability to differentiate self from nonself, to bind to a variety of microbes, to generate secondary effector mechanisms, and to be widely distributed throughout the body including mucosal secretions.

Interest in the collectin conglutinin has perked up recently with the demonstration, first, that it is found in humans and not just in cows, and second, that it can bind to *N*-acetylglucosamine; being polyvalent, this implies an ability to coat bacteria with C3b by cross-linking the available sugar residue in the complement fragment with the bacterial proteoglycan. Although it is not clear whether conglutinin is a member of the acute phase protein family, we mention it here because it embellishes the general idea that the evolution of lectin-like molecules which bind to microbial rather than self polysaccharides, and which can then hitch themselves to the complement system or to phagocytic cells, has proved to be such a useful form of protection for the host (figure 1.18).

Interferons inhibit viral replication

These are a family of broad-spectrum antiviral agents present in birds, reptiles and fishes as well as the higher animals, and first recognized by the phenomenon of viral interference in which an animal infected with one virus resists superinfection by a second unrelated virus. Different molecular forms of interferon have been identified, all of which have been gene cloned. There are at least 14 different α-interferons (IFNα) produced by leukocytes, while fibroblasts, and probably all cell types, synthesize IFNβ. We will keep a third type (IFNγ), which is not directly induced by viruses, up our sleeves for the moment.

Cells synthesize interferon when infected by a virus and secrete it into the extracellular fluid where it binds to specific receptors on uninfected neighboring cells. The bound interferon now exerts its antiviral effect in the following way. At least two genes are thought to be derepressed in the interferon-treated cell allowing the synthesis of two new enzymes. The first, a protein kinase, catalyses the phosphorylation of a ribosomal protein and an initiation factor necessary for protein synthesis, so greatly reducing mRNA translation. The other catalyses the formation of a short polymer of adenylic acid which activates a latent endonuclease; this in turn degrades both viral and host mRNA.

Figure 1.18. A major defensive strategy by soluble factors. The recognition elements link the microorganism to a microbicidal system through the adaptor region. PAMP, pathogen-associated molecular pattern.

Whatever the precise mechanism of action ultimately proves to be, the net result is to establish a cordon of uninfectable cells around the site of virus infection so restraining its spread. The effectiveness of interferon *in vivo* may be inferred from experiments in which mice injected with an antiserum to murine interferons could be killed by several hundred times less virus than was needed to kill the controls. However, it must be presumed that interferon plays a significant role in the recovery from, as distinct from the prevention of, viral infections.

As a group, the interferons may prove to have a wider biologic role than the control of viral infection. It will be clear, for example, that the induced enzymes described above would act to inhibit host cell division just as effectively as viral replication. The interferons may also modulate the activity of other cells, such as the natural killer cells, to be discussed in the following section.

EXTRACELLULAR KILLING

Natural killer (NK) cells

Viruses lack the apparatus for self renewal and so it is essential for them to penetrate the cells of the infected host in order to take over its replicative machinery. It is clearly in the interest of the host to find a way to kill such infected cells before the virus has had a chance to reproduce. NK cells appear to do just that when studied *in vitro*.

They are large granular lymphocytes (figure 2.6a) with a characteristic morphology (figure 2.7b). Killer and target are brought into close opposition (figure 1.19a) through recognition by lectin-like (i.e. carbohydrate-binding) and other receptors on the NK cell (cf. p. 69) of structures on high molecular weight glycoproteins on the surface of virally infected cells. Activation of the NK cell ensues and leads to polarization of granules between nucleus and target within minutes and extracellular release of their contents into the space between the two cells followed by target cell death.

One of the most important of the granule components is a **perforin** or cytolysin bearing some structural homology to C9; like that protein, but without any help other than from Ca^{2+}, it can insert itself into the membrane of the target, apparently by binding to phosphorylcholine through its central amphipathic domain. It then polymerizes to form a transmembrane pore with an annular structure, comparable to the complement membrane attack complex (figure 1.19a).

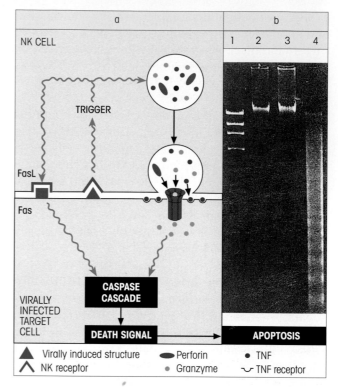

Figure 1.19. Extracellular killing of virally infected cell by natural killer (NK) cell. (a) Binding of the NK receptors to the surface of the virally infected cell triggers the extracellular release of perforin molecules from the granules; these polymerize to form transmembrane channels which may facilitate lysis of the target by permitting entry of granzymes which induce apoptotic cell death through activation of the caspase protease cascade and ultimate fragmentation of nuclear DNA. (Model resembling that proposed by Hudig D., Ewoldt G.R. & Woodward S.L. (1993) *Current Opinion in Immunology* **5**, 90.). Another granule component, TNF, activates caspase-dependent apoptosis through the 'death domains' of the surface TNF receptors on the target cell. Engagement of the NK receptor also activates a parallel killing mechanism mediated through the binding of the Fas-ligand (FasL) on the effector to the target cell Fas receptor whose cytoplasmic death domains activate procaspase-8. (b) Fragmentation of nucleosome DNA into 200 kb 'ladder' fragments following programed cell death (kindly provided by Professor S. Martin). Lane 1: standards obtained by digestion of λ DNA by *Hind*III; lanes 2 and 3: undegraded DNA from normal control cells; lane 4: characteristic breakdown of DNA from apoptotic cells. Because this is such a fundamental 'default' mechanism in every cell, it is crucial for there to be heavy regulation: thus a large group of regulatory proteins, the Bcl-2 subfamily, inhibit apoptosis while the Bax and BH3 subfamilies promote it. The word 'apoptosis' in ancient Greek describes the falling of leaves from trees or of petals from flowers and aptly illustrates apoptosis in cells where they detach from their extracellular matrix support structures. (See figure 12.7 for morphologic appearance of apoptotic cells.)

Target cells are told to commit suicide

Whereas C9-induced cell lysis is brought about through damage to outer membranes followed later by nuclear changes, NK cells kill by activating **apoptosis** (programed cell death), a mechanism present in every cell which leads to self immolation. Apoptosis is mediated by a cascade of proteolytic enzymes termed **caspases**. Like other multicomponent cascades, such as the blood clotting and complement systems, it depends upon the activation by proteolytic cleavage of a proenzyme next in the chain, and so on. The sequence terminates with very rapid nuclear fragmentation effected by a Ca-dependent endonuclease which acts on the vulnerable DNA between nucleosomes to produce the 200 kb 'nucleosome ladder' fragments (figure 1.19b); only afterwards can one detect release of ^{51}Cr-labeled cytoplasmic proteins through defective cell surface membranes. These nuclear changes are not produced by C9. Thus, although perforin and C9 appear to produce comparable membrane 'pores', there is a dramatic difference in their killing mechanisms.

In addition to perforin, the granules contain tumor necrosis factor-α (TNFα), lymphotoxin-β and a family of serine proteases termed **granzymes**, one of which, granzyme B, can function as an NK cytotoxic factor by passing through the perforin membrane pore into the cytoplasm where it can split procaspase-8 and activate the apoptotic process. Tumor necrosis factor can induce apoptotic cell death through reaction with cell surface TNF receptors whose cytoplasmic 'death domains' can also activate procaspase-8. Chondroitin sulfate A, a protease-resistant highly negatively charged proteoglycan present in the granules, may subserve the function of protecting the NK cell from autolysis by its own lethal agents.

Killing by NK cells can still occur in perforin-deficient mice, probably through a parallel mechanism involving **Fas** receptor molecules on the target cell surface. Engagement of Fas by the so-called **Fas-ligand (FasL)** on the effector cell provides yet another pathway for the induction of an apoptotic signal in the unlucky target.

The various interferons augment NK cytotoxicity and, since interferons are produced by virally infected cells, we have a nicely integrated feedback defense system.

Eosinophils

Large parasites such as helminths cannot physically be phagocytosed and extracellular killing by eosinophils would seem to have evolved to help cope with this situation. These polymorphonuclear 'cousins' of the neutrophil have distinctive granules which stain avidly with acid dyes (figure 1.4c) and have a characteristic appearance in the electron microscope (figure 13.22). A major basic protein is localized in the core of the granules while an eosinophilic cationic protein together with a peroxidase have been identified in the granule matrix. Other enzymes include arylsulfatase B, phospholipase D and histaminase. They have surface receptors for C3b and on activation produce a particularly impressive respiratory burst with concomitant generation of active oxygen metabolites. Not satisfied with that, nature has also armed the cell with granule proteins capable of producing a transmembrane plug in the target membrane like C9 and the NK perforin. Quite a nasty cell.

Most helminths can activate the alternative complement pathway, but although resistant to C9 attack, their coating with C3b allows adherence of eosinophils through their C3b receptors. If this contact should lead to activation, the eosinophil will launch its extracellular attack which includes the release of the major basic protein and especially the cationic protein which damages the parasite membrane.

SUMMARY

A wide range of innate immune mechanisms operate which do not improve with repeated exposure to infection.

Barriers against infection
• Microorganisms are kept out of the body by the skin, the secretion of mucus, ciliary action, the lavaging action of bactericidal fluids (e.g. tears), gastric acid and microbial antagonism.

• If penetration occurs, bacteria are destroyed by soluble factors such as lysozyme and by phagocytosis with intracellular digestion.

Phagocytic cells kill microorganisms
• The main phagocytic cells are polymorphonuclear neutrophils and macrophages.
• The phagocytic cells use their pattern recognition

(continued p. 20)

receptors (PRRs) to recognize and adhere to pathogen-associated molecular patterns (PAMPs) on the microbe surface.

- Organisms adhering to the phagocyte surface activate the engulfment process and are taken inside the cell where they fuse with cytoplasmic granules.
- A formidable array of microbicidal mechanisms then come into play: the conversion of O_2 to reactive oxygen intermediates, the synthesis of nitric oxide and the release of multiple oxygen-independent factors from the granules.

Complement facilitates phagocytosis

- The complement system, a multicomponent triggered enzyme cascade, is used to attract phagocytic cells to the microbes and engulf them.
- The most abundant component, C3, is split by a convertase enzyme formed from its own cleavage product C3b and factor B and stabilized against breakdown caused by factors H and I, through association with the microbial surface. As it is formed, C3b becomes linked covalently to the microorganism.
- The next component, C5, is activated yielding a small peptide, C5a; the residual C5b binds to the surface and assembles the terminal components C6–9 into a membrane attack complex which is freely permeable to solutes and can lead to osmotic lysis.
- C5a is a potent chemotactic agent for neutrophils and greatly increases capillary permeability.
- C3a and C5a act on mast cells causing the release of further mediators, such as histamine, leukotriene B_4 and tumor necrosis factor (TNF), with effects on capillary permeability and adhesiveness, and neutrophil chemotaxis; they also activate neutrophils.

The complement-mediated acute inflammatory reaction

- Following the activation of complement with the ensuing attraction and stimulation of neutrophils, the activated phagocytes bind to the C3b-coated microbes by their surface C3b receptors and may then ingest them. The influx of polymorphs and the increase in vascular permeability constitute the potent antimicrobial **acute inflammatory response** (figure 2.18).
- Inflammation can also be initiated by tissue macrophages which subserve a similar role to the mast cell, since signaling by bacterial toxins, C5a or iC3b-coated bacteria adhering to surface complement receptors causes release of neutrophil chemotactic and activating factors.

Humoral mechanisms provide a second defensive strategy

- In addition to lysozyme, peptide defensins and the complement system, other humoral defenses involve the acute phase proteins, such as C-reactive and mannose-binding proteins, whose synthesis is greatly augmented by infection. Mannose-binding protein is a member of the collectin family including conglutinin and surfactants SP-A and SP-D, notable for their ability to distinguish microbial from 'self' surface carbohydrate groups by their pattern recognition molecules.
- Recovery from viral infections can be effected by the interferons which block viral replication.

Extracellular killing

- Virally infected cells can be killed by large granular lymphocytes with NK activity through a perforin/granzyme and a separate Fas-mediated pathway, leading to programed cell death (apoptosis) mediated by activation of the caspase protease cascade which fragments the nuclear DNA.
- Extracellular killing by C3b-bound eosinophils may be responsible for the failure of many large parasites to establish a foothold in potential hosts.

See the accompanying website (**www.roitt.com**) for multiple choice questions.

Specific acquired immunity

INTRODUCTION

Our microbial adversaries have tremendous opportunities through mutation to evolve strategies which evade our innate immune defenses. For example, most of the *successful* parasites activate the alternative complement pathway and bind C3b, yet eosinophils which adhere are somehow not triggered into offensive action. The same holds true for many bacteria, while some may so shape their exteriors as to avoid complement activation completely. The body obviously needed to 'devise' defense mechanisms which could be dovetailed individually to each of these organisms no matter how many there were. In other words *a very large number* of **specific immune defenses** needed to be at the body's disposal. Quite a tall order!

ANTIBODY—THE SPECIFIC ADAPTOR

Evolutionary processes came up with what can only be described as a brilliant solution. This was to fashion an adaptor molecule which was intrinsically capable not only of activating the complement system *and* of stimulating phagocytic cells, but also of sticking to the offending microbe. The adaptor thus had three main regions, two concerned with communicating with complement and the phagocytes (the biological functions) and one devoted to binding to an individual microorganism (the external recognition function). In

most biological systems like hormones and receptors, and enzymes and substrates, recognition usually occurs through fairly accurate complementarity in shape allowing the ligands to approach so close to each other as to permit the normal intermolecular forces to become relatively strong. In the present case, each adaptor would have a recognition portion complementary in shape to some microorganism to which it could then bind reasonably firmly. The part of the adaptor with biological function would be constant, but for each of hundreds of thousands of different organisms, a special recognition portion would be needed.

Thus the body has to make hundreds of thousands, or even millions, of **adaptors with different recognition sites**. The adaptor is of course the molecule we know affectionately as **antibody** (figure 2.1).

Antibody initiates a new complement pathway ('classical')

Antibody, when bound to a microbe, will link to the first molecule in the so-called **classical complement sequence**, C1q, and trigger the latent proteolytic activity of the C1 complex (figure 2.2). This then dutifully plays its role in the amplifying cascade by acting on components C4 and C2 to generate many molecules of $\overline{C4b2a}$, a new **C3-splitting enzyme** (figure 2.3).

The molecular events responsible for this seem to be rather clear. C1q is polyvalent with respect to antibody binding and consists of a central collagen-like stem branching into six peptide chains each tipped by an

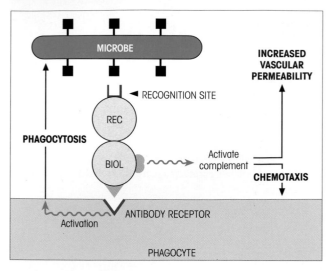

Figure 2.1. The antibody adaptor molecule. The constant part with biological function (BIOL) activates complement and the phagocyte. The portion with the recognition unit for the foreign microbe (REC) varies from one antibody to another.

Figure 2.3. Comparison of the alternative and classical complement pathways. The classical pathway is activated by antibody whereas the alternative pathway is not. The molecular units with protease activity are highlighted, the enzymic domains showing considerable homology. Beware confusion with nomenclature; the large C2 fragment which forms the C3 convertase is designated as C2a, but to be consistent with C4b, C3b and C5b, it would have been more logical to call it C2b. Note that C-reactive protein (p. 16), on binding to microbial phosphorylcholine, can trigger the classical pathway. Mannose-binding lectin, when combined with microbial surface carbohydrate, associates with the serine proteases MASP-1 and 2 (p. 17) which activate the classical pathway; under these conditions, MASP-1 cleaves C3 directly and MASP-2 splits C4 and C2.

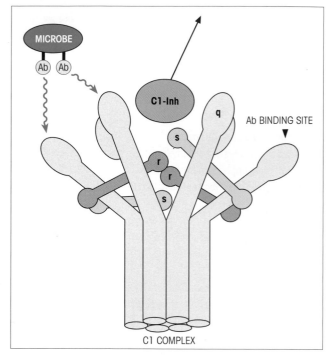

Figure 2.2. Activation of the classical complement pathway. C1 is composed of C1q associated with the flexible rod-like Ca-dependent complex, $C1r_2$–$C1s_2$ (⬭○◯—◗ r r ◖—◯○⬭); s and r indicate potential serine protease active sites), which interdigitates with the six arms of C1q, either as indicated or as 'W' shapes on the outer side of these arms. The C1-inhibitor normally prevents spontaneous activation of $C1r_2$–$C1s_2$. If the complex of a microbe or antigen with antibodies attaches two or more of the globular Ab-binding sites on C1q, the molecule presumably undergoes conformational change which releases the C1–Inh and activates $C1r_2$–$C1s_2$.

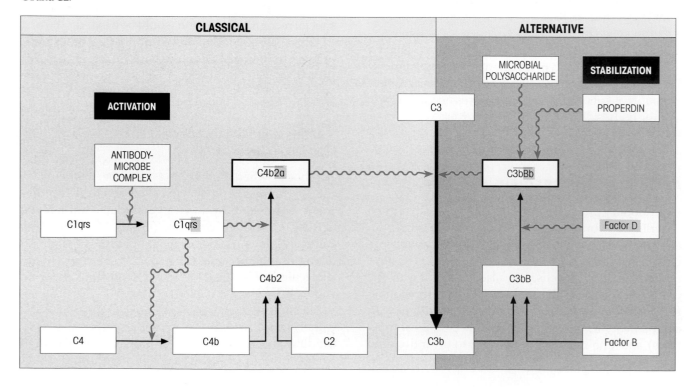

antibody-binding subunit (resembling the blooms on a bouquet of flowers). C1q is associated with two further subunits, C1r and C1s, in a Ca^{2+}-stabilized trimolecular complex (figure 2.2). Both these molecules contain repeats of a 60-amino acid unit folded as a globular domain and referred to as a complement control protein (CCP) repeat since it is a characteristic structural feature of several proteins involved in control of the complement system. Changes in C1q consequent upon binding the antigen–antibody complex bring about the sequential activation of proteolytic activity in C1r and then C1s.

The next component in the chain, C4 (unfortunately components were numbered before the sequence was established), now binds to C1 through these CCPs and is cleaved enzymatically by $C\overline{1s}$. As expected in a multienzyme cascade, several molecules of C4 undergo cleavage, each releasing a small C4a fragment and revealing a nascent labile internal thiolester bond in the residual $C\overline{4b}$ like that in C3 (cf. figure 1.11) which may then bind either to the antibody–C1 complex or the surface of the microbe itself. Note that C4a, like C5a and C3a, has anaphylatoxin activity, although feeble, and C4b resembles C3b in its opsonic activity. In the presence of Mg^{2+}, C2 can complex with the $C\overline{4b}$ to become a new substrate for the $C\overline{1s}$, the resulting product $C\overline{4b2a}$ now has the vital C3 convertase activity required to cleave C3.

This classical pathway C3 convertase has the same specificity as the $C\overline{3bBb}$ generated by the alternative pathway, likewise producing the same C3a and C3b fragments. Activation of a single C1 complex can bring about the proteolysis of literally thousands of C3 molecules. From then on things march along exactly in parallel to the post-C3 pathway with one molecule of C3b added to the $C\overline{4b2a}$ to make it into a C5-splitting enzyme with eventual production of the **membrane attack complex** (figures 1.13 and 2.4). Just as the alternative pathway C3 convertase is controlled by factors H and I, so the breakdown of $C\overline{4b2a}$ is brought about by either a C4-binding protein (C4bp) or a cell surface C3b receptor (CR1) in the presence of factor I.

The similarities between the two pathways are set out in figure 2.3 and show how antibody can supplement and even improve on the ability of the innate immune system to initiate **acute inflammatory reactions**. Antibody provides yet a further bonus in this respect; the class known as immunoglobulin E (see legend to figure 2.4) can sensitize mast cells through binding to their surface so that combination with antigen triggers mediator release independently of C3a or C5a, adding yet more flexibility to our defenses.

Complexed antibody activates phagocytic cells

We drew attention to the fact that some C3b-coated organisms may adhere to phagocytic cells and yet avoid provoking their uptake. If small amounts of antibody are added the phagocyte springs into action. It does so through the recognition of two or more antibody molecules bound to the microbe, using specialized receptors on the cell surface.

A single antibody molecule complexed to the microorganism is not enough because it cannot cause the cross-linking of antibody receptors in the phagocyte surface membrane which is required to activate the cell. There is a further consideration connected with what is often called **the bonus effect of multivalency**; for thermodynamic reasons, which will be touched on in Chapter 5, the association constant of ligands, which use several rather than a single bond to react with receptors, is increased geometrically rather than arithmetically. For example, three antibodies bound close together on a bacterium could be attracted to a macrophage a thousand times more strongly than a single antibody molecule (figure 2.5).

Figure 2.4. Multiple lesions in cell wall of *Escherichia coli* bacterium caused by interaction with IgM antibody and complement. (Human antibodies are divided into five main classes: immunoglobulin M (shortened to IgM), IgG, IgA, IgE and IgD, which differ in the specialization of their 'rear ends' for different biological functions such as complement activation or mast cell sensitization.) Each lesion is caused by a single IgM molecule and shows as a 'dark pit' due to penetration by the 'negative stain'. This is somewhat of an illusion since in reality these 'pits' are like volcano craters standing proud of the surface, and are each single 'membrane attack' complexes. Comparable results may be obtained in the absence of antibody since the cell wall endotoxin can activate the alternative pathway in the presence of higher concentration of serum (×400000). (Courtesy of Drs R. Dourmashkin and J.H. Humphrey.)

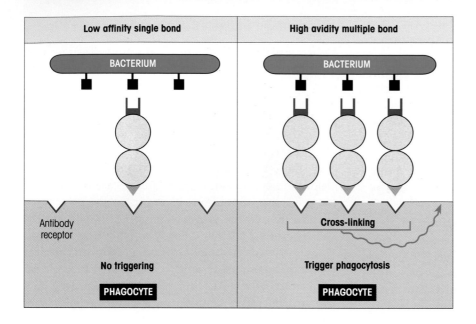

Figure 2.5. Binding of bacterium to phagocyte by multiple antibodies gives strong association forces and triggers phagocytosis by cross-linking the surface receptors for antibody.

CELLULAR BASIS OF ANTIBODY PRODUCTION

Antibodies are made by lymphocytes

The majority of resting **lymphocytes** are small cells with a darkly staining nucleus due to condensed chromatin and relatively little cytoplasm containing the odd mitochondrion required for basic energy provision. Figures 2.6 and 2.7 compare the morphology of these cells with that of the minority population of **large granular lymphocytes** which includes the natural killer (NK) set referred to in Chapter 1.

The central role of the **small lymphocyte** in the production of antibody was established largely by the work of Gowans. He depleted rats of their lymphocytes by chronic drainage of lymph from the thoracic duct by an indwelling cannula, and showed that they had a grossly impaired ability to mount an antibody response to microbial challenge. The ability to form antibody could be restored by injecting thoracic duct lymphocytes obtained from another rat. The same effect could be obtained if, before injection, the thoracic duct cells were first incubated at 37°C for 24 hours under conditions which kill off large- and medium-sized cells and leave only the small lymphocytes. This shows that the small lymphocyte is necessary for the **antibody response**.

The small lymphocytes can be labeled if the donor rat is previously injected with tritiated thymidine; it then becomes possible to follow the fate of these lymphocytes when transferred to another rat of the same strain which is then injected with microorganisms to produce an antibody response (figure 2.8). It transpires that after contact with the injected microbes, some of the transferred labeled lymphocytes develop into **plasma cells** (figures 2.6d and 2.9) which can be shown to contain (figure 2.6e) and secrete antibody.

Antigen selects the lymphocytes which make antibody

The molecules in the microorganisms which evoke and react with antibodies are called **antigens** (**gen**erates **anti**bodies). We now know that antibodies are formed before antigen is ever seen and that they are **selected** for by antigen.

It works in the following way. Each lymphocyte of a subset called the **B-lymphocytes**, because they differentiate in the *bone marrow*, is programed to make one, and only one, antibody and it places this antibody on its outer surface to act as a receptor. This can be detected by using fluorescent probes and, in figure 2.6c, one can see the molecules of antibody on the surface of a human B-lymphocyte stained with a fluorescent rabbit antiserum raised against a preparation of human antibodies. Each lymphocyte has of the order of 10^5 identical antibody molecules on its surface.

When an antigen enters the body, it is confronted by a dazzling array of lymphocytes all bearing different antibodies each with its own individual recognition site. The antigen will only bind to those receptors with which it makes a good fit. Lymphocytes whose recep-

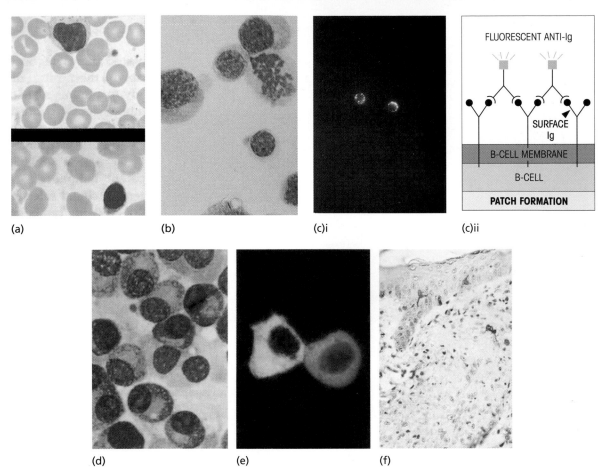

(a) (b) (c)i (c)ii

(d) (e) (f)

Figure 2.6. Cells involved in the acquired immune response. (a) Small lymphocytes. Condensed chromatin gives rise to heavy staining of the nucleus. The cell on the bottom is a typical resting agranular T-cell with a thin rim of cytoplasm. The upper nucleated cell is a large granular lymphocyte; it has more cytoplasm and azurophilic granules are evident. Isolated platelets are visible. B-lymphocytes range from small to intermediate in size and lack granules. Giemsa stain. (b) Transformed T-lymphocytes (lymphoblasts) following stimulation of lymphocytes in culture with a polyclonal activator, such as the lectins phytohemagglutinin, concanavalin A and pokeweed mitogen which stimulate a wide range of cells independently of their specificity for antigen. The large lymphoblasts with their relatively high ratio of cytoplasm to nucleus may be compared in size with the isolated small lymphocyte. One cell is in mitosis. May–Grünwald–Giemsa. (c) Immunofluorescent staining of B-lymphocyte surface immunoglobulin using fluorescein-conjugated (■) anti-Ig. Provided the reaction is carried out in the cold to prevent pinocytosis, the labeled antibody cannot penetrate to the interior of the viable lymphocytes and reacts only with surface components. Patches of aggregated surface Ig are seen which are beginning to form a cap in the right-hand lymphocyte. During cap formation, submembranous myosin becomes redistributed in association with the surface Ig and induces locomotion of the previously sessile cell in a direction away from the cap. (d) Plasma cells. The nucleus is eccentric. The cytoplasm is strongly basophilic due to high RNA content. The juxtanuclear lightly stained zone corresponds with the Golgi region. May–Grünwald–Giemsa. (e) Plasma cells stained to show intracellular immunoglobulin using a fluorescein-labeled anti-IgG (green) and a rhodamine-conjugated anti-IgM (red). (f) Langerhans' cells in human epidermis in leprosy, increased in the subepidermal zone, possibly as a consequence of the disease process. Stained by the immunoperoxidase method with S-100 antibodies. (Material for (a) was kindly supplied by Mr M. Watts of the Department of Haematology, Middlesex Hospital Medical School; (b) and (c) by Professor P. Lydyard; (d) and (e) by Professor C. Grossi; and (f) by Dr Marian Ridley.)

tors have bound antigen receive a triggering signal and develop into antibody-forming plasma cells and, since the lymphocytes are programed to make only one antibody, that secreted by the plasma cell will be identical with that originally acting as the lymphocyte receptor, i.e. it will bind well to the antigen. In this way, antigen selects for the antibodies which recognize it effectively (figure 2.10).

The need for clonal expansion means humoral immunity must be acquired

Because we can make hundreds of thousands, maybe even millions, of different antibody molecules, it is not feasible for us to have too many lymphocytes producing each type of antibody; there just would not be enough room in the body to accommodate them. To

(a)

(b)

Figure 2.7. Lymphocyte ultrastructure. (a) Small agranular T-lymphocyte. Indented nucleus with condensed chromatin, sparse cytoplasm: single mitochondrion shown and many free ribosomes but otherwise few organelles (×13 000). B-lymphocytes are essentially similar with slightly more cytoplasm and occasional elements of rough-surfaced endoplasmic reticulum. (b) Large granular lymphocyte (×7500). The more abundant cytoplasm contains several mitochondria (M), free ribosomes (R) with some minor elements of rough-surfaced endoplasmic reticulum (ER), prominent Golgi apparatus (Go) and characteristic membrane-bound electron-dense granules (Gr). The nuclear chromatin is less condensed than that of the agranular T-cell. (Courtesy of Professors A. Zicca and C.E. Grossi.)

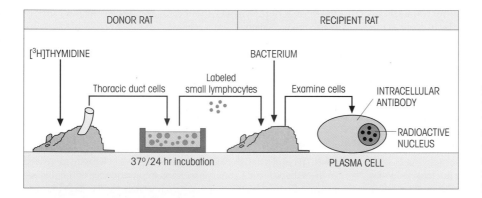

Figure 2.8. Labeled small lymphocytes become antibody-forming plasma cells when transferred to a recipient rat which is immunized with a bacterium. Transferred cell with radioactive nucleus shown by autoradiography. Intracellular antibody revealed by staining with fluorescent probes (cf. figure 2.6e).

compensate for this, lymphocytes which are triggered by contact with antigen undergo successive waves of proliferation (figure 2.6b) to build up a large clone of plasma cells which will be making antibody of the kind for which the parent lymphocyte was programed. By this system of **clonal selection**, large enough concentrations of antibody can be produced to combat infection effectively (Milestone 2.1; figure 2.11).

The importance of proliferation for the development of a significant antibody response is high-lighted by the ability of antimitotic drugs to abolish antibody production to a given antigen stimulus completely.

Because it takes time for the proliferating clone to build up its numbers sufficiently, it is usually several days before antibodies are detectable in the serum following primary contact with antigen. The newly formed antibodies are a consequence of antigen exposure and it is for this reason that we speak of the **acquired immune response**.

Figure 2.9. Plasma cell (×10 000). Prominent rough-surfaced endo-plasmic reticulum associated with the synthesis and secretion of Ig.

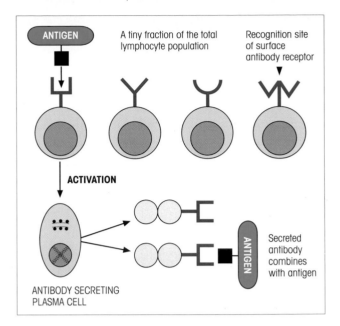

Figure 2.10. Antigen activates those B-cells whose surface anti-body receptors it can combine with firmly.

Figure 2.11. The cellular basis for the generation of effector and memory cells by clonal selection after primary contact with antigen. The cell selected by antigen undergoes many divisions during the clonal proliferation and the progeny mature to give an expanded population of antibody-forming cells. The antibody response is particularly vulnerable to antimitotic agents at the proliferation stage. A fraction of the progeny of the original antigen-reactive lymphocytes become nondividing memory cells and others the effector cells of either humoral, i.e. antibody-mediated, or, as we shall see subsequently, cell-mediated immunity. Memory cells require fewer cycles before they develop into effectors and this shortens the reaction time for the secondary response. The expanded clone of cells with memory for the original antigen provides the basis for the greater secondary relative to the primary immune response. Priming with low doses of antigen can often stimulate effective memory without producing very adequate antibody synthesis.

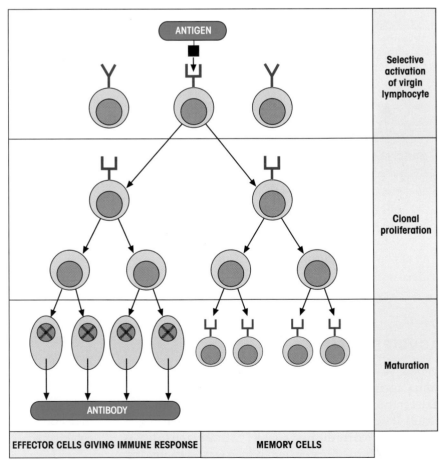

Milestone 2.1 — Clonal Selection Theory

Antibody production according to Ehrlich

In 1894, well in advance of his time as usual, the remarkable Paul Ehrlich proposed the side-chain theory of antibody production. Each cell would make a large variety of surface receptors which bound foreign antigens by complementary shape 'lock and key' fit. Exposure to antigen would provoke overproduction of receptors (antibodies) which would then be shed into the circulation (figure M2.1.1).

Template theories

Ehrlich's hypothesis implied that antibodies were preformed prior to antigen exposure. However, this view was difficult to accept when later work showed that antibodies could be formed to almost any organic structure synthesized in the chemist's laboratory (e.g. azobenzene arsonate; figure 5.1) despite the fact that such molecules would never be encountered in the natural environment. Thus was born the idea that antibodies were synthesized by using the antigen as a template. Twenty years passed before this idea was 'blown out of the water' by the observation that, after an antibody molecule is unfolded by guanidinium salts in the absence of antigen, it spontaneously refolds to regenerate its original specificity. It became clear that each antibody has a different amino acid sequence which governs its final folded shape and hence its ability to recognize antigen.

Selection theories

The wheel turns full circle and we once more live with the idea that, since different antibodies must be encoded by separate genes, the information for making these antibodies must pre-exist in the host DNA. In 1955, Nils Jerne perceived that this could form the basis for a selective theory of antibody production. He suggested that the complete antibody repertoire is expressed at a low level and that, when antigen enters the body, it selects its complementary antibody to form a complex which in some way provokes further synthesis of that particular antibody. But how?

Mac Burnet now brilliantly conceived of a cellular basis for this selection process. Let each lymphocyte be programed to make its own singular antibody which is inserted like an Ehrlich 'side-chain' into its surface membrane. Antigen will now form the complex envisaged by Jerne, on the surface of the lymphocyte, and by triggering its activation and clonal proliferation, large amounts of the specific antibody will be synthesized (figure 2.11). Bow graciously to that soothsayer Ehrlich—he came so close in 1894!

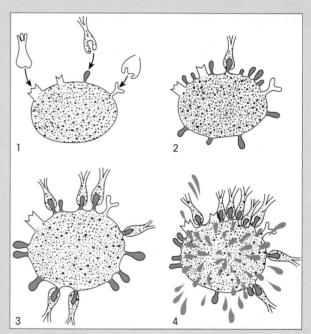

Figure M2.1.1. Ehrlich's side-chain theory of Ab production. (Reproduced from *Proceedings of the Royal Society B* (1900), **66**, 424.)

ACQUIRED MEMORY

When we make an antibody response to a given infectious agent, by definition that microorganism must exist in our environment and we are likely to meet it again. It would make sense then for the immune mechanisms alerted by the first contact with antigen to leave behind some memory system which would enable the response to any subsequent exposure to be faster and greater in magnitude.

Our experience of many common infections tells us that this must be so. We rarely suffer twice from such diseases as measles, mumps, chickenpox, whooping cough and so forth. The first contact clearly imprints some information, imparts some **memory**, so that the body is effectively prepared to repel any later invasion by that organism and a state of immunity is established.

Secondary antibody responses are better

By following the production of antibody on the first

and second contacts with antigen, we can see the basis for the development of immunity. For example, when we inject a bacterial product such as tetanus toxoid into a rabbit, for the reasons already discussed, several days elapse before antibodies can be detected in the blood; these reach a peak and then fall (figure 2.12). If we now allow the animal to rest and then give a second injection of toxoid, the course of events is dramatically altered. Within 2–3 days the antibody level in the blood rises steeply to reach much higher values than were observed in the **primary response**. This **secondary response** then is characterized by a more rapid and more abundant production of antibody resulting from the 'tuning up' or priming of the antibody-forming system.

With our knowledge of lymphocyte function, it is perhaps not surprising to realize that these are the cells which provide memory. This can be demonstrated by **adoptive transfer** of lymphocytes to another animal, an experimental system frequently employed in immunology (cf. figure 2.8). In the present case, the immunologic potential of the transferred cells is expressed in a recipient treated with X-rays which destroy its own lymphocyte population; thus any immune response will be of donor not recipient origin. In the experiment described in figure 2.13, small lymphocytes are taken from an animal given a primary injection of tetanus toxoid and transferred to an irradiated host which is then boosted with the antigen; a rapid, intense production of antibody characteristic of a secondary response is seen. To exclude the possibility that the first antigen injection might exert a *nonspecific* stimulatory effect on the lymphocytes, the boosting injection includes influenza hemagglutinin as a control antigen. Furthermore, a 'criss-cross' control group primed with influenza hemagglutinin must also be included to ensure that this antigen is capable of giving a secondary booster response. We have explained the design of the experiment at some length to call attention to the need for careful selection of controls.

The higher response given by a primed lymphocyte population can be ascribed mainly to an expansion of the numbers of cells capable of being stimulated by the antigen (figure 2.11), although we shall see later that there are some qualitative differences in these memory cells as well (pp. 195–197).

Figure 2.12. **Primary and secondary response.** A rabbit is injected on two separate occasions with tetanus toxoid. The antibody response on the second contact with antigen is more rapid and more intense.

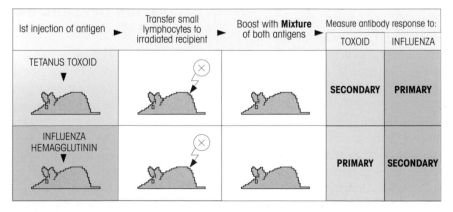

Figure 2.13. **Memory for a primary response can be transferred by small lymphocytes.** Recipients are treated with a dose of X-rays which directly kill lymphocytes (highly sensitive to radiation) but only affect other body cells when they divide; the recipient thus functions as a living 'test-tube' which permits the function of the donor cells to be followed. The reasons for the design of the experiment are given in the text. In practice, because of the possibility of interference between the two antigens, it would be wiser to split each of the primary antigen-injected groups into two, giving a separate boosting antigen to each to avoid using a mixture.

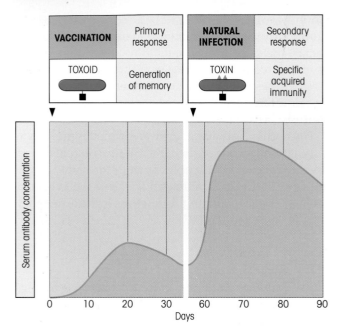

Figure 2.14. The basis of vaccination illustrated by the response to tetanus toxoid. Treatment of the bacterial toxin with formaldehyde destroys its toxicity (associated with ▲▲) but retains antigenicity. Exposure to toxin in a subsequent natural infection boosts the memory cells, producing high levels of neutralizing antibody which are protective.

ACQUIRED IMMUNITY HAS ANTIGEN SPECIFICITY

Discrimination between different antigens

The establishment of memory or immunity by one organism does not confer protection against another unrelated organism. After an attack of measles we are immune to further infection but are susceptible to other agents such as the polio or mumps viruses. Acquired immunity then shows **specificity** and the immune system can differentiate specifically between the two organisms. A more formal experimental demonstration of this discriminatory power was seen in figure 2.13 where priming with tetanus toxoid evoked memory for that antigen but not for influenza and vice versa.

The basis for this lies of course in the ability of the recognition sites of the antibody molecules to distinguish between antigens; antibodies which react with the toxoid do not bind to influenza and, *mutatis mutandis* as they say, anti-influenza is not particularly smitten with the toxoid.

Discrimination between self and nonself

This ability to recognize one antigen and distinguish it from another goes even further. The individual must also recognize what is foreign, i.e. what is 'nonself'. The failure to discriminate between **self** and **nonself** could lead to the synthesis of antibodies directed against components of the subject's own body (**auto-antibodies**), which in principle could prove to be highly embarrassing. On purely theoretical grounds it seemed to Burnet and Fenner that the body must develop some mechanism whereby 'self' and 'nonself' could be distinguished, and they postulated that those circulating body components which were able to reach the developing lymphoid system in the perinatal period could in some way be 'learnt' as 'self'. A permanent unresponsiveness or **tolerance** would then be created so that as immunologic maturity was reached there would normally be an inability to respond to 'self' components. At this stage it is salutory to note that Burnet had the sagacity to realize that his clonal selection theory could readily provide the cellular basis for such a mechanism to operate. He argued that if each lymphocyte were preoccupied with making its own individual antibody, those cells programed to express antibodies reacting with circulating self components could be rendered unresponsive without affecting those lymphocytes specific for foreign antigens. In other words, self-reacting lymphocytes could be selectively suppressed or tolerized without undermining the ability of the host to respond immunologically to infectious agents. As we shall see in Chapter 12, these predictions have been amply verified, although we will learn that, as new lymphocytes differentiate throughout life, they will all go through this self-tolerizing screening process. However, self tolerance is not absolute and normally innocuous but potentially harmful anti-self lymphocytes exist in all of us.

VACCINATION DEPENDS ON ACQUIRED MEMORY

Some 200 years ago, Edward Jenner carried out the remarkable studies which mark the beginning of immunology as a systematic subject. Noting the pretty pox-free skin of the milkmaids, he reasoned that deliberate exposure to the pox virus of the cow, which is not virulent for the human, might confer protection against the related human smallpox organism. Accordingly, he inoculated a small boy with cowpox and was delighted—and presumably breathed a sigh of relief—to observe that the boy was now protected against a subsequent exposure to smallpox (what would today's ethical committees have said about that?!). By injecting a harmless form of a disease organism, Jenner had utilized the specificity and memory of the acquired immune response to lay the foundations for modern **vaccination** (Latin *vacca*, cow).

The essential strategy is to prepare an *innocuous* form of the infectious organism or its toxins which still substantially retains the antigens responsible for establishing protective immunity. This has been done by using killed or live attenuated organisms, purified microbial components or chemically modified antigens (figure 2.14).

CELL-MEDIATED IMMUNITY PROTECTS AGAINST INTRACELLULAR ORGANISMS

Many microorganisms live inside host cells where it is impossible for humoral antibody to reach them. Obligate intracellular parasites like viruses have to replicate inside cells; facultative intracellular parasites like *Mycobacteria* and *Leishmania* can replicate within cells, particularly macrophages, but do not have to; they like the intracellular life because of the protection it affords. A totally separate acquired immunity system has evolved to deal with this situation based on a distinct lymphocyte subpopulation made up of **T-cells**, designated thus because, unlike the B-lymphocytes, they differentiate within the milieu of the **thymus gland**. Because they are specialized to operate against cells bearing intracellular organisms, T-cells only recognize antigen when it is on the surface of a body cell. Accordingly, the **T-cell surface receptors**, which are different from the antibody molecules used by B-lymphocytes, recognize antigen plus a surface marker which informs the T-lymphocyte that it is making contact with another cell. These cell markers belong to an important group of molecules known as the **major histocompati-** bility complex (MHC), identified originally through their ability to evoke powerful transplantation reactions in other members of the same species. Now naive or virgin T-cells must be introduced to the antigen and MHC by a special dendritic antigen-presenting cell (figures 2.6f and 8.13) before they can be initiated into the rites of a primary response. However, once primed, they are activated by antigen and MHC present on the surface of other cell types such as macrophages as we shall now see.

Cytokine-producing T-cells help macrophages to kill intracellular parasites

These organisms only survive inside macrophages through their ability to subvert the innate killing mechanisms of these cells. Nonetheless, they cannot prevent the macrophage from processing small antigenic fragments (possibly of organisms which have spontaneously died) and placing them on the host cell surface. A subpopulation of T-lymphocytes called **T-helper cells**, if primed to that antigen, will recognize and bind to the combination of antigen with so-called **class II** MHC molecules on the macrophage surface and produce a variety of soluble factors termed **cytokines** which include the interleukins IL-2, etc. (p. 177). Different cytokines can be made by various cell types and generally act at a short range on neighboring cells. Some T-cell cytokines help B-cells to make antibodies, while others such as γ-interferon (IFNγ) act as **macrophage activating factors** which switch on the previously subverted microbicidal mechanisms of the macrophage and bring about the death of the intracellular microorganisms (figure 2.15).

Figure 2.15. Intracellular killing of microorganisms by macrophages. (1) Surface antigen (💲) derived from the intracellular microbes is complexed with class II MHC molecules (🔲). (2) The primed T-helper cell binds to this surface complex and is triggered to release the cytokine γ-interferon (IFNγ). This activates microbicidal mechanisms in the macrophage. (3) The infectious agent meets a timely death.

1	2	3
Infection by intracellular facultative organisms	Macrophage activation	Death of intracellular microbes

Virally infected cells can be killed by cytotoxic T-cells and ADCC

We have already discussed the advantage to the host of killing virally infected cells before the virus begins to replicate and have seen that large granular lymphocytes with NK activity (p. 18) can subserve a cytotoxic function. However, NK cells have a limited range of specificities and, in order to improve their efficacy, this range needs to be expanded.

One way in which this can be achieved is by coating the target cell with antibodies specific for the virally coded surface antigens because NK cells have receptors for the constant part of the antibody molecule, rather like phagocytic cells. Thus antibodies will bring the NK cell very close to the target by forming a bridge, and the NK cell being activated by the complexed antibody molecules is able to kill the virally infected cell by its extracellular mechanisms (figure 2.16). This system, termed **antibody-dependent cellular cytotoxicity (ADCC)**, is very impressive when studied *in vitro* but it has proved difficult to establish to what extent it operates within the body.

On the other hand, a **subset** of **T-cells with cytotoxic potential** has evolved for which there is clear evidence

of *in vivo* activity. Like the T-helpers, these cells have a very wide range of antigen specificities because they clonally express a large number of different surface receptors similar to, but not identical with, the surface antibody receptors on the B-lymphocytes. Again, each lymphocyte is programed to make only one receptor and, again like the T-helper cell, recognizes antigen only in association with a cell marker, in this case the **class I** MHC molecule (figure 2.16). Through this recognition of surface antigen, the cytotoxic cell comes into intimate contact with its target and administers the 'kiss of apoptotic death'. It also releases **IFNγ** which would help to reduce the spread of virus to adjacent cells, particularly in cases where the virus itself may prove to be a weak inducer of IFNα or β.

In an entirely analogous fashion to the B-cell, T-cells are selected and activated by combination with antigen, expanded by clonal proliferation and mature to give T-helpers and cytotoxic T-effectors, together with an enlarged population of memory cells. Thus both T- and B-cells provide **specific acquired immunity** with a variety of mechanisms, which in most cases operate to extend the range of effectiveness of innate immunity and confer the valuable advantage that a first infection

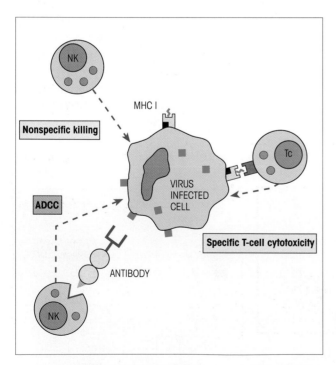

Figure 2.16. Killing virally infected cells. The nonspecific killing mechanism of the NK cell can be focused on the target by antibody to produce antibody-dependent cellular cytotoxicity (ADCC). The cytotoxic T-cell homes onto its target specifically through receptor recognition of surface antigen in association with MHC class I molecules.

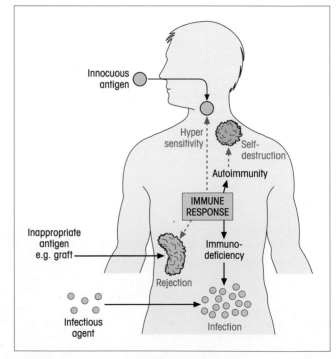

Figure 2.17. Inappropriate immune responses can produce damaging reactions such as the hypersensitivity response to inhaled otherwise innocuous allergens, the destruction of self tissue by autoimmune attack, the rejection of tissue transplants, and the susceptibility to infection in immunodeficient individuals.

prepares us to withstand further contact with the same microorganism.

IMMUNOPATHOLOGY

The immune system is clearly 'a good thing', but like mercenary armies, it can turn to bite the hand that feeds it, and cause damage to the host (figure 2.17).

Thus where there is an especially heightened response or persistent exposure to exogenous antigens, tissue damaging or **hypersensitivity** reactions may result. Examples are allergy to grass pollens, blood dyscrasias associated with certain drugs, immune complex glomerulonephritis occurring after streptococcal infection, and chronic granulomas produced during tuberculosis or schistosomiasis.

In other cases, hypersensitivity to autoantigens may arise through a breakdown in the mechanisms which control self tolerance, and a wide variety of **autoimmune diseases**, such as insulin-dependent diabetes and multiple sclerosis and many of the rheumatologic disorders, have now been recognized.

Another immunopathologic reaction of some consequence is **transplant rejection**, where the MHC antigens on the donor graft may well provoke a fierce reaction. Lastly, one should consider the by no means infrequent occurrence of inadequate functioning of the immune system—**immunodeficiency**. We would like to think that at this stage the reader would have no difficulty in predicting that the major problems in this condition relate to persistent infection, the type of infection being related to the elements of the immune system which are defective.

SUMMARY

Antibody—the specific adaptor

• The antibody molecule evolved as a specific adaptor to attach to microorganisms which either fail to activate the alternative complement pathway or prevent activation of the phagocytic cells.

• The antibody fixes to the antigen by its specific recognition site and its constant structure regions activate complement through the classical pathway (binding C1 and generating a $\overline{C4b2a}$ convertase to split C3) and phagocytes through their antibody receptors.

• This supplementary route into the acute inflammatory reaction is enhanced by antibodies which sensitize mast cells and by immune complexes which stimulate mediator release from tissue macrophages (figure 2.18).

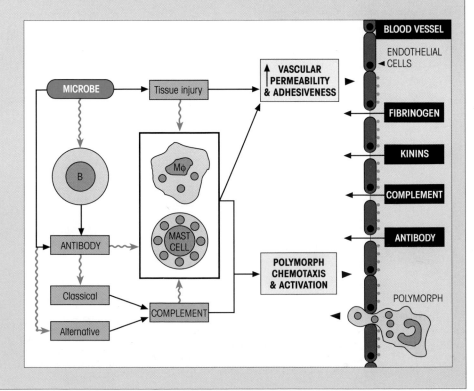

Figure 2.18. Production of a protective acute inflammatory reaction by microbes either: (i) through tissue injury (e.g. bacterial toxin) or direct activation of the alternative complement pathway, or (ii) by antibody-dependent triggering of the classical complement pathway or mast cell degranulation (a special class of antibody, IgE, does this).

(continued p. 34)

Cellular basis of antibody production

• Antibodies are made by plasma cells derived from B-lymphocytes, each of which is programed to make antibody of a single specificity which is placed on the cell surface as a receptor.

• Antigen binds to the cell with a complementary antibody, activates it and causes clonal proliferation and finally maturation to antibody-forming cells and memory cells. Thus the antigen brings about clonal selection of the cells making antibody to itself.

Acquired memory and vaccination

• The increase in memory cells after priming means that the acquired secondary response is faster and greater, providing the basis for vaccination using a harmless form of the infective agent for the initial injection.

Acquired immunity has antigen specificity

• Antibodies differentiate between antigens because recognition is based on molecular shape complementarity. Thus memory induced by one antigen will not extend to another unrelated antigen.

• The immune system differentiates self components from foreign antigens by making immature self-reacting lymphocytes unresponsive through contact with host molecules; lymphocytes reacting with foreign antigens are unaffected since they only make contact after reaching maturity.

Cell-mediated immunity protects against intracellular organisms

• Another class of lymphocyte, the T-cell, is concerned with control of intracellular infections. Like the B-cell, each T-cell has its individual antigen receptor (although it differs structurally from antibody) which recognizes antigen and the cell then undergoes clonal expansion to form effector and memory cells providing specific acquired immunity.

• The T-cell recognizes cell surface antigens in association with molecules of the MHC. Naive T-cells are only stimulated to undergo a primary response by specialized dendritic antigen-presenting cells.

• Primed T-helper cells, which see antigen with class II MHC on the surface of macrophages, release cytokines which in some cases can help B-cells to make antibody and in others activate macrophages and enable them to kill intracellular parasites.

• Cytotoxic T-cells have the ability to recognize specific antigen plus class I MHC on the surface of virally infected cells which are killed before the virus replicates. They also release γ-interferon which can make surrounding cells resistant to viral spread (figure 2.19).

• NK cells have lectin-like 'nonspecific' receptors for cells infected by viruses but do not have antigen-specific receptors; however, they can recognize antibody-coated virally infected cells through their Fcγ receptors and kill the target by antibody-dependent cellular cytotoxicity (ADCC).

• Although the innate mechanisms do not improve with repeated exposure to infection as do the acquired, they play a vital role since they are intimately linked to the acquired systems by **two different pathways** which all but **encapsulate the whole of immunology**. Antibody, complement and polymorphs give protection against most extracellular organisms, while T-cells, soluble cytokines, macrophages and NK cells deal with intracellular infections (figure 2.20).

Figure 2.19. T-cells link with the innate immune system to resist intracellular infection. Class I (⊟) and class II (⊟) major histocompatibility molecules are important for T-cell recognition of surface antigen. The T-helper cells (Th) cooperate in the development of cytotoxic T-cells (Tc) from precursors. The macrophage (Mφ) microbicidal mechanisms are switched on by macrophage activating lymphokines. Interferon inhibits viral replication and stimulates NK cells which, together with Tc, kill virus-infected cells.

(continued)

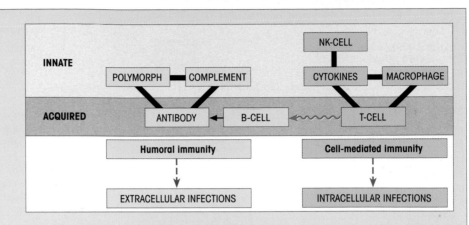

Figure 2.20. The two pathways linking innate and acquired immunity which provide the basis for humoral and cell-mediated immunity, respectively.

Immunopathology

• Immunopathologically mediated tissue damage to the host can occur as a result of:

inappropriate hypersensitivity reactions to exogenous antigens;

loss of tolerance to self giving rise to autoimmune disease;

reaction to foreign grafts.

• Immunodeficiency leaves the individual susceptible to infection.

See the accompanying website (**www.roitt.com**) for multiple choice questions.

FURTHER READING

General reading

Aderem A. & Underhill D.M. (1999) Mechanisms of phagocytosis in macrophages. *Annual Review of Immunology* **17**, 593.

Alt F. & Marrack P. (eds) (2001) *Current Opinion in Immunology* **13**. (Appears bimonthly; Issue No. 1 deals with 'Innate Immunity'.)

Gudmundsson G.H. & Agerberth B. (1999) Neutrophil antibacterial peptides, multifunctional effector molecules in the mammalian immune system. *Journal of Immunological Methods* **232**, 45.

Levy O. (1996) Antibiotic proteins of polymorphonuclear leukocytes. *European Journal of Haematology* **56**, 263.

Matzinger P. (1998) An innate sense of danger. *Seminars in Immunology* **10**, 399.

Morgan B.P. (1991) *Complement. Clinical Aspects and Relevance to Disease*. Academic Press, London.

Neth O. *et al.* (2000) Mannose-binding lectin binds to a range of clinically relevant micro-organisms and promotes complement deposition. *Infection and Immunity* **68**, 688.

Reid K.B.M. (1995) The complement system—a major effector mechanism in humoral immunity. *The Immunologist* **3**, 206.

Segal A.W. & Abo A. (1993) The biochemical basis of the NADPH oxidase of phagocytes. *Trends in Biochemical Sciences* **18**, 43.

Shi L., Krant R.P., Aebersold R. & Greenberg A.H. (1992) An NK cell granule protein that induces DNA fragmentation and apoptosis (in perforin permeabilized cells). *Journal of Experimental Medicine* **175**, 553.

Sitaram N. & Nagaraj R. (1999) Interaction of antimicrobial peptides with biological and model membranes: structural and charge requirements for activity. *Biochimica et Biophysica Acta—Biomembranes* **1462**, 29.

Reference work

Delves P.J. & Roitt I.M. (eds) (1998) *Encyclopedia of Immunology*, 2nd edn. Academic Press, London. (Covers virtually all aspects of the subject and describes immune responses to most infections.)

Historical

Clarke W.R. (1991) *The Experimental Foundations of Modern Immunology*, 4th edn. John Wiley & Sons, New York. (Important for those wishing to appreciate the experiments leading up to many of the major discoveries.)

Ehrlich P. (1890) On immunity with special reference to cell life. In Melchers F. *et al.* (eds) *Progress in Immunology* **VII**. Springer-Verlag, Berlin. (Translation of a lecture to the Royal Society (London) on the side-chain theory of antibody formation, showing this man's perceptive genius. A must!)

Landsteiner K. (1946) *The Specificity of Serological Reactions*. Harvard University Press (reprinted 1962 by Dover Publications, New York).

Mazumdar P.M.M. (ed.) (1989) *Immunology 1930–1980*. Wall & Thompson, Toronto.

Metchnikoff E. (1893) *Comparative Pathology of Inflammation*. Kegan Paul, Trench, Trubner, London (translated by F.A. & E.H. Starling).

Palmer R. (ed.) (1993) *Outstanding Papers in Biology*. Current Biology, London. (A delight to browse through some of the seminal papers which have shaped modern biology; wonderful material for teaching.)

Silverstein A.M. (1989) *A History of Immunology*. Academic Press, San Diego.

Tauber A.I. (1991) *Metchnikoff and the Origins of Immunology*. Oxford University Press, Oxford.

Table 2.1. The major immunologic journals and their impact factors.

GENERAL JOURNALS OF PARTICULAR INTEREST TO IMMUNOLOGISTS	*IMPACT FACTOR
Cell	36.2
EMBO J.	14.0
Lancet	10.2
Nature	29.5
Nature Medicine	26.6
New England Journal of Medicine	28.9
Proceedings of the National Academy of Sciences of the USA	10.3
Science	24.6

IMMUNOLOGICAL JOURNALS	*IMPACT FACTOR
Autoimmunity	1.1
Cancer Immunology Immunotherapy	2.3
Cellular Immunology	2.3
Clinical and Experimental Allergy	2.7
Clinical and Experimental Immunology	2.8
European Journal of Immunology	5.6
Human Immunology	2.6
Immunity	20.6
Immunogenetics	2.9
Immunology	2.6
Immunopharmacology	1.4
Infection and Immunity	4.2
International Archives of Allergy and Applied Immunology	1.9
International Immunology	2.9
Journal of Allergy and Clinical Immunology	4.6
Journal of Autoimmunity	2.2
Journal of Clinical Immunology	2.4
Journal of Experimental Medicine	15.7
Journal of Immunology	7.1
Journal of Immunological Methods	1.9
Journal of Immunotherapy	3.1
Journal of Reproductive Immunology	1.5
Molecular Immunology	2.1
Nature Immunology	N/A
Parasite Immunology	2.0
Scandinavian Journal of Immunology	1.7
Tissue Antigens	3.0
Transplantaion	3.5
Vaccine	3.2

*IMPACT FACTOR = relative frequency with which the journal's 'average article' has been cited in other publications

N/A, not available.

In-depth series for the advanced reader
Advances in Immunology (Annual). Academic Press, London.
Advances in Neuroimmunology (edited by G.B. Stefano & E.M. Smith). Pergamon, Oxford.
Annual Review of Immunology. Annual Reviews Inc., California.
Immunological Reviews (edited by P. Parham). Munksgaard, Copenhagen. (Specialized, authoritative and thoughtful.)
Progress in Allergy. Karger, Basle.
Seminars in Immunology. Academic Press, Cambridge. (In-depth treatment of single subjects.)

Current information
Current Biology. Current Biology, London. (What the complete biologist needs to know about significant current advances.)
Current Opinion in Immunology. Current Science, London. (Important personal opinions on focused highlights of the advances made in the previous year; most valuable for the serious immunologist.)
Trends in Molecular Medicine. Elsevier Science Publications, Amsterdam. (Frequent articles of interest to immunologists with very good perspective.)
The Immunologist. Hogrefe & Huber Publishers, Seattle. (Official organ of the International Union of Immunological Societies—IUIS. Excellent, didactic and compact articles on current trends in immunology.)
Trends in Immunology. Elsevier Science Publications, Amsterdam. (The immunologist's 'newspaper'. Excellent.)

Multiple choice questions
Roitt I.M. & Delves P.J. 400 MCQs each with five annotated learning responses. See **Website**.

Website (linked to Roitt's Essential Immunology) http://www.roitt.com
The Website contains (i) 400 *Multiple Choice Revision Questions*, (ii) continual *update* providing abstracts and comments on important current immunologic publications, (iii) a series of *Interactive Core Tutorials in Immunology*. Blackwell Science Ltd, Oxford (CD ROM Mac/Windows: 110 fundamental immunologic principles using animations accompanied by spoken explanations to clarify and guide. Reference to standard and advanced text in *Essential Immunology* and a selection of multiple choice questions), (iv) *Further Reading* and reference archive, and (v) *Image archive* with over 400 illustrations from *Essential Immunology*.

Major journals
The major journals of interest and their impact factors are noted in table 2.1.

Antibodies

INTRODUCTION

The antibody molecule is made up of two identical heavy and two identical light chains held together by interchain disulfide bonds (figure M3.1.1). These chains can be separated by reduction of the S–S bonds and acidification. In the most abundant type of antibody in the circulation, **immunoglobulin G**, the exposed hinge region is extended in structure due to the high proline content and is therefore vulnerable to proteolytic attack; thus the molecule can be easily split in the laboratory using papain to yield two identical **Fab** fragments, each with a single combining site for antigen, and a third fragment, **Fc**, which lacks the ability to bind antigen. Pepsin strikes at a different point and cleaves the Fc from the remainder of the molecule to leave a large 5S fragment which is designated F(ab')$_2$ since it is still divalent with respect to antigen binding just like the parent antibody (Milestone 3.1).

ANTIBODIES HAVE DISCREET SITES FOR BINDING ANTIGEN

The location of the antigen combining sites was elegantly demonstrated by a study of purified antibodies to the dinitrophenyl (DNP) group mixed with the compound:

The two DNP groups are far enough apart not to interfere with each other's combination with antibody so that they can bring the antigen combining sites on two different antibodies together end to end. When viewed by negative staining in the electron microscope, a series of geometric forms is observed which represents the different structures to be expected if a flexible Y-shaped hinged molecule with a combining site at the end of each of the two arms of the Y were to complex with this divalent antigen. Triangular trimers, square tetramers and pentagonal pentamers may be readily discerned (figure 3.1). The way in which these polymeric forms arise is indicated in figure 3.2. The position of the Fc fragment and its lack of involvement in the combination with antigen are apparent from the shape of the polymers formed using the pepsin F(ab')$_2$ fragment (figure 3.1C).

AMINO ACID SEQUENCES REVEAL VARIATIONS IN IMMUNOGLOBULIN STRUCTURE

For good reasons, the antibody population in any

Milestone 3.1—Four-polypeptide Structure of Immunoglobulin Monomers

Early studies showed the bulk of the antibody activity in serum to be in the slow electrophoretic fraction termed γ-globulin (subsequently immunoglobulin). The most abundant antibodies were divalent, i.e. had two combining sites for antigen and could thus form a precipitating complex (cf. figure 6.2).

To Rodney Porter and Gerald Edelman must go the credit for unlocking the secrets of the basic structure of the immunoglobulin molecule. If the internal disulfide bonds are reduced, the component polypeptide chains still hang together by strong noncovalent attractions. However, if the reduced molecule is held under acid conditions, these attractive forces are lost as the chains become positively charged and can now be separated by gel filtration into larger so-called heavy chains of approximately 55 000 Da (for IgG, IgA and IgD) or 70 000 Da (for IgM and IgE) and smaller light chains of about 24 000 Da.

The clues to how the chains are assembled to form the antibody molecule came from selective cleavage using proteolytic enzymes. Papain destroyed the precipitating power of the intact molecule but produced two univalent Fab fragments still capable of binding to antigen (Fab = *fragment antigen binding*); the remaining fragment had no affinity for antigen and was termed Fc by Porter (*fragment crystallizable*). After digestion with pepsin a molecule called F(ab')₂ was isolated; it still precipitated antigen and so retained both binding sites, but the Fc portion was further degraded. The structural basis for these observations is clearly evident from figure M3.1.1. In essence, with minor changes, all immunoglobulin molecules are constructed from one or more of the basic four-chain monomer units.

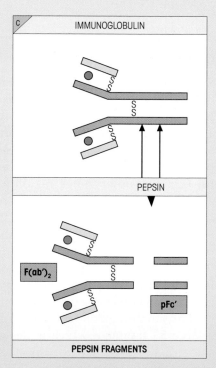

Figure M3.1.1. The antibody basic unit, consisting of two identical heavy and two identical light chains held together by interchain disulfide bonds, can be broken down into its constituent polypeptide chains and to proteolytic fragments, the pepsin F(ab')₂ retaining two binding sites for antigen and the papain Fab with one. After pepsin digestion the pFc' fragment representing the C-terminal half of the Fc region is formed and is held together by noncovalent bonds. The portion of the heavy chain in the Fab fragment is given the symbol Fd. The N-terminal residue is on the left for each chain.

Figure 3.1. (A) and (B) Electron micrograph (×1 000 000) of complexes formed on mixing the divalent DNP hapten with rabbit anti-DNP antibodies. The 'negative stain' phosphotungstic acid is an electron-dense solution which penetrates into the spaces between the protein molecules. Thus the protein stands out as a 'light' structure in the electron beam. The hapten links together the Y-shaped antibody molecules to form trimers (A) and pentamers (B) (cf. figure 3.2). The flexibility of the molecule at the hinge region is evident from the variation in angle of the arms of the 'Y'. (C) As in (A); but the trimers were formed using the F(ab')₂ antibody fragment from which the Fc structures have been digested by pepsin (× 500 000). The trimers can be seen to lack the Fc projections at each corner evident in (A). (After Valentine R.C. & Green N.M. (1967) *Journal of Molecular Biology* **27**, 615; courtesy of Dr Green and with the permission of Academic Press, New York.)

Figure 3.2. Three DNP antibody molecules held together as a trimer by the divalent antigen (●—●). Compare figure 3.1A. When the Fc fragments are first removed by pepsin, the corner pieces are no longer visible (figure 3.1C).

given individual is just incredibly heterogeneous, and this has meant that the determination of amino acid sequences was utterly useless until it proved possible to obtain the homogeneous product of a single clone. The opportunity to do this first came from the study of **myeloma proteins**.

In the human disease known as multiple myeloma, one cell making one particular individual immunoglobulin divides over and over again in the uncontrolled way a cancer cell does, without regard for the overall requirement of the host. The patient then possesses enormous numbers of identical cells derived as a clone from the original cell and they all synthesize the same immunoglobulin—the myeloma or M-protein—which appears in the serum, sometimes in very high concentrations. By purification of the myeloma protein we can obtain a preparation of an immunoglobulin having a unique structure. **Monoclonal antibodies** can also be obtained by fusing individual antibody-forming cells with a B-cell tumor to produce a constantly dividing clone of cells dedicated to making the one antibody (cf. figures 2.11 and 6.20).

The sequencing of a number of such proteins has revealed that the N-terminal portions of both heavy and light chains show considerable variability, whereas the remaining parts of the chains are relatively constant, being grouped into a restricted number of structures. It is conventional to speak of variable and constant regions of both heavy and light chains (figure 3.3).

Certain sequences in the variable regions show quite remarkable diversity and systematic analysis localizes these hypervariable sequences to three segments on the light chain (figure 3.4) and three on the heavy chain.

IMMUNOGLOBULIN GENES

Immunoglobulins are encoded by multiple gene segments

Clusters of genes on three different chromosomes code for κ light chains, λ light chains and for heavy chains, respectively. Since a wide range of antibodies with differing amino acid sequences can be produced, there must be corresponding nucleotide sequences to encode them. However, the complete gene encoding each heavy and light chain is not present as such in the inherited (germ-line) DNA, but is created during early development of the B-cell by the joining together of minisegments of the gene. Take the human κ light chain for example; the variable region is made up of two gene

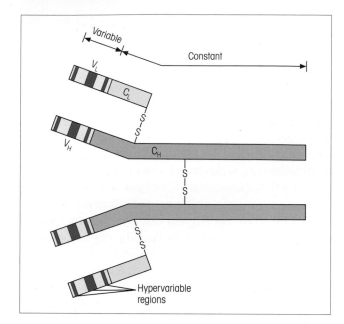

Figure 3.3. Amino acid sequence variability in the antibody molecule. The terms 'V region' and 'C region' are used to designate the variable and constant regions, respectively; 'V_L' and 'C_L' are generic terms for these regions on the light chain and 'V_H' and 'C_H' specify variable and constant regions on the heavy chain. Certain segments of the variable region are hypervariable but adjacent framework regions are more conserved. As stressed previously, each pair of heavy chains is identical, as is each pair of light chains.

Figure 3.4. Wu and Kabat plot of amino acid variability in the variable region of immunoglobulin heavy and light chains. The sequences of chains from a large number of myeloma monoclonal proteins are compared and the variability at each position is computed as the number of different amino acids found divided by the frequency of the most common amino acid. Obviously, the higher the number the greater the variability; for a residue at which all 20 amino acids occur randomly, the number will be 400 (20 ÷ 0.05), and at a completely invariant residue, the figure will be 1 (1 ÷ 1). The three hypervariable regions (blue) in the (a) heavy and (b) light chains, usually referred to as **complementarity determining regions (CDRs)**, are clearly defined. The intervening peptide sequences (gray) are termed framework regions (Fr1–4). (Courtesy of Professor E. A. Kabat.)

segments, a large V_κ and a small J_κ, while a single gene encodes the constant region (figure 3.5). There is a cluster of ~40 V_κ genes and just five functional J_κ genes. In the immature B-cell, a translocation event leads to the joining of one of the V_κ genes to one of the J_κ segments. Each V segment has its own leader sequence and a number of upstream promoter sites, including a characteristic octamer sequence, to which transcription factors bind (figure 3.6). When the Ig gene is transcribed, splicing of the nuclear RNA brings the $V_\kappa J_\kappa$ sequence into contiguity with the constant region C_κ sequence, the whole being read off as a continuous κ chain polypeptide within the endoplasmic reticulum.

The same general principles apply to the arrangement of λ light chain and the heavy chain genes, although the latter constellation shows additional features: the different constant region genes form a single cluster and there is a group of around 25 highly variable D segments located between the V and J regions (figure 3.7). The D segment together with its junctions to the V and J segments encodes almost the entire third hypervariable region, the first two hypervariable regions being encoded entirely within the V sequence.

A special mechanism effects *VDJ* recombination

In essence, the translocation involves the mutual recognition of conserved heptamer–spacer–nonamer recombination signal sequences which flank each germ-line V, D and J segment (figure 3.8). The products of the recombination activating genes *RAG-1* and *RAG-2* catalyse the introduction of double-strand breaks between the elements to be joined and their respective flanking sequences. At this stage, nucleotides may either be deleted or inserted between the *VD*, *DJ* or *VJ* joining elements before they are ultimately ligated.

Figure 3.5. Genetic basis for synthesis of human κ chains. The V_κ genes are arranged in a series of families or sets of a closely related sequence. Each V_κ gene has its own leader sequence (*L*). As the cell becomes immunocompetent, the variable region is formed by the random combination of one out of the 40 V_κ genes with one of the five joining segments *J*, a gene rearrangement process facilitated by base sequences in the intron following the 3′ end of the V_κ segment pairing up with sequences in the intron 5′ to *J*. The final joining occurs when the intervening intron sequence between *J* and C_κ is spliced out of the RNA transcript. By convention, the genes are represented in italics and the antigens they encode in normal type.

STRUCTURAL VARIANTS OF THE BASIC IMMUNOGLOBULIN MOLECULE

Isotypes

Based upon the structure of their heavy chain constant regions, immunoglobulins are classed into major groups termed **classes** which may be further subdivided into **subclasses**. In the human, for example, there are five classes: immunoglobulin G (IgG), IgΛ, IgM, IgD and IgE. They may be differentiated not only by their sequences but also by the antigenic structures to which these sequences give rise. Thus, by injecting a human IgG myeloma protein into a rabbit, it is possible to raise an antiserum which can be absorbed by mixtures of myelomas of other classes to remove cross-reacting antibodies and which will then be capable of reacting with IgG, but not IgA, IgM, IgD or IgE (figure 3.9).

Since all the heavy chain constant region (C_H) structures which give rise to classes and subclasses are expressed together in the serum of a normal subject, they are termed **isotypic variants** (table 3.1). Likewise, the light chain constant regions (C_L) exist in isotypic forms known as κ and λ which are associated with all heavy chain isotypes. Because the light chains in a given antibody are identical, immunoglobulins are either κ or λ but never mixed. Thus IgG exists as IgGκ or IgGλ, IgM as IgMκ or IgMλ, and so on.

Allotypes

This type of variation depends upon the existence of allelic forms (encoded by alleles or alternative genes at a single locus) which therefore provide genetic markers (table 3.1). In somewhat the same way as the red cells in genetically different individuals can differ in terms of the blood group antigen system A, B, O, so the Ig heavy chains differ in the expression of their allotypic groups. Typical allotypes are the **Gm specificities** on IgG

Figure 3.6. Genes controlling immunoglobulin heavy chain transcription. Each *VDJ* segment encoding the variable region is associated with a leader sequence. Closely upstream is the TATA box of the promoter which binds RNA polymerase II and the octamer motif which is one of a number of short sequences which bind transacting regulatory transcription factors. The *V*-region promoters are relatively inactive and only association with enhancers, which are also composites of short sequence motifs capable of binding nuclear pro-

teins, will increase the transcription rate to levels typical of actively secreting B-cells. The enhancers are near to the regions which control switching from one Ig class constant region to another, e.g. IgM to IgG. Primary transcripts are initiated 20 nucleotides downstream of the TATA box and extend beyond the end of the constant region. These are spliced, cleaved at the 3′ end and polyadenylated to generate the translatable mRNA.

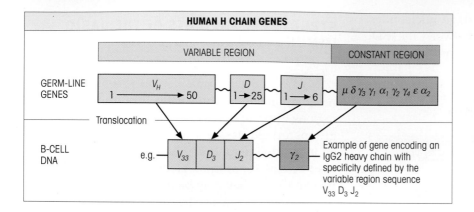

Figure 3.7. Human *V*-region genes shuffled by gene rearrangement to generate the single heavy chain specificity characteristic of each B-cell. The V_H genes can be grouped into seven different families (V_H1–V_H7) based upon sequence homology of > 80%, with V_H3 being by far the largest family. Individual members of a family are interspersed throughout the locus, i.e. there is no significant grouping together of V_H family genes. Note the additional *D* segment minigenes that are present in the heavy chain locus.

Table 3.1. Summary of immunoglobulin variants.

V_H/V_L		CONSTANT
IDIOTYPE ISOTYPE		ISOTYPE

Hypervariable
(Ag combining site)   ALLOTYPE

TYPE OF VARIATION	DISTRIBUTION	VARIANT	LOCATION	EXAMPLES
ISOTYPIC	All variants present in serum of a normal individual	Classes Subclasses Types Subgroups Families	C_H C_H C_L C_L V_H/V_L	IgM, IgE IgA1, IgA2 κ, λ $\lambda Oz^+, \lambda Oz^-$ $V_{\kappa I}\ V_{\kappa II}\ V_{\kappa III}$ $V_{HI}\ V_{HII}\ V_{HIII}$
ALLOTYPIC	Alternative forms: genetically controlled so not present in all individuals	Allotypes	Mainly C_H/C_L sometimes V_H/V_L	Gm groups (human) b4, b5, b6, b9 (rabbit light chains) Igh-1^a, Igh-1^b (mouse γ_{2a} heavy chains)
IDIOTYPIC	Individually specific to each immuno-globulin molecule	Idiotypes	Variable regions	One or more hypervariable regions forming the antigen-combining site

(Gm = *marker* on IgG). Allotypic differences at a given Gm locus usually involve one or two amino acids in the peptide chain. Take, for example, the G1m(a) locus on IgG1 (table 3.1). An individual with this allotype would have the peptide sequence Asp.Glu.Leu.Thr.Lys on each of his or her IgG1 molecules. An individual possessing the a-negative allotype would have the sequence Glu.Glu.Met.Thr.Lys, i.e. two amino acids different. To date, 20 Gm groups have been found on the γ heavy chains and a further three (the Km—previously Inv groups) on the κ constant region.

As in other allelic systems, individuals may be homozygous or heterozygous for the genes encoding the markers; these are expressed codominantly and are inherited in simple Mendelian fashion. Take, for example, the b4, b5 allotypes on rabbit light chains: an animal of b^4b^4 genotype would express the b4 allotype, whereas a rabbit of b^4b^5 genotype derived from b^4b^4 and b^5b^5 parents would express the b4 marker on one fraction and b5 on another fraction of its immunoglobulin molecules.

Idiotypes

We have seen that it is possible to obtain antibodies that recognize isotypic and allotypic variants; one can also raise antiserums which are specific for individual antibody molecules and discriminate between one monoclonal antibody and another independently of isotypic or allotypic structures (figure 3.9). Such antiserums define the individual determinants character-

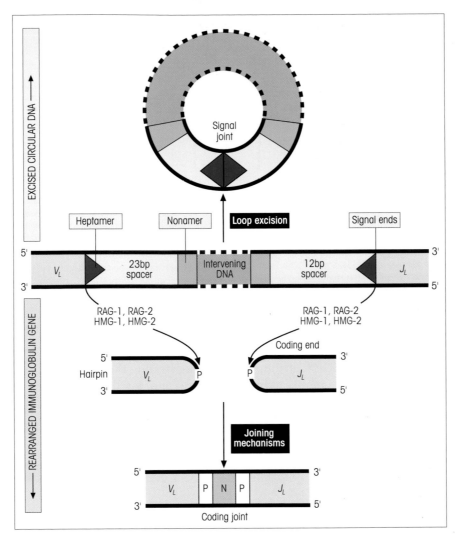

Figure 3.8. The joining of *V*, *D* and *J* segments. Joining is masterminded by the recombination activating genes *RAG-1* and *RAG-2*, the products of which cleave the DNA at the signal ends. RAG-1 and RAG-2 together produce several thousand times more efficient *VDJ* recombination than either alone. The introns adjoining the *V*, *D* and *J* gene segments contain specialized **recombination signal sequences (RSSs)** which include conserved heptamers and nonamers separated by spacers of either 12 or 23 base pairs. The two joining segments, in this example V_L and J_L, are brought into proximity by interaction between their respective RSSs mediated by the DNA bending and looping high mobility group-1 and -2 proteins (HMG-1 and HMG-2). RAG-1 and RAG-2 cleave the DNA to produce double-strand breaks at the border of the RSS. The excised signal sequences are ligated to form the signal joint resulting in a piece of circular DNA containing the excised sequences. This is probably maintained in the cell for a period of time before eventually being lost from the cell. The double strands of each coding segment form 'hairpin' ends.

The enzyme Ku (a dimer of Ku70 and Ku86) binds to the DNA ends and stimulates DNA-dependent protein kinase (DNA-PK, mutation of which gives rise to mice with severe combined immunodeficiency (SCID)) which facilitates the opening of the hairpin. Terminal deoxynucleotidyl transferase (TdT) adds nucleotides to the ends of the DNA strands in order to generate N-region diversity. Unlike the precision of the signal joint, the coding joint is variable because it can involve the addition of base pairs resulting from both the resolution of the hairpin loop (P-elements) and the TdT-mediated N-region diversity. Nucleases remove any excess nucleotides and polymerases fill in any gaps before the DNA ligase IV and XRCC4 enzymes carry out ligation of the two sequences. Since the coding elements are joined at random with respect to the reading frames, two out of three events have two coding elements out of frame. Although apparently wasteful, this is evolutionarily tolerated because it confers so much benefit in the form of antigen receptor diversity. *VDJ* recombination products define the major antigen-binding domains.

istic of each antibody, collectively termed the **idiotype** (Kunkel & Oudin). Not surprisingly, it turns out that the idiotypic determinants are located in the variable part of the antibody associated with the hypervariable regions (figure 3.10).

Anti-idiotypes which react with one antibody and no other are said to recognize **private** idiotypes and provide further support for the idea that each antibody has a unique structure. Frequently, antibody molecules of closely similar amino acid structure may, in ad-

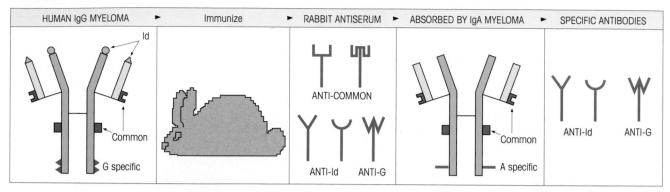

Figure 3.9. How to use monoclonal myeloma proteins to produce antibodies specific for different Ig structures. The rabbit makes antibodies directed to different parts of the human IgG myeloma. Antibodies to those parts which are common to other Ig classes can be absorbed out with myelomas of those classes leaving other antibodies reacting with class-specific G and variable region-specific (idiotype=Id) structures on the original molecule. By the same token, further absorption with other IgG myelomas will remove the common IgG-specific antibodies leaving an antiserum directed to the id-iotypic determinants alone. (In an attempt to simplify, we have ignored subclasses and allotypes, but the same principles can be extended to the generation of antisera specific for these variants.) The rabbit produces a mixture of polyclonal antibodies directed against each structural site on the antigen, i.e. they are produced by clones derived from a variety of antigen-specific parent cells which each react stereochemically in a slightly different way with the same structure (cf. p. 62).

dition, share idiotypes (e.g. M104 and HDEX 2 in figure 3.10) and we then speak of **public** or **cross-reacting** idiotypes.

Anti-idiotypic serums provide useful reagents for demonstrating the same V region on different heavy chains and on different cells, for identification of specific immune complexes in patients' serums, for recognition of V_L type amyloid in subjects excreting

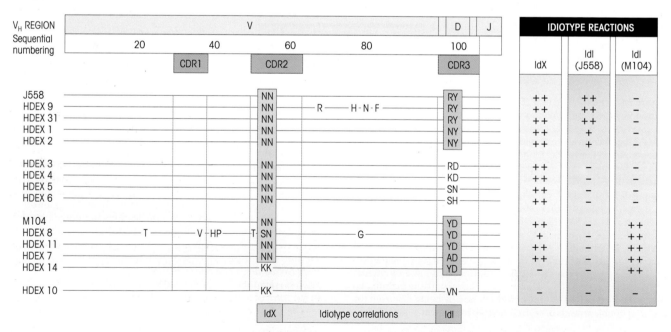

Figure 3.10. Structural correlates of idiotopes (individual determinants on an idiotype) on antidextran antibodies. Amino acid sequences of variable heavy chain regions of mouse monoclonal antidextran antibodies are shown. All antibodies have λ_1 L chains. Horizontal lines indicate identity to the sequence of the first protein, J558; letters (Dayhoff code) show differences or regions correlated with idiotopes (central boxed areas). The cross-reacting idiotope (IdX) is associated with the second complementarity determining region (CDR2) structures, while the private idiotopes (IdI) are fea-tures of the CDR3 region in these antibodies. The presence of the idiotopes on each antibody molecule is assessed by reaction with antisera specific for IdX, J558 IdI and M104 IdI (on the right). Cross-reacting idiotopes may also be associated with the CDR3 region in other systems. The hatched boxes either side of the D segment represent N-region diversity and P-elements. (Reproduced from Davie J.M. *et al.* (1986) *Annual Review of Immunology* **4**, 147 with permission. © by Annual Reviews Inc.)

Bence-Jones proteins, for detection of residual monoclonal protein after therapy and perhaps for selecting lymphocytes with certain surface receptors. The reader will (or should) be startled to learn that it is possible to raise autoanti-idiotypic sera since this means that individuals can make antibodies to their own idiotypes. This has quite momentous consequences, as will become apparent when we discuss the Jerne network theory in Chapter 11.

IMMUNOGLOBULINS ARE FOLDED INTO GLOBULAR DOMAINS WHICH SUBSERVE DIFFERENT FUNCTIONS

Immunoglobulin domains have a characteristic structure

In addition to the *interchain* disulfide bonds shown by Edelman to link the heavy and light chains, there are internal *intrachain* disulfide bonds which stabilize each of the globular **immunoglobulin domains** (figure 3.11). Each domain has a characteristic β-pleated sheet structure and comprises approximately 110 amino acids, of which 65–70 are between the two cysteines which form the intrachain disulfide bond of each domain (see figure 3.13a). Significantly, the hypervariable sequences appear at one end of the variable domain where they form parts of the β-turn loops and are clustered close to each other in space.

The variable domain binds antigen

The clustering of the hypervariable loops at the tips of the variable regions where the antigen-binding site is localized makes them the obvious candidates to subserve the function of antigen recognition (figures 3.11 and 3.12). That this is indeed the case was confirmed when X-ray crystallographic analysis of complexes formed between the Fab fragments of monoclonal antibodies and their respective antigens was carried out. Indeed, the antigen specificity of a mouse monoclonal antibody can be conferred on a human immunoglobulin molecule by replacing the human hypervariable sequences with those of the mouse (cf. figure 6.21). The sequence heterogeneity of the three heavy and three light chain hypervariable loops ensures tremendous diversity in combining specificity for antigen through variation in the shape and nature of the surface they create. Thus each hypervariable region may be looked upon as an independent structure contributing to the complementarity of the binding site for antigen and one speaks of **complementarity determining regions (CDRs)**.

That these variable regions of heavy and light chains both contribute to antibody specificity is suggested by experiments in which isolated chains were examined for their antigen combining power. In general, varying degrees of residual activity were associated with the heavy chains but relatively little with the light chains; on recombination, however, there was always a significant increase in antigen-binding capacity. Interestingly though, the majority of immunoglobulins in camels and llamas lack light chains, although this does not seem to leave them unduly inconvenienced.

Constant region domains determine secondary biological function

The classes of antibody differ from each other in many respects: in their half-life, their distribution throughout the body, their ability to fix complement and their binding to cell surface Fc receptors. Since the classes all have the same κ and λ light chains, and heavy and light variable region domains, these differences must lie in the heavy chain constant regions.

These biological activities (effector functions) were originally localized to the various heavy chain domains by using myeloma proteins which have spontaneous domain deletions, or enzymic fragments produced by papain (which generates Fab and Fc fragments) or pepsin (which gives F(ab')$_2$ and pFc', the C-terminal portion of Fc). More recently, the critical amino acids involved in individual functions have in many cases been identified using site-specific mutagenesis.

A model of the IgG molecule is presented in figure 3.13b which indicates the spatial disposition and interaction of the domains in IgG, while figure 3.13c ascribes the various biological functions to the relevant structures. In principle, the V-region domains form the recognition unit (cf. figure 2.1) and constant region domains mediate the secondary biological functions.

To enable the Fab arms to have the freedom to move and twist so that they can align their hypervariable regions with the antigenic sites on large immobile carriers, and to permit the Fc structures to adjust spatially in order to trigger their effector functions, it is desirable for IgG to have a high degree of flexibility. And it has just that (figure 3.13d). Structural analysis shows that the Fab can 'elbow-bend' at its V–C junction and twist about the hinge, which itself can more properly be described as a *loose tether*, allowing the Fab and the Fc to drift relative to each other with remarkable suppleness (cf. figure 3.1). It could be said that movements like that make it a very sexy molecule!

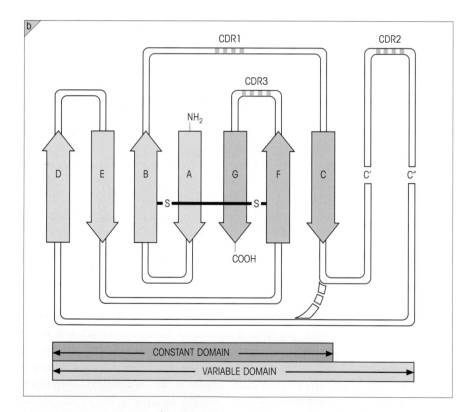

Figure 3.11. Ig domain structure. (a) Structure of the globular domains of a light chain (from X-ray crystallographic studies of a Bence-Jones protein by Schiffler *et al.* (1973) *Biochemistry* **12**, 4620). One surface of each domain is composed essentially of four strands (light blue arrows) arranged in an antiparallel β-pleated sheet structure stabilized by interstrand H bonds between the amide CO· and NH· groups running along the peptide backbone, and the other surface of a second β-pleated sheet of three strands (darker blue arrows); the black bar represents the intrachain disulfide bond. This structure is characteristic of all immunoglobulin domains. Of particular interest is the location of the hypervariable regions (▪ ▪ ▪ ▪) in three separate loops which are closely disposed relative to each other and form the light chain contribution to the antigen-binding site (cf. figure 3.12). One numbered residue from each complementarity determining region is identified. To generate a Fab fragment (cf. left side of figure 3.13d), imagine a V_H–C_H1 segment just like the V_L–C_L in the diagram, rotate it 180° around the axis of the arrow on the right of the figure and lay it on top of the V_L–C_L segment (Dr A. Feinstein). (b) Schematic view of folding pattern of constant and variable light chain domains showing the β-strands (A–G). The extra sequence C'C" in the variable structure includes the CDR2 region and, in some variable region sequences, H bonding patterns occur which produce two extra β-strands, giving a five-stranded β-pleated sheet instead of a three-stranded one. Lettering and colors as in (a).

IMMUNOGLOBULIN CLASSES AND SUBCLASSES

The physical and biological characteristics of the five major immunoglobulin classes in the human are summarized in tables 3.2 and 3.3. The following comments are intended to supplement this information.

Immunoglobulin G has major but varied roles in extracellular defenses

Its relative abundance in the circulation and in most tissues, its ability to develop high affinity binding for antigen and its wide spectrum of secondary biological properties make IgG the prime workhorse of the Ig stable. IgG, together with IgA, is the major immunoglobulin to be synthesized during the secondary response. Because IgG diffuses

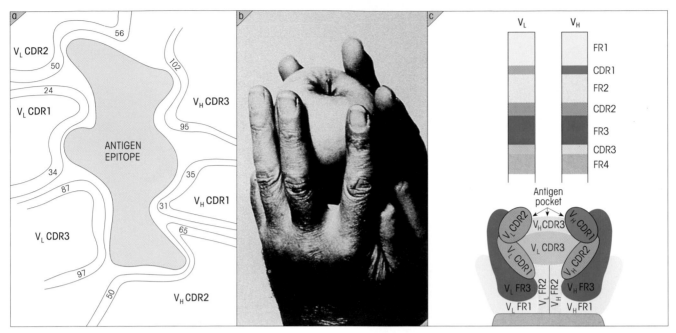

Figure 3.12. The binding site. (a) Idealized two-dimensional representation of an antigen-binding site formed by spatial apposition of polypeptide loops containing the hypervariable regions on light and heavy chains. Numbers refer to amino acid residues. In the heavy chain CDR1 is composed of amino acids 31–35, CDR2 50–65 and CDR3 95–102. For the light chain CDR1 is found at position 24–34, CDR2 at 50–56 and CDR3 at 87–97. Glycine residues are nearly always present at certain positions in or around the CDRs, allowing peptide chains to fold back and form β-pleated sheet structures which enable the hypervariable regions to lie close to each other (figure 3.11a ■). Wu and Kabat have suggested that the flexibility of the bond angle in this amino acid contributes to the effective formation of a binding site. By using different combinations of hypervariable regions and different residues within each of these regions, each antibody molecule may be able to form a complex with a variety of antigenic determinants (with a comparable variety of affinities). (b) A simulated combining site for a hapten formed by apposing the three middle fingers of each hand, each finger representing a hypervariable loop. With protein epitopes the area of contact is usually greater and tends to involve more superficial residues (cf. figure 5.5). There appears to be a small repertoire of main chain conformations for at least five of the six CDRs, the particular configuration adopted being determined by a few key conserved residues (Chothia C. *et al.* (1989) *Nature* **342**, 877). (Photograph by B.N.A. Rice; inspired by A. Munro!) (c) An idealized space-filling model indicating the relative locations of the six CDR loops (taken from Silverman G.J. (1994) *The Immunologist* **2**, 52, with permission.)

more readily than the other immunoglobulins into the extravascular body spaces, it is the predominant species in nonmucosal tissues, where it carries the major burden of neutralizing bacterial toxins and of binding to microorganisms to enhance their phagocytosis.

Activation of the classical complement pathway

Complexes of bacteria with IgG antibody trigger the C1 complex when a minimum of two Fcγ regions in the complex bind C1q (see figure 2.2). As shown by site-specific mutagenesis of the Cγ2 domain, the common core motif for binding to C1q is Glu.318-X-Lys.320-X-Lys.322 where X, the residue separating these charged amino acids, can vary. In keeping with this analysis, it is comforting to note that synthetic peptides with this structure can block C1q binding to IgG. Activation of the next component, C4, tends to produce attachment of C4b to the Cγ1 domain. Thereafter, one observes C3 convertase formation, covalent coupling of C3b to the bacteria and release of C3a and C5a leading to the chemotactic attraction of our friendly polymorphonuclear phagocytic cells (cf. p. 2). These adhere to the bacteria through surface receptors for complement and the Fc portion of IgG (Fcγ) and then ingest the microorganisms through phagocytosis. In a similar way, the extracellular killing of target cells coated with IgG antibody is mediated largely through recognition of the surface Fcγ by NK (natural killer) cells bearing the appropriate receptors (cf. p. 18). The thesis that the **biological individuality of different immunoglobulin classes is dependent on the heavy chain constant regions, particularly the Fc**, is amply borne out in relationship to activities such as transplacental passage, complement fixation and binding to various cell types, where function has been shown to be mediated by the Fc part of the molecule.

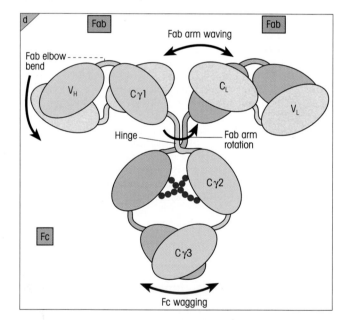

Figure 3.13. The disposition, interaction and biological properties of the Ig domains in IgG. (a) Stylized representation of IgG indicating typical positions of the intrachain and interchain disulfide bonds and the location of the hinge region. The number of interheavy chain disulfide bonds varies with the subclass of IgG; although for simplicity only one is shown, there are actually two in IgG1 and IgG4, four in IgG2 and a massive 11 in IgG3. (b) Computer-generated model of IgG. One heavy chain is depicted in light blue, the other in darker blue and the light chains in gray. Carbohydrate bound to and separating the Cγ2 domains is in red. The molecule analysed was a mutant with a truncated hinge region since the flexibility associated with the hinge (see (d) below) makes the X-ray pictures fuzzy and difficult to interpret. (The structure was determined by Silverton E.W., Navia M.A. & Davies J.R. (1977) *Proceedings of the National Academy of Sciences of the USA* **74**, 5140, and the figure generated by computer graphics using R.J. Feldmann's system (National Institute of Health).) (c) Diagram based on the model indicating domain location of biological function. The combined Cγ2 and Cγ3 domains bind to Fc receptors on phagocytic cells, NK cells and placental syncytiotrophoblast; also to staphylococcal protein A. (Note the IgG heavy chain is designated γ and the constant region domains Cγ1, Cγ2 and Cγ3.) (d) Diagram indicating IgG flexibility (cf. Brekke O.H. *et al.* (1995) *Immunology Today* **16**, 85) and showing apposing domains making contact through hydrophobic regions (after Dr A. Feinstein). The structures of these contact frameworks are highly conserved, an essential feature if different V_H and V_L domains are to associate in order to generate a wide variety of antibody specificities. These hydrophobic regions on the two complement-fixing C_H2 (Cγ2) domains are partly masked by carbohydrate and remain independent, so allowing the formation of a hinge region which is extremely flexible both with respect to variation in the angle of the Fab fragments (waving) and their rotation about the hinge peptide chain. This flexibility enables combining sites in IgG to be readily adapted to spatial variations in the presentation of the antigenic epitopes; Fc 'wagging' permits optimal orientation to receptors on effector cells.

Table 3.2. Physical properties of major human immunoglobulin classes.

DESIGNATION	IgG	IgA	IgM	IgD	IgE
Sedimentation coefficient	7S	7S,9S,11S*	19S	7S	8S
Molecular weight	150 000	160 000 and dimer	970 000	175 000	190 000
Number of basic four-peptide units	1	1,2*	5	1	1
Heavy chains	γ	α	μ	δ	ε
Light chains	κ or λ	κ or λ	κ or λ	κ or λ	κ or λ
Molecular formula†	$\gamma_2\kappa_2,\gamma_2\lambda_2$	$(\alpha_2\kappa_2)_{1-2}$ $(\alpha_2\lambda_2)_{1-2}$ $(\alpha_2\kappa_2)_2 S*$ $(\alpha_2\lambda_2)_2 S*$	$(\mu_2\kappa_2)_5$ $(\mu_2\lambda_2)_5$	$\delta_2\kappa_2$ $\delta_2\lambda_2$?	$\varepsilon_2\kappa_2,\varepsilon_2\lambda_2$
Valency for antigen binding	2	2,4	5(10)	2	2
Concentration range in normal serum	8-16 mg/ml	1.4-4 mg/ml	0.5-2 mg/ml	0.003-0.04 mg/ml	17-450 ng/ml‡
% Total immunoglobin	75	15	5-10	0-1	0.002
% Carbohydrate content	3	8	12	9	12

*7S monomer, 9S dimer, and 11S dimer in external secretions which carries secretory component (S).

†IgA dimer and IgM contain J chain.

‡ng = 10^{-9} g.

Table 3.3. Biological properties of major immunoglobulin classes in the human.

	IgG	IgA	IgM	IgD	IgE
Major characteristics	Most abundant Ig of internal body fluids particularly extravascular where it combats micro-organisms and their toxins	Major Ig in seromucous secretions where it defends external body surfaces	Very effective agglutinator; produced early in immune response – effective first-line defence against bacteremia	Mostly present on lymphocyte surface	Protection of external body surfaces. Recruits anti-microbial agents. Raised in parasitic infections. Responsible for symptoms of atopic allergy
Complement fixation					
Classical	++	–	+++	–	–
Alternative	–	+	–	–	–
Cross placenta	++	–	–	–	–
Sensitizes mast cells and basophils	–	–	–	–	+++
Binding to macrophages and polymorphs	+++	+	–	–	+

The diversity of Fcγ receptors

Since a wide variety of interactions between IgG complexes and different effector cells have been identified, we really should spend a little time looking at the membrane receptors for Fcγ which mediate these phenomena (figure 3.14). But first let us reiterate a point made earlier in figure 2.5 (p. 24). Simple occupancy of the receptor by its IgG ligand does *not* activate the cell; cellular activation is only triggered when the receptors are cross-linked by immune complexes containing more than one IgG molecule.

Leukocyte receptors for the Fc region of IgG						
FcγRI	FcγRIIA	FcγRIIB1	FcγRIIB2	FcγRIIC	FcγRIIIA	FcγRIIIB
α γ₂ Cytoplasmic peptide tail					α γ₂	Glycosyl phosphatidylinositol anchor
Affinity (M^{-1})						
hi 10^9	lo<10^7	lo<10^7	lo<10^7	lo<10^7	med 3×10^7	lo<10^7
Bind monomeric IgG						
++	–	–	–	–	–	–
Bind aggregated IgG						
+++	++	++	++	++	++	++
Present on:						
Monocytes +	+	–	+	–	i	–
Macrophages +	+	–	+	–	+	–
Dendritic cells +	+	–	+	–	+	–
Neutrophils i	+	–	+	–	+	+
Eosinophils i	+	–	+	–	+	–
NK cells –	–	–	–	+	+	–
B-cells –	–	+	+	–	+	–
Mast cells –	–	+	+	–	+	–

Figure 3.14. The structures and characteristics of leukocyte surface receptors for IgG Fc regions. bars = disulfide bridge; i = inducible. Although three separate genes and several different transcripts have been described for the high affinity FcγRI, only one of these, the FcγRIA transcript, has been convincingly demonstrated to produce an FcγRI protein. This possesses three immunoglobulin-like domains, and provides a higher affinity binding for IgG than the other types of FcγR which have only two immunoglobulin-like domains. Recent evidence suggests that FcγRI may also bind C-reactive protein. There are also three separate genes for the low affinity FcγRII. These all encode proteins and, due to splice variants, collectively produce a total of six expressed isoforms of FcγRII. They each possess two immunoglobulin-like domains but have diverse cytoplasmic domains which contain signaling motifs. The FcγRIIA isoform additionally exhibits genetic polymorphism, with either a histidine or arginine at position 131, which influences the affinity of the receptor for the different IgG subclasses. The His 131 variant is the only FcR on leukocytes which is capable of interacting with IgG2 and, perhaps because of this, polymorphisms of FcγRIIA appear to be risk factors for certain infectious and autoimmune diseases. The FcγRII family members have signaling motifs in their cytoplasmic tails which undergo phosphorylation by tyrosine kinases, either a stimulatory ITAM (*immunoreceptor tyrosine-based activation motif*; ●) in the case of FcγRIIA and FcγRIIC, or an inhibitory ITIM (*immunoreceptor tyrosine-based inhibitory motif*; ●) in the cytoplasmic tails of the FcγRIIB molecules. The other Fcγ receptors lack signaling motifs of their own and, in the case of FcγRI and FcγRIIIA, are therefore associated with the γ signaling homodimer which bears the necessary ITAMs. FcγRIIIA in NK cells can alternatively associate with the ITAM-containing ζ chain signaling molecule also used by the T-cell receptor (TCR). Homologous ITAMs are present in the cytoplasmic regions of the Ig α/β heterodimer (see figure 4.3), the CD3 γ, δ, ε molecules and in the β chain of one of the versions of the high affinity IgE receptor. It is not known how FcγRIIIB transmits signals into the cell, but this GPI anchored molecule may associate with so-called cell membrane 'rafts' which contain signaling molecules. Genetically inherited polymorphisms of both FcγRIIIA and FcγRIIIB may be associated with the autoimmune disease systemic lupus erythematosus (SLE) (cf. p. 425).

Specific Fc receptors may exist for all the classes of antibody, although receptors for IgD and IgM are not particularly well characterized. For IgG a quite extensive family of Fc receptors has emerged, the nine known genes encoding four major groups of receptors FcγRI, FcγRII, FcγRIII and FcγRn (or, more simply, FcRn). Within these groups there are a number of splice variants and inherited polymorphic forms. All the Fcγ receptors display immunoglobulin-like domains (p. 45) on the extracellular surface and the leukocyte Fcγ receptors (FcγRI, FcγRII, FcγRIII) utilize these for binding Ig Fc regions, just as other molecules of related structure (the immunoglobulin 'superfamily', p. 245) are mutually attracted through domain interactions.

FcγRI (CD64) is constitutively present on monocytes, macrophages and dendritic cells, and is induced on neutrophils following their activation by IFNγ and G-CSF (*granulocyte colony-stimulating factor*). Conversely, FcγRI can be downregulated in response to IL-

4 and IL-13. Structurally, it consists of an IgG-binding α chain which lacks cytoplasmic signaling domains and a γ chain homodimer containing *immunoreceptor tyrosine-based activation motifs* (ITAMs) used to transmit an activation signal into the cell. It binds monomeric IgG avidly to the surface of the cell thus sensitizing it for subsequent encounter with antigen. Its main roles are probably in facilitating phagocytosis, antigen presentation and in mediating extracellular killing of target cells coated with IgG antibody, a process referred to as *antibody-dependent cellular cytotoxicity* (ADCC; p. 332). It might also be concerned with the overall regulation of IgG levels in the body, since the *catabolic rate* appears to depend directly upon the total IgG concentration and one might speculate that endocytosis of IgG attached to FcγRI, the only leukocyte Fc receptor to have a high affinity for monomeric IgG, could contribute significantly to this degradation. On the other hand, *synthesis* is largely governed by antigen stimulation, so that in germ-free animals, for example, IgG levels are extremely low but rise rapidly on transfer to a normal environment.

Unlike the single isoform of FcγRI, there are six expressed isoforms of **FcγRII (CD32)** which collectively are present on the surface of most types of leukocyte (figure 3.14). Binding of monomeric IgG to these receptors is insignificant. This lends itself to a cheeky play of outstanding simplicity for the uptake of immune complexes: because of the geometric increase in binding strength of polymeric vs monomeric ligands (cf. the 'bonus effect of multivalency', p. 87), complexes bind really well to these receptors and are selectively adsorbed to the cell surface in the face of competition from the dauntingly high concentrations of monomeric IgG in the body fluids. Furthermore, because of their fixed spatial relationship within the immune complex, the bound IgG molecules bring about the cross-linking of Fc receptors mandatory for cell signaling. Thus the binding of IgG complexes triggers phagocytic cells and may provoke thrombosis through their reaction with platelets. The FcγRIIA mediates phagocytosis and ADCC whilst the FcγRIIB2 (and FcγRIII) efficiently mediates endocytosis leading to antigen presentation. FcγRIIB1 on B-cells does not endocytose immune complexes and therefore B-cells principally present only their cognate antigen following ligation and endocytosis of the *B-cell receptor* (BCR). In fact, the FcγRIIB molecules have cytoplasmic domains which contain *immunoreceptor tyrosine-based inhibitory motifs* (ITIMs) and their occupation leads to *downregulation* of cellular responsiveness. In the case of the B-cell this mediates the negative-feedback effect of

IgG on antibody production (cf. p. 201). Thus, whereas the isoforms on phagocytic cells are associated with ligand internalization, that on the B-cell fails to internalize but concentrates instead on lymphocyte regulation.

The two *FcγRIII (CD16)* genes encode the isoforms FcγRIIIA and FcγRIIIB which have a medium and low affinity for IgG, respectively. FcγRIIIA is found on most types of leukocyte, whereas FcγRIIIB is restricted mainly to neutrophils and is unique amongst the Fc receptors in being attached to the cell membrane by a glycosylphosphatidylinositol (GPI) anchor rather than a transmembrane segment. FcγRIIIA is known to be associated with the γ chain signaling dimer on monocytes and macrophages, and with either ζ and/or γ chain signaling molecules in NK cells, and its expression is upregulated by transforming growth factor β (TGFβ) and downregulated by IL-4. With respect to their functions, FcγRIIIA is largely responsible for mediating ADCC by NK cells and the clearance of immune complexes from the circulation by macrophages. For example, the clearance of IgG-coated erythrocytes from the blood of chimpanzees was essentially inhibited by the monovalent Fab fragment of a monoclonal anti-FcγIII (work out why the Fab fragment was used). FcγRIIIB cross-linking stimulates the production of superoxide by neutrophils.

The fourth major type of FcγR is not present on leukocytes but instead is found on epithelial cells. It is referred to as **FcRn** due to its original description as a **n**eonatal receptor, although it is now known to be present also in the adult. This molecule has a *major histocompatibility complex* (MHC)-like structure and its α chain associates with β_2-microglobulin. It acts as an intracellular trafficking receptor and at least four major activities have been proposed for this molecule. It is fairly well established that it transfers maternal circulating IgG across the placenta to the fetus (figure 3.15a) and, at least in rodents, colostral and maternal milk IgG from the intestine to the circulation of the neonate (figure 3.15b). IgG is alone amongst the Ig classes in its ability to cross the human placenta, thereby providing a major life-line of defense not only for the fetus *in utero* but also for the first few weeks of the newborn baby's life. Transfer of IgG across the gut mucosa in the neonate may further reinforce this protection. FcRn may additionally be involved in maintaining steady state levels of circulating IgG and in the bidirectional transport of IgG across the adult intestinal epithelium and possibly across mucosal surfaces at other sites in the body. Binding of IgG to FcRn is regulated by pH,

Figure 3.15. The epithelial cell surface receptor for IgG Fc regions. (a) The FcRn receptor is present in the placenta where it fulfils the important task of transferring maternal IgG to the fetal circulation. This will provide important protection prior to the generation of immunocompetence in the fetus. Furthermore, it is self-evident that any infectious agent which might reach the fetus *in utero* will have had to have passed through the mother first, and the fetus will rely upon the mother's immune system to have produced IgG with appropriate binding specificities. This maternal IgG also provides protection for the neonate, because it takes some weeks following birth before the transferred IgG is eventually all catabolized. (b) It has been clearly demonstrated in rodents, although remains speculative in humans, that there is epithelial transport of IgG from maternal milk across the intestinal cells of the newborn. IgG binds to FcRn at pH 6.0, is taken into the cell within a clathrin-coated vesicle and released at the pH of the basal surface. The directional movement of IgG is achieved by the asymmetric pH effect on Ig–receptor interac-tion. FcRn has homology to MHC class I molecules and contains β_2-microglobulin (cf. p. 70). Knockout mice lacking FcRn are incapable of acquiring maternal Ig as neonates. Furthermore, they have a grossly shortened IgG half-life, suggesting that FcRn may also serve a role as a protective receptor which prevents degradation of IgG and then recycles it to the circulation. The IgG half-life is unusually long compared with that of IgA and IgM and this enables the response to antigen to be sustained for many months following infection. (c) An additional, and still to be proven, role of FcRn may be as a bidirectional shuttle receptor. IgG binding on the nonluminal side of the epithelial cell may occur, following endocytosis, within the more favorable pH of acidic endosomes. This receptor may thus provide a mechanism for mucosal immunosurveillance, traveling back and forth across the epithelial cell, delivering IgG to the intestinal lumen and then returning the same antibodies in the form of immune complexes for the stimulation of B-cells by follicular dendritic cells.

with high affinity binding at acidic pH but very little at neutral or alkali pH. Unlike the transcytosis across epithelial cells mediated by the pIgA-R (see below), FcRn does not undergo proteolytic cleavage and therefore has the potential for generating bidirectional traffic (figure 3.15c).

Nonprecipitating 'univalent' antibodies

IgG has two combining sites for antigen. However, 5–15% of the IgG in all antiserums appears to consist of nonprecipitating asymmetric molecules with a single effective binding site. The other site is blocked stereochemically by a mannose-rich carbohydrate in the Fab region.

Immunoglobulin A guards the mucosal surfaces

IgA appears selectively in the seromucous secretions, such as saliva, tears, nasal fluids, sweat, colostrum, and secretions of the lung, genitourinary and gastrointestinal tracts, where it clearly has the job of defending the exposed external surfaces of the body against attack by microorganisms. This responsibility is clearly taken seriously since approximately 40 mg of secretory IgA/kg body weight is transported daily through the human intestinal crypt epithelium to the mucosal surface as compared with a *total* daily production of IgG of 30 mg/kg.

The IgA is synthesized locally by plasma cells and dimerized intracellularly together with a cysteine-rich polypeptide called J chain, of molecular weight 15 000. The dimeric molecule is effectively tetravalent and will have a much higher binding avidity for polymeric antigens than the monomeric form due to the bonus effect of multivalency (cf. p. 87). If dimerization occurred randomly *after* secretion, dimers of mixed specificity would be formed which would be no more effective in combining with antigen than the monomers. The dimeric IgA binds strongly through its J chain to a receptor for polymeric Ig (**poly-Ig receptor, pIgR,** which also binds polymeric IgM) present in the membrane of mucosal epithelial cells. The complex is then actively endocytosed, transported across the cytoplasm and secreted into the external body fluids after cleavage of the pIgR peptide chain. The fragment

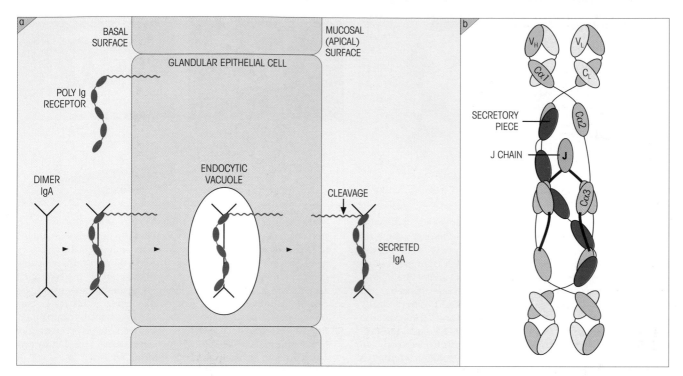

Figure 3.16. Secretory IgA. (a) The mechanism of IgA secretion at the mucosal surface. The mucosal cell synthesizes a receptor for polymeric Ig (pIgR) which is inserted into the basal membrane. Dimeric IgA binds to this receptor and is transported via an endocytic vacuole to the apical surface. Cleavage of the receptor releases secretory IgA still attached to part of the receptor termed the secretory piece. Note how the receptor cleavage introduces an asymmetry which drives the transport of IgA dimers to the mucosal surface (in quite the opposite direction to the transcytosis of milk IgG in figure 3.15). (b) Schematic view of the structure of secreted IgA. The J chain, which is an integral part of secreted polymeric Ig (IgA and IgM), forms disulfide bonds with the penultimate residue of the Cα3 domain which is a cysteine (Cys 495). Covalent linkage of the J chain seems to be critical for the initial binding to the polymeric Ig receptor.

of the receptor remaining bound to the IgA is termed secretory component and the whole molecule, **secretory IgA** (figure 3.16). The reader is strongly recommended to turn to figure 8.9 (p. 156) for a dramatic demonstration of secretory IgA held in the surface mucus of intestinal mucosal epithelial cells.

The function of the secretory piece may be to protect the IgA hinge from bacterial proteases. It would also be nice to think that it acted as a molecular Teflon to endow the IgA dimer with 'nonstick' potential, since IgA antibodies function by inhibiting the adherence of coated microorganisms to the surface of mucosal cells, thereby preventing entry into the body tissues. They will also combine with the myriad soluble antigens of dietary and microbial origin to block their access to the body. Aggregated IgA binds to polymorphs and can also activate the alternative (figure 2.3), as distinct from the classical, complement pathway, largely through its abundant carbohydrate groups. This may account for reports of a synergism between IgA, complement and lysozyme in the killing of certain coliform organisms, where it is supposed that complement-induced disruption of the outer surface permits access of the enzyme to the peptidoglycan wall.

Plasma IgA is predominantly monomeric and, since this form is a relatively poor activator of complement, it seems likely that the body uses it for the direct neutralization of any antigens which breach the epithelial barrier to enter the circulation in appreciable quantities. However, it has additional functions which are mediated through the FcαR (CD89) for IgA present on monocytes, macrophages, neutrophils and subpopulations of both T- and B-lymphocytes. Structurally, this receptor most closely resembles FcγRIIIA in that it has two immunoglobulin domains and associates with a γ chain signaling homodimer. Following cross-linking, the receptor can activate endocytosis, phagocytosis, inflammatory mediator release and ADCC. Expression of the FcαR on monocytes is strongly upregulated by bacterial lipopolysaccharide.

Figure 3.17. The structure of IgM. (a) The arrangement of domains in one of the five subunits showing how the pentamer is built up through the disulfide linkages between the Cys 414 in the Cμ3 domains and between the Cys 575, the penultimate C-terminal residue in the 19-amino acid tailpiece which follows Cμ4 (after Hilschman & Feinstein). Without too much aggravation, we hope the reader will appreciate that the hinge region in IgG (cf. figure 3.13) is replaced by a rigid pair of extra domains (Cμ2), while Cμ3 and Cμ4 domains in IgM are structurally equivalent to the Cγ2 and Cγ3 regions, respectively, in IgG. (b) The structure as shown by electron microscopy of a human Waldenström's macroglobulin in free solution adopting a 'star'-shaped configuration. (c) The structure as revealed in an electron microscope preparation of specific sheep IgM antibody bound to *Salmonella paratyphi* flagellum where the immunoglobulin has assumed a 'crab-like' conformation in establishing its links with antigen. With the F(ab')$_2$ arms bent out of the plane of the central Fc$_5$ region, the Cμ3 complement binding domains are now readily accessible to the first component of complement (cf. p. 22). The Fc$_5$ constellation obtained by papain cleavage can activate complement directly. (Electron micrographs are negatively stained preparations of magnification ×2 000 000, i.e. 1 mm represents 0.5 nm; kindly provided by Dr A. Feinstein and Dr E.A. Munn.)

Immunoglobulin M provides a defense against bacteremia

In the past referred to as the macroglobulin antibodies because of their high molecular weight, IgM molecules are polymers of five four-peptide subunits each bearing an extra C$_H$ domain. As with IgA, a single J chain is incorporated into the pentamer which has the structure shown in figure 3.17a. Under negative staining in the electron microscope, the free molecule in solution assumes a 'star' shape but, when combined as an antibody with an antigenic surface membrane, it can adopt a 'crab-like' configuration (figure 3.17b and c) in which multiple Fc regions are now accessible to C1q which is bound most firmly. A small proportion of circulating IgM exists in a hexameric form which lacks J chain but is up to 20 times more effective in activating complement-mediated lysis than the pentamer. Circulating monomeric IgM (i.e. a single four-peptide unit) is present during chronic infections but is unable to activate complement. The theoretical combining valency of the pentamer is of course 10 but this is only observed on interaction with small haptens; with larger antigens the effective valency falls to 5 and this must be attributed to some form of steric restriction due to lack of flexibility in the molecule. IgM antibodies tend to be of relatively low affinity as measured against single determinants (haptens) but, because of their high valency, they bind with quite respectable avidity to antigens with multiple epitopes (bonus effect of multivalency, p. 87). For the same reason, these antibodies are extremely efficient agglutinating and cytolytic agents and, since they appear early in the response to infection and are largely confined to the bloodstream, it is likely that they play a role of particular importance in cases of bacteremia. The isohemagglutinins (anti-A, anti-B) and many of the 'natural' antibodies to microorganisms are usually IgM; antibodies to the typhoid 'O' antigen (endotoxin) and the 'WR' antibodies in syphilis are also found in this class. IgM would appear to precede IgG in the phylogeny of the immune response in vertebrates.

Monomeric IgM, with a hydrophobic sequence stitched into the C-terminal end of the heavy chain to anchor the molecule in the cell membrane, is the major antibody receptor used by B-lymphocytes to recognize antigen (cf. figure 2.10).

Immunoglobulin D is a cell surface receptor

This class was recognized through the discovery of a myeloma protein which did not have the antigenic specificity of IgG, A or M, although it reacted with antibodies to immunoglobulin light chains and had the

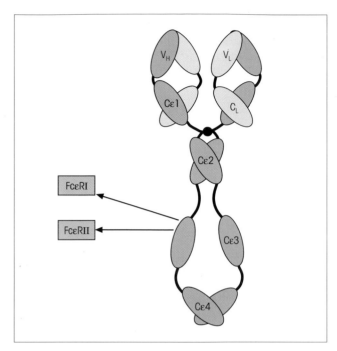

Figure 3.18. Domain structure of IgE. Note the general similarity in structure to the IgM basic unit in figure 3.17 with the IgG hinge replaced by the extra Cε2 paired domains, but also the lack of association of the penultimate C-terminal domains (in this case Cε3) which is a consistent feature of all Ig classes. The α chain of the high affinity mast cell receptor for IgE (FcεRI) binds very avidly to a single site located in positions 301–304 of the Cε3 domain. The low affinity FcεRII on inflammatory cells and B-lymphocytes requires the presence of both Cε3 domains for significant binding to IgE. 'Knockout' mice lacking the FcεRI α chain do not express the receptor and cannot produce anaphylactic reactions; conclusion, the low affinity FcεRII receptor which is expressed does not contribute significantly to IgE/mast cell-mediated anaphylaxis.

basic four-peptide structure. The hinge region is particularly extended and, although protected to some degree by carbohydrate, it may be this feature which makes IgD, among the different immunoglobulin classes, uniquely susceptible to proteolytic degradation, and account for its short half-life in plasma (2.8 days). Nearly all the IgD is present, together with IgM, on the surface of a proportion of B-lymphocytes where it seems likely that they may operate as mutually interacting antigen receptors for the control of lymphocyte activation and suppression.

Immunoglobulin E triggers inflammatory reactions

Only very low concentrations of IgE are present in serum and only a very small proportion of the plasma cells in the body are synthesizing this immunoglobu-

lin. It is not surprising, therefore, that so far only a handful of IgE myelomas have been recognized compared with tens of thousands of IgG paraproteinemias. IgE antibodies (figure 3.18) remain firmly fixed for an extended period when injected into human skin, bound to the high affinity FcεRI receptor on mast cells (figure 3.19). Contact with antigen leads to degranulation of the mast cells with release of preformed vasoactive amines and cytokines, and the synthesis of a variety of inflammatory mediators derived from arachidonic acid (cf. figure 1.15). This process is responsible for the symptoms of hay fever and of extrinsic asthma when patients with atopic allergy come into contact with the allergen, e.g. grass pollen.

The main *physiological* role of IgE would appear to be protection of anatomic sites susceptible to trauma and pathogen entry by local recruitment of plasma factors and effector cells through the **triggering of an acute inflammatory reaction**. Infectious agents penetrating the IgA defenses would combine with specific IgE on the mast cell surface and trigger the release of vasoactive agents and factors chemotactic for granulocytes, so leading to an influx of plasma IgG, complement, neutrophils and eosinophils (cf. p. 272). In such a context, the ability of eosinophils to damage IgG-coated helminths and the generous IgE response to such parasites would constitute an effective defense.

The low affinity FcεRII receptor, CD23, is present on many different types of hematopoietic cells (figure 3.19c). Its primary function appears to be in the regulation of IgE synthesis by B-cells, with a stimulatory role at low concentrations of IgE and an inhibitory role at high concentrations. It can also facilitate phagocytosis of IgE opsonized antigens.

Immunoglobulins are further subdivided into subclasses

Antigenic analysis of IgG myelomas revealed further variation and showed that they could be grouped into four isotypic **subclasses** termed IgG1, IgG2, IgG3 and IgG4. The differences all lie in the heavy chains which have been labeled γ1, γ2, γ3 and γ4, respectively. These heavy chains show considerable homology and have certain structures in common with each other — the ones which react with specific anti-IgG antisera — but each has one or more additional structures characteristic of its own subclass arising from differences in primary amino acid composition and in interchain disulfide bridging. These give rise to differences in biological behavior which are summarized in table 3.4.

Figure 3.19. The structures and characteristics of surface receptors for IgE Fc regions. Bars signify disulfide bridges. The high affinity receptor for IgE, FcεRI, is found only on basophils and mast cells (and some non-T-, non-B-lymphocytes) in the mouse. However, humans also express a version of FcεRI that lacks an associated four-transmembrane region β chain, and this receptor is expressed, albeit at lower levels than on mast cells, on a number of different cell types. More recently acquired data on FcεRI structure are presented in Figure 16.1. The high affinity binding site for IgE on these receptors involves a hydrophobic patch of four tryptophans at the top of the molecule. The low affinity receptor for IgE, FcεRII (CD23), differs from most other types of Fc receptors in that it utilizes C-type lectin domains rather than Ig-type domains. It is present on the cell surface as a trimer, but the details of how it transduces signals into the cell are incompletely understood. There are two versions of FcεRII which differ by seven amino acids in their cytoplasmic tails. Whilst FcεRIIA is essentially restricted to B-cells and eosinophils, FcεRIIB shows a much broader distribution.

	FcεRIαβγ2	FcεRIαγ2	FcεRIIA (CD23)	FcεRIIB (CD23)
Affinity (M^{-1})	v.hi 10^{10}	v.hi 10^{10}	lo $< 10^7$	lo $< 10^7$
Bind monomeric IgG	–	–	–	–
Bind aggregated IgG	–	–	–	–
Bind monomeric IgE	++	++	+	+
Present on:				
Monocytes	–	+	–	+
Macrophages	–	+	–	+
Dendritic cells	–	+	–	+
Neutrophils	–	–	–	+
Eosinophils	–	+	+	+
NK cells	–	–	–	?
T-cells	–	–	–	+
B-cells	–	–	+	+
Mast cells	++	++	–	?

	IgG1	IgG2	IgG3	IgG4
Serum concentration (mg/ml)	9	3	1	0.5
% Total IgG in normal serum	67	22	7	4
Serum half-life (days)	23	23	8	23
Complement activation (classical pathway)*	++	+	+++	±
Binding to monocyte/macrophage Fc receptors	+++	±	+++	+
Ability to cross placenta	+++	±	+++	+++
Spontaneous aggregation	–	–	+++	
Binding to staphyloccal protein A	+++	+++	±	+++
Binding to staphyloccal protein G	+++	+++	+++	+++
Gm allotypes	a,z,f,x	n	b0,b1,b3, g,s,t, etc.	4a,4b

Table 3.4. Comparison of human IgG subclasses. *The very poor complement-fixing ability of IgG4 cannot be ascribed to its rigid hinge region since substitution of serine 331 with proline (as in IgG1 and IgG3) endows the molecule with excellent C1q-binding and complement-mediated lytic capability. Intriguingly, substitution of proline 331 with serine in IgG1 maintains C1q-binding ability but grossly diminishes lytic activity, a puzzle still to be resolved.

Two subclasses of IgA have also been found, of which IgA1 constitutes 80–90% of the total. The IgA2 subclass exists in two allotypic forms, one of which (IgA2m(1)) is unusual in that it lacks interchain disulfide bonds between heavy and light chains. Class and subclass variation is not restricted to human immunoglobulins but is a feature of all the mammals so far studied: monkey, sheep, rabbit, guinea-pig, rat and mouse.

SUMMARY

The basic structure is a four-peptide unit

• Immunoglobulins (Ig) have a basic four-peptide structure of two identical heavy and two identical light chains joined by interchain disulfide links.

• Papain splits the molecule at the exposed flexible hinge region to give two identical univalent antigen-binding fragments (Fab) and a further fragment (Fc). Pepsin proteolysis gives a divalent antigen-binding fragment F(ab')$_2$ lacking the Fc.

Amino acid sequences reveal variations in immunoglobulin structure

• There are perhaps 10^8 or more different Ig molecules in normal serum.

• Analysis of myeloma proteins, which are homogeneous Ig produced by single clones of malignant plasma cells, has shown the N-terminal region of heavy and light chains to have a variable amino acid structure and the remainder to be relatively constant in structure.

Immunoglobulin genes

• Clusters of genes on three different chromosomes encode κ, λ and heavy Ig chains, respectively. In each cluster in humans there are approximately 30–50 functional variable region (*V*) genes and around four to six small *J* minisegments. Heavy chain clusters in addition contain of the order of 25 *D* minigenes. There is a single gene encoding each of the nine different class and subclass constant regions.

• A special splicing mechanism involving mutual recognition of 5' and 3' flanking sequences, catalysed by recombinase enzymes, effects the *DJ*, *VD* and *VJ* translocations.

Structural variants of the basic Ig molecule

• Isotypes are Ig variants based on different heavy chain constant structures, all of which are present in each individual; examples are the Ig classes IgG, IgA, etc.

• Allotypes are heavy chain variants encoded by allelic (alternative) genes at single loci and are therefore genetically distributed; examples are Gm groups.

• An idiotype is the collection of antigenic determinants on an antibody, usually associated with the hypervariable regions, recognized by other antigen-specific receptors, either antibody (the anti-idiotype) or T-cell receptors.

• The variable region domains bind antigen, and three hypervariable loops (termed complementarity determining regions) on the heavy chain and three on the light chain form the antigen-binding site.

• The constant region domains of the heavy chain (particularly the Fc) carry out a secondary biological function after the binding of antigen, e.g. complement fixation and macrophage binding.

Immunoglobulin classes and subclasses

• In the human there are five major types of heavy chain giving five classes of Ig. IgG is the most abundant Ig in the extravascular fluids where it neutralizes toxins and combats microorganisms by fixing complement via the C1 pathway and facilitating the binding to phagocytic cells by receptors for C3b and Fcγ. It crosses the placenta in late pregnancy and the intestine in the neonate.

• Various Fcγ receptors are specialized for different functions such as phagocytosis, antibody-dependent cellular cytotoxicity, placental transport and B-lymphocyte regulation.

• IgA exists mainly as a monomer (basic four-polypeptide unit) in plasma, but in the seromucous secretions, where it is the major Ig concerned in the defense of the external body surfaces, it is present as a dimer linked to a secretory component.

• IgM is most commonly a pentameric molecule although a minor fraction is hexameric. It is essentially intravascular and is produced early in the immune response. Because of its high valency it is a very effective bacterial agglutinator and mediator of complement-dependent cytolysis and is therefore a powerful first-line defense against bacteremia.

• IgD is largely present on the lymphocyte and functions together with IgM as the antigen receptor on naive B-cells.

• IgE binds firmly to mast cells and contact with antigen leads to local recruitment of antimicrobial agents through degranulation of the mast cells and release of inflammatory mediators. IgE is of importance in certain parasitic infections and is responsible for the symptoms of atopic allergy.

• Further diversity of function is possible through the subdivision of classes into subclasses based on structural differences in heavy chains all present in each normal individual.

See the accompanying website (**www.roitt.com**) for multiple choice questions.

FURTHER READING

Amigorena S. & Bonnerot C. (1999) Fc receptor signaling and trafficking: a connection for antigen processing. *Immunological Reviews* **172**, 279.

Brown D.A. & London E. (1998) Functions of lipid rafts in biological membranes. *Annual Review of Cellular and Developmental Biology* **14**, 111.

Cedar H. & Bergman Y. (1999) Developmental regulation of immune system gene rearrangement. *Current Opinion in Immunology* **11**, 64.

Daeron M. (1997) Fc receptor biology. *Annual Review of Immunology* **15**, 203.

Delves P.J. & Roitt I.M. (eds) (1998) *Encyclopedia of Immunology*, 2nd edn. Academic Press, London. (Articles on IgG, IgA, IgM, IgD and IgE and immunoglobulin function and domains.)

Dickinson B.L. *et al.* (1999) Bidirectional FcRn-dependent IgG transport in a polarized human intestinal epithelial cell line. *Journal of Clinical Investigation* **104**, 903.

Grawunder U. & Harfst E. (2001) How to make ends meet in V(D)J recombination. *Current Opinion in Immunology* **13**, 186.

Grawunder U., West R.B. & Lieber M.R. (1998) Antigen receptor gene rearrangement. *Current Opinion in Immunology* **10**, 172.

Kinet J-P. (1999) The high-affinity IgE receptor (FcεRI): from physiology to pathology. *Annual Review of Immunology* **17**, 931.

Ravetch J.V. & Bolland S. (2001) IgG Fc receptors. *Annual Review of Immunology* **19**, 275.

Reddy P.S. & Corley R.B. (1999) The contribution of ER quality control to the biologic functions of secretory IgM. *Immunology Today* **20**, 582.

Membrane receptors for antigen

INTRODUCTION

The interaction of lymphocytes with antigen takes place through binding to specialized cell surface antigen-specific receptors functioning as recognition units. Since B- and T-cells use quite distinct receptors to bind antigen, they will have to be discussed separately.

THE B-CELL SURFACE RECEPTOR FOR ANTIGEN (BCR)

The B-cell inserts a transmembrane immunoglobulin into its surface

In Chapter 2 we discussed the cunning system by which an antigen can be led inexorably to its doom by selecting the lymphocytes capable of making antibodies complementary in shape to itself through its ability to combine with a copy of the antibody molecule on the lymphocyte surface. It will be recalled that combination with the surface receptor can activate the cell to proliferate before maturing into a clone of plasma cells secreting antibody specific for the inciting antigen (cf. figure 2.11).

Immunofluorescent staining of live B-cells with labeled anti-immunoglobulin (anti-Ig) (e.g. figure 2.6c)

reveals the earliest membrane Ig to be of the IgM class. The cell is committed to the production of just one antibody specificity and so transcribes its individual rearranged $VJC\kappa$ (or λ) and $VDJC\mu$ genes. The solution to the problem of secreting antibody with the same specificity as that present on the cell surface as a membrane Ig is found in a **differential splicing** mechanism. The initial nuclear μ chain RNA transcript includes sequences coding for **hydrophobic transmembrane regions** which enable the IgM to sit in the membrane where it acts as the B-cell receptor (BCR), but if these are spliced out, the antibody molecules can be secreted in a soluble form (figure 4.1).

As the B-cell matures, it coexpresses a BCR utilizing surface IgD of the same specificity. This surface IgM+surface IgD B-cell phenotype is abundant in the mantle zone lymphocytes of secondary lymphoid follicles (cf. figure 8.7f) and is achieved by differential splicing of a single transcript containing VDJ, Cμ and Cδ segments producing either membrane IgM or IgD (figure 4.2). As the B-cell matures further, other isotypes such as IgG may be utilized in the BCR (cf. p. 238).

The surface immunoglobulin is complexed with associated membrane proteins

The cytoplasmic tail of the surface IgM is a miserable

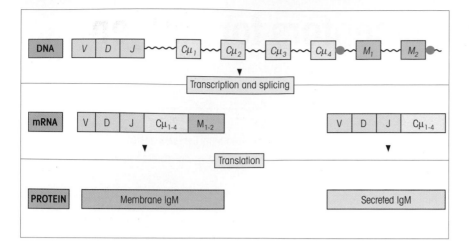

Figure 4.1. Splicing mechanism for the switch from the membrane to the secreted form of IgM. Alternative processing determines whether a secreted or membrane-bound form of the μ heavy chain is produced. If transcription termination or cleavage occurs in the intron between $C\mu_4$ and M_1, the $C\mu_4$ poly-A addition signal (AAUAAA) is used and the secreted form is produced. If transcription continues through the membrane exons, then $C\mu4$ can be spliced to the M sequences resulting in the M_2 poly-A addition signal being utilized. The hydrophobic sequence encoded by the exons M_1 and M_2 then anchors the receptor IgM to the membrane. For simplicity, the leader sequence has been omitted. $\sim\!\sim$ = introns.

Figure 4.2. Surface membrane IgM and IgD receptors of identical specificity appear on the same cell through differential splicing of the composite primary RNA transcript (leader sequences again omitted for simplicity).

three amino acids long. In no way could this accommodate the structural motifs required for interaction with intracellular protein tyrosine kinases which mediate the activation of signal transduction cascades. With some difficulty, it should be said, it eventually proved possible to isolate a disulfide-linked heterodimer which copurifies with the membrane Ig. This consists of two glycoprotein chains called Ig-α (CD79a) and Ig-β (CD79b) (figure 4.3). Both Ig-α and Ig-β have an extracellular immunoglobulin-type domain, but it is their C-terminal cytoplasmic domains which are obligatory for signaling and which become phosphorylated on cell activation by antigen-induced cross-linking of the BCR, an event also associated with rapid Ca^{2+} mobilization. Tyrosine-containing structural motifs (*i*mmunoreceptor *t*yrosine-based *a*ctivation *m*otifs,

ITAMs) are present in the cytoplasmic domains of the Ig-α/β heterodimer (figure 4.3) and it is these that undergo phosphorylation by tyrosine kinases.

THE T-CELL SURFACE RECEPTOR FOR ANTIGEN (TCR)

The receptor for antigen is a transmembrane heterodimer

When it was eventually tracked down (Milestone 4.1), the antigen-specific **T-cell receptor** was identified as a membrane-bound molecule composed of two disulfide-linked chains, α and β. Each chain folds into two Ig-like domains, one having a relatively invariant structure and the other exhibiting a high degree of

Milestone 4.1—The T-cell Receptor

Since T-lymphocytes respond by activation and proliferation when they contact antigen presented by cells such as macrophages, it seemed reasonable to postulate that they do so by receptors on their surface. In any case, it would be difficult to fit T-cells into the clonal selection club if they lacked such receptors. Guided by Ockam's razor (the *Law of Parsimony*, which contends that it is the aim of science to present the facts of nature in the simplest and most economical conceptual formulations), most investigators plumped for the hypothesis that nature would not indulge in the extravagance of evolving two utterly separate molecular recognition species for B- and T-cells, and many fruitless years were spent looking for the Holy Grail of the T-cell receptor with anti-immunoglobulin serums or monoclonal antibodies (cf. p. 120). Success only came when a monoclonal antibody directed to the idiotype of a T-cell was used to block the response to antigen. This was identified by its ability to block one individual T-cell clone out of a large number, and it was correctly assumed

that the structure permitting this selectivity would be the combining site for antigen on the T-cell receptor. Immunoprecipitation with this antibody brought down a disulfide-linked heterodimer composed of 40–44 kDa subunits (figure M4.1.1).

The other approach went directly for the genes, arguing as follows. The T-cell receptor should be an integral membrane protein not present in B-cells. Hence, T-cell polysomal mRNA from the endoplasmic reticulum, which should provide an abundant source of the appropriate transcript, was used to prepare cDNA from which genes common to B- and T-cells were subtracted by hybridization to B-cell mRNA. The resulting T-specific clones were used to probe for a T-cell gene which is rearranged in all functionally mature T-cells but is in its germ-line configuration in all other cell types (figure M4.1.2). In such a way were the genes encoding the β-subunit of the T-cell receptor uncovered.

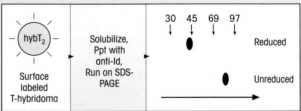

Ab to T-cell receptor immunoprecipitates 2 chains

Figure M4.1.1. Ab to T-cell receptor (anti-idiotype) blocks Ag recognition. Based on Haskins K., Kubo R., White J., Pigeon M., Kappler J. & Marack P. (1983) *Journal of Experimental Medicine* **157**, 1149. (Simplified a little.)

Figure M4.1.2. Isolation of T-cell receptor genes. Different sized DNA fragments produced by a restriction enzyme are separated by electrophoresis and probed with the T-cell gene. The T-cells show rearrangement of one of the two germ-line genes found in liver or B-cells. Based on Hendrick S.M., Cohen D.I., Nielsen E.A. & Davis M.M. (1984) *Nature* **308**, 149.

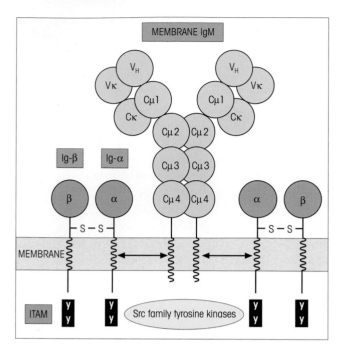

Figure 4.3. Model of B-cell receptor (BCR) complex. The Ig-α/ Ig-β heterodimer is encoded by the B-cell-specific genes *mb-1* and *B29*, respectively. Two of these heterodimers are shown with the Ig-α associating with the membrane-spanning region of the IgM μ chain. The Ig-like extracellular domains are colored blue. Each tyrosine (Y)-containing box possesses a sequence of general structure Tyr.X₂.Leu.X₇.Tyr.X₂.Ile (where X is not a conserved residue), re ferred to as the immunoreceptor tyrosine-based activation motif (ITAM). On activation of the B-cell, these ITAM sequences act as signal transducers through their ability to associate with and be phosphorylated by a series of tyrosine kinases. Note that whilst a κ light chain is illustrated for the surface IgM, some B-cells utilize a λ light chain.

variability, so that the αβ TCR has a structure really quite closely resembling an Ig Fab fragment. This analogy stretches even further—each of the two variable regions has three hypervariable regions which X-ray diffraction data have defined as incorporating the amino acids which make contact with the peptide–major histocompatibility complex (MHC) ligand.

Both α and β chains are required for antigen specificity as shown by transfection of the T-receptor genes from a cytotoxic T-cell clone specific for fluorescein to another clone of different specificity; when it expressed the new α and β genes, the transfected clone acquired the ability to lyse the fluoresceinated target cells. Another type of experiment utilized T-cell hybridomas formed by fusing single antigen-specific T-cells with T-cell tumors to achieve 'immortality'. One hybridoma recognizing chicken ovalbumin, presented by a macrophage, gave rise spontaneously

to two variants, one of which lost the chromosome encoding the α chain, and the other, the β chain. Neither variant recognized antigen but, when they were physically fused together, each supplied the complementary receptor chain and reactivity with antigen was restored.

There are two classes of T-cell receptors

Not long after the breakthrough in identifying the αβ T-cell receptor, came reports of the existence of a second type of receptor composed of γ and δ chains. Since it appears earlier in thymic ontogeny, the γδ receptor is sometimes referred to as **TCR1** and the αβ receptor as **TCR2** (cf. p. 227).

In the human, γδ cells make up only 0.5–15% of the T-cells in peripheral blood but they show greater dominance in the intestinal epithelium and in skin. In contrast, between 30% and 80% of blood T-cells in ruminants are γδ, reflecting a somewhat different physiological life-style, but it does make the point that these cells can play an important role in immune responses. In general, γδ T-cells seem to be strongly biased towards the recognition of certain types of microbial antigens, a number of which are components of mycobacteria, including lipid and glycolipid molecules and heat-shock proteins.

The encoding of T-cell receptors is similar to that of immunoglobulins

The gene segments encoding the T-cell receptor β chains follow a broadly similar arrangement of *V, D, J* and constant segments to that described for the immunoglobulins (figure 4.4). In a parallel fashion, as an immunocompetent T-cell is formed, rearrangement of *V, D* and *J* genes occurs to form a continuous *VDJ* sequence. The firmest evidence that B- and T-cells use similar recombination mechanisms comes from mice with severe combined immunodeficiency (SCID) which have a single autosomal recessive defect preventing successful recombination of *V, D* and *J* segments (cf. p. 42). Homozygous mutants fail to develop immunocompetent B- and T-cells and identical sequence defects in *VDJ* joint formation are seen in both pre-B- and pre-T-cell lines.

Looking first at the β chain cluster, one of the two *Dβ* genes rearranges next to one of the *Jβ* genes. Note that, because of the way the genes are organized, the first *Dβ* gene, *Dβ₁*, can utilize any of the 13 *Jβ* genes, but *Dβ₂* can only choose from the seven *Jβ₂* genes (figure 4.4). Next one of the 50 or so *Vβ* genes is rearranged to the pre-

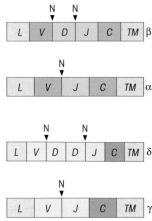

Figure 4.4. Genes encoding αβ and γδ T-cell receptors. Genes encoding the δ chains lie between the Vα and Jα clusters and some V segments in this region can be used in either δ or α chains, i.e. as either Vα or Vδ. TCR genes rearrange in a manner analogous to that seen with immunoglobulin genes, including N-region diversity at the V(D)J junctions (cf. figures 3.8 and 3.10). One of the Vδ genes is found downstream (3') of the Cδ gene and rearranges by an inversional mechanism.

formed DβJβ segment. **Variability in junction formation** and the **random insertion of nucleotides** to create N-region diversity either side of the D segment mirror the same phenomenon seen with Ig gene rearrangements. Sequence analysis emphasizes the analogy with the antibody molecule; each V segment contains two hypervariable regions, while the **DJ** junctional sequence provides the **very hypervariable** CDR3 structure, making a total of six potential complementarity determining regions for antigen binding in each TCR (figure 4.5). As in the synthesis of antibody, the intron between VDJ and C is spliced out of the mRNA before translation with the restriction that rearrangements involving genes in the $D\beta_2J\beta_2$ cluster can only link to $C\beta_2$.

All the other chains of the TCRs are encoded by genes formed through similar translocations. The α chain gene pool lacks D segments but possesses a prodigious number of J segments. The number of Vγ and Vδ genes is small in comparison with Vα and Vβ. Like the α chain pool, the γ chain cluster has no D segments. The awkward location of the δ locus embedded within the α gene cluster results in T-cells which have undergone Vα–Jα combination having no δ genes on the rearranged chromosome; in other words, the δ genes are completely excised.

The CD3 complex is an integral part of the T-cell receptor

The T-cell antigen recognition complex and its B-cell counterpart can be likened to specialized army platoons whose job is to send out a signal when the enemy has been sighted. When the TCR 'sights the enemy', i.e. ligates antigen, it relays a signal through an associated complex of transmembrane polypeptides (**CD3**) to the interior of the T-lymphocyte, instructing it to awaken from its slumbering G0 state and do something useful—like becoming an effector cell. In all immunocompetent T-cells, the antigen receptor is noncovalently but still intimately linked with CD3 in a complex which, as current wisdom has it, may contain two heterodimeric TCR αβ or γδ recognition units closely apposed to one molecule of the invariant CD3 polypeptide chains γ and δ, two molecules of CD3ε, plus the disulfide-linked ζ–ζ dimer. The total complex therefore has the structure TCR_2-$CD3\gamma\delta\epsilon_2$-$\zeta_2$ (figure 4.5b). The ITAM tyrosine motifs (cf. legend figure 4.3) associate with protein tyrosine kinases thereby transducing signals generated by ligand binding to the TCR. In mice, either or both of the ζ chains can be replaced by a splice variant from the ζ gene termed η. The ζ chain also associates with the FcγRIIIA receptor in natural killer (NK) cells where it functions as part of the signal transduction mechanism in that context also.

THE GENERATION OF DIVERSITY FOR ANTIGEN RECOGNITION

We know that the immune system has to be capable of recognizing virtually any pathogen that has arisen or might arise. The awesome genetic solution to this problem of anticipating an unpredictable future

Figure 4.5. The T-cell receptor/CD3 complex. The TCR resembles the immunoglobulin Fab antigen-binding fragment in structure. The variable and constant segments of the TCR α and β chains (VαCα/VβCβ), and of the corresponding γ and δ chains of the γδ TCR, belong structurally to the immunoglobulin-type domain family. (a) In the model the α chain CDRs are colored magenta (CDR1), purple (CDR2) and yellow (CDR3), whilst the β chain CDRs are cyan (CDR1), navy blue (CDR2) and green (CDR3). The fourth hypervariable region of the β chain (CDR4), which constitutes part of the binding site for some superantigens (cf. p. 103), is colored orange. (Reproduced from Garcia, K. *et al.* (1998) *Science* **279**, 1166, with permission.) The TCR α and β CDR3 loops encoded by *(D)J* genes are both short; the TCR γ CDR3 is also short with a narrow length distribution, but the δ loop is long with a broad length distribution, resembling the Ig light and heavy chain CDR3s, respectively. (b) The TCRs may be expressed in pairs linked to the CD3 complex. Negative charges on transmembrane segments of the invariant chains of the CD3 complex contact the opposite charges on the TCR Cα and Cβ chains conceivably as depicted. (c) The cytoplasmic domains of the CD3 peptide chains contain *immunoreceptor tyrosine-based activation motifs* (ITAM; cf. B-cell receptor, figure 4.3) which contact src protein tyrosine kinases. Try not to confuse the TCR γδ and the CD3 γδ chains.

involves the generation of millions of different specific antigen receptors, probably vastly more than the lifetime needs of the individual. Since this greatly exceeds the estimated number of 31 000 or so genes in the body, there must be some clever ways to generate all this diversity, particularly since the total number of *V*, *D*, *J* and *C* genes in an individual human coding for antibodies and T-cell receptors is only around 400. Well, of course there are, and we can now profitably examine the mechanisms which have evolved to generate tremendous diversity from such limited gene pools.

Intrachain amplification of diversity

Random VDJ combination increases diversity geometrically

Just as we can use a relatively small number of different building units in a child's construction set such as Lego to create a rich variety of architectural masterpieces, so the individual receptor gene segments can be viewed as building blocks to fashion a multiplicity of antigen-specific receptors for both B- and T-cells.

The light chain variable regions are created from V and J segments, and the heavy chain variable regions from V, D and J segments. As already described in the previous chapter, the enzymes RAG-1 and RAG-2 recognize recombination signal sequences (RSSs) adjacent to the coding sequences of these gene segments. The RSSs consist of conserved heptamers and nonamers separated by spacers of either 12 or 23 base pairs (cf. p. 43) and are found at the 3' of each V segment, on both the 5' and 3' sides of each D segment, and at the 5' of each J segment (see figure 4.8). Those associated with the V_H and J_H segments have 23 base pair spacers; those flanking the D_H segments have 12 base pair spacers. An RSS with a 23 base pair spacer can only recombine with an RSS containing a 12 base pair spacer, the so-called '12/23 rule'. Thus the arrangement of the RSSs of the immunoglobulin heavy chain genes ensures that a D segment is always included in the rearrangement; V_H cannot join directly to J_H as they both have 23 base pair spacers. A comparable enforcement exists for the V, D and J segments of the TCR β chain.

To see how sequence diversity is generated, let us take the immunoglobulin heavy chain genes as an example (table 4.1). Although the precise number of gene segments varies from one individual to another, there are typically around 25 D and six J functional segments. If there were entirely **random joining** of any one D to any one J segment (cf. figure 3.8), we would in this individual have the possibility of generating 150 DJ combinations (25×6). Let us go to the next stage. Since each of these 150 DJ segments could join with any one of the approximately 50 V_H functional sequences, the net potential repertoire of VDJ genes encoding the heavy chain variable region would be $50 \times 150 = 7500$. In other words, just taking the V, D and J genes, which in this example add up arithmetically to 81, we have produced a range of some 7500 different variable regions by **geometric recombination** of the basic elements. But that is only the beginning.

Playing with the junctions

Another ploy to squeeze more variation out of the germ-line repertoire involves variable boundary recombinations of V, D and J to produce different junctional sequences (figure 4.6).

As discussed earlier, further diversity results from the generation of palindromic sequences (P-elements, figure 4.7a) arising from the formation of hairpin structures during the recombination process and from the insertion of nucleotides at the N region between the V, D and J segments, a process associated with the expression of terminal deoxynucleotidyl transferase (figure 4.7b). Whilst these mechanisms add nucleotides to the sequence, yet more diversity can be created by nucleases chewing away at the exposed strand ends to remove nucleotides. These maneuvers greatly increase the repertoire, especially important for the T-cell receptor γ and δ genes which are otherwise rather limited in number.

Table 4.1. Calculations of human V gene diversity. It is known that the precise number of gene segments varies from one individual to another, perhaps between 40 and 70 in the case of the V_H genes for example, so that these calculations represent 'typical' numbers. The number of specificities generated by straightforward random combination of germ-line segments is calculated. These will be increased by the further mechanisms listed: *minimal assumption of approximately 10 variants for chains lacking D segments and 100 for chains with D segments. The calculation for the T-cell receptor β chain requires further explanation. The first of the two D segments, $D\beta_1$, can combine with 50 V genes and with all 13 $J\beta_1$ and $J\beta_2$ genes. $D\beta_2$ behaves similarly but can only combine with the seven downstream $J\beta_2$ genes.

	γδTCR (TCR1)		αβTCR (TCR2)		Ig		
	γ	δ	α	β	H	L κ	λ
V gene segments	12	~8	75	50	50	40	30
D gene segments	-	3	-	1,1	25	-	-
J gene segments	3,2	3	60	6,7	6	5	4
Random Combinatorial joining (without junctional diversity)	$V \times J$ 12 x 5	$V \times D \times J$ 8 x 3 x 3	$V \times J$ 75 x 60	$V \times D \times J$ 50(13+7)	$V \times D \times J$ 50 x 25 x 6	$V \times J$ 40 x 5	$V \times J$ 30 x 4
Total	60	72	4500	1000	7500	200	120
Combinatorial heterodimers	60 x 72		4500 x 1000		7500 x 200		7500 x 120
Total (rounded)	4.3×10^3		4.5×10^6		1.5×10^6		0.9×10^6
Other mechanisms: D's in 3 reading frames, junctional diversity, N region insertion;* x 10^3	4.3×10^6		4.5×10^9		1.5×10^9		0.9×10^9
Somatic mutation	-		-		+++		+++

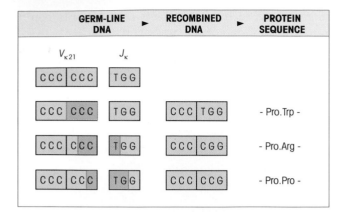

Figure 4.6. Junctional diversity between two germ-line segments producing three variant protein sequences. The nucleotide triplet which is spliced out is colored the darker blue.

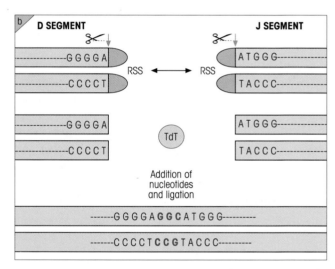

Figure 4.7. P-elements and N-region diversity. In addition to junctional diversity (cf. figure 4.6), additional nucleotides can be incorporated into the final sequence. (a) This can occur when hairpin loop structures are created between the two strands of the DNA following cleavage at the RSS, and a subsequent cleavage of one strand creates an overhang which acts as a template for the addition of nucleotides, creating a **P**alindromic sequence (**P**-element, here GATC/CTAG and TA/AT, with the newly added sequence in bold). (b) Nucleotides can be added in a **N**ontemplated fashion (**N**-region diversity, indicated by the red nucleotides) by the enzyme terminal deoxynucleotidyl transferase (TdT).

Additional mechanisms relate specifically to the *D*-region sequence: particularly in the case of the TCR δ genes, where the *D* segment can be read in three different reading frames and two *D* segments can join together, such *DD* combinations produce a longer third complementarity determining region (CDR3) than is found in other TCR or antibody molecules.

Since the CDR3 in the various receptor chains is essentially composed of the regions between the *V(D)J* segments, where junctional diversity mechanisms can introduce a very high degree of amino acid variability, one can see why it is that this hypervariable loop usually contributes the most to determining the fine antigen-binding specificity of these molecules.

Receptor editing

Recent observations have established that lymphocytes are not necessarily stuck with the antigen receptor they initially make; if they don't like it they can change it. The replacement of an undesired receptor with one which has more acceptable characteristics is referred to as receptor editing. This process has been described for both immunoglobulins and for TCR, allowing the replacement of either nonfunctional rearrangements or autoreactive specificities. Furthermore, receptor editing in the periphery may rescue low affinity B-cells from apoptotic cell death by replacing a low affinity receptor with a selectable one of higher affinity. That this does indeed occur in the periphery is strongly supported by the finding that mature B-cells in germinal centers can express RAG-1 and RAG-2 which mediate the rearrangement process.

But how does this receptor editing work? Well, in the case of the receptor chains which lack *D* gene segments, namely the immunoglobulin light chain and the TCR α chain, a secondary rearrangement may occur by a *V* gene segment upstream of the previously rearranged *VJ* segment recombining to a 3' *J* gene sequence, both of these segments having intact RSSs that are compatible (figure 4.8a). However, for immunoglobulin heavy chains and TCR β chains the process of *VDJ* rearrangement deletes all of the *D*

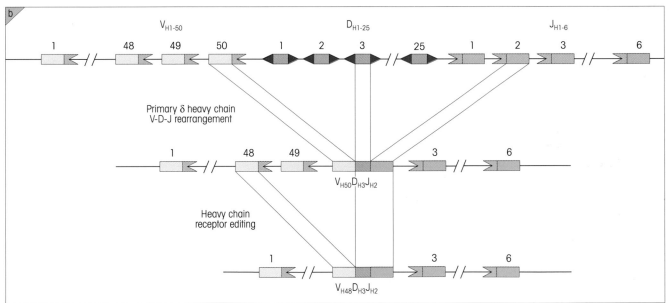

Figure 4.8. Receptor editing. (a) For immunoglobulin light chain or TCR α chain the recombination signal sequences (RSSs; heptamer–nonamer motifs) at the 3′ of each variable (V) segment and the 5′ of each joining (J) segment are compatible with each other and therefore an entirely new rearrangement can potentially occur as shown. This would result in a receptor with a different light chain variable sequence (in this example $V\kappa_{37}J\kappa_4$ replacing $V\kappa_{39}J\kappa_3$) together with the original heavy chain. (b) With respect to the immunoglobulin heavy chain or TCR β chain the organization of the heptamer–nonamer sequences in the RSS precludes a V segment directly recombining with the J segment. This is the so-called 12/23 rule whereby the heptamer–nonamer sequences associated with a 23 base pair spacer (colored violet) can only base pair with heptamer–nonamer sequences containing a 12 base pair spacer (colored red). The heavy chain V and J both have an RSS with a 23 base pair spacer and so this is a nonstarter. Furthermore, all the unrearranged D segments have been deleted so that there are no 12 base pair spacers remaining. This apparent bar to secondary rearrangement is probably overcome by the presence of an RSS-like sequence near the 3′ end of the V gene coding sequences, so that only the V gene segment is replaced (in the example shown, the sequence $V_{H48}D_{H3}J_{H2}$ replaces $V_{H50}D_{H3}J_{H2}$).

segment-associated RSSs (figure 4.8b). Because V_H and J_H both have 23 base pair spacers in their RSSs, they cannot recombine: that would break the 12/23 rule. This apparent obstacle to receptor editing of these chains may be overcome by the presence of a sequence near the 3′ end of the V coding sequences that can function as a surrogate RSS, such that the new V segment would simply replace the previously rearranged V, maintaining the same D and J sequence (figure 4.8b). This is probably a relatively inefficient process and

Figure 4.9. Mutations in a germ-line gene. The amino acid sequences of the V_H regions of five IgM and five IgG monoclonal phosphorylcholine antibodies generated during an antipneumococcal response in a single mouse are compared with the primary structure of the T15 germ-line sequence. A line indicates identity with the T15 prototype and an orange circle a single amino acid difference. Mutations have only occurred in the IgG molecules and are seen in both hypervariable and framework segments. (After Gearhart P.J. (1982) *Immunology Today* **3**, 107.) Whilst in some other studies somatic hypermutation has been seen in IgM antibodies, the amount of mutation usually greatly increases following class switching.

receptor editing may therefore occur more readily in immunoglobulin light chains and TCR α chains than in immunoglobulin heavy chains and TCR β chains. Indeed, it has been suggested that the TCR α chain may undergo a series of rearrangements, continuously deleting previously functionally rearranged *VJ* segments until a selectable TCR is produced.

Interchain amplification

The immune system took an ingenious step forward when two different types of chain were utilized for the recognition molecules because the combination produces not only a larger combining site with potentially greater affinity, but also new variability. Heavy–light chain pairing amongst immunoglobulins appears to be largely random and therefore two B-cells can employ the same heavy chain but different light chains. This route to producing antibodies of differing specificity is easily seen *in vitro* where shuffling different recombinant light chains against the same heavy chain can be used to either fine tune or sometimes even alter the specificity of the final antibody. In general, the available evidence suggests that *in vivo* the major contribution to diversity and specificity comes from the heavy chain, perhaps not unrelated to the fact that the heavy chain CDR3 gets off to a head start in the race for

diversity being, as it is, encoded by the junctions between three gene segments: *V, D* and *J*.

This random association between TCR γ and δ chains, TCR α and β chains, and Ig heavy and light chains yields a further geometric increase in diversity. From table 4.1 it can be seen that approximately 230 functional T-cell receptor and 160 functional Ig germ-line segments can give rise to 4.5 million and 2.4 million different combinations, respectively, by straightforward associations *without* taking into account all of the fancy junctional mechanisms described above. Hats off to evolution!

Somatic hypermutation

There is inescapable evidence that immunoglobulin *V*-region genes can undergo significant **somatic hypermutation**. Analysis of 18 murine λ myelomas revealed 12 with identical structure, four showing just one amino acid change, one with two changes and one with four changes, all within the hypervariable regions and indicative of somatic hypermutation of the single mouse λ germ-line gene. In another study, following immunization with pneumococcal antigen, a single germ-line T15 V_H gene gave rise by mutation to several different V_H genes all encoding phosphorylcholine antibodies (figure 4.9).

A number of features of this somatic diversification phenomenon deserve a mention. The mutations are the result of single nucleotide substitutions, they are restricted to the variable as distinct from the constant region and occur in both framework and hypervariable regions. The mutation rate is remarkably high, approximately 10^{-4}–10^{-3} per base pair per generation, which is approximately a million times higher than for other mammalian genes. In addition, the mutational mechanism is bound up in some way with class switch since hypermutation is more frequent in IgG and IgA than in IgM antibodies, affecting both heavy (figure

4.9) and light chains. However, V_H genes are on average more mutated than V_L genes. This might be a consequence of receptor editing acting more frequently on light chains, as this would have the effect of wiping the slate clean with respect to light chain V gene mutations whilst maintaining already accumulated heavy chain V gene point mutations.

Somatic hypermutation does not appear to add significantly to the repertoire available in the early phases of the primary response, but occurs during the generation of memory and is probably responsible for tuning the response towards higher affinity. The mechanism behind the greatly enhanced mutation frequency in immunoglobulin genes is unknown, but, intriguingly, it has recently been shown that the *bcl-6* proto-oncogene also undergoes somatic hypermutation in around one-third of normal germinal center B-cells and memory B-cells. The rate of mutation is only around 10% of that seen in the immunoglobulin genes, but nonetheless is way above that seen in other genes in the B-cell. Furthermore, the types of mutation are extremely similar to those seen in the immunoglobulin V genes, suggesting a common mechanism. The present favored idea is that somatic hypermutation is associated with an error-prone DNA polymerase which is coupled to RNA transcription.

Recently data have been put forward suggesting that there is yet another mechanism for creating further diversity. This involves the insertion or deletion of short stretches of nucleotides within the immunoglobulin V gene sequence of both heavy and light chains. This mechanism would have an intermediate effect on antigen recognition, being more dramatic than single point mutation, but considerably more subtle than receptor editing. In one study, a *reverse transcriptase-polymerase chain reaction* (RT-PCR) was employed to amplify the expressed V_H and V_L genes from 365 IgG$^+$ B-cells and it was shown that 6.5% of the cells contained nucleotide insertions or deletions. The transcripts were left in-frame and no stop codons were introduced by these modifications. The percentage of cells containing these alterations is likely to be an underestimate. All the insertions and deletions were in, or near to, CDR1 and/or CDR2. N-region diversity of the CDR3 meant that it was not possible to analyse the third hypervariable region for insertions/deletions of this type and therefore these would be missed in the analysis. The fact that the alterations were associated with CDRs does suggest that the B-cells had been subjected to selection by antigen. It was also notable that the insertions/deletions occurred at known hot spots for somatic point mutation, and the same error-prone DNA polymerase responsible for somatic hypermuta-

tion may also be involved here. The sequences were often a duplication of an adjacent sequence in the case of insertions or a deletion of a known repeated sequence. This type of modification may, like receptor editing, play a major role in eliminating autoreactivity and also in enhancing antibody affinity.

T-cell receptor genes, on the other hand, **do not generally undergo somatic hypermutation**. It has been argued that this would be a useful safety measure since T-cells are positively selected in the thymus for weak reactions with self MHC (cf. p. 226), so that mutations could readily lead to the emergence of high affinity autoreactive receptors and autoimmunity.

One may ask how it is that this array of germ-line genes is protected from genetic drift. With a library of 390 or so functional V, D and J genes, selection would act only weakly on any single gene which had been functionally crippled by mutation and this implies that a major part of the library could be lost before evolutionary forces operated. One idea is that each subfamily of related V genes contains a prototype coding for an antibody indispensable for protection against some common pathogen, so that mutation in this gene would put the host at a disadvantage and would therefore be selected against. If any of the other closely related genes in its set became defective through mutation, this indispensable gene could repair them by gene conversion, a mechanism in which it will be remembered that two genes interact in such a way that the nucleotide sequence of part or all of one becomes identical to that of the other. Although gene conversion has been invoked to account for the diversification of MHC genes, it can also act on other families of genes to maintain a degree of sequence homogeneity. Certainly it is used extensively by, for example, chickens and rabbits, in order to generate immunoglobulin diversity. In the rabbit only a single germ-line V_H gene is rearranged in the majority of B-cells; this then becomes a substrate for gene conversion by one of the large number of V_H pseudogenes. There are also large numbers of V_H pseudogenes and orphan genes (genes located outside the gene locus, often on a completely different chromosome) in humans which actually outnumber the functional genes, although there is no evidence to date that these are used in gene conversion processes.

NK RECEPTORS

One of the main functions of natural killer (NK) cells is to patrol the body looking for cells which have lost expression of the normally ubiquitously present MHC class I molecules. Such abnormal cells are usually either malignant or infected with a microorganism that interferes with class I expression. The NK cells carry out their task using two sets of receptors, *activating receptors* that recognize molecules collectively present on all cell surfaces and *inhibitory receptors* that recognize MHC class I molecules. Upon ligation, the activating receptors signal the NK cell to kill the target cell and/or to secrete cytokines. This potentially anarchic situation in which the NK cells would attack all cells in the body is normally prevented due to the recognition of MHC class I by the inhibitory receptors (figure 4.10). Any nucleated cell lacking MHC class I will not engage the inhibitory receptors and will only trigger the activating receptors, resulting in its execution by the NK cell.

A second mode of killing which NK cells enjoy is *a*ntibody-*d*ependent *c*ellular *c*ytotoxicity (ADCC, cf. p. 32) for which they are equipped with FcγRIII receptors in order to recognize antibody-coated target cells (figure 4.10).

THE MAJOR HISTOCOMPATIBILITY COMPLEX (MHC)

Molecules within this complex were originally defined by their ability to provoke vigorous rejection of grafts exchanged between different members of a species (Milestone 4.2). In Chapter 2, brief mention was made of the necessity for antigens to be associated with class I or class II MHC molecules in order that they may be recognized by T-lymphocytes. The intention now is to give more insight into the nature of these molecules.

Class I and class II molecules are membrane-bound heterodimers

MHC class I

Class I molecules consist of a heavy polypeptide chain of 44 kDa noncovalently linked to a smaller 12 kDa polypeptide called β$_2$-**microglobulin**. The largest part of the heavy chain is organized into three globular domains (α_1, α_2 and α_3; figure 4.11) which protrude from the cell surface; a hydrophobic section anchors the molecule in the membrane and a short hydrophilic sequence carries the C-terminus into the cytoplasm.

X-ray analysis of crystals of a human class I molecule provided an exciting leap forwards in our understanding of MHC function. Both β$_2$-microglobulin and the α_3 region resemble classic Ig domains in their folding pattern (cf. figure 4.11c). However, the α_1 and α_2 domains, which are most distal to the membrane, form two

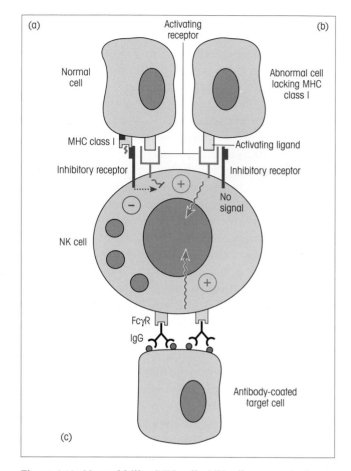

Figure 4.10. Natural killer (NK) cells. NK cells possess both activating and inhibitory receptors. Engagement of an activating receptor by its ligand sends a stimulatory signal into the NK cell but this is normally subverted by a signal transmitted upon recognition of MHC class I molecules by an inhibitory receptor (a). Any nucleated cell lacking class I is deemed abnormal and is killed following unimpeded transmission of the activation signal (b). Many NK receptors belong to either the *killer cell immunoglobulin-like receptor* (KIR) family or the C-type lectin domain family. Both families contain some members that are activating and others that are inhibitory. The inhibitory receptors bear *immunoreceptor tyrosine-based inhibition motifs* (ITIMs) in their cytoplasmic domain. Activating receptors lack ITIMs and possess a charged residue in their transmembrane sequence which permits their association with *immunoreceptor tyrosine-based activation motif* (ITAM)-containing adaptor proteins such as DAP12, CD3 ζ chain or FcR γ-chain. With respect to the KIR family, isoforms with a long cytoplasmic domain (KIR2DL and KIR3DL, depending on whether they possess 2 or 3 Ig-type extracellular domains) bear ITIMs and are therefore inhibitory, whilst those with a short cytoplasmic domain (KIR2DS and KIR3DS) lack ITIMs, associate with DAP12, and are therefore activating. Inhibitory KIRs recognize HLA-A, -B and -C irrespective of the peptide bound, whilst some of the inhibitory C-type lectin NK receptors interact with HLA-E presenting signal sequence peptides derived from other HLA class I molecules. C-type lectin family members which are inhibitory include CD94/NKG2A and, in the mouse, NKR-P1B and Ly-49C, whilst those that are activating include CD94/NKG2C, CD94/NKG2D, and the murine Ly-49D. The stress-inducible nonclassical MHC molecule MICA is a major ligand for NKG2D. NK cells usually possess several different inhibitory and activating receptors and it is the balance of signals from these that determines whether the cell becomes activated. Like several other cell types, NK cells can utilize their Fcγ receptors to mediate ADCC on target cells coated with antibody (c).

Milestone 4.2—The Major Histocompatibility Complex

Peter Gorer raised rabbit antiserums to erythrocytes from pure strain mice (resulting from >20 brother–sister matings) and, by careful cross-absorption with red cells from different strains, he identified the strain-specific antigen II, now known as H-2 (table M4.2.1).

He next showed that the rejection of an albino (A) tumor by black (C57) mice was closely linked to the presence of the antigen II (table M4.2.2) and that tumor rejection was associated with the development of antibodies to this antigen.

Subsequently, George Snell introduced the term **histocompatibility (H)** antigen to describe antigens provoking graft rejection and demonstrated that, of all the potential H antigens, differences at the H-2 (i.e. antigen II) locus provoked the strongest graft rejection seen between various mouse strains. *Poco a poco*, the painstaking studies gradually uncovered a remarkably complicated situation. Far

from representing a single gene locus, H-2 proved to be a large complex of multiple genes, many of which were highly polymorphic, hence the term **major histocompatibility complex (MHC)**. The major components of the current genetic maps of the human HLA and mouse H-2 MHC are drawn in figure M4.2.1 to give the reader an overall grasp of the complex make-up of this important region (to immunologists we mean!—presumably all highly transcribed regions are important to the host in some way).

Table M4.2.2. Relationship of antigen II to tumor rejection.

Antigen II phenotype of recipient strain	Rejection of tumor inoculum (A strain) by:			
	*Pure strain		**(A x C57) F1 backcross to C57	
	−	+	−	+
Ag II +ve (A)	39	0	17 (19.3)	17 (19.5)
Ag II -ve (C57)	0	45	0	44 (39)

*A tumor inoculum derived from A strain bearing antigen II is rejected by the C57 host (+ = rejection; − = acceptance).
**Offspring of A × C57 mating were backcrossed to the C57 parent and the resulting progeny tested for antigen II (Ag II) and their ability to reject the tumor. The figures in brackets = number expected if tumor growth is influenced by two dominant genes, one of which determines the presence of antigen II.

Table M4.2.1. Identification of H-2 (antigen II).

Rabbit antiserum to:	Antigens detected on Albino red cells		
	I	II	III
Albino (A)	+++	+++	++
Black (C57)	++	−	++

MAIN GENETIC REGIONS OF THE MAJOR HISTOCOMPATIBILITY COMPLEX											
HUMAN	MHC CLASS		II			III			I		CHROMOSOME 6
	HLA	DP	DQ	DR	C′	HSP	TNF	etc	B	C	A

	MHC CLASS	I	II		III				I		CHROMOSOME 17
MOUSE	H-2	K	A	E	C′	HSP	TNF	etc	D	L	

Figure M4.2.1. Main genetic regions of the major histocompatibility complex.

extended α-helices above a floor created by strands held together in a β-pleated sheet, the whole forming an undeniable **groove** (figure 4.11b and c). The appearance of these domains is so striking, we doubt whether the reader needs the help of gastronomic analogies such as 'two sausages on a barbecue' to prevent any

class I structural amnesia. Another curious feature emerged. The groove was occupied by a linear molecule, now known to be a peptide, which had cocrystallized with the class I protein. The significance of these unique findings for T-cell recognition of antigen will be revealed in the following chapter.

Figure 4.11. Class I and class II MHC molecules. (a) Diagram showing domains and transmembrane segments; the α-helices and β-sheets are viewed end on. (b) Schematic bird's eye representation of the top surface of human class I molecule (HLA-A2) based on the X-ray crystallographic structure. The strands making the β-pleated sheet are shown as thick gray arrows in the amino to carboxy direction; α-helices are represented as dark red helical ribbons. The inside-facing surfaces of the two helices and the upper surface of the β-sheet form a cleft. The two black spheres represent an intrachain disulfide bond. (c) Side view of the same molecule clearly showing the anatomy of the cleft and the typical Ig-type folding of the α₃- and β₂-microglobulin domains (four antiparallel β-strands on one face and three on the other). (Reproduced from Bjorkman P.J. *et al.* (1987) *Nature* **329**, 506, with permission.)

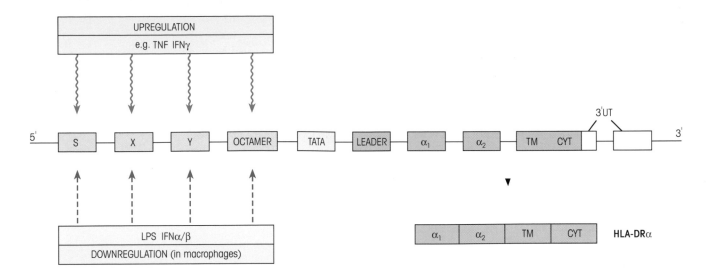

Figure 4.12. Genes encoding human HLA-DRα chain (darker blue) and their controlling elements (regulatory sequences in light blue and TATA box promoter in yellow). α_1/α_2 encode the two extracellular domains; TM and CYT encode the transmembrane and cytoplasmic segments, respectively. 3′ UT represents the 3′ untranslated sequence. Octamer motifs are also found in virtually all heavy and light chain immunoglobulin *V* gene promoters (cf. figure 3.6) and in the promoters of other B-cell-specific genes such as *B29* and *CD20*.

MHC class II

Class II MHC molecules are also transmembrane glycoproteins, in this case consisting of α and β polypeptide chains of molecular weight 34 kDa and 29 kDa, respectively.

There is considerable sequence homology with class I and structural studies have shown that the α_2 and β_2 domains, the ones nearest to the cell membrane, assume the characteristic Ig fold, while the α_1 and β_1 domains mimic the class I α_1 and α_2 in forming a groove bounded by two α-helices and a β-pleated sheet floor (figure 4.11a).

The organization of the genes encoding the α chain of the human class II molecule HLA-DR and the main regulatory sequences which control their transcription are shown in figure 4.12.

Several immune response-related genes contribute to the remaining class III region of the MHC

A variety of other genes which congregate within the MHC chromosome region are grouped under the heading of class III. Broadly, one could say that many are directly or indirectly related to

immune defense functions. A notable cluster involves four genes coding for complement components, two of which are for the C4 isotypes C4A and C4B and the other two for C2 and factor B. The cytokines, tumor necrosis factor (TNF, sometimes referred to as TNFα) and lymphotoxin (LTα and LTβ), are encoded under the class III umbrella as are three members of the human 70 kDa heat-shock proteins. As ever, things don't quite fit into the nice little boxes we would like to put them in. Even if it were crystal clear where one region of the MHC ends and another begins (and it isn't), some genes located in the middle of the 'classical' (cf. figure 4.13) class I or II regions should more correctly be classified as part of the class III cohort. For example, the *LMP* and *TAP* genes concerned with the intracellular processing and transport of T-cell epitope peptides are found in the class II region (see below), but do not have the classical class II structure nor are they expressed on the cell surface.

Gene map of the MHC

The complete sequence of a human MHC was published at the very end of the last millennium after a gargantuan collaborative effort involving groups in England, France, Japan and the USA. The entire sequence, which represents a composite of different MHC haplotypes, comprises 224 gene loci. Of the 128 of these genes which are predicted to be expressed, it is estimated that about 40% of them have functions related to the immune system. The region between class II and class I in the human contains 60 or so class III genes. An overall view of the main clusters of class I, II

HUMAN	HLA GENE	MICB	MICA	B	C	E	A	G	F
	GENE PRODUCT	MICB	MICA	HLA-B	HLA-C	HLA-E	HLA-A	HLA-G	HLA-F

MOUSE	H-2 GENE	TAPASIN	K	D	L	Q	T	M
	GENE PRODUCT	TAPASIN	H-2K	H-2D	H-2L	Q	T	H-2M

Figure 4.13. MHC class I gene map. The 'classical' polymorphic class I genes, *HLA-A, -B, -C* in humans and *H-2K, -D, -L* in mice, are highlighted with orange shading and encode peptide chains which, together with β$_2$-microglobulin, form the complete class I molecules originally identified in earlier studies as antigens by the antibodies they evoked on grafting into another member of the same species. Note that only some strains of mice possess an *H-2L* gene. The genes expressed most abundantly are *HLA-A* and *-B* in the human and *H-2K* and *-D* in the mouse. The other class I genes ('class Ib') are termed 'nonclassical' or 'class I chain-related'. They are oligo- rather than polymorphic or sometimes invariant, and many are silent or pseudogenes. In the mouse there are approximately 15 *Q* (also referred to as *Qa*) genes, 25 *T* (also referred to as *TL* or *Tla*) genes and 10 *M* genes. MICA and MICB are ligands for NK cell receptors. Tapasin is involved in peptide transport (cf. p. 94). The gene encoding this molecule is at the centromeric end of the MHC region and therefore is shown in this gene map with respect to the mouse, but in figure 4.14, the class II gene map with respect to the human—look at figure M4.2.1 to see why.

HUMAN	HLA GENE	TAPASIN	DPB	DPA	DOA	DMA	DMB	LMP2	TAP1	LMP7	TAP2	DOB	DQB	DQA	DRB	DRA
	GENE PRODUCT	TAPASIN	DPβ	DPα	DOα	DMα	DMβ	PROTEASOME COMPLEX		PEPTIDE TRANSPORTER		DOβ	DQβ	DQα	DRβ	DRα
			HLA-DP		HLA-DO	HLA-DM						HLA-DO	HLA-DQ		HLA-DR	

MOUSE	H-2 GENE	Oa	Ma	Mb2	Mb1	LMP2	TAP2	LMP7	TAP1	Ob	Ab	Aa	Eb	Ea
	GENE PRODUCT	Oα	DMα	DMβ2	DMβ1	PROTEASOME COMPLEX		PEPTIDE TRANSPORTER		β	Aβ	Aα	Eβ	Eα
		H-2O	H-2DM							H-2O	H-2A		H-2E	

Figure 4.14. MHC class II gene map with 'classical' *HLA-DP, -DQ, -DR* in the human and *H-2A (I-A)* and *H-2E (I-E)* in mice more heavily shaded. Both α and β chains of the class II heterodimer are transcribed from closely located genes. There are usually two expressed *DRB* genes, *DRB1* and one of either *DRB3, DRB4* or *DRB5*. A similar situation of a single α chain pairing with different β chains is found in the mouse I-E molecule. The *LMP2* and *LMP7* genes encode part of the proteasome complex which cleaves cytosolic proteins into small peptides which are transported by the *TAP* gene products into the endoplasmic reticulum. *HLA-DMA* and *-DMB* (mouse *H-2DMa, -DMb1* and *-DMb2*) encode the DM αβ heterodimer which removes class II-associated invariant chain peptide (CLIP) from classical class II molecules to permit the binding of high affinity peptides. The mouse H-2DM molecules are often referred to as H-2M1 and H-2M2, although this is a horribly confusing designation because the term *H-2M* is also used for a completely different set of genes which lie distal to the *H-2T* region and encode members of the class Ib family (cf. figure 4.13). The *HLA-DOA* (alternatively called *HLA-DNA*) and *-DOB* genes (*H-2Oa* and *-Ob* in the mouse) also encode an αβ heterodimer which may play a role in peptide selection or exchange with classical class II molecules.

and III genes in the MHC of the mouse and human may be gained from figure M4.2.1 in Milestone 4.2. More detailed maps of each region are provided in figures 4.13–4.15. A number of pseudogenes have been omitted from these gene maps in the interest of simplicity.

The cell surface class I molecule based on a transmembrane chain with three extracellular domains associated with β$_2$-microglobulin has clearly proved to be an advantageous model for evolution to mould as evidenced by the variety of molecular species which utilize this structure. It is helpful to subdivide them, first into the **classical class I molecules** (sometimes referred to as class Ia), HLA-A, -B and -C in the human and H-2K, -D and -L in the mouse. These were defined serologically by the antibodies arising in grafted individuals using methods developed from Gorer's pioneering studies (Milestone 4.2). Other molecules, sometimes referred to as class Ib, have related structures and are either encoded within the MHC locus itself ('**nonclassical**' MHC molecules, for example the human HLA-E, -F and -G, HFE, MICA and MICB, the murine H-2T, -Q and -M), or elsewhere in the genome ('**class I chain-related**', including the CD1 family and FcRn). Nonclassical MHC genes are far less polymorphic than the classical MHC, are often invariant, and many are pseudogenes.

HUMAN	CYP21B	C4B	CYP21A	C4A	BF	C2	HSPA1B	HSPA1A	HSPA1L	LTB	TNF	LTA

MOUSE	CYP21A1	C4	CYP21A2	Slp	BF	C2	HSP70-1	HSP70-3	Hsc70t	LTB	TNF	LTA

Figure 4.15. MHC class III gene map. This region is something of a 'rag bag'. Aside from immunologically 'respectable' products like C2, C4, factor B (encoded by the *BF* gene), tumor necrosis factor (*TNF*), lymphotoxin-α and lymphotoxin-β (encoded by *LTA* and *LTB*, respectively) and three 70 kDa heat-shock proteins (the *HSPA1A*, *HSPA1B* and *HSPA1L* genes in humans, *HSP70-1*, *HSP70-3* and *Hsc70t* genes in mice), genes not shown in this figure but nonetheless present in this locus include those encoding valyl tRNA synthetase (*G7a*), NOTCH4, which has a number of regulatory activities, and tenascin, an extracellular matrix protein. Of course many genes may have drifted to this location during the long passage of evolutionary time without necessarily having to act in concert with their neighbors to subserve some integrated defensive function. The 21-hydroxylases (21OHA and B, encoded by *CYP21A* and *CYP21B*, respectively) are concerned with the hydroxylation of steroids such as cortisone. *Slp* (sex-limited protein) encodes a murine allele of C4, expressed under the influence of testosterone.

The genes of the MHC display remarkable polymorphism

Unlike the immunoglobulin system where, as we have seen, variability is achieved in each individual by a **multigenic** system, the MHC has evolved in terms of variability between individuals with a highly **polymorphic** (literally 'many shaped') system based on **multiple alleles** (i.e. alternative genes at each locus). The class I and class II genes are the most polymorphic genes in the human genome; for some of these genes over 200 allelic variants have been identified. Class I HLA-A, -B and -C molecules are highly polymorphic and so are the class II β chains (HLA-DRβ most, -DPβ next and -DQβ third) and, albeit to a lesser extent than the β chains, the α chains of -DP and -DQ. HLA-DRα and β_2-microglobulin are invariant in structure. The amino acid changes responsible for this polymorphism are restricted to the α_1 and α_2 domains of class I and to the α_1 and β_1 domains of class II. It is of enormous significance that they occur essentially in the β-sheet floor and on the inner surfaces of the α-helices which line the central cavity (figure 4.11a) and also on the upper surfaces of the helices.

The MHC region represents an outstanding hotspot with mutation rates two orders of magnitude higher than non-MHC loci. These multiple allelic forms can be generated by a variety of mechanisms: point mutations, recombination, homologous but unequal crossing over and **gene conversion**.

The degree of sequence homology and an increased occurrence of the dinucleotide motif 5′-cytosine-guanine-3′ (to produce what are referred to as CpG islands) seem to be important for gene conversion, and it has been suggested that this might involve a DNA-nicking activity which targets CpG-rich DNA sequences. MHC genes that lack these sequences, for example H-2Ea^d and HLA-DRA, do not appear to undergo gene conversion, whereas those that possess CpG islands act as either donors (e.g. H-2Eb^b, H-2Q2^k, H-2Q10^b), acceptors (e.g. H-2A^b) or both (e.g. H-2K^k, HLA-DQB1). The large number of pseudogenes within the MHC may represent a stockpile of genetic information for the generation of polymorphic diversity in the 'working' class I and class II molecules.

Nomenclature

Since much of the experimental work relating to the MHC is based on experiments in our little laboratory friend, the mouse, it may be helpful to explain the nomenclature used to describe the allelic genes and their products. If someone says to you in an obscure language 'we are having free elections', you fail to understand, not because the idea is complicated but because you do not comprehend the language. It is much the same with the shorthand used to describe the H-2 system which looks unnecessarily frightening to the uninitiated. In order to identify and compare allelic genes within the H-2 complex in different strains, it is usual to start with certain pure homozygous inbred strains, obtained by successive brother–sister matings, to provide the prototypes. The collection of genes in the H-2 complex is called the **haplotype** and the haplotype of each prototypic inbred strain will be allotted a given superscript. For example, the DBA strain haplotype is designated *H-2^d* and the genes constituting the complex are therefore *H-2K^d*, *H-2Aa^d*, *H-2Ab^d*, *H-2D^d* and so on; their products will be H-2K^d, H-2A^d and H-2D^d and so forth (figure 4.16). When new strains are derived from these by genetic recombination during breeding, they are assigned new haplotypes, but the individual genes are designated by the haplotype of the prototype strain from which they were derived. Thus the A/J strain produced by genetic cross-over during interbreeding between (*H-2^k×H-2^d*) F1 mice

Strain	Haplotype	MHC Designation	I	II				III		I	
C57BL	*b*	*H-2^b*	*K^b*	*Ab^b*	*Aa^b*	*Eb^b*	*Ea^b*	*C4^b*	*etc*	*D^b*	*etc*
CBA	*k*	*H-2^k*	*K^k*	*Ab^k*	*Aa^k*	*Eb^k*	*Ea^k*	*C4^k*	*etc*	*D^k*	*etc*

Figure 4.16. How the definition of *H-2* haplotype works. Pure strain mice homozygous for the whole *H-2* region through prolonged brother–sister mating for at least 20 generations are each arbitrarily assigned a **haplotype** designated by a superscript. Thus the particular set of alleles which happens to occur in the strain named C57BL is assigned the haplotype *H-2^b* and the particular nucleotide sequence of each allele in its MHC is labeled as **gene^b**, e.g. ***H-2K^b***, etc. It is obviously more convenient to describe a given allele by the haplotype than to trot out its whole nucleotide sequence, and it is easier to follow the reactions of cells of known *H-2* make-up by using the haplotype terminology—see, for example, the interpretation of the experiment in figure 4.17.

Figure 4.17. Inheritance and codominant expression of MHC genes. Each homozygous (pure) parental strain animal has two identical chromosomes bearing the *H-2* haplotype, one paternal and the other maternal. Thus in the present example we designate a strain which is *H-2^k* as *k/k*. The first familial generation (F1) obtained by crossing the pure parental strains CBA (*H-2^k*) and DBA/2 (*H-2^d*) has the *H-2* genotype *k/d*. Since 100% of F1 lymphocytes are killed in the presence of complement by antibodies to H-2^k or to H-2^d (raised by injecting H-2^k lymphocytes into an H-2^d animal and vice versa), the MHC molecules encoded by both parental genes must be expressed on every lymphocyte. The same holds true for other tissues in the body.

Table 4.2. The haplotypes of the *H-2* complex of some commonly used mouse strains and recombinants derived from them. A/J was derived by interbreeding (*k×d*) F1 mice, recombination occurring between E (class II) and S (class III) regions*.

STRAIN	HAPLOTYPE	ORIGIN OF INDIVIDUAL REGIONS				
		K	A	E	S	D
C57BL	*b*	*b*	*b*	*b*	*b*	*b*
CBA	*k*	*k*	*k*	*k*	*k*	*k*
DBA/2	*d*	*d*	*d*	*d*	*d*	*d*
A/J	*a*	*k*	*k*	*k**	*d*	*d*
B.10A(4R)	*h4*	*k*	*k*	*b*	*b*	*b*

(figure 4.17) is arbitrarily assigned the haplotype *H-2^a*, but table 4.2 shows that individual genes in the complex are identified by the haplotype symbol of the original parents.

Inheritance of the MHC

Pure strain mice derived by prolonged brother–sister mating are homozygous for each pair of homologous chromosomes. Thus, in the present context, the haplotype of the MHC derived from the mother will be identical to that from the father; animals of the C57BL strain, for example, will each bear two chromosomes with the *H-2^b* haplotype (cf. table 4.2).

Let us see how the MHC behaves when we cross two pure strains of haplotypes *H-2^k* and *H-2^d*, respectively. We find that the lymphocytes of the offspring (the F1 generation) all display *both* H-2^k and H-2^d molecules on their surface, i.e. there is **codominant expression** (figure 4.17). If we go further and breed F1s together, the progeny have the genotypes *k*, *k/d* and *d* in the proportions to be expected if the **haplotype segregates as a single Mendelian trait**. This happens because the H-2 complex spans 0.5 centimorgans, equivalent to a recombination frequency between the *K* and *D* ends of 0.5%, and the haplotype tends to be inherited *en bloc*. Only the relatively infrequent recombinations caused by meiotic cross-over events, as described for the A/J strain above, reveal the complexity of the system.

Figure 4.18. Comparison of the crystal structures of CD1 and MHC class I. (a) Backbone ribbon diagram of mouse CD1d1 (red, α-helices; blue, β-strands). (b) Ribbon diagram of the mouse MHC class I molecule H-2K^b (cyan, α-helices; green, β-strands). (c) Super-position using alignment of β_2-microglobulin highlights some of the differences between CD1d1 and H-2K^b. Note in particular the shifting of the α-helices. This produces a deeper and more voluminous groove in CD1d1, which is narrower at its entrance compared with H-2K^b. (Reprinted with permission from Porcelli S.A. *et al.* (1998) *Immunology Today* **19**, 362.)

The tissue distribution of MHC molecules

Essentially, all nucleated cells carry classical class I molecules. These are abundantly expressed on both lymphoid and myeloid cells, less so on liver, lung and kidney and only sparsely on brain and skeletal muscle. In the human, the surface of the placental extravillous cytotrophoblast lacks HLA-A and -B, although there is now some evidence that it may express HLA-C. What is well established is that the extravillous cytotrophoblast and other placental tissues bear HLA-G, a molecule which generally lacks allodeterminants and which does not appear on most other body cells, except for medullary and subcapsular epithelium in the thymus, and on blood monocytes following activation with γ-interferon. The role of HLA-G in the placenta is unclear, but it may function as a replacement for allodeterminant-bearing classical class I molecules and/or may play a role in shifting potentially harmful Th1 responses towards a Th2-type response. Class II molecules, on the other hand, are highly restricted in their expression, being present only on B-cells, dendritic cells, macrophages and thymic epithelium.

However, when activated by agents such as γ-interferon, capillary endothelia and many epithelial cells in tissues other than the thymus express surface class II and increased levels of class I.

MHC function

Although originally discovered through transplantation reactions, as we will see in subsequent chapters, the MHC molecules act as cell surface markers which enable infected cells to signal cytotoxic and helper T-cells. There is no doubt that this role in immune responsiveness is immensely important, and in this respect the rich **polymorphism of the MHC** region represents a species response to **maximize protection against diverse microorganisms**. An apparent example is the malaria-driven selection at the HLA-B locus whereby resistance to severe malaria resulting from strains of *Plasmodium falciparum* in East Africa is associated with HLA-DRB1*0101, whereas HLA-DRB1*1302 confers resistance to West African strains of the parasite.

The nonclassical MHC and class I chain-related molecules

These molecules include the **CD1** family which utilize β_2-microglobulin and have a similar overall structure to the classical class I molecules (figure 4.18). They are, however, encoded by a set of genes on a different chromosome to the MHC, namely on chromosome 1 in humans and chromosome 3 in the mouse. Like its true

MHC counterparts, CD1 is involved in the presentation of antigens to T-cells, but the antigen-binding groove is to some extent covered over, contains mainly hydrophobic amino acids, and is accessible only through a narrow entrance. Instead of binding peptide antigens, the CD1 molecules generally present lipids or glycolipids. At least four different CD1 molecules are found expressed on human cells; CD1a, b and c are present on cortical thymocytes, dendritic cells and a subset of B-cells, whilst CD1d is expressed on intestinal epithelium, hepatocytes and all lymphoid and myeloid cells. Mice appear to only express two different CD1 molecules which are both similar to the human CD1d in structure and tissue distribution and are referred to as CD1d1 and CD1d2 (or CD1.1 and CD1.2).

Genes in the MHC itself which encode nonclassical MHC molecules include the H-2T, -Q and -M loci in mice, each of which encodes a number of different molecules. The T22 and T10 molecules, for example, are induced by cellular activation and are recognized directly by γδ TCR without a requirement for antigen, possibly suggesting that they are involved in triggering immunoregulatory γδ T-cells. Other nonclassical class I molecules do bind peptides, such as H-2M3 which presents N-formylated peptides produced either in mitochondria or by bacteria.

In the human, HLA-E binds a nine-amino acid peptide derived from the signal sequence of HLA-A, -B, -C and -G molecules, and is recognized by the CD94/NKG2 receptors on NK cells and cytotoxic T-cells, as well as by the αβ TCR on some cytotoxic T-cells. HLA-E is upregulated when other HLA alleles provide the appropriate leader peptides, thereby perhaps allowing NK cells to monitor the expression of polymorphic class I molecules using a single receptor. The murine homolog, Qa-1, has a similar function.

The stress-inducible MICA and MICB (*MHC class I chain-related molecules*) have the same domain structure as classical class I and display a relatively high level of polymorphism. They are present on epithelial cells, mainly in the gastrointestinal tract and in the thymic cortex, and are recognized by the NKG2D activating molecule. One possible role for this interaction is in the promotion of NK and T-cell antitumor responses.

The function of HLA-F is unclear. In contrast, although HLA-G shows extremely limited polymorphism, it is known to bind a range of self peptides with a defined binding motif and there is evidence for HLA-G restricted T-cells.

HFE, previously referred to as HLA-H, possesses an extremely narrow groove which is unable to bind peptides, and it may serve no role in immune defense. However, it binds to the transferrin receptor and appears to be involved in iron uptake. A point mutation (C282Y) in HFE is found in 70–90% of patients with hereditary hemochromatosis.

SUMMARY

The B-cell surface receptor for antigen

• The B-cell inserts its Ig gene product containing a transmembrane segment into its surface where it acts as a specific receptor for antigen.

• The surface Ig is complexed with the membrane proteins Ig-α and Ig-β which become phosphorylated on cell activation and transduce signals received through the Ig antigen receptor.

The T-cell surface receptor for antigen

• The receptor for antigen is a transmembrane dimer, each chain consisting of two Ig-like domains.

• The outer domains are variable in structure, the inner ones constant, rather like a membrane-bound Fab.

• Both chains are required for antigen recognition.

• Most T-cells express a receptor (TCR) with α and β chains (TCR2). A separate lineage (TCR1) bearing γδ receptors is transcribed strongly in early thymic ontogeny but is associated mainly with epithelial tissues in the adult.

• The encoding of the TCR is similar to that of immunoglobulins. The variable region coding sequence in the differentiating T-cell is formed by random translocation from clusters of *V*, *D* (for β and δ chains) and *J* segments to give a single recombinant *V(D)J* sequence for each chain.

• Like the Ig chains, each variable region has three hypervariable sequences which function in antigen recognition.

• The CD3 complex, composed of γ, δ, ε and either ζ_2, ζη or η_2 covalently linked dimers, forms an intimate part of the receptor and has a signal transducing role following ligand binding by the TCR.

The generation of antibody diversity for antigen recognition

• Ig heavy and light chains and TCR α and β chains generally are represented in the germ-line by between 30 and 75 variable region genes, between 2 and 25 *D* segment minigenes (Ig heavy and TCR β and δ only) and 4–60 short *J* segments.

(continued)

- TCR γ and δ chains are encoded by far fewer genes.
- Random recombination of any single V, D and J from each gene cluster generates approximately 7.5×10^3 Ig heavy chain VDJ sequences, 200 light chains, 4.5×10^3 TCR α, 1×10^3 TCR β, but only 60 TCR γ and 72 TCR δ.
- Random interchain combination produces roughly 1.5×10^6 Ig, 4.5×10^6 TCR αβ and 4.3×10^3 TCR γδ receptors.
- Further diversity is introduced at the junctions between V, D and J segments by variable combination as they are spliced together by recombinase enzymes and by the N-region insertion of random nontemplated nucleotide sequences. These mechanisms may be particularly important in augmenting the number of specificities which can be squeezed out of the relatively small γδ pool.
- Useless or self-reactive receptors can be replaced by receptor editing.
- In addition, after a primary response, B-cells but not T-cells undergo high rate somatic mutation affecting the V regions.

NK receptors

- NK cells bear a number of receptors with Ig-type domains and other receptors with C-type lectin domains. Members of both types of receptor family can function as inhibitory or activatory receptors to determine if the target cell is killed.

MHC

- Each vertebrate species has an MHC identified originally through its ability to evoke very powerful transplantation rejection.
- Each contains three classes of genes. Class I encodes 44 kDa transmembrane polypeptides associated at the cell surface with β2-microglobulin. Class II molecules are transmembrane heterodimers. Class III products are heterogeneous but include complement components linked to the formation of C3 convertases, heat-shock proteins and tumor necrosis factors.
- The genes display remarkable polymorphism. A given MHC gene cluster is referred to as a 'haplotype' and is usually inherited en bloc as a single Mendelian trait, although its constituent genes have been revealed by cross-over recombination events.
- Classical class I molecules are present on virtually all cells in the body and signal cytotoxic T-cells.
- Class II molecules are particularly associated with B-cells, dendritic cells and macrophages but can be induced on capillary endothelial cells and epithelial cells by γ-interferon. They signal T-helpers for B-cells and macrophages.
- The two domains distal to the cell membrane form a peptide binding cavity bounded by two parallel α-helices sitting on a floor of β-sheet strands; the walls and floor of the cavity and the upper surface of the helices are the sites of maximum polymorphic amino acid substitutions.
- Silent class I genes may increase polymorphism by gene conversion mechanisms.
- Nonclassical MHC molecules and MHC-like molecules have a number of functions, and include CD1 which presents lipid and glycolipid antigens to T-cells, and HLA-E which presents signal sequence peptides from classical class I molecules to the CD94/NKG2 receptor of NK cells.

See the accompanying website (**www.roitt.com**) for multiple choice questions.

FURTHER READING

Braud V.M., Allan D.S.J. & McMichael A.J. (1999) Functions of nonclassical MHC and non-MHC-encoded class I molecules. *Current Opinion in Immunology* **11**, 100.

Clark D.A. (1999) Human leukocyte antigen-G: new roles for old? *American Journal of Reproductive Immunology* **41**, 117.

Fernandez-Miguel G. et al. (1999) Multivalent structure of an αβ T cell receptor. *Proceedings of the National Academy of Sciences of the United States of America* **96**, 1547.

Grawunder U. & Harfst E. (2001) How to make ends meet in V(D)J recombination. *Current Opinion in Immunology* **13**, 186.

Kelsoe G. (1999) V(D)J hypermutation and receptor revision: coloring outside the lines. *Current Opinion in Immunology* **11**, 70.

Lanier L.L. (ed.) (2000) Human NK cell receptors. *Seminars in Immunology* **12** (2).

Lanier L.L. (2001) On guard—activating NK cell receptors. *Nature Immunology* **2**, 23.

Mak T.W. (1998) T-cell receptor, αβ. In Delves P.J. & Roitt I.M. (eds) *Encyclopedia of Immunology*, 2nd edn, p. 2264. Academic Press. (See also article by Hayday A. & Pao W. on the γδ TCR; *ibid.*, p. 2268.)

Matsuda F. et al. (1999) The complete nucleotide sequence of the human immunoglobulin heavy chain variable region locus. *Journal of Experimental Medicine* **188**, 2151.

MHC Sequencing Consortium (1999) Complete sequence and gene map of a human major histocompatibility complex. *Nature* **401**, 921.

Nemazee D. (2000) Receptor editing in B cells. *Advances in Immunology* **74**, 89.

Parham P. (ed.) (1999) Genomic organisation of the MHC: structure, origin and function. *Immunological Reviews* **167**.

Porcelli S.A. & Modlin R.L. (1999) The CD1 system: antigen-presenting molecules for T cell recognition of lipids and glycolipids. *Annual Review of Immunology* **17**, 297.

Raulet D.H., Vance R.E. & McMahon C.W. (2001) Regulation of the natural killer cell receptor repertoire. *Annual Review of Immunology* **19**, 291.

de Wildt R.M.T. et al. (1999) Somatic insertions and deletions shape the human antibody repertoire. *Journal of Molecular Biology* **294**, 701.

The primary interaction with antigen

INTRODUCTION

A man cannot be a husband without a wife and a molecule cannot be an antigen without a corresponding antiserum or antibody or T-cell receptor. The term **antigen** is used in two senses, the first to describe a molecule which *gen*erates an immune response (also called an **immunogen**) and the second, a molecule which reacts with antibodies or primed T-cells irrespective of its ability to generate them. If this last situation sounds a trifle confusing, an example may help. A mouse injected with its own red cells, not too surprisingly, will not make any antibodies; if it is now given rat erythrocytes,

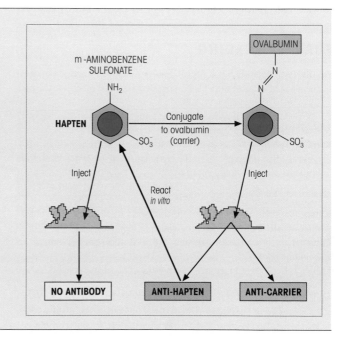

Figure 5.1. A hapten on its own will not induce antibodies. However, it will react *in vitro* with antibodies formed to a conjugate with an immunogenic carrier.

(continued)

antibodies are formed to both rat and *mouse* red cells and the latter bind to the animal's own cells *in vivo*, i.e. the mouse red cell acts as antigen in binding antibodies even though unable to evoke their formation. Similarly, **haptens**, which are small well-defined chemical groupings such as dinitrophenyl (DNP; cf. p. 37) or *m*-aminobenzene sulfonate, are not immunogenic on their own but will react with preformed antibodies induced by injection of the hapten linked to a 'carrier' molecule which is itself an immunogen (figure 5.1).

The parts of the hypervariable regions on the antibody which contact the antigen are termed the **paratope** and the part of the antigen which is in contact with the paratope is designated the **epitope**. To get some idea of size, if the antigen is a linear peptide or carbohydrate, the combining site can usually accommodate up to five or six amino acid residues or hexose units. With a globular protein, typically 14–21 amino acid residues are in contact on both the antibody and the antigen (cf. figure 5.5).

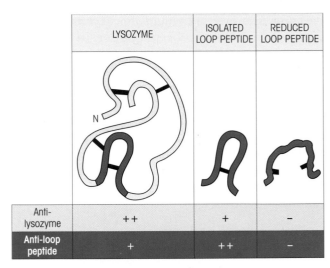

Figure 5.2. **Specificity and three-dimensional configuration in a globular protein, lysozyme.** Antibodies to the whole molecule and to the isolated loop peptide do not react with the peptide after reduction of its disulfide bond, showing that the linear reduced peptide has lost the antigenic configuration it had when held as a loop even though the amino acid sequence is unchanged. (From Maron E., Shiowa C., Arnon R. & Sela M. (1971) *Biochemistry* **10**, 763.)

THE NATURE OF B-CELL EPITOPES

Of epitopes and antigen determinants

Antibodies formed in response to immunization with a native globular protein (as distinct from a fibrillar protein) do not tend to react well with denatured preparations, and this is consistent with the view that the majority recognize topographic (surface) structures (i.e. epitopes) which depend upon the conformation of the native molecule. For this reason, antibodies to native proteins do not usually react as strongly with peptides having the same primary sequence (figure 5.2). When individual epitopes are mapped using homogeneous monoclonal antibodies (cf. p. 120), they are frequently seen to involve amino acid residues far apart in the primary sequence, but brought together by the folding of the peptide chains in the native protein (figures 5.3 and 5.5). It seems reasonable to talk of **discontinuous** or assembled rather than **continuous** or sequential epitopes in these cases.

If one were to take each individual antibody within an antiserum raised to a protein antigen and plot the approximate center of the corresponding epitope on

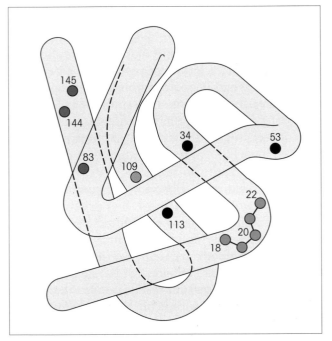

Figure 5.3. **Epitope residues on the folded peptide chain of sperm whale myoglobin.** Amino acid residues 34, 53 and 113 (●) contribute to the epitope recognized by one homogeneous monoclonal antibody, 83, 144 and 145 (●), to another. These are clearly discontinuous epitopes. Amino acids 18–22 (●—●) are postulated to form part of a continuous epitope based on reactions with the isolated peptides. Much of the myoglobin chain is in the α-helical form. Residue 109 (●) is critical for T-cell recognition and so far no antibodies reacting with this site have been demonstrated. (Based on Benjamin D.C. *et al.* (1986) *Annual Review of Immunology* **2**, 67.)

the antigen surface, one would almost certainly finish up with a 'contour map' of epitope density indicating regions on the antigen surface of **dominant epitope clusters** (figure 5.4a and b). Each of these clusters is as near as we can get to defining an antigen **determinant**. It is important to be aware that each antigen usually bears several determinants on its surface, which may well be structurally distinct from each other; thus a monoclonal antibody reacting with one determinant will usually not react with any other determinants on the same antigen unless the molecule has axes of symmetry (figure 5.4c).

Identification of B-cell epitopes

This is a subject of particular interest to those wishing to make simple peptide substitutes for complex protein antigens. In general, large proteins, because they have more potential determinants, are better antigens than small ones. The more foreign an antigen, that is the less similar to self configurations which induce tolerance, the more effective it is in provoking an immune response.

Parts of the peptide chains which protrude significantly from the globular surface tend to be sites of high epitope density. The least antigenic segments of the surface are associated with neighboring concave regions containing water molecules which may be more difficult to displace. However, prediction of B-cell epitopes, even when one knows the three-dimensional structure of an antigen, is still a pretty hopeless task, not least because each immunized host has its own way of recognizing the different regions of a given antigen. In fact, the only recognition unit that can be deployed to identify an epitope is that which defines it, namely the antibody bearing the complementary paratope.

The greatest precision is undoubtedly provided by X-ray crystallographic analysis of a complex of a monoclonal antibody (or fragment thereof) with the antigen (cf. figure 5.5). Whilst over 100 such structures have been solved, this approach is not for the run of the mill scientist, being difficult, time-consuming and very 'high tech'. An alternative strategy, applicable to protein antigens, is to carry out a series of mutations to locate the residues which provide the dominant binding to antibody—useful but not without its limitations. Attempts to mimic the epitope by building synthetic peptides will be described later (p. 292). To anticipate, this is good for linear epitopes and frustrating for those which are discontinuous.

Figure 5.4. A globular protein antigen usually bears a mosaic of determinants (dominant epitope clusters) on its surface, defined by the heterogeneous population of antibody molecules in a given antiserum. (a) Highly idealized diagram illustrating the idea that individual antibodies in a polyclonal antiserum with different combining sites (paratopes) can react with overlapping epitopes forming a determinant on the surface of the antigen. The numbers refer to the imagined relative frequency of each antibody specificity. (b) Hypothetical 'contour' map of surface showing how determinants represent regions of clustering but overlapping epitopes, whose positions are plotted as the center of the area making contact with antibody. The actual size of a single epitope may be gauged by looking at figure 5.5. (c) Cross-section of a theoretical antigen with an axis of symmetry displaying six determinants including two pairs which are identical. The clusters of overlapping antibodies to each determinant (one representative of each antibody cluster is shown) do not react with the other structurally unrelated determinants.

ANTIGENS AND ANTIBODIES INTERACT BY SPATIAL COMPLEMENTARITY NOT BY COVALENT BONDING

Variation in hapten structure shows importance of shape

Once a method had been found for raising antibodies to small chemically defined haptens (figure 5.1), it then became possible to relate variations in the chemical structure of a hapten to its ability to bind to a given antibody. In one experiment, antibodies raised to *m*-aminobenzene sulfonate were tested for their ability to combine with *ortho*, *meta* and *para* isomers of the hapten and related molecules in which the sulfonate group was substituted by arsonate or carboxylate (table 5.1). The hapten with the sulfonate group in the *ortho* position combines somewhat less well with the antibody than the original *meta* isomer, but the *para*-substituted compound (chemically similar to the *ortho*) shows very poor reactivity. The substitution of arsonate for sulfonate leads to weaker combination with the antibody; both groups are negatively charged and have a tetrahedral structure but the arsonate group is larger in size and has an extra H atom. The aminobenzoates in which the sulfonate is substituted by the negatively charged but planar carboxylate group show even less affinity for the antibody. It would appear that the **overall** configuration of the hapten is even more important than its **chemical** nature, i.e. the hapten is recognized by the overall three-dimensional shape of its outer electron cloud as distinct from its chemical reactivity. The production of antibodies against such strange moieties as benzene sulfonate and arsonate becomes more comprehensible if they are thought to be directed against a particular electron-cloud shape rather than a specific chemical structure.

Spatial complementarity of epitope and paratope can be demonstrated

It eventually proved possible, with not a little difficulty, to crystallize a complex of the Fab fragment of monoclonal antilysozyme with its antigen. X-ray analysis of these crystals was convincing; antigen and antibody fitted strongly together due to complementarity in shape over a wide area of contact (figure 5.5). Similar studies with further monoclonal antibodies reacting with the same antigen confirmed the 'lock and key' type fit between paratope and epitope. It is important not to regard the 'lock and key' as inflexible entities like two pieces of rock, since this might make it very difficult for an animal to produce an antibody with such a unique complementary surface. In fact, most monoclonal antilysozyme antibodies studied in this way revealed significant changes in the polypeptide backbone of up to 1.0 Å as the antibody complexed with its antigen (cf. figure 5.6), and if one adds into the equation the possibility of rotational movement of the amino acid side-chains and alterations in the relative positions of the variable domains of light and heavy chains (V_L/V_H) in the Fab, it would seem more correct to think of antigen and antibody as surfaces which are to some extent mutually deformable — more like clouds than rocks as Lerner has so graphically expressed it. In this context, it is pertinent to draw attention to the association between those parts of a protein antigen which provide the dominant epitopes for antibody binding, and their peptide chain flexibility as measured by the temperature factors derived from X-ray crystallography. This mutual

Table 5.1. Effect of variations in hapten structure on strength of binding to antibodies raised against *m*-aminobenzene sulfonate. The reaction of the antibody with the original hapten against which it was raised is highlighted by the box. (From Landsteiner K. & van der Scheer J. (1936) *Journal of Experimental Medicine* **63**, 325.)

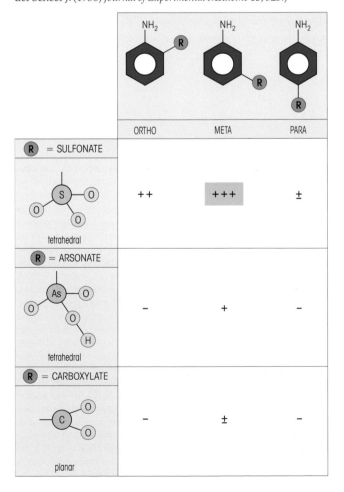

	ORTHO	META	PARA
R = SULFONATE (tetrahedral)	++	+++	±
R = ARSONATE (tetrahedral)	–	+	–
R = CARBOXYLATE (planar)	–	±	–

accommodation of structures on antigen and antibody obviously permits the maximum contact, but there must be a price to pay in that energy has to be expended in inducing these conformational changes. In general, though, this will be more than compensated by the intrinsic free energy change associated with the formation of the new binding sites (figure 5.7a and b). This input of energy to produce conformational change leading to strong binding appears to be the factor behind the frequent occurrence of normally 'buried' hydrophobic side-chains as contact residues for antibody.

With globular protein antigens, the area of contact between epitope and paratope is quite large, of the order of 600–800 Å^2. Tyrosines and tryptophans tend to occur with greater frequency in the combining site than they do in the remainder of the antibody molecule. Both can form H bonds with solvent or antigen, yet have large hydrophobic surfaces, undeniably useful characteristics for residues exposed to water when the antibody is free but buried (i.e. excluded from solvent contact) when interacting closely with antigen.

Antigen–antibody bonds are readily reversible

If the link between epitope and paratope is entirely dependent on spatial complementarity and does not involve the formation of covalent chemical bonds, it should not be too difficult to pull them apart. This can easily be put to the test. If one puts a mixture of the hapten with antibody inside a dialysis bag, the hapten will be found to diffuse out into the surrounding fluid until an equilibrium is reached in which some hapten is bound to antibody and some is free; if this exterior fluid is continually renewed, all the hapten will be lost from the bag showing that it can be completely dissociated from the antibody (figure 5.8). With larger antigens, the complexes can be dissociated by a change in

Figure 5.5. Structure of the contact regions between a monoclonal Fab antilysozyme and lysozyme. (a) Space-filling model showing Fab and lysozyme molecules fitting snugly together. Antibody heavy chain, blue; light chain, yellow; lysozyme, green with its glutmine 121 in red. (b) Fab and lysozyme models pulled apart to show how the protuberances and depressions of each are complementary to each other. (c) End-on views of antibody combining site (left) and the lysozyme epitope (right) obtained from (b) by rotating each molecule 90° about a vertical axis. Contact residues are red, except Gln121 in light purple. The Gln121 fits into an antibody surface cavity surrounded by V_L residues 32, 91, 92 and 93 and V_H residue 101. The sixteen contact residues in the lysozyme epitope comprise: eight amino acids from a stretch of 10 amino acids at positions 18–27, seven amino acids from a stretch of nine amino acids at positions 116–124, together with amino acid residue 129, i.e. this is clear evidence for a discontinuous epitope. All the CDRs make contact with the antigen: in the heavy chain residues 30–32 (CDR1), 52–54 (CDR2) and 99–102 (CDR3) and in the light chain residues 30 and 32 (CDR1), 49 and 50 (CDR2) and 91–93 (CDR3). All contacting residues may not contribute positively to the attractive forces between antigen and antibody; the striking influence of the Gln121 is revealed by the poor binding of lysozymes from other species in which the Gln121 is replaced by histidine. (Reproduced with permission from Amit A. *et al.* (1986) *Science* **233**, 747. Copyright © 1986 by the AAAS.)

Figure 5.6. Antibody structural flexibility on complexing with the antigen. (a) Significant conformational changes (0.5–1.0 Å) occur in the Cα backbone of the complementarity determining regions (CDRs) of an autoantibody Fab specific for single-stranded DNA on complexing with a fragment of antigen (thymidine trimer). Only the Fv ($V_H + V_L$) domains of the antibody are shown. The unliganded Fv is yellow and the ligand (antigen) red. In the complexed form, the V_L is blue and the V_H purple. (b) Movements in the contacting amino acid side-chains as a result of binding antigen. (Reproduced with permission from Herron J.N., He X.M., Ballard D.W., Blier P.R., Pace P.E., Bothwell A.L.M., Voss E.W. Jr. & Edmundson A.B. (1991) *Proteins* **11**, 150. Reprinted by permission of Wiley-Liss, a division of John Wiley and Sons, Inc.)

pH which brings about alterations in protein conformation and destroys the complementarity of the two reactants. As will be seen subsequently (p. 125), this principle can be used for the purification of either antigens or antibodies by affinity chromatography.

THE FORCES BINDING ANTIGEN TO ANTIBODY BECOME LARGE AS INTERMOLECULAR DISTANCES BECOME SMALL

The forces involved in antibody binding to antigen are noncovalent and therefore reversible, and are gener-

ally only effective over short distances. They may be classified under four headings.

1 *Electrostatic.* The attraction between oppositely charged ionic groups (figure 5.9a). The opposing electrostatic forces need to approximately match each other if the antibody is to substantially bind the antigen.

2 *Hydrogen bonding.* The sharing of a hydrogen between two electronegative atoms (figure 5.9b). Hydrogen bonding can occur between atoms such as oxygen, nitrogen or sulfur. In addition, water molecules can fill cavities in the interface which would otherwise have a destabilizing effect on the complex and these water molecules can form hydrogen bonds to bridge the antibody and antigen.

3 *Hydrophobic.* Hydrophobic groups can preferentially interact with each other rather than with water molecules (figure 5.9c). Such hydrophobic interactions very often play a major role in antibody–antigen binding.

4 *Van der Waals.* The forces between molecules which depend upon interaction between the external 'electron clouds' (figure 5.9d). Van der Waals forces account for a minority, between 2% and 20%, of the total interaction energy in the binding of a typical antibody to its antigen.

One essential feature common to all four types of force is that they depend upon the close approach of both molecules before the forces become of significant magnitude, the more so if water molecules are excluded. And this is at the heart of the combination of antigen and antibody. The **complementary** electron-cloud shapes on the combining site of the antibody and the surface determinant of the antigen enable the two molecules to fit snugly together (cf. figure 5.5) so that the **intermolecular distance becomes very small** and the **noncovalent protein interaction forces are considerably increased**; the greater the areas of antigen and antibody which fit together, the greater the force of attraction, particularly if there is apposition of opposite charges and hydrophobic groupings.

By contrast, when the electron clouds of the two molecules effectively overlap, powerful repulsive forces are generated and energy must be expended in displacing the overlapping residues from their normal equilibrium positions.

AFFINITY MEASURES STRENGTH OF BINDING OF ANTIGEN AND ANTIBODY

We saw from the electron microscope studies on the interaction between a divalent DNP conjugate and antibody that each DNP group fitted into one antibody

Figure 5.7. Flexibility of antigen and antibody contributes to binding affinity. In the illustration we show: (a) three types of energy-consuming reactions required to deform both molecules, thereby allowing (b) positive interaction between residues in the paratope and epitope — (1) bond rotation exposing a hydrophobic side-chain normally buried within the interior, (2) flexing of the α-carbon backbone to bring interacting residues close together, and (3) lateral displacement of a residue whose electron clouds would overlap with those of its opposite partner. Provided that the total deformation energy is less than the energy of attraction of the deformed molecules, complex formation will be favored. Expressed mathematically:

Free energy of deformation $= (\Delta G_1 + \Delta G_2 + \Delta G_3) = \Delta G_{\text{def}}$

where ΔG_1 is the Gibbs free energy change of reaction (1) and so on.

Energy of association of deformed antigen and antibody = the sum of the individual binding energies $= \Delta G_{\text{binding}}$ (an attractive force gives a negative ΔG).

Overall energy changes for complex formation
$= \Delta G_{\text{def}} + \Delta G_{\text{binding}} = -RT \ln K_{\text{a}}$

Provided that $-\Delta G_{\text{binding}} > \Delta G_{\text{def}}$, antigen and antibody will associate at equilibrium with a reasonable association affinity constant K_{a}. (R, gas constant; T, absolute temperature; ln, natural logarithm.)

If the antigen were completely rigid, it would be unable to approach close enough to the antibody to generate significant binding energy.

combining site (figures 3.1 and 3.2). This means that small haptens by themselves are monovalent with respect to reaction with antibody. The experiment on mixing hapten with antibody in a dialysis bag (figure 5.8) showed that the combination with antibody was reversible and that the complex so formed could readily dissociate depending upon the strength of binding, which we call **affinity**. In the simplistic situation of one Fab arm binding in isolation to one epitope on the antigen, the binding strength can be defined through the **equilibrium constant (K_{a})** of the **association reaction**:

Ab + Ag $\rightleftharpoons$ AbAg

given by the mass action equation

$$K_{\text{a}} = \frac{[\text{AbAg}]}{[\text{Ab}][\text{Ag}]}$$

where [Ab] is the concentration of free antibody combining sites and [Ag] is the concentration of free antigen at equilibrium. If the antibody and antigen fit together very closely, the equilibrium will lie well over to the right of the association reaction; we refer to such antibodies which bind strongly to the antigen as **high affinity antibodies**. At a certain free antigen concentration $[\text{Ag}_c]$ where half of the antibody sites are bound:

$$[\text{AbAg}] = [\text{Ab}] \text{ and } K_{\text{a}} = 1/[\text{Ag}_c]$$

i.e. the affinity constant K_{a} is equal to the reciprocal of the concentration of free antigen at the equilibrium point where half the antibody sites are in the bound form. In other words, when an antibody has a high affinity constant and binds antigen strongly, it only needs a low antigen concentration to half-saturate the antibody. An individual epitope on the surface of a complex antigen is by definition monovalent, and the

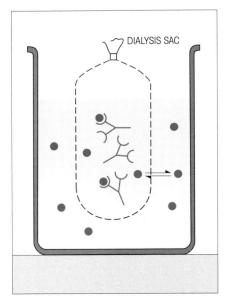

Figure 5.8. Reversibility of the interaction between antibody (✧) **and hapten (●).** Within the dialysis sac the hapten is partly in the free form and partly bound to antibody according to the affinity of the antibody. Only hapten can diffuse through the dialysis membrane, and the external concentration then will equal the concentration of unbound hapten within the sac. Measurement of total hapten in the dialysis sac then enables the amount bound to antibody to be calculated. Constant renewal of the external buffer will lead to total dissociation and loss of hapten from inside the dialysis sac showing the reversible nature of the antigen–antibody bond.

strength of its combination with one antigen-binding arm (Fab) of an antibody is therefore defined by an affinity constant.

Affinity can equally well be formulated in terms of the **dissociation constant (K_d)** of the reaction:

$$AbAg \rightleftharpoons Ab + Ag$$

Expressing concentrations in moles per liter:

$$K_d = \frac{[Ab \ moles/l][Ag \ moles/l]}{[AbAg \ moles/l]}$$

Clearly, K_d is the reciprocal of K_a, i.e. $1/K_a$, and has the units moles/l or M. Conversely, K_a is expressed in the units 1/mole or M^{-1} and has the advantage that the stronger the binding, the higher the number.

The value of K_a is determined by the difference in free energy (ΔG) between the antigen and antibody in the free state on the one hand and in the complexed form on the other, according to the equation:

$$\Delta G = -RT \ln K_a$$

where R is the universal gas constant, T is the absolute temperature and ln is the natural logarithm.

One can study the interaction of hapten and antibody by the dialysis method described in figure 5.8 and use the data to calculate the affinity constant from the mass action equation (figure 5.10). K_a values may sometimes be as high as $10^{12} M^{-1}$.

Analysis of the binding at different hapten concentrations generally shows a heterogeneity (figure 5.10) which indicates that most antiserums, even those raised against haptens with a simple structure, contain a variety of different antibodies with a range of binding affinities which depend upon the area of contact between the antibody and the hapten or epitope, the closeness of fit, conformational changes necessitated by electron-cloud overlap and the distribution of charged and hydrophobic groups.

The avidity of antiserum for antigen — the bonus effect of multivalency

While the term affinity describes the binding of antibody to a monovalent hapten or single antigen determinant, in most practical circumstances we are concerned with the interaction of an antiserum (i.e. the serum from an immunized individual) with a multivalent antigen. The term employed to express this binding is **avidity** or **functional affinity**.

The factors which contribute to avidity are complicated, including as they do the heterogeneity of antibodies in a given serum which are directed against each determinant on the antigen, and the heterogeneity of the determinants themselves (figures 5.4 and 5.10). But yet a further factor must be considered. The multivalency of most antigens leads to an interesting **bonus** effect in which the binding of antigen to antibody by multiple links is always greater, usually many-fold greater, than the arithmetic sum of the individual antibody bonds. This is illustrated in figure 5.11. The mechanism of this effect may be interpreted by considering an analogy. Let us fabricate an unheard of disease in which we cannot stop our hands opening and closing continuously. If we now try to hold an object in one hand, it will fall the moment we open that hand. However, if we use both hands to hold the object, provided that we open and close our hands at different times, there is much less chance of the object falling. The reversible combination of antigen and antibody is like the opening and closing of the hands; the more valencies holding the antigen, the less likely it is to be lost when the complex dissociates at any one binding site (figure 5.12).

Figure 5.9. Protein–protein interactions. (a) Coulombic attraction between oppositely charged ionic groups on the two protein side-chains as illustrated by an ionized amino group (NH_3^+) on a lysine of one protein and an ionized carboxyl group ($—COO^-$) of glutamate on the other. The force of attraction is inversely proportional to the square of the distance between the charges. Thus, as the charges come closer together, the attractive force increases considerably: if we halve the distance apart, we quadruple the attraction. Furthermore, since the dielectric constant of water is extremely high, the exclusion of water molecules through the contiguity of the interacting residues would greatly increase the force of attraction. Dipoles on antigen and antibody can also attract each other. In addition, electrostatic forces may be generated by charge transfer reactions between antibody and antigen; for example, an electron-donating protein residue such as tryptophan could part with an electron to a group such as dinitrophenyl (DNP) which is electron accepting, thereby creating an effective +1 charge on the antibody and −1 on the antigen. (b) Hydrogen bonding between two proteins involving the formation of reversible hydrogen bridges between hydrophilic groups, such as ·OH, ·NH$_2$ and ·COOH, depends very much upon the close approach of the two molecules carrying these groups. Although H bonds are relatively weak, because they are essentially electrostatic in nature, exclusion of water between the reacting side-chains would greatly enhance the binding energy through the gross reduction in dielectric constant. (c) Nonpolar, hydrophobic groups such as the side-chains of valine, leucine and isoleucine tend to associate in an aqueous environment. The driving force for this hydrophobic interaction derives from the fact that water in contact with hydrophobic molecules (——), with which it cannot H bond, will associate with other water molecules, but the number of configurations which allow H bonds to form will not be as great as that occurring when they are surrounded completely by other water molecules, i.e. the entropy is lower. The greater the area of contact between water and hydrophobic surfaces, the lower the entropy and the higher the energy state. Thus, if hydrophobic groups on two proteins come together so as to exclude water molecules between them (– – –), the net surface in contact with water is reduced and the proteins take up a lower energy state than when they are separated (in other words, there is a force of attraction between them). (d) Van der Waals force: the interaction between the electrons in the external orbitals of two different macromolecules may be envisaged (for simplicity!) as the attraction between induced oscillating dipoles in the two electron clouds. The nature of this interaction is difficult to describe in non-mathematical terms, but it has been likened to a temporary perturbation of electrons in one molecule effectively forming a dipole which induces a dipolar perturbation in the other molecule, the two dipoles then having a force of attraction between them; as the displaced electrons swing back through the equilibrium position and beyond, the dipoles oscillate. The force of attraction is inversely proportional to the seventh power of the distance and, as a result, this rises very rapidly as the interacting molecules come closer together.

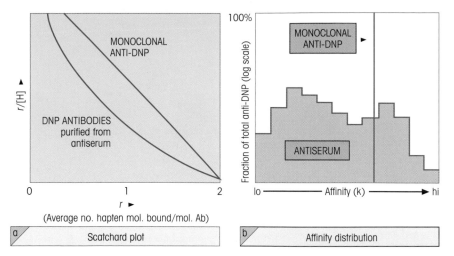

a — Scatchard plot

b — Affinity distribution

Figure 5.10. Heterogeneity of IgG antihapten (dinitrophenyl, DNP) antibodies from the serum of an immunized animal contrasting with the homogeneity of a monoclonal IgG anti-DNP. (a) A Scatchard plot of hapten binding to antibodies purified from the serum. If r represents the average number of DNP molecules bound to each antibody molecule, of affinity constant k and number of binding sites n, in the presence of a free hapten concentration [H], then from the mass action equation of equilibrium relationships (p. 86) it can be shown that:

$$r/[H] = nk - rk$$

Thus, a Scatchard plot of $r/[H]$ against r for a single antibody species will be a straight line of slope $-k$ as seen for the monoclonal antibody; the deviation from a straight line given by anti-DNP from the antiserum clearly indicates the existence of antibodies with different affinities, as may be confirmed by the binding of labeled DNP to many different bands after separation of the individual antibodies by isoelectric focusing of the serum. Extrapolation to $r/[H] = 0$ (at infinitely high concentration of antigen) gives the number of binding sites on each IgG molecule as two (cf. figure 3.2). For IgM antibodies, the value would be 10. Because the slope of the Scatchard plot varies with $r/2$ (the fractional occupancy of the antibody combining sites for a bivalent Ab), the affinity (which = −slope) will vary depending upon the range of values of r utilized in the experiments: thus affinity must be defined in terms of standard conditions of antibody dilution and concentration of hapten. (b) Histogram showing a typical distribution of antibody affinities in the anti-DNP serum. Measurable affinities tend to range between 10^4 and 10^{10} or 10^{11} M^{-1} and have skewed and not necessarily unimodal distributions. The monoclonal antibody of course gives a single affinity value since it is a homogeneous protein.

The same considerations apply to the binding of antibody to a polymeric antigen with repeating determinants, such as ovalbumin substituted by several DNP groups, or most bacterial polysaccharides or red cells with repeating blood-group determinants. As one moves from a univalent Fab fragment to a divalent IgG to a pentameric IgM, the bonus effect of multivalency produces striking increases in the strength of antigen–antibody complex formation.

Avidity, being a measure of the functional affinity of an antiserum for the whole antigen, is of obvious relevance to the reaction with antigen in the body. High avidity is superior to low for a wide variety of functions *in vivo*, e.g. immune elimination of antigen, virus neutralization, protective role against bacteria, and so on.

THE SPECIFICITY OF ANTIGEN RECOGNITION BY ANTIBODY IS NOT ABSOLUTE

The ability of antibodies to discriminate between different antigens was well illustrated by the range of reactivity of an antihapten for a series of structurally related molecules as described in table 5.1. Since the strength of the reaction can be quantified by the affinity or avidity, we would relate the **specificity** of an antiserum to its relative avidity for the antigens which are being discriminated.

In so far as we recognize that an antiserum may have a relatively greater avidity for one antigen rather than another, by the same token we are saying that the antiserum is displaying relative rather than absolute specificity; in practice we speak of degrees of **cross-reactivity**. An antiserum raised against a given antigen can cross-react with a partially related antigen which bears one or more identical or similar determinants. In figure 5.13 it can be seen that an antiserum to antigen$_1$ (Ag$_1$) will react less strongly with Ag$_2$, which bears just one identical determinant, because only certain of the antibodies in the serum can bind. Ag$_3$, which possesses a similar but not identical determinant, will not fit as well with the antibody and the binding is even weaker. Ag$_4$, which has no structural similarity at all, will not react significantly with the antibody. Thus, based upon stereochemical considerations, we can see why the

Figure 5.11. The 'bonus' effect of multivalent attachment on binding strength. The force binding the two antigen molecules in (c) with two antibody bridges is many-fold greater than (a)+(b). Thus, the binding of the two antibodies to determinants 1 and 2 on the antigen can each be described by the individual change in free energy state on forming the epitope–paratope bond with its corresponding affinity constant, i.e.:

$$\Delta G_1 = -RT \ln k_1 \text{ and } \Delta G_2 = -RT \ln k_2$$

For both antibodies operating in conjunction, the overall free energy change giving the avidity (K_{avid}) would be:

$$\Delta G = \Delta G_1 + \Delta G_2 = -RT \ln k_1 - RT \ln k_2$$
$$= -RT(\ln k_1 + \ln k_2) = -RT(\ln k_1 \times k_2)$$

Since $\Delta G = -RT \ln K_{avid}$, $K_{avid} = k_1 \times k_2$

The tremendous increase in equilibrium constant resulting from **multiplying the contributing affinities** is responsible for the bonus effect. To give a concrete example, if k_1 is 10^4 and k_2 is 10^3, K_{avid} would be 10^7 M^{-1}. In practice, this bonus effect would be reduced by entropy losses resulting from any restriction of the flexibility of the antibody molecules required by adaptation to the spatial demands of the epitopes and from the restriction in translational movement of the individual components.

Figure 5.13. Specificity and cross-reaction. The avidity of the serum antibodies ($\rfloor\lfloor$ and $)\!($) for $Ag_1 > Ag_2 > Ag_3 \gg Ag_4$.

avidity of the antiserum for Ag_2 and Ag_3 is less than for the homologous antigen, while for the unrelated Ag_4 it is negligible. It would be customary to describe the antiserum as being highly specific for Ag_1 in relation to Ag_4, but cross-reacting with Ag_2 and Ag_3 to different extents.

By being directed towards single epitopes on the antigen, monoclonal antibodies frequently show high specificity in terms of their low cross-reactivity with other antigens. Occasionally, however, one sees quite unexpected binding to antigens which react poorly, if at all, with a specific antiserum. It is an instructive exercise to see how it is that a polyclonal antiserum containing a heterogeneous collection of antibodies can be more specific in discriminating between two antigens than can a monoclonal antibody. The six hypervariable regions of an antibody encompass a relatively large molecular area composed of highly diverse amino acid side-chains and it is self evident that a number of different epitopic structures could fit into different parts of this hypervariable 'terrain', albeit with a spectrum of combining affinities.

Thus, each antibody will react not only with the antigen which stimulated its production, but also with some possibly quite unrelated molecules. Figure 5.14 explains (we hope) how this may translate into a higher specificity for the polyclonal serum.

WHAT THE T-CELL SEES

We have on several occasions alluded to the fact that the T-cell receptor sees antigen on the surface of cells associated with an MHC class I or II molecule. Now is the time for us to go into the nuts and bolts of this relationship.

Figure 5.12. The mechanism of the bonus effect. Each antigen–antibody bond is reversible and, with a single antibody bridge between two antigen molecules (a), dissociation of either bond could enable an antigen molecule to 'escape' as in (b). If there are two antibody bridges, even when one dissociates the other prevents the antigen molecule from escaping and holds it in position ready to reform the broken bond (c). In effect, the orientation of the broken bond greatly increases the effective combining concentration of antibody and thereby speeds up the velocity of the association reaction: $V_a = k_a[Ag][Ab\uparrow]$.

Figure 5.14. The specificity of an antiserum derives from the reactivity common to the component antibodies. Antigen A stimulates lymphocytes whose polyfunctional receptors bind A but could also bind other determinants as indicated (small letters). All antibodies in the resulting antiserum will have anti-A as a common specificity, but the other specificities will be so diverse that none of them will reach appreciable concentrations to cross-react significantly with another antigen bearing a or b, etc., i.e. the antiserum shows specificity for A. On the other hand, a monoclonal antibody cannot dilute out its alternative specificity and so in the example shown with an asterisk there would be strong cross-reaction with an unrelated antigen a. (With acknowledgment to Talmage D.W. (1959) *Science* **129**, 1643.)

Haplotype restriction reveals the need for MHC participation

It has been established in tablets of stone that T-cells bearing αβ receptors, with some exceptions (cf. p. 100), only respond when the antigen-presenting cells express the same MHC haplotype as the host from which the T-cells were derived (Milestone 5.1). This **haplotype restriction** on T-cell recognition tells us unequivocally that MHC molecules are intimately and necessarily involved in the interaction of the antigen-bearing cell with its corresponding antigen-specific T-lymphocyte. We also learn that, generally speaking, cytotoxic T-cells recognize antigen in the context of class I MHC, and helper T-cells which interact with macrophages respond when the antigen is associated with class II molecules.

Accepting then the participation of MHC in T-cell recognition, what of the antigen? For some time it was perplexing that, in so many systems, antibodies raised to the native antigen failed to block cytotoxicity (cf. figure M5.1.1b), despite consistent success with anti-MHC class I sera. We now know why.

T-cells recognize a linear peptide sequence from the antigen

In Milestone 5.1, we commented on experiments involving influenza nucleoprotein-specific T-cells which could kill cells infected with influenza virus. Killing occurs after the cytotoxic T-cell adheres strongly to its target through recognition of specific surface molecules. It is curious then that the nucleoprotein, which lacks a signal sequence or transmembrane region and so cannot be expressed on the cell surface, can nonetheless function as a target for cytotoxic T-cells, particularly since we have already noted that antibodies to native nucleoprotein have no influence on the killing reaction (figure M5.1.1b). Furthermore, uninfected cells do not become targets for the cytotoxic T-cells when whole nucleoprotein is added to the culture system. However, if, instead, we add a series of short peptides with sequences derived from the primary structure of the nucleoprotein, the uninfected cells now become susceptible to cytolytic T-cell attack (figure 5.15).

Thus was the secret revealed! The startling reality is that T-cells recognize linear peptides derived from the antigen, and that is why antibodies raised against nucleoprotein in its native three-dimensional conformation (cf. figure 5.2) do not inhibit killing. Note that only certain nucleoprotein peptides were recognized by the polyclonal T-cells in the donor population and these are to be regarded as T-cell epitopes. When clones of identical specificity are derived from these T-cells, each clone reacts with only one of the peptides; in other words, like B-cell clones, each clone is specific for one corresponding epitope.

Entirely analogous results are obtained when *T-helper* clones are stimulated by antigen-presenting cells to which certain peptides derived from the original antigen have been added. Again, by synthesizing a series of such peptides, the T-cell epitope can be mapped with some precision.

The conclusion is that the **T-cell recognizes both MHC and peptide** and we now know that the peptide which acts as a T-cell epitope lies along the groove formed by the α-helices and the β-sheet floor of the

Milestone 5.1 — MHC Restriction of T-cell Reactivity

b			
TARGET CELLS			**% KILLING OF TARGET BY NP-SPECIFIC T-CELLS**
Infected	Haplotype	Ab added	
–	HLA-A2	–	
+	HLA-A2	–	
+	HLA-A1	–	
+	HLA-A2	anti-HLA-A2	
+	HLA-A2	anti-HLA-A1	
+	HLA-A2	anti-HLA-DR	
+	HLA-A2	anti-NP	

Figure M5.1.1. T-cell killing is restricted by the MHC haplotype of the virus-infected target cells. (a) Haplotype-restricted killing of lymphocytic choriomeningitis (LCM) virus-infected target cells by cytotoxic T-cells. Killer cells from H-2^d hosts only killed H-2^d-infected targets, not those of H-2^k haplotype and vice versa. (b) Killing of influenza-infected target cells by influenza nucleoprotein (NP)-specific T-cells from an HLA-A2 donor (cf. p. 356 for human MHC nomenclature). Killing was restricted to HLA-A2 targets and only inhibited by antibodies to A2, not to A1, nor to the class II HLA-DR framework or native NP antigen.

The realization that the MHC, which had figured for so long as a dominant controlling element in tissue graft rejection, should come to occupy the center stage in T-cell reactions has been a source of fascination and great pleasure to immunologists—almost as though a great universal plan had been slowly unfolding.

One of the seminal observations which helped to elevate the MHC to this lordly position was the dramatic Nobel prize-winning revelation by Doherty and Zinkernagel that cytotoxic T-cells taken from an individual recovering from a viral infection will only kill virally infected cells which share an MHC haplotype with the host. They found that cytotoxic T-cells from mice of the H-2^d haplotype infected with lymphocytic choriomeningitis virus could kill virally infected cells derived from any H-2^d strain but not cells of H-2^k or other H-2 haplotype. The reciprocal experiment with H-2^k mice shows that this is not just a special property associated with H-2^d (figure M5.1.1a). Studies with recombinant strains (cf. table 4.2) pin-pointed class I MHC as the restricting element and this was confirmed by showing that antibodies to class I MHC block the killing reaction.

The same phenomenon has been repeatedly observed in the human. HLA-A2 individuals recovering from influenza have cytolytic T-cells which kill HLA-A2 target cells infected with influenza virus, but not cells of a different HLA-A tissue-type specificity (figure M5.1.1b). Note how

Figure M5.1.2. The T-cell clone only responds by proliferation *in vitro* when the antigen-presenting cells (e.g. macrophages) pulsed with ovalbumin express the same class II MHC.

cytotoxicity could be inhibited by antiserum specific for the donor HLA-A type, but not by antisera to the allelic form HLA-A1 or the HLA-DR class II framework. Of striking significance is the inability of antibodies to the nucleoprotein to block T-cell recognition even though the T-cell specificity in these studies was known to be directed towards this antigen. Since the antibodies react with

(continued)

nucleoprotein in its native form, the conformation of the antigen as presented to the T-cell must be quite different.

In parallel, an entirely comparable series of experiments has established the role of MHC class II molecules in antigen presentation to helper T-cells. Initially, it was shown by Shevach and Rosenthal that lymphocyte proliferation to antigen *in vitro* could be blocked by antisera raised between two strains of guinea-pig which would have included antibodies to the MHC of the responding lymphocytes. More stringent evidence comes from the type of experiment in which a T-cell clone proliferating in response to ovalbumin on antigen-presenting cells with the H-2A[b] phenotype fails to respond if antigen is presented in the context of H-2A[k]. However, if the H-2A[k] antigen-presenting cells are transfected with the genes encoding H-2A[b], they now communicate effectively with the T-cells (figure M5.1.2).

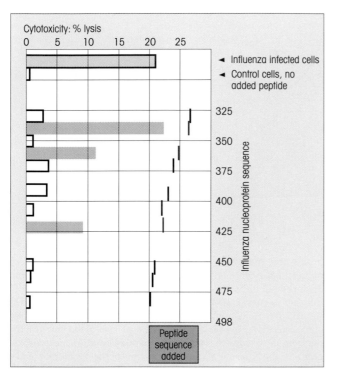

Figure 5.15. Cytotoxic T-cells, from a human donor, kill uninfected target cells in the presence of short influenza nucleoprotein peptides. The peptides indicated were added to ^{51}Cr-labeled syngeneic (i.e. same as T-cell donor) mitogen-activated lymphoblasts and cytotoxicity was assessed by ^{51}Cr release with a killer to target ratio of 50:1. The three peptides indicated in red induced good killing. Blasts infected with influenza virus of a different strain served as a positive control. (Reproduced from Townsend A.R.M. *et al.* (1986) *Cell* **44**, 959, with permission. Copyright ©1986 by Cell Press.)

class I and class II outermost domains (figure 4.11). Just how does it get there?

PROCESSING OF INTRACELLULAR ANTIGEN FOR PRESENTATION BY CLASS I MHC

Within the cytosol lurk proteolytic structures, the proteasomes, involved in the routine turnover and cellular degradation of proteins (figure 5.16). Cytosolic proteins destined for antigen presentation, including viral proteins, are degraded to peptides via a pathway involving these structures, although other cytosolic proteases including leucine- and aspartyl-aminopeptidases may also contribute to this antigen processing. In addition to cytosol-resident proteins, a proportion of membrane-bound and secretory proteins are transported from the endoplasmic reticulum (ER) back into the cytosol by the SEC61 molecular complex, and such proteins can then also undergo processing for class I presentation, as can proteins derived from mitochondria. Prior to processing, proteins are covalently linked to several ubiquitin molecules in an ATP-dependent process. The polyubiquitination targets the polypeptides to the proteasome (figure 5.16).

Only about 10% of the peptides produced by proteasomes are the optimal length (octamers or nonamers) to fit into the MHC class I groove; about 70% are likely to be too small to function in antigen presentation; and the remaining 20% would require further trimming by, for example, cytosolic aminopeptidases. The cytokine IFNγ increases the production of three catalytic proteosomal subunits, the polymorphic *low molecular weight proteins* LMP2 and LMP7, and the nonpolymorphic LMP10. These molecules replace the homologous catalytic subunits (β_1, β_5 and β_2, respectively) in the housekeeping proteasome to produce what has been termed the **immunoproteasome**, a process thought to modify the cleavage specificity in order to tailor peptide production for class I binding.

Both proteasome- and immunoproteasome-generated peptides are translocated into the ER by the *transporters associated with antigen processing* (TAP1 and TAP2) (figure 5.17), a process which might also involve heat-shock protein family members. The newly synthesized class I heavy chain is retained in the ER by the molecular chaperone calnexin which is thought to assist in folding, disulfide bond formation and

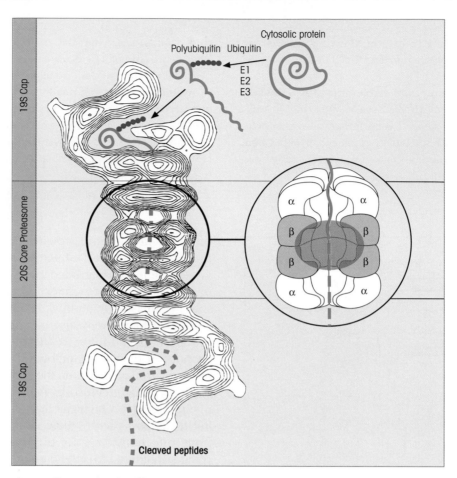

Figure 5.16. Cleavage of cytosolic proteins by the proteasome. Cytosolic proteins become polyubiquitinated in an ATP-dependent reaction in which the enzyme E1 forms a thiolester with the C-terminus of ubiquitin and then transfers the ubiquitin to one of 10–15 different E2 ubiquitin-carrier proteins. The C-terminus of the ubiquitin is then conjugated by one of a dozen or so E3 ubiquitin-protein ligase enzymes to a lysine residue on the polypeptide. There is specificity in these processes in that the individual E2 and E3 enzymes have preferences for different proteins. The ubiquitinated cytosolic protein binds to the ATPase-containing cap where ATP drives the unfolded protein chain through the hydrophobic conducting channels of the α-subunits into the central hydrolytic chamber where it is exposed to a variety of proteolytic activities associated with the different β-subunits. The whole 26S proteasome, which is a 2000 kDa complex of about 50 different subunits consisting of the 20S 650 kDa core proteasome with twin 19S 700 kDa regulatory caps, is displayed as a contour plot derived from electron microscopy and image analysis. The core proteasome is a cylindrical structure made up of 28 subunits arranged in four stacked rings. The cross-section of the proteasome reveals the site of proteolytic activity (red shading) within the two central rings, each comprising seven homologous but distinct β-subunits, three of which in each ring contain proteolytically active sites. The outer two α-rings are again each made up of seven different but homologous α-subunits, but these all lack proteolytic activity. A novel catalytic mechanism is involved in which the nucleophilic residue that attacks the peptide bonds is the hydroxyl group on the N-terminal threonine residue of the β-subunits. Three distinct peptidase activities have been associated with specific β-subunits. One is 'chymotrypsin-like' in that it hydrolyses peptides after large hydrophobic residues, one is 'trypsin-like' and cleaves after basic residues, and one hydrolyses after acidic residues. The LMP2, LMP7 and LMP10 (the latter often called MECL1; *m*ulticatalytic *e*ndopeptidase *c*omplex *l*ike-1) immunoproteasome-associated molecules show similar specificities but have enhanced chymotrypsin and trypsin activity and reduced postacidic cleavage compared to their counterparts in the housekeeping proteasome. (Based on Peters J.-M. *et al.* (1993) *Journal of Molecular Biology* **234**, 932 and Rubin D.M. & Finley D. (1995) *Current Biology* **5**, 854.)

promotion of assembly with β_2-microglobulin. In the human, but not in the mouse, calnexin is then replaced by calreticulin. The ER-resident protein, Erp57, which has thiol reductase, cysteine protease and chaperone functions, becomes associated with the complex of calreticulin–calnexin and class I heavy chain which now folds together with β_2-microglobulin. The empty class I molecule bound to these chaperones becomes linked to TAP1/2 by tapasin. Upon peptide loading, the class I molecule can dissociate from the various accessory molecules, and the now stable peptide–class I heavy chain–β_2-microglobulin complex traverses the Golgi stack and reaches the surface where it is a sitting target for the cytotoxic T-cell.

Figure 5.17. Processing and presentation of endogenous antigen by class I MHC. Cytosolic proteins are degraded by the proteasome complex into peptides which are transported into the endoplasmic reticulum (ER). TAP1 and TAP2 are members of the ABC family of ATP-dependent transport proteins and, under the influence of these transporters, the peptides are loaded into the groove of the membrane-bound class I MHC. The peptide–MHC complex is then released from all its associated transporters and chaperones, traverses the Golgi system, and appears on the cell surface ready for presentation to the T-cell receptor. Mutant cells deficient in TAP1/2 do not deliver peptides to class I and cannot function as cytotoxic T-cell targets. However, if they are transfected with a gene encoding the antigenic peptide linked to a cleavable signal sequence, the peptide is delivered to the ER without the need for TAP1/2 and the cells once again can become targets.

PROCESSING OF ANTIGEN FOR CLASS II MHC PRESENTATION FOLLOWS A DIFFERENT PATHWAY

Class II MHC complexes with antigenic peptide are generated by a fundamentally different intracellular mechanism, since the antigen-presenting cells which interact with T-helper cells need to sample the antigen from both the *extra*cellular and *intra*cellular compartments. In essence, a trans-Golgi vesicle containing class II has to intersect with a late endosome containing exogenous protein antigen taken into the cell by an endocytic mechanism.

Regarding the class II molecules themselves, these are assembled from α and β chains in the endoplasmic reticulum in association with the transmembrane **invariant chain (Ii)** (figure 5.18) which has several functions. Firstly, it acts as a dedicated chaperone to ensure correct folding of the nascent class II molecule. Secondly, an internal sequence of the luminal portion of Ii sits in the MHC groove to inhibit the precocious binding of peptides in the ER before the class II molecule reaches the endocytic compartment containing antigen. Additionally, combination of Ii with the αβ class II heterodimer inactivates a retention signal and allows transport to the Golgi. Finally, targeting motifs in the N-terminal cytoplasmic region of Ii ensure delivery of the class II-containing vesicle to the endocytic pathway.

Meanwhile, exogenous protein is taken up by endocytosis and, as the early endosome undergoes progressive acidification, is processed into peptides by endosomal proteases such as asparaginyl endopeptidase. The late endosomes, which ultimately mature into lysosomes, characteristically acquire *l*ysosomal-*a*ssociated *m*embrane *p*roteins (LAMPs), although the function of these molecules is still unclear. These late endosomes fuse with the vacuole containing the class II–Ii complex. Under the acidic conditions within these *M*HC class *II*-enriched *c*ompartments (MIICs), proteases degrade Ii except for the part sitting in the MHC groove which, for the time being, remains there as a peptide referred to as CLIP (*c*lass II-associated *i*nvariant chain *p*eptide). An MHC-related dimeric molecule, DM, then catalyses the removal of CLIP and keeps the groove open so that peptides generated in the endosome can be inserted (figure 5.19). This process may be assisted by members of the hsp70 family which promiscuously bind unfolded peptides. Initial peptide binding is determined by the concentration of the peptide and its on-rate, but DM may subsequently assist in the removal of lower affinity peptides to allow their replacement by high affinity peptides, i.e. act as a peptide editor permitting the incorporation of peptides with the most stable binding characteristics, namely those with a slow off-rate. Particularly in B-cells an additional MHC-related molecule, DO, associates with DM bound to class II and modifies its function in a pH-dependent fashion. Its effect may be to favor the presentation of antigens internalized via the BCR over those taken up by fluid phase endocytosis. The tetraspanin family member CD82 is also present in the MIIC, though its role is unclear at present. The class II–peptide complexes are eventually transported to the membrane for presentation to T-helper cells.

Thus, in general, endogenous protein antigens are processed for class I presentation whilst exogenous protein antigens are processed for class II presentation. Processing of antigens for class II presentation is not, however, confined to soluble proteins taken up from the exterior, but can also encompass microorganisms whose antigens reach the lysosomal structures, either after direct phagocytosis or prolonged intracellular cohabitation. Proteins and peptides within the ER are also potential clients for the class II groove and could also make the journey to the MIIC. Conversely, class I-restricted responses can be generated against exogenous antigens, a process sometimes referred to as **cross-priming**. This may occur either by a TAP-dependent pathway in phagocytic cells where proteins are transferred from the phagosome to the cytosol, or by endocytosis of cell surface MHC class I molecules which then arrive in the class II-enriched compartments where peptide exchange occurs with sequences derived from the endocytic processing pathway.

THE NATURE OF THE 'GROOVY' PEPTIDE

The MHC grooves impose some well-defined restrictions on the nature and length of the peptides they ac-

Figure 5.18. Processing and presentation of exogenous antigen by class II MHC. Class II molecules with Ii are assembled in the endoplasmic reticulum (ER) and transported through the Golgi to the trans-Golgi reticulum (actually as a nonamer consisting of three invariant, three α and three β chains—not shown). There it is sorted to a late endosomal vesicle with lysosomal characteristics known as MIIC (meaning MHC class II-enriched compartment) containing partially degraded protein derived from the endocytic uptake of exogenous antigen. Degradation of the invariant chain leaves the CLIP (class II-associated invariant chain peptide) lying in the groove but, under the influence of the DM molecule, this is replaced by other peptides in the vesicle including those derived from exogenous antigen, and the complexes are transported to the cell surface for presentation to T-helper cells. This version of events is supported by the finding of high concentrations of invariant chain CLIP associated with class II in the MIIC vacuoles of DM-deficient mutant mice which are poor presenters of antigen to T-cells.

| MHC II/invariant chain (Ii) heterononamer transport | Degradation of Ii in MIIC | DM-catalysed replacement of CLIP with antigenic peptide |

Figure 5.19. MHC class II transport and peptide loading illustrated by Tulp's gently vulgar cartoon. (Reproduced from Benham A. *et al.* (1995) *Immunology Today* **16**, 361, with permission of the authors and Elsevier Science Ltd.)

commodate and the pattern varies with different MHC alleles. Otherwise, at the majority of positions in the peptide ligand, a surprising degree of redundancy is permitted and this relates in part to residues interacting with the T-cell receptor rather than the MHC.

Binding to MHC class I

X-ray analysis reveals the peptides to be tightly mounted along the length of the groove in an extended configuration with no breathing space for α-helical structures (figure 5.20). The N- and C-termini are tightly H bonded to conserved residues at each end of the groove, independently of the MHC allele.

The naturally occurring peptides can be extracted from purified MHC class I and sequenced. They are predominantly 8–9 residues long; longer peptides bulge upwards out of the cleft. Analysis of the peptide pool sequences usually gives strong amino acid signals at certain key positions (table 5.2). These are called **anchor positions** and represent the preferred amino acid side-chains which fit into allele-specific pockets in the MHC groove (figure 5.21a). There are usually two, sometimes three, such major anchor positions for class

I-binding peptides, one at the C-terminal end and the other frequently at position 2 (P2), but it may also occur at P3, P5 or P7. Sometimes, a major anchor pocket may be replaced by two or three more weakly binding secondary binding pockets. Even with the constraints of two or three anchor motifs, each MHC class I allele can accommodate a considerable number of different peptides.

Except in the case of viral infection, the natural class I ligands will be self peptides derived from proteins endogenously synthesized by the cell, histones, heat-shock proteins, enzymes, leader signal sequences, and so on. It turns out that 75% or so of these peptides originate in the cytosol (figure 5.22) and most of them will be in low abundance, say 100–400 copies per cell. Thus proteins expressed with unusual abundance, such as oncofetal proteins in tumors and viral antigens in infected cells, should be readily detected by resting T-cells.

Binding to MHC class II

Unlike class I, where the allele-independent H bonding to the peptide is focused at the N- and C-termini, the class II groove residues H bond along the entire length of the peptide with links to the atoms forming the main chain. With respect to class II allele-specific binding pockets for peptide side-chains, motifs based on three or four major anchor residues seem to be the order of the day (figure 5.21b). Secondary binding pockets with less strict preference for individual side-

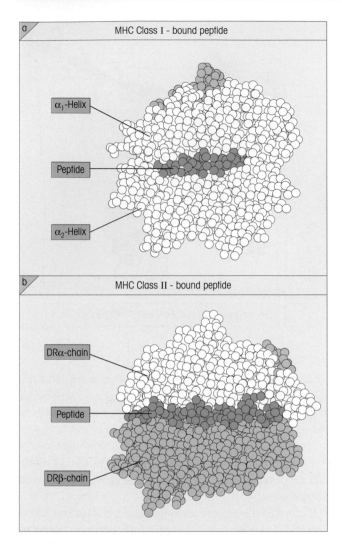

Figure 5.20. Binding of peptides to the MHC cleft. T-cell receptor 'view' looking down on the α-helices lining the cleft (cf. figure 4.11b) represented in space-filling models. (a) Peptide 309–317 from HIV-1 reverse transcriptase bound tightly within the class I HLA-A2 cleft. In general, one to four of the peptide side-chains point towards the TCR, giving a solvent accessibility of 17–27%. (b) Influenza hemagglutinin 306–318 lying in the class II HLA-DR1 cleft. In contrast with class I, the peptide extends out of both ends of the binding groove and from four to six out of an average of 13 side-chains point towards the TCR, increasing solvent accessibility to 35%. (Based on Vignali D.A.A. & Strominger J.L. (1994) *The Immunologist* **2**, 112, with permission of the authors and publisher.)

Table 5.2. Natural MHC class I peptide ligands contain two allele-specific anchor residues. (Based on Rammensee H.G., Friede T. & Stevanovic S. (1995) *Immunogenetics* **41**, 178.) Letters represent the Dayhoff code for amino acids; where more than one residue predominates at a given position, the alternative(s) is given; • = any residue.

Class I allele	Amino acid position								
	1	2	3	4	5	6	7	8	9
H-2K^d	•	Y	•	•	•	•	•	•	I/L
H-2K^b	•	•	•	•	Y/F	•	•	L/M	
H-2D^b	•	•	•	•	N	•	•	•	L/M/I
HLA-A*0201	•	L/M/I	•	•	•	•	•	•	L/V/I/M
HLA-B*2705	•	R	•	•	•	•	•	•	R/K/L/F

Figure 5.21. Allele-specific pockets in the MHC-binding grooves bind the major anchor residue motifs of the peptide ligands. Cross-section through the longitudinal axis of the MHC groove. The two α-helices forming the lateral walls of the groove lie horizontally above and below the plane of the paper. (a) The class I groove is closed at both ends. The anchor at the carboxy terminus is invariant but the second anchor very often at P2 may also be at P3, P5 or P7 depending on the MHC allele (cf. table 5.2). (b) In contrast, the class II groove is open at both ends and does not constrain the length of the peptide. There are usually three major anchor pockets at P1, P4, P6, P7 or P9 with P1 being the most important.

chains can still modify the affinity of the peptide–MHC complex, while 'nonpockets' may also influence preferences for particular peptide sequences, especially if steric hindrance becomes a factor. Unfortunately, we cannot establish these preferences for the individual residues within a given peptide because the open nature of the class II groove places no constraint on the length of the peptide, which can dangle nonchalantly from each end of the groove, quite unlike the straitjacket of the class I ligand site (figures 5.20 and 5.21). Thus, as noted earlier, each class II molecule binds a collection of peptides with a spectrum of lengths rang-

| Class I | Class II |

Cytosolic   **Exogenous**
Membrane-associated   **MHC-related**

Figure 5.22. The origins of class I- and class II-bound peptides. Virtually all class I peptides are derived from endogenous proteins and, even after viral infections, it is the intracellular antigens which are processed. Processing in the endosomal compartments ensures that proteins of endogenous origin and those derived from membranes constitute over 90% of the peptides bound to the class II grooves. (Diagram reproduced from Vignali D.A.A. & Strominger J.L. (1994) *The Immunologist* **2**, 112, with permission of the authors and publisher.)

ing from eight to 30 amino acid residues, and analysis of such a naturally occurring pool isolated from the MHC would not establish which amino acid side-chains were binding preferentially to the nine available sites within the groove. A modern approach is to study the binding of soluble class II molecules to very large libraries of random-sequence peptides expressed on the surface of bacteriophages (cf. the combinatorial phage libraries, p. 124). The idea is emerging that each amino acid in a peptide contributes independently of the others to the total binding strength, and it should be possible to compute each contribution quantitatively from this random binding data, so that ultimately we could predict which sequences in a given protein antigen would bind to a given class II allele.

Because of the accessible nature of the groove, as the native molecule is unfolded and reduced, but before any degradation need occur, the high affinity epitopes could immediately bury themselves in the class II-binding groove where they are protected from proteolysis. At least for the HLA-DR1 molecule it has been shown that peptide binding leads to a transition from a more open conformation to one with a more compact structure extending throughout the peptide-binding groove. Trimming can take place after peptide binding, leaving peptides 8–30 amino acids long. Several factors will influence the relative concentration of pep-

tide–MHC complex formed: the affinity for the groove as determined by the fit of the anchors, enhancement or hindrance by internal residues (sequences outside the binding residues have little or no effect on peptide-binding specificity), sensitivity to proteases and disulfide reduction, and downstream competition from determinants of higher affinity.

The range of concentration of the different peptide complexes which result will engender a hierarchy of epitopes with respect to their ability to interact with T-cells; the most effective will be **dominant**, the less so **subdominant**. Dominant, and presumably subdominant, **self** epitopes will generally induce tolerance during T-cell ontogeny in the thymus (see p. 231). Complexes with some self peptides which are of relatively low abundance will not tolerize their T-cell counterparts and these autoreactive T-cells constantly pose an underlying threat of potential autoimmunity. Sercarz has labeled these **cryptic** epitopes, and we will discuss their possible relationship to autoimmune disease in Chapter 19.

THE αβ T-CELL RECEPTOR FORMS A TERNARY COMPLEX WITH MHC AND ANTIGENIC PEPTIDE

The forces involved in peptide binding to MHC and in TCR binding to peptide–MHC are similar to those seen between antibody and antigen, i.e. noncovalent. When soluble TCR preparations produced using recombinant DNA technology are immobilized on a sensor chip, they can bind MHC–peptide complex specifically with rather low affinities (K_a) in the 10^4 to 10^7 M^{-1} range. This low affinity and the relatively small number of atomic contacts (27–68 in the structures so far solved) formed between the TCRs and their MHC–peptide ligands when T-cells contact their target cell make the contribution of TCR recognition to the binding energy of this cellular interaction fairly trivial. The brunt of the attraction rests on the antigen-independent major adhesion molecules, such as ICAM-1/2, LFA-1/2 and CD2, but any subsequent triggering of the T-cell by MHC–peptide antigen must involve signaling through the T-cell receptor.

Topology of the ternary complex

Of the three complementarity determining regions present in each TCR chain, CDR1 and CDR2 are much less variable than CDR3 which, like its immunoglobulin counterpart, has (D)J sequences which result from a multiplicity of combinatorial and nucleotide insertion mechanisms (cf. p. 65). Since the MHC elements in a given individual are fixed, but great variability is expected in the antigenic peptide, a logical model would have CDR1 and CDR2 of each TCR chain contacting the α-helices of the MHC, and the CDR3 concerned in binding to the peptide. In accord with this view, several studies have shown that T-cells which recognize small variations in a peptide in the context of a given MHC restriction element differ only in their CDR3 hypervariable regions.

The combining sites of the TCRs which have been crystallized to date are relatively flat (figure 5.23), which would be expected given the need for complementarity to the gently undulating surface of the peptide–MHC combination. For recognition of peptides presented by MHC class I (figure 5.24a), the TCR lies diagonally across the peptide–MHC with the TCR Vα domain overlying the MHC α$_2$-helix and the N-terminus of the peptide and the Vβ domain overlying the α$_1$-helix and the C-terminal portion of the peptide (figure 5.24b). Until many more crystal structures are solved, it is impossible to put forward any hard and fast rules for binding, but it is already clear that the CDR3 loops, which have the greatest variability, make the major contacts with the peptide, particularly focusing in on the middle of the peptide (P4 to P6). The CDR1s can make contacts with both the peptide and the α-helices of the MHC, whilst so far it seems that the CDR2s interact largely with the MHC α-helices (figure 5.24a and b). Significant conformational changes are induced in the CDR3s by these interactions. The recent crystal structure of a TCR recognizing a peptide presented by MHC class II indicates that here there is a different orientation, with the TCR crossing the bound peptide in an orthogonal orientation (figure 5.24c). Whilst the peptides presented by MHC class II molecules are longer, the size of the TCR combining site limits recognition to a maximum of nine sequential peptide residues, and it is again the central residues of the peptide within the MHC groove which are the focus of the TCR's attention. The TCR Vα domain contacts the class II β$_1$-helix and the Vβ domain the α$_1$-helix.

One idea is that the TCR 'scans' the MHC and that the binding energy between TCR and the MHC is sufficient to allow the TCR to temporarily dock onto the peptide–MHC complex and interrogate the peptide. If there are sufficient energetically favorable contacts between the TCR and the peptide–MHC, then signaling through the TCR complex can occur. It now seems likely that complexes of two TCR molecules with two MHC–peptide moieties can form and this formation of complexes may be linked to T-cell signaling.

T-CELLS WITH A DIFFERENT OUTLOOK

Nonclassical class I molecules can also present antigen

MHC class I-like molecules

In addition to the highly polymorphic classical MHC class I molecules (HLA-A, B and C in the human and H-2K, D and L in the mouse), there are other loci en-

Figure 5.23. T-cell receptor antigen combining site. Although the surface is relatively flat, there is a clearly visible cleft between the CDR3α and CDR3β which can accommodate a central upfacing side-chain of the peptide bound into the groove of an MHC molecule. The surface and loop traces of the Vα CDR1 and CDR2 are colored magenta, Vβ CDR1 and CDR2 blue, Vα CDR3 and Vβ CDR3 yellow, and the Vβ fourth hypervariable region, which makes contact with some superantigens, orange. (Reproduced from Garcia K.C. *et al.* (1996) *Science* **274**, 209, with permission.)

(a)

Figure 5.24. Complementarity between MHC–peptide and T-cell receptor. (a) Backbone structure of a TCR (designated 2C) recognizing a peptide (dEV8) presented by the MHC class I molecule H-2K^b. The TCR is in the top half of the picture, with the α chain in pink and its CDR1 colored magenta, CDR2 purple and CDR3 yellow. The β chain is colored light blue with its CDR1 cyan, CDR2 navy blue, CDR3 green and the fourth hypervariable loop orange. Below the TCR is the MHC α chain in green and β$_2$-microglobulin in dark green. The peptide with its side-chains is colored yellow. (Reproduced from Garcia K.C. *et al.* (1998) *Science* **279**, 1166, with permission.) (b) The same complex looking down onto a molecular surface representation of the H-2K^b in yellow, with the diagonal docking mode of the TCR in a backbone worm representation colored brown. The dEV8 peptide is drawn in a ball and stick format. (c) In contrast, here we see the orthogonal docking mode of a TCR recognizing a peptide presented by MHC class II. The TCR (scD10) backbone worm representation shows the Vα in green and Vβ in blue, and the I-A^k class II molecular surface representation has the α chain in light green and the β chain in orange, holding its conalbumin-derived peptide. (Reproduced from Reinherz E.L. *et al.* (1999) *Science* **286**, 1913, with permission.)

coding MHC molecules containing β$_2$-microglobulin with relatively nonpolymorphic heavy chains. These are **H-2M**, **Q** and **T** in mice and **HLA-E**, **F** and **G** in *Homo sapiens*.

The best studied molecule encoded by the H-2M locus is **H-2M3**, which is unusual in its ability to present bacterial *N*-formyl methionine peptides to T-cells. Expression of H-2M3 is limited by the availability of these peptides so that high levels are only seen during prokaryotic infections. The demonstration of H-2M3-restricted CD8-positive αβ T-cells specific for *Listeria monocytogenes* encourages the view that this class I-like molecule could underwrite a physiological function in infection. Discussion of the role of HLA-G expression in the human syncytiotrophoblast will arise in Chapter 17 (p. 369).

The family of CD1 non-MHC class I-like molecules can present exotic antigens

After MHC class I and class II, the CD1 family (p. 77) represents a third lineage of antigen-presenting molecules recognized by T-lymphocytes. The CD1 polypeptide chain associates with β_2-microglobulin as becomes an honest class I-like moiety, and the overall structure is similar to that of classical class I molecules, although the topology of the binding groove is altered (see figure 4.18).

CD1 molecules can act as **restriction elements** for the presentation of **lipid and glycolipid** microbial antigens to T-cells. A common structural motif facilitates CD1-mediated antigen presentation and comprises a hydrophobic region of a branched or dual acyl chain and a hydrophilic portion formed by the polar or charged groups of the lipid and/ or its associated carbohydrate. The hydrophobic regions are buried in the binding groove of CD1, whilst the hydrophilic regions, such as the carbohydrate structures, are recognized by the TCR. Because antigen recognition by CD1-restricted T-cells involves clonally diverse αβ and γδ TCRs, it is likely that CD1 can present a broad range of such antigens. One group of major ligands for CD1b are glycophosphatidylinositols, such as the mycobacterial cell wall component lipoarabinomannan.

Just like their proteinaceous colleagues, exogenously derived lipid and glycolipid antigens are delivered to the acidic endosomal compartment. Localization of CD1 molecules to the endocytic pathway is mediated by a targeting sequence in the cytoplasmic tail. There is evidence that human CD1a, which lacks the targeting motif, does not localize to this pathway and therefore presumably must follow a different route for peptide loading. The acidic environment of the endosome induces a conformational change in CD1, thereby increasing accessibility to the lipid-binding site in the hydrophobic groove of the molecule. Antigens derived from endogenous pathogens can also be presented by the CD1 pathway, but in a process that,

unlike class I-mediated presentation, is independent of TAP and DM.

Some T-cells have NK markers

NK T-cells possess the NK1.1$^+$ marker, characteristic of NK cells, together with a T-cell receptor. However, the TCR bears an invariant α chain (Vα14-Jα281 in mice, Vα24-JαQ in humans) with no N-region modifications and a limited β chain repertoire. These cells are a major component of the T-cell compartment, accounting for 20–30% of T-cells in bone marrow and liver, and up to 1% of spleen cells. NK1.1$^+$ T-cells rapidly secrete interleukin-4 (IL-4) and IFNγ following stimulation and therefore may have important regulatory functions. Although substantial numbers of NK T-cells are CD1-restricted, others are restricted by classical MHC molecules.

γδ TCRs have some features of antibody

Unlike αβ T-cells, γδ T-cells recognize antigens directly without a requirement for antigen processing. Whilst some T-cells bearing a γδ receptor are capable of recognizing MHC molecules, neither the polymorphic residues associated with peptide binding nor the peptide itself are involved. Thus, a γδ T-cell clone specific for the herpes simplex virus glycoprotein-1 can be stimulated by the native protein bound to plastic, suggesting that the cells are triggered by cross-linking of their receptors by antigen which they recognize in the intact native state just as antibodies do. There are structural arguments to give weight to this view. The CDR3 loops, which are critical for foreign antigen recognition by T-cells and antibodies, are comparable in length and relatively constrained with respect to size in the α and β chains of the αβ TCR, presumably reflecting a relative constancy in the size of the MHC–peptide complexes to which they bind. CDR3 regions in the immunoglobulin light chains are short and similarly constrained in length, but in the heavy chains they are longer on average and more variable in length, related perhaps to their need to recognize a wide range of epitopes. Quite strikingly, the γδ TCRs resemble antibodies in that the γ chain CDR3 loops are short with a narrow length distribution, while in the δ chain they are long with a broad length distribution. Therefore, in this respect, the γδ **TCR resembles antibody** more than the αβ TCR. The X-ray crystallographic structure of a TCR Vδ domain highlighted that the γδ TCR indeed incorporates key structural elements of both immunoglobulin and TCR V regions. Overall, the framework regions are more like antibody V_H than TCR $V\alpha$, whilst the conformations and relative positions of the CDRs share features with both $V\alpha$ and V_H domains. The binding site of the $V\delta$ in this particular crystal structure is a relatively flat surface similar to that seen in $\alpha\beta$ TCRs. However, the CDR3 loop of this $V\delta$ is 10 amino acid residues long and, whilst this is approximately the median length of $V\delta$ CDR3s, the broad length distribution already alluded to means that many $\gamma\delta$ receptors will bear longer or shorter $V\delta$ CDR3s. These will have topographically more adventurous binding sites, thereby facilitating the ability of $\gamma\delta$ T-cells to interact with intact rather than processed antigen.

More secrets are being teased out of the $\gamma\delta$ T-cell sect. In the mouse, $\gamma\delta$ T-cells have been isolated which directly recognize the MHC class I molecule I-E^k and the nonclassical MHC molecules T10 and T22 in a peptide-independent fashion. T10 and T22 are expressed by $\alpha\beta$ T-cells following their activation, and it has been suggested that $\gamma\delta$ T-cells specific for these nonclassical MHC molecules may exert a regulatory function. Stressed or damaged cells appear to be powerful activators of $\gamma\delta$ cells, and there is evidence for molecules such as heat-shock proteins as stimulators of $\gamma\delta$ T-cells. Low molecular weight **phosphate-containing nonproteinaceous** antigens, such as isopentenyl pyrophosphate and ethyl phosphate, which occur in a range of microbial and mammalian cells, have been identified as potent stimulators.

A particular subset of $\gamma\delta$ cells, which possess a diverse range of TCRs utilizing different *D* and *J* gene segments but always using the same *V* gene segments, $V\gamma2$ and $V\delta2$, expand *in vivo* to comprise a large proportion (8–60%) of all peripheral blood T-cells during a diverse range of infections. These $V\gamma2V\delta2$ T-cells recognize a newly appreciated group of antigens, the alkylamines, which have chemical and biological properties distinct from lipid and phosphate antigens, further extending the variety of nonprotein antigens which can be recognized by T-cells. A number of alkylamine antigens are produced by human pathogens, including *Salmonella typhimurium*, *Listeria monocytogenes*, *Yersinia enterocolitica* and *Escherichia coli*. Individual $V\gamma2V\delta2$ T-cells can recognize both positively charged alkylamines and negatively charged molecules such as ethyl phosphate, but this should be fairly straightforward for the receptor given the small hapten-like size of these antigens.

The above characteristics provide the $\gamma\delta$ cells with a distinctive role complementary to that of the $\alpha\beta$ population and enable them to function in the recognition of microbial pathogens and of damaged or stressed host cells.

SUPERANTIGENS STIMULATE WHOLE FAMILIES OF LYMPHOCYTE RECEPTORS

Bacterial toxins represent one major group of T-cell superantigens

Whereas an individual peptide complexed to MHC will react with antigen-specific T-cells which represent a relatively small percentage of the T-cell pool because of the requirement for specific binding to particular CDR3 regions, a special class of molecule has been identified which stimulates the 5–20% of the total T-cell population expressing the same TCR $V\beta$ family structure. These molecules do this irrespective of the antigen specificity of the receptor. They have been described as **superantigens** by Kappler and Marrack.

The pyogenic toxin superantigen family can cause food poisoning, vomiting and diarrhea and includes *Staphylococcus aureus* enterotoxins (SEA, SEB and several others), staphylococcal toxic shock syndrome toxin-1 (TSST-1), streptococcal superantigen (SSA) and several streptococcal pyogenic exotoxins (SPEs). Although these molecules all have a similar structure, they stimulate T-cells bearing different $V\beta$ sequences. They are strongly mitogenic for these T-cells in the presence of MHC class II accessory cells. SEA must be one of the most potent T-cell mitogens known, causing marked proliferation in the concentration range 10^{-13} to 10^{-16} M. Like the other superantigens it can cause the release of copious amounts of cytokines, including IL-2 and lymphotoxin, and of mast cell leukotrienes, which probably form the basis for its ability to produce toxic shock syndrome. Other superantigens which do not belong to the pyogenic toxin superantigen family include staphylococcal exfoliative toxins (ETs), *Mycoplasma arthritidis* mitogen (MAM) and *Yersinia pseudotuberculosis* mitogen.

Superantigens are not processed by the antigen-presenting cell, but cross-link the class II and $V\beta$ independently of direct interaction between MHC and TCR molecules (figure 5.25).

Endogenous mouse mammary tumor viruses (MMTV) act as superantigens

Very many years ago, Festenstein made the curious observation that B-cells from certain mouse strains could produce powerful proliferative responses in roughly 20% of unprimed T-cells from another strain of identical MHC. The so-called Mls gene product responsible for inciting proliferation turns out to be encoded by the open reading frame (ORF) located in the 3′ long terminal repeat of **MMTV**. They are type B retroviruses transmitted as infectious agents in milk and are specific for B-cells. They associate with class II MHC in the B-cell membrane and act as superantigens through their affinity for certain TCR Vβ families in a similar fashion to the bacterial toxins. Other proposed viral superantigens capable of polyclonally activating T-cells include the nucleocapsid protein of rabies virus, and antigens associated with cytomegalovirus and with Epstein–Barr virus.

Microbes can also provide B-cell superantigens

Staphylococcal protein A reacts not only with the Fcγ region of IgG but also with 15–50% of polyclonal IgM,

IgA and IgG F(ab′)$_2$, all of which belong to the V$_H$3 family. This superantigen is mitogenic for B-cells through its recognition by a discontinuous binding sequence composed of amino acid residues from FR1, CDR2 and FR3 of the V$_H$ domain. The human immunodeficiency virus (HIV) glycoprotein gp120 also reacts with immunoglobulins which utilize V$_H$3 family members. The binding site appears to partially overlap with that for protein A and utilizes amino acid residues from FR1, CDR1, CDR2 and FR3.

THE RECOGNITION OF DIFFERENT FORMS OF ANTIGEN BY B- AND T-CELLS IS ADVANTAGEOUS TO THE HOST

It is our conviction that this section deals with a subject of the utmost importance, which is at the epicenter of immunology.

Antibodies combat microbes and their products in the extracellular body fluids where they exist essen-

Figure 5.25. Interaction of superantigen with MHC and TCR. In this composite model, the interaction with the superantigen staphylococcal enterotoxin B (SEB) involves SEB wedging itself between the TCR Vβ chain and the MHC, effectively preventing interaction between the TCR and the peptide in the groove, and between the TCR β chain and the MHC. Thus direct contact between the TCR and the MHC is limited to Vα amino acid residues. (Reproduced from Li H. *et al.* (1999) *Annual Review of Immunology* **17**, 435, with permission.) Other superantigens are likely to disrupt direct TCR interactions with peptide–MHC to varying extents.

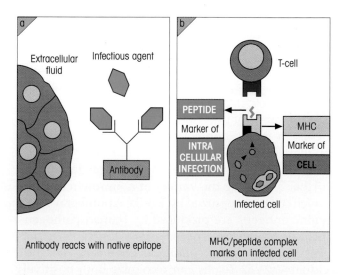

Figure 5.26. (a) Antibodies are formed against the native, not denatured, form of infectious agents which are attacked in the extracellular fluids. (b) Effector T-cells recognize infected cells by two surface markers: the MHC is a signal for the cell, and the foreign peptide is present in the MHC groove since it is derived from the proteins of an intracellular infectious agent. Further microbial cell surface signals can be provided by undegraded antigens and low molecular weight phosphate-containing antigens (seen by γδ T-cells), and lipids and glycolipids presented by CD1 molecules.

tially in their native form (figure 5.26a). Clearly it is to the host's advantage for the B-cell receptor to recognize epitopes on the **native molecules**.

αβ T-cells have quite a different job. In the case of cytotoxic T-cells, and the T-cells which secrete cytokines that activate infected macrophages, they have to seek out and bind to the infected cells and carry out their effector function face to face with the target. First, with respect to proteins produced by intracellular infectious agents, the MHC molecules tell the effector T-lymphocyte that it is encountering a cell. Second, the T-cell does not want to attack an uninfected cell on whose surface a native microbial molecule is sitting adventitiously nor would it wish to have its antigenic target on the appropriate cell surface blocked by an ex-

cess of circulating antibody. Thus it is of benefit for the infected cell to express the microbial antigen on its surface in a form distinct from that of the native molecule. As will now be more than abundantly clear, the evolutionary solution was to make the T-cell recognize a processed peptide derived from the intracellular antigen and to hold it as a complex with the surface MHC molecules. The single T-cell receptor then recognizes both the **MHC cell marker** and the **peptide infection marker** in one operation (figure 5.26b).

A comparable situation arises when CD1 molecules substitute for MHC in antigen presentation to T-cells, in this case associating with processed microbial lipids and glycolipids. The physiological role of the γδ cells has yet to be fully unraveled.

SUMMARY

The nature of antigen recognition by antibody
• An antigen is defined by its antibody. The contact area with an antibody is called an **epitope** and the corresponding area on an antibody, a **paratope**.
• Antisera recognize a series of dominant epitope clusters on the surface of an antigen; each cluster is called a determinant.
• Most epitopes on globular proteins are **discontinuous** rather than **linear**, involving amino acids far apart in the primary sequence.
• The protruding regions and probably the 'flexible' segments of globular proteins tend to be associated with higher epitope densities.

Antigens and antibodies interact by spatial complementarity, not by covalent binding
• The forces of interaction include electrostatic, hydrogen bonding, hydrophobic and van der Waals.
• The forces become large as the separation of antigen and antibody diminishes, especially when water molecules are excluded.
• Antigen–antibody bonds are readily **reversible**.
• Antigens and antibodies are mutually deformable.

Affinity
• The strength of binding to a single antibody combining site is measured by the **affinity**.

• The reaction of multivalent antigens with the heterogeneous mixture of antibodies in an antiserum is defined by **avidity (functional affinity)** and is usually much greater than affinity due to the 'bonus effect of multivalency'.
• The **specificity** of antibodies is not absolute and they may cross-react with other antigens to different extents, measured by their relative avidities.

T-cell recognition
• αβ T-cells see antigen in association with MHC molecules.
• They are restricted to the haplotype of the cell which first primed the T-cell.
• Protein antigens are processed by antigen-presenting cells to form small linear peptides which associate with the MHC molecules, binding to the central groove formed by the α-helices and the β-sheet floor.

Processing of antigen for presentation by class I MHC
• Endogenous cytosolic antigens such as viral proteins are cleaved by **immunoproteasomes** and the peptides so formed are **transported** to the ER by the TAP1/2 system.
• The peptide then dissociates from TAP1/2 and forms a stable heterotrimer with newly synthesized class I MHC heavy chain and β_2-microglobulin.
• This **peptide–MHC complex** is then transported to the surface for presentation to cytotoxic T-cells.

(continued p. 106)

Processing of antigen for presentation by class II MHC

- The αβ **class II molecule** is synthesized in the ER and complexes with membrane-bound **invariant chain (Ii)**.
- This facilitates transport of the vesicles containing class II across the Golgi and directs them to an acidified late endosome or lysosome containing exogenous protein taken into the cell by endocytosis or phagocytosis.
- Proteolytic degradation of Ii in the endosome leaves a peptide referred to as CLIP which protects the MHC groove.
- Processing by endosomal proteases degrades the antigen to peptides which replace the CLIP.
- The **class II–peptide** complex now appears on the cell surface for presentation to T-helper cells.

The nature of the peptide

- Class I peptides are held in extended conformation within the MHC groove.
- They are usually 8–9 residues in length and have two or three key **anchor**, relatively invariant residues which bind to allele-specific pockets in the MHC.
- Class II peptides are between 8 and 30 residues long, extend beyond the groove and usually have three or four anchor residues.
- The other amino acid residues in the peptide are greatly variable and are recognized by the T-cell receptor (TCR).

Complex between TCR, MHC and peptide

- The first and second hypervariable regions (CDR1 and CDR2) of each TCR chain mostly contact the MHC α-helices, while the CDR3s, having the greatest variability, interact with the antigenic peptide. Complexes of TCR_2 with $(MHC–peptide)_2$ are probably formed.

Some T-cells are independent of classical MHC molecules

- MHC class I-like molecules, such as H-2M, are rela-tively nonpolymorphic and can present antigens such as bacterial *N*-formyl methionine peptides.
- The CD1 family of non-MHC class I-like molecules can present antigens such as lipid and glycolipid mycobacterial antigens.
- γδ T-cells resemble antibodies in recognizing whole unprocessed molecules such as low molecular weight phosphate-containing nonproteinaceous molecules.

Superantigens

- These are potent mitogens which stimulate whole lymphocyte subpopulations sharing the same TCR Vβ or immunoglobulin V_H family independently of antigen specificity.
- *Staphylococcus aureus* enterotoxins are powerful human superantigens which cause food poisoning and toxic shock syndrome.
- T-cell superantigens are not processed but cross-link MHC class II and TCR Vβ independently of their direct interaction.
- Mouse mammary tumor viruses are B-cell retroviruses which are superantigens in the mouse.

Recognition of different forms of antigen by B- and T-cells is an advantage

- B-cells recognize epitopes on the native antigen; this is important because antibodies react with native antigen in the extracellular fluid.
- T-cells must contact infected cells and, to avoid confusion between the two systems, the infected cell signals itself to the T-cell by the combination of MHC and degraded antigen.

See the accompanying website (**www.roitt.com**) for multiple choice questions.

FURTHER READING

Alfonso C. *et al.* (1999) The role of H2-O and HLA-DO in major histocompatibility complex class II-restricted antigen processing and presentation. *Immunological Reviews* **172**, 255.

Benlagha K. & Bendelac A. (2000) CD1d-restricted mouse Vα14 and human Vα24 T cells: lymphocytes of innate immunity. *Seminars in Immunology* **12**, 537.

Bukowski J.F., Morita C.T. & Brenner M.B. (1999) Human γδ T cells recognize alkylamines derived from microbes, edible plants, and tea: implications for innate immunity. *Immunity* **11**, 57.

Eisen H.N. (2001) Specificity and degeneracy in antigen recognition: Yin and Yang in the immune system. *Annual Review of Immunology* **19**, 1.

van den Eynde B.J. & Morel S. (2001) Differential processing of class I-restricted epitopes by the standard proteasome and the immunoproteasome. *Current Opinion in Immunology* **13**, 147.

Früh K. & Yang Y. (1999) Antigen presentation by MHC class I and its regulation by interferon γ. *Current Opinion in Immunology* **11**, 76.

Garcia K.C., Teyton L. & Wilson I. (1999) Structural basis of T cell recognition. *Annual Review of Immunology* **17**, 369.

Getzoff E.D., Tainer J.A., Lerner R.A. & Geysen H.M. (1988) The chemistry and mechanism of antibody binding to protein antigens. *Advances in Immunology* **43**, 1.

Grommé M. *et al.* (1999) Recycling MHC class I molecules and endosomal peptide loading. *Proceedings of the National Academy of Sciences of the United States of America* **96**, 10326.

Hennecke J. & Wiley D.C. (2001) T cell receptor–MHC interactions up close. *Cell* **104**, 1.

Karray S., Juompan L., Maroun R.C., Isenberg D., Silverman G.J. & Zouali M. (1998) Structural basis of the gp120 superantigen-binding site on human immunoglobulins. *Journal of Immunology* **161**, 6681.

Karush F. (1976) Multivalent binding and functional affinity. In Inman F.P. (ed.) *Contemporary Topics in Molecular Immunology*, Vol. 5, p. 217. Plenum Press, New York. (Bonus effect of multivalency.)

Li H., Lebedeva M.I., Liera A.S., Fields B.A., Brenner M.B. & Mariuzza, R.A. (1998) Structure of the Vδ domain of a human γδ T-cell antigen receptor. *Nature* **391**, 502.

Li H., Llera A., Malchiodi E.L. & Mariuzza R.A. (1999) The structural basis of T cell activation by superantigens. *Annual Review of Immunology* **17**, 435.

MacCallum R.M., Martin A.C.R. & Thornton J.M. (1996) Antibody–antigen interactions: contact analysis and binding site topography. *Journal of Molecular Biology* **262**, 732.

Manoury B., Hewitt E.W., Morrice N., Dando P.M., Barrett A.J. & Watts C. (1998) An asparaginyl endopeptidase processes a microbial antigen for class II MHC presentation. *Nature* **396**, 695.

Nisonoff A. & Pressman D. (1957) Closeness of fit and forces involved in the reactions of antibody homologous to the *p-(p'-N-*azophenylazo)-benzoate ion group. *Journal of the American Chemistry Society* **79**, 1616.

Rammensee H.-G. & Lanzavecchia A. (eds) (1999) Quantitative aspects of T-cell recognition. *Seminars in Immunology* **11** (6).

Reinherz E.L. *et al.* (1999) The crystal structure of a T cell receptor in complex with peptide and MHC class II. *Science* **286**, 1913.

Rock K.L. & Goldberg A.L. (1999) Degradation of cell proteins and the generation of MHC class I-presented peptides. *Annual Review of Immunology* **17**, 739.

Sato A.K. *et al.* (2000) Determinants of the peptide-induced conformational change in the human class II major histocompatibility complex protein HLA-DR1. *Journal of Biological Chemistry* **275**, 2165.

Sigal L.J., Crotty S., Andino R. & Rock K.L. (1999) Cytotoxic T-cell immunity to virus-infected non-haematopoietic cells requires presentation of exogenous antigen. *Nature* **398**, 77.

Immunochemical techniques

INTRODUCTION

Since antigens and antibodies are defined by their mutual interactions, they can each be used to quantify each other. Before we get down to details, it is worth posing the question 'What does serum "antibody content" mean?'

If we have a solution of a monoclonal antibody, we can define its affinity and specificity with considerable confidence and, if pure and in its native conformation, we will know that the concentration of antibody is the same as that of the measurable immunoglobulin in ng/ml or whatever. When it comes to measuring the antibody content of an antiserum, the problem is of a different order because the immunoglobulin fraction is composed of an enormous array of molecules of varying abundance and affinity (figure 6.1a).

An **average** K_a for the whole IgG can be obtained by analysing the overall interaction with antigen as a mass action equation. But how can the **antibody content** of the IgG be defined in a meaningful way? The answer is of course that one would usually wish to describe antibody in practical functional terms: does a serum protect against a given infectious dose of virus, does it promote effective phagocytosis of bacteria, does it permit complement-mediated bacteriolysis, does it neutralize toxins, and so on? For such purposes, very low affinity molecules would be useless because they form such inadequate amounts of complex with the antigen.

At the practical level in a diagnostic laboratory, the functional tests are labor intensive and therefore expensive, and a compromise is usually sought by using immunochemical assays which measure a composite of medium to high affinity antibodies and their abundance. The majority of such tests usually measure the total amount of antibody binding to a given amount of antigen; this could be a modest amount of high affinity antibody or much more antibody of lower affinity, or all combinations in between. Sera are compared for high or low 'antibody content' either by seeing how much antibody binds to antigen at a fixed serum dilution, or testing a series of serum dilutions to see at which level a standard amount of antibody just sufficient to give a positive result is bound. This is the so-called **antibody titer**. To take an example, a serum might be diluted, say, 10 000 times and still just give a positive agglutination test (cf. figure 6.9). This titer of 1:10 000 enables comparison to be made with another much 'weaker' serum which has a titer of only, say, 1:100. Note that the titer of a given serum will vary with the sensitivity of the test, since much smaller amounts of antibody are needed to bind to antigen for a highly sensitive test, such as agglutination, than for a test of low sensitivity, such as precipitation, which requires high concentrations of antibody–antigen product (figure 6.1b).

To summarize: the '**effective antibody contents**' of different sera can be compared by seeing **how**

(continued)

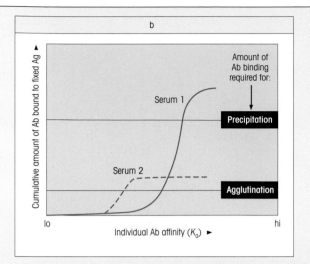

Figure 6.1. Distribution of affinity and abundance of IgG molecules in an individual serum. (a) Distribution of affinities of IgG molecules for a given antigen in the serum of a hypothetical individual. There is a great deal of low affinity antibody which would be incapable of binding to antigen effectively, and much lower amounts of high affinity antibody whose skewed distribution is assumed to arise from exposure to infection. (b) Relationship of affinity distribution to positivity in tests for antigen binding. Rearranging the mass action equation, for all molecules of the same affinity K_x and concentration of unbound antibody $[Ab_x]$:

the amount of complex formed $[AgAb] \propto K_x[Ab_x]$ for
    fixed $[Ag]$.

Starting with the lowest affinity molecules in the serum, we have charted the cumulative total of antibody bound for each antibody species up to and including the one being plotted. As might be expected, the very low affinity antibodies make no contribution to the tests. Serum 2 has more low affinity antibody and virtually no high affinity, but it can produce just enough complex to react in the sensitive agglutination test although, unlike serum 1, it forms insufficient to give a positive precipitin. Because of its relatively high 'content' of antibody, serum 1 can be diluted to a much greater extent than serum 2 and yet still give positive agglutination, i.e. it has a higher titer. The precipitin test is less sensitive, requiring more complex formation, and serum 1 cannot be diluted much before this test becomes negative, i.e. the precipitin titer will be far lower than the agglutination titer for the same serum.

much antibody binds to the fixed amount of test antigen, or the titer can be determined, i.e. how far the serum can be diluted before the test becomes negative. This is a compromise between abundance and affinity and for practical purposes is used as an approximate indicator of biological effectiveness.

ESTIMATION OF ANTIBODY

Antigen–antibody interactions in solution

The classical precipitin reaction

When an antigen solution is added progressively to a potent antiserum, antigen–antibody precipitates are formed (figure 6.2a and b). The cross-linking of antigen and antibody gives rise to three-dimensional lattice structures, as suggested by John Marrack, which coalesce, largely through Fc–Fc interaction, to form large precipitating aggregates. As more and more antigen is added, an optimum is reached (figure 6.2b) after which consistently less precipitate is formed. At this stage the supernatant can be shown to contain soluble complexes of antigen (Ag) and antibody (Ab), many of composition Ag_4Ab_3, Ag_3Ab_2 and Ag_2Ab (figure 6.2c). In extreme antigen excess (figure 6.2c), ultracentrifugal analysis reveals the complexes to be mainly of the form Ag_2Ab, a result directly attributable to the two combining sites (divalence) of the IgG antibody molecule (cf. electron microscope study, figure 3.1, and Scatchard analysis, figure 5.10a).

Serums frequently contain up to 10% of nonprecipitating antibodies which are effectively monovalent because of the asymmetric presence of oligosaccharide on one antigen-binding arm of the antibody molecule which stereochemically blocks the combining site. Also, frank precipitates are only observed when antigen, and particularly antibody, are present in fairly hefty concentrations. Thus, when complexes are formed which do not precipitate spontaneously, more devious methods must be applied to detect and estimate the antibody level.

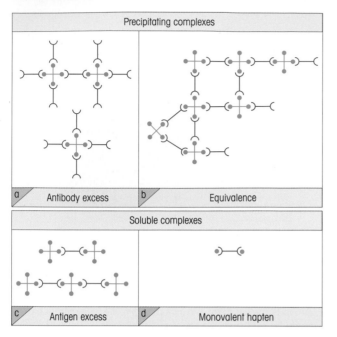

Figure 6.2. Diagrammatic representation of complexes formed between a hypothetical tetravalent antigen ( ) and bivalent antibody ( ) mixed in different proportions. In practice, the antigen valencies are unlikely to lie in the same plane or to be formed by identical determinants as suggested in the figure. (a) In extreme antibody excess, the antigen valencies are saturated and the molar ratio Ab : Ag approximates to the valency of the antigen. (b) At equivalence, most of the antigen and antibody combines to form large lattices which aggregate to produce typical immune precipitates. (c) In extreme antigen excess, where the two valencies of each antibody molecule become rapidly saturated, the complex Ag$_2$Ab tends to predominate. (d) A monovalent hapten binds but is unable to cross-link antibody molecules.

Nonprecipitating antibodies can be detected by nephelometry

The small aggregates formed when dilute solutions of antigen and antibody are mixed create a cloudiness or turbidity which can be measured by forward angle scattering of an incident light source (nephelometry). Greater sensitivity can be obtained by using monochromatic light from a laser and by adding polyethyl-ene glycol to the solution so that aggregate size is increased. In practice, nephelometry is applied more to the detection of antigen than antibody and this will be dealt with in a later section.

Complexes formed by nonprecipitating antibodies can be precipitated

The relative antigen-binding capacity of an antiserum which forms soluble complexes can be estimated using radiolabeled antigen. The complex can be brought out of solution either by changing its solubility or by adding an anti-immunoglobulin reagent as in figure 6.3.

Enhancement of precipitation by countercurrent immunoelectrophoresis

This technique may be applied to antigens which migrate towards the positive pole on electrophoresis in agar (if necessary antigens can be substituted with negatively charged groups to achieve this end). Antigen and antiserum are placed in wells punched in the agar gel and a current applied (figure 6.4). The antigen migrates steadily into the antibody zone where it successively binds more and more antibody molecules, in essence artificially increasing the effective antibody concentration and thus forming a precipitin line.

Measurement of antibody affinity

As discussed in earlier chapters (cf. p. 85), the binding strength of antibody for antigen is measured in terms of the association constant (K_a) or its reciprocal, the dissociation constant (K_d), governing the reversible interaction between them and defined by the mass action equation at equilibrium:

$$K_a = \frac{[\text{AgAb complex}]}{[\text{free Ag}][\text{free Ab}]}$$

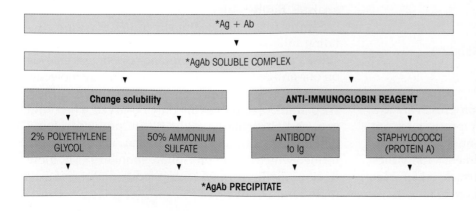

Figure 6.3. Binding capacity of an antiserum for labeled antigen (*Ag) by precipitation of soluble complexes either: (i) by changing the solubility so that the complexes are precipitated while the uncombined Ag and Ab remain in solution, or (ii) by adding a precipitating anti-immunoglobulin antibody or staphylococcal organisms which bind immunoglobulin Fc to the protein A on their surface; the complex can then be spun down. The level of label (e.g. radioactivity) in the precipitate will be a measure of antigen-binding capacity.

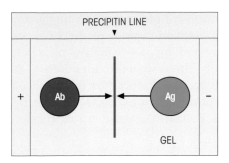

Figure 6.4. Countercurrent immunoelectrophoresis. Antibody moves towards the negative pole in the gel on electrophoresis due to endosmosis; an antigen which is negatively charged at the pH employed will move towards the positive pole and precipitate on contact with antibody.

With small haptens, the equilibrium dialysis method can be employed to measure K_a (see p. 87), but usually one is dealing with larger antigens and other techniques must be used. One approach is to add increasing amounts of radiolabeled antigen to a fixed amount of antibody, and then separate the free from bound antibody by precipitating the soluble complex as described above (e.g. by an anti-immunoglobulin). The reciprocal of the bound, i.e. complexed, antibody concentration can be plotted against the reciprocal of the free antigen concentration, so allowing the affinity constant to be calculated (figure 6.5a). For an antiserum this will give an affinity constant representing

Figure 6.5. Determination of affinity with large antigens. The equilibria between Ab and Ag at different concentrations are determined as follows:
(a) For a polyclonal antiserum one can use the Steward–Petty modification of the Langmuir equation:

$1/b = 1/(Ab_t.c.K_a) + 1/Ab_t$

where Ab_t = total Ab combining sites, b = bound Ab concentration, c = free Ag concentration and K_a = average affinity constant. At infinite Ag concentration, all Ab sites are bound and $1/b = 1/Ab_t$. When half the Ab sites are bound, $1/c = K_a$ (cf. p. 86).
(b) The method of Friguet et al. for monoclonal antibodies. First, a calibration curve for free antibody is established by estimating the proportion binding to solid-phase antigen, bound antibody being measured by enzyme-labeled anti-Ig (ELISA: see text). Using the calibration curve, the amount of free Ab in equilibrium with Ag in solution is determined by seeing how much of the Ab binds to solid-phase Ag (the amount of solid-phase antigen is insufficient to affect the solution equilibrium materially). Combination of the Klotz and Scatchard equations gives:

$A_o/A_o - A = 1 + K_d/a_o$

where A_o = ELISA optical density (OD) for Ab in the absence of Ag, A = OD in the presence of Ag concentration a_o where a_o is approximately $10\times$ concentration of Ab. The slope of the plot gives K_d. (Labeled molecules are marked with an asterisk.)

an average of the heterogeneous antibody components and a measure of the effective number of antigen-binding sites operative at the highest levels of antigen used.

Various types of ELISA (see below) have been developed which provide a measure of antibody affinity. In one system the antibody is allowed to first bind to its antigen, and then a chaotropic agent such as thiocyanate is added in increasing concentration in order to disrupt the antibody binding; the higher the affinity of the antibody, the more agent that is required to reduce the binding. Another type of ELISA for measuring affinity is the indirect competitive system devised by Friguet and associates (figure 6.5b). A constant amount of antibody is incubated with a series of antigen concentrations and the free antibody at equilibrium is assessed by secondary binding to solid-phase antigen. In this way, values for K_a are not affected by any distortion of antigen by labeling. This again stresses the superiority of determining affinity by studying the **primary reaction** with antigen in the **soluble state** rather than conformationally altered through binding to a solid phase.

Increasingly, affinity measurements are obtained using **surface plasmon resonance**. A sensor chip consisting of a monoclonal antibody coupled to dextran overlying a gold film on a glass prism will totally internally reflect light at a given angle (figure 6.6a). Antigen present in a pulse of fluid will bind to the sensor chip and, by increasing its size, alter the angle of reflection. The system provides data on the kinetics of association and dissociation (and hence K) (figure 6.6b) and permits comparisons between monoclonal antibodies and also assessment of subtle effects of mutations.

Agglutination of antigen-coated particles

Whereas the cross-linking of multivalent protein antigens by antibody leads to precipitation, cross-linking of cells or large particles by antibody directed against surface antigens leads to agglutination. Since most cells are electrically charged, a reasonable number of antibody links between two cells are required before the mutual repulsion is overcome. Thus agglutination of cells bearing only a small number of determinants may be difficult to achieve unless special methods such as further treatment with an antiglobulin reagent are used. Similarly, the higher avidity of multivalent IgM antibody relative to IgG (cf. p. 89) makes the former more effective as an agglutinating agent, molecule for molecule (figure 6.7).

Agglutination reactions are used to identify bacteria and to type red cells; they have been observed with

Figure 6.6. Surface plasmon resonance. (a) The principle: as antigen binds to the antibody-coated sensor chip it alters the angle of reflection. (b) This signals the rates of association during the antigen pulse and dissociation. In this example, the same antigen was injected over three immobilized monoclonal antibodies. The arrows point to the beginning and end of the antigen injection, which is followed by buffer flow. Note the differences between the antibodies in the association and dissociation rates. (Data kindly provided by Dr R. Karlsson, Biacore AB, and reproduced from Panayotou G. (1998) Surface plasmon resonance. In Delves P.J. & Roitt I.M. (eds) *Encyclopedia of Immunology*, 2nd edn. Academic Press, with permission.) The system can be used with antigen immobilized on the sensor chip and antibody in the fluid phase, or can be applied to any other single ligand-binding assay.

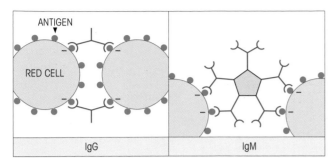

Figure 6.7. Mechanism of agglutination of antigen-coated particles by antibody cross-linking to form large macroscopic aggregates. If red cells are used, several cross-links are needed to overcome the electrical charge at the cell surface. IgM is superior to IgG as an agglutinator because of its multivalent binding and because the charged cells are further apart.

(a)   (b)

Figure 6.8. Macroscopic agglutination of latex coated with human IgG by serum from a patient with rheumatoid arthritis. This contains rheumatoid factor, an autoantibody directed against determinants on IgG. (a) Normal serum. (b) Patient's serum.

Figure 6.9. Red cell hemagglutination test for thyroglobulin autoantibodies. Thyroglobulin-coated cells were added to dilutions of patients' serums. Uncoated cells were added to a 1:10 dilution of serum as a control. In a positive reaction, the cells settle as a carpet over the bottom of the cup. Because of the 'V'-shaped cross-section of these cups, in negative reactions the cells fall into the base of the 'V', forming a small, easily recognizable button. The reciprocal of the highest serum dilution giving an unequivocally positive reaction is termed the titer. The titers reading from left to right are: 640, 20, >5120, neg, 40, 320, neg, >5120. The control for serum no. 46 was slightly positive and this serum should be tested again after absorption with uncoated cells.

leukocytes and platelets, and even with spermatozoa in certain cases of male infertility due to sperm agglutinins. Because of its sensitivity and convenience, the test has been extended to the identification of antibodies to soluble antigens which have been artificially coated on to erythrocytes, latex or gelatin particles. Agglutination of IgG-coated latex is used to detect rheumatoid factors (figure 6.8). Similar tests using antigen-coated particles can be carried out in U-bottom microtiter plates where the settling pattern on the bottom of the well may be observed (figure 6.9); this provides a more sensitive indicator than macroscopic clumping. Quantification of more subtle degrees of agglutination can be achieved by nephelometry or Coulter counting.

Immunoassay for antibody using solid-phase antigen

The principle

The antibody content of a serum can be assessed by the ability to bind to antigen which has been immobilized by physical adsorption to a plastic tube or microtiter plate with multiple wells; the bound immunoglobulin may then be estimated by addition of a labeled anti-Ig raised in another species (figure 6.10). Consider, for example, the determination of DNA autoantibodies in SLE (cf. p. 401). When a patient's serum is added to a microwell coated with antigen (in this case DNA), the autoantibodies will bind to the antigen and the remaining serum proteins can be readily washed away. Bound antibody can now be estimated by addition of ^{125}I-labeled purified rabbit anti-human IgG; after rinsing out excess unbound reagent, the radioactivity of the tube will clearly be a measure of the autoantibody content of the patient's serum. The distribution of antibody in different classes can be determined by using specific antisera. Take the radio-allergosorbent test (RAST) for IgE antibodies in allergic patients. The allergen (e.g. pollen extract) is covalently coupled to an immunoabsorbent, in this case a

Add Ag | Add patient's serum | Add labeled anti-Ig

wash   wash   wash   ▶   MEASURE LABEL

Plastic tube

Figure 6.10. Solid-phase immunoassay for antibody. To reduce nonspecific binding of IgG to the solid phase after adsorption of the first reagent, it is usual to add an irrelevant protein, such as dried skimmed milk powder or bovine serum albumin, to block any free sites on the plastic. Note that the conformation of a protein often alters on binding to plastic, e.g. a monoclonal antibody which distinguishes between the apo and holo forms of cytochrome c in solution combines equally well with both proteins on the solid phase. Covalent coupling to carboxy-derivatized plastic or capture of the antigen substrate by solid-phase antibody can sometimes lessen this effect.

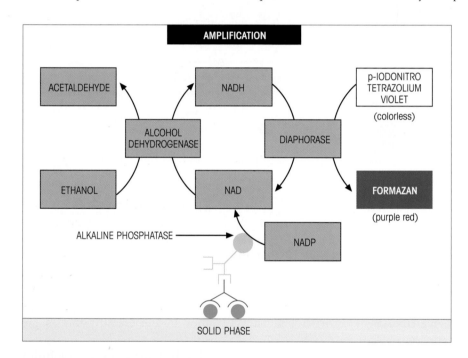

AMPLIFICATION

ACETALDEHYDE ← ALCOHOL DEHYDROGENASE → NADH

ETHANOL → ALCOHOL DEHYDROGENASE → NAD

NADH → DIAPHORASE → NAD

p-IODONITRO TETRAZOLIUM VIOLET (colorless) → DIAPHORASE → FORMAZAN (purple red)

ALKALINE PHOSPHATASE → NADP → NAD

SOLID PHASE

Figure 6.11. Coenzyme-geared amplification of the phosphatase reaction to reveal solid-phase anti-immunoglobulin label.

paper disk, which is then treated with patient's serum. The amount of specific IgE bound to the paper can now be estimated by the addition of labeled anti-IgE.

A wide variety of labels are available

Whilst providing extremely good sensitivity, radiolabels have a number of disadvantages, including loss of sensitivity during storage due to radioactive decay, the deterioration of the labeled reagent through radiation damage, and the precautions needed to minimize human exposure to radioactivity. Therefore, other types of label are often employed in immunoassays.

ELISA (enzyme-linked immunosorbent assay). Enzymes which give a colored soluble reaction product are cur-

rently the most commonly used labels, with horseradish peroxidase (HRP) and calf intestine alkaline phosphatase (AP) being by far the most popular. *Aspergillus niger* glucose oxidase, soy bean urease and *Escherichia coli* β-galactosidase provide further alternatives. One clever ploy for amplifying the phosphatase reaction is to use nicotinamide adenine dinucleotide phosphate (NADP) as a substrate to generate NAD which now acts as a coenzyme for a second enzyme system (figure 6.11).

Other labels. Enzyme-labeled streptococcal protein G or staphylococcal protein A will bind to IgG. Conjugation with the vitamin biotin is frequently used since this can readily be detected by its reaction with enzyme-linked avidin or streptavidin (the latter gives

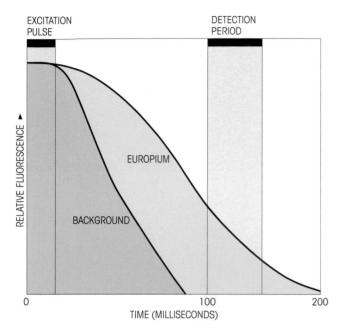

Figure 6.12. The principle of time-resolved fluorescence assay. The problem with conventional methods of detection of low fluorescent signals is interference from reflection of incident light and background instrument fluorescence. By using just a short excitation pulse and measuring the signal after background has fallen to zero but before the europium with its long fluorescence half-life has decayed completely, good discrimination between a weak signal and background becomes possible.

lower background binding), both of which bind with ferocious specificity and affinity ($K = 10^{15}\,\text{M}^{-1}$).

Chemiluminescent systems based on the HRP-catalysed enhanced luminol reaction, where light from the oxidized luminol substrate is intensified and the signal duration increased by the use of an enhancing reagent, provide increased sensitivity and dynamic range. Special mention should be made of time-resolved fluorescence assays based upon chelates of rare earths such as europium 3^+ (figure 6.12), although these have a more important role in antigen assays.

DETECTION OF IMMUNE COMPLEX FORMATION

Many techniques for detecting circulating complexes have been described and because of variations in the size, complement-fixing ability and Ig class of different complexes, it is useful to apply more than one method. Two fairly robust methods for general use are:

1 precipitation of complexed IgG from serum at concentrations of polyethylene glycol which do not bring down significant amounts of IgG monomer, followed by estimation of IgG in the precipitate by single radial immunodiffusion (SRID) or laser nephelometry, and

2 binding of C3b-containing complexes to beads coated with bovine conglutinin (cf. p. 17) and estimation of the bound Ig with enzyme-labeled anti-Ig.

Other techniques include: (i) estimation of the binding of ^{125}I-C1q to complexes by coprecipitation with polyethylene glycol, (ii) inhibition by complexes of rheumatoid factor-induced aggregation of IgG-coated particles, and (iii) detection with radiolabeled anti-Ig of serum complexes capable of binding to the C3b (and to a lesser extent the Fc) receptors on the Raji cell line. Sera from patients with immune complex disease often form a cryoprecipitate when allowed to stand at 4°C. Measurement of serum C3 and its conversion product C3c is sometimes useful.

Tissue-bound complexes are usually visualized by the immunofluorescent staining of biopsies with conjugated anti-immunoglobulins and anti-C3 (cf. figure 16.17).

IDENTIFICATION AND MEASUREMENT OF ANTIGEN

Precipitation reaction can be carried out in gels

Characterization of antigens by electrophoresis and immunofixation

This technique is most often applied to the detection of an abnormal protein in serum or urine, usually a monoclonal paraprotein secreted by a B-cell tumor. The paraprotein localizes as a dense compact 'M' band of defined electrophoretic mobility and its antigenic identity is then revealed by immunofixation with specific precipitating antiserums applied in paper strips overlying parallel lanes in the electrophoresis gel (figure 6.13).

Quantification by single radial immunodiffusion (SRID)

When antigen diffuses from a well into agar containing suitably diluted antiserum, initially it is present in a relatively high concentration and forms soluble complexes; as the antigen diffuses further the concentration continuously falls until the point is reached at which the reactants are nearer optimal proportions and a ring of precipitate is formed. The higher the concentration of antigen, the greater the diameter of this ring (figure 6.14). By incorporating, say, three standards of known antigen concentration in the plate, a calibration curve can be obtained and used to determine the amount of antigen in the unknown samples tested (figure 6.15). The method was used routinely in

Figure 6.13. Electrophoresis and immunofixation of a paraprotein in serum. The sample is separated into its component bands by electrophoresis in agarose gel and these are visualized by direct staining after drying down the gel. The test sample is also run on a parallel gel which is then overlaid with strips of paper soaked in a specific antiserum. The antibodies diffuse into the gel and 'fix' the antigen by precipitation; after washing to remove the nonprecipitated soluble proteins, the gel is dried and stained to reveal the location of the paraprotein–antibody complex. N, normal serum; P, patient's serum showing compact paraprotein band; G, M, κ and λ represent immunofixations with antiserum specific for each immunoglobulin chain. In the example chosen, the paraprotein is an IgGλ. (Material kindly supplied by Mr T. Heys.)

Figure 6.14. Single radial immunodiffusion: relation of antigen concentration to size of precipitation ring formed. Antigen at the higher concentration $[Ag_1]$ diffuses further from the well before it falls to the level giving precipitation with antibody near optimal proportions.

Figure 6.15. Measurement of IgG concentration in serum by single radial immunodiffusion. The diameter of the standards (●) enables a calibration curve to be drawn and the concentration of IgG in the serum under test can be read off:

T_1—serum from patient with IgG myeloma; 15 mg/ml;
T_2—serum from patient with hypogammaglobulinemia; 2.6 mg/ml;
T_3—normal serum; 9.6 mg/ml.
(Courtesy of Professor F.C. Hay.)

clinical immunology, particularly for immunoglobulin determinations, and also for substances such as the third component of complement, transferrin, C-reactive protein (CRP) and the embryonic protein, α-fetoprotein, which is associated with certain liver tumors. More affluent laboratories now tend to use nephelometry (see below).

The nephelometric assay for antigen

If antigen is added to a solution of excess antibody, the amount of complex which can be assessed by forward light scatter in a nephelometer (cf. p. 110) is linearly related to the concentration of antigen. With the ready availability of a wide range of monoclonal antibodies which facilitate the standardization of the method, nephelometry is replacing SRID for the estimation of immunoglobulins, C3, C4, haptoglobin, ceruloplasmin and CRP in those favored laboratories which can sport the appropriate equipment. Very small samples down in the range 1–10 µl can be analysed. Turbidity of the sample can be a problem; blanks lacking antibody can be deducted but a more satisfactory solution is to

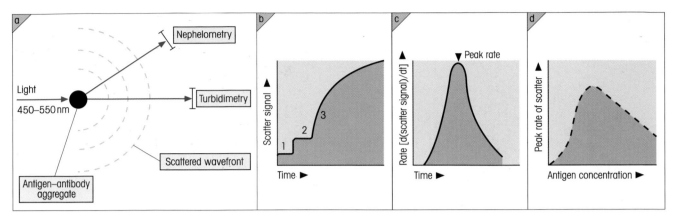

Figure 6.16. Rate nephelometry. (a) On addition of antiserum, small antigen–antibody aggregates form (cf. figure 6.2) which scatter incident light filtered to give a wavelength band of 450–550 nm. For nephelometry, the light scattered at a forward angle of 70° or so is measured. (b) After addition of the sample (1) and then the antibody (2), the rate at which the aggregates form (3) is determined from the scatter signal. (c) The software in the instrument then computes the maximum rate of light scatter which is related to the antigen concentration as shown in (d). (Copied from the operating manual for the 'Array' rate reaction automated immunonephelometer with permission from Beckman Coulter Ltd.)

follow the **rate of formation** of complexes which is proportional to antigen concentration since this obviates the need for a separate blank (figure 6.16). Because soluble complexes begin to be formed in antigen excess, it is important to ensure that the value for antigen was obtained in antibody excess by running a further control in which additional antigen is included.

Sodium dodecyl sulfate–polyacrylamide gel electrophoresis (SDS–PAGE) for analysis of immunoprecipitates and immunoblotting

When proteins are denatured by SDS, the larger they are the more SDS they bind and the more negatively charged they become. Thus proteins of different size can be separated by electrophoresis in a gel such as polyacrylamide on the basis of their overall charge.

If one or more antigens are radiolabeled and the complex with added antibody is precipitated with an anti-Ig reagent such as staphylococci bearing protein A, SDS–PAGE of the complex followed by autoradiography should define the **number** and **molecular weights of the antigens** concerned (figure 6.17).

A **Western blot (immunoblot)** of antigens separated from a complex mixture by SDS–PAGE (or by isoelectric focusing) can be carried out. This employs transverse electrophoresis on to polyvinylidene difluoride (PVDF) or nitrocellulose membranes, where the proteins bind nonspecifically and are subsequently identified by staining with appropriately labeled antibodies. Obviously, such a procedure will not work with antigens which are irreversibly denatured by this detergent, and it is best to use polyclonal antisera for blotting to increase the chance of including antibodies to whichever epitopes do survive the denaturation

Figure 6.17. Immunoprecipitation of membrane antigen. Analysis of membrane-bound class I MHC antigens (cf. p. 70). The membranes from human cells pulsed with ^{35}S-methionine were solubilized in a detergent, mixed with a monoclonal antibody to HLA-A and B molecules and immunoprecipitated with staphylococci. An autoradiograph (A) of the precipitate run in SDS–PAGE shows the HLA-A and B chains as a 43 000 molecular weight doublet (the position of a 45 000 marker is arrowed). If membrane vesicles are first digested with proteinase K before solubilization, a labeled band of molecular weight 39 000 can be detected (B) consistent with a transmembrane orientation of the HLA chain: the 4000 Da hydrophilic C-terminal fragment extends into the cytoplasm and the major portion, recognized by the monoclonal antibody and by tissue typing reagents, is present on the cell surface (cf. figure 4.11). (From data and autoradiographs kindly supplied by Dr M.J. Owen.)

procedure; a surprising number do (figure 6.18). Conversely, the spectrotype of an antiserum can be revealed by isoelectric focusing, blotting and then staining with labeled antigen.

94
67
43
30
20
14

94
67
43
30
20

a   b   ←——————— Patients' serums ——————→ ←— Con —→

Figure 6.18. Western blot analysis of human polymorph primary granules with sera from patients with systemic vasculitis. Human polymorph postnuclear supernatant was run on SDS–PAGE. (a) Gel stained for protein with Coomassie Blue. Numbers refer to molecular weight markers (kDa). (b) Blots from gel stained with serums from five patients and one control and visualized with alkaline phosphatase-conjugated goat anti-human IgG. Three different patterns of autoantibody reaction are evident. (Kindly supplied by Drs J. Cambridge & B. Leaker.) The antibodies used for immunoblotting are usually labeled with enzymes or biotin (followed by enzyme-labeled avidin).

The immunoassay of antigens

The ability to establish the concentration of an analyte (i.e. a substance to be measured) through fractional occupancy of its specific binding reagent is a feature of any ligand-binding system (Milestone 6.1), but because antibodies can be raised to virtually any structure, its application is most versatile in immunoassay.

Large analytes, such as protein hormones, are usually estimated by a noncompetitive two-site assay in which the original ligand binder and the labeled detection reagent are both antibodies (figure M6.1.1). By using monoclonal antibodies directed to two different epitopes on the same analyte, the system has greater power to discriminate between two related analytes; if the fractional cross-reactivity of the first antibody for a related analyte is 0.1 and of the second also 0.1, the final readout for cross-reactivity will be as low as 0.1×0.1, i.e. 1%. Using chemiluminescent and time-resolved fluorescent probes, highly sensitive assays are available for an astonishing range of analytes.

For small molecules like drugs or steroid hormones, where two-site binding is impractical, competitive assays (figure M6.1.1) are appropriate.

Immunoassay on multiple microspots

Paradoxically, minute spots of solid-phase antibody are not completely saturated by analyte in the range of concentrations normally worked with in most immunoassays. Rather, analysis has shown that the fractional occupancies expected permit immunoassay technology, or any other ligand-specific binding system, to be practical options (Ekins), particularly with the advent of modern highly sensitive probes. Furthermore, when the amount of antibody on the microspot is very small, the fractional occupancy is independent of antibody level and also of analyte volume (**the ambient analyte principle**). Sensitivities compare very favorably with the best immunoassays and, with such miniaturization, arrays of microspots which capture antibodies of different specificities can be placed on a single chip, opening the door to multiple analyte screening in a single test, with each analyte being identified by its grid coordinates in the array.

Epitope mapping

T-cell epitopes

Where the primary sequence of the whole protein is known, the identification of T-cell epitopes is comparatively straightforward. Since these epitopes are linear in nature, multipin solid-phase synthesis can be employed to generate a series of overlapping peptides, 8–9-mers for cytotoxic T-cells and usually 10–14-mers for T-helpers (figure 6.19), and their ability to react

Milestone 6.1 — Ligand-binding Assays

The appreciation that a ligand could be measured by the fractional occupancy (*F*) of its specific binding agent heralded a new order of sensitive wide-ranging assays. Ligand-binding assays were first introduced for the measurement of thyroid hormone by thyroxine-binding protein (Ekins) and for the estimation of hormones by antibody (Berson & Yalow). These findings spawned the technology of radioimmunoassay, so called because the antigen had to be trace-labeled in some way and the most convenient candidates for this were radioisotopes.

The relationship between fractional occupancy and analyte concentration [An] is given by the equation:

$$F = 1 - (1/1 + K[An])$$

where *K* is the association constant of the ligand-binding reaction. *F* can be measured by noncompetitive or competitive assays (figure M6.1.1) and related to a calibration curve constructed with standard amounts of analyte.

For competitive assays, the maximum theoretical sensitivity is given by the term ε/K where ε is the experimental error (coefficient of variation). Suppose the error is 1% and *K* is $10^{11}\,\text{M}^{-1}$, the maximum sensitivity will be $0.01 \times 10^{-11}\,\text{M} = 10^{-13}\,\text{M}$ or 6×10^7 molecules/ml. For noncompetitive assays, labels of very high specific activity could give sensitivities down to 10^2–10^3 molecules/ml under ideal conditions. In practice, however, since the sensitivity represents the lowest analyte concentration which can be measured against a background containing zero analyte, the error of the measurement of background poses an ultimate constraint on sensitivity.

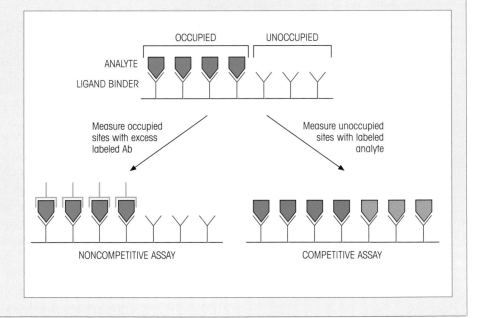

Figure M6.1.1. The principle of ligand-binding assays. The ligand-binding agent may be in the soluble phase or bound to a solid support as shown here, the advantage of the latter being the ease of separation of bound from free analyte. After exposure to analyte, the fractional occupancy of the ligand-binding sites can be determined by competitive or noncompetitive assays using labeled reagents (in orange) as shown.

with antigen-specific T-cell lines or clones can be deciphered to characterize the active epitopes.

Dissecting out T-cell epitopes where the antigen has not been characterized is a more daunting task. Randomized peptide libraries can be produced but strategies need to be devised in order to keep these within manageable numbers. Information from the accumulated data deposited in various databanks can be used to identify key anchor residues and libraries constructed that maintain the relevant amino acids at

these positions. Thus, a positional scanning approach employs a peptide library in which one amino acid at a particular position is kept constant and all the different amino acids are used at the other positions.

B-cell epitopes

If they are linear protein epitopes formed directly from the primary amino acid sequence, then binding of antibody to individual overlapping peptides synthesized

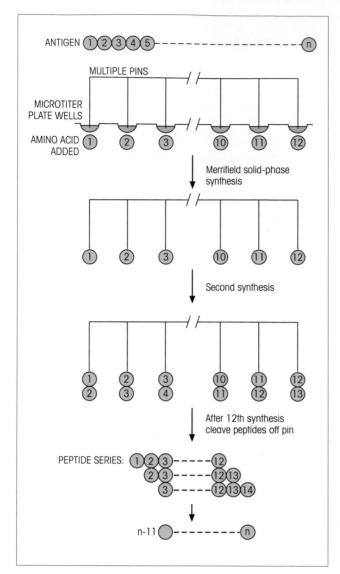

Figure 6.19. Synthesis of overlapping peptide sequences for (PEPSCAN) epitope analysis. A series of pins which sit individually in the wells of a 96-well microtiter plate each provide a site for solid-phase synthesis of peptide. A sequence of such syntheses as shown in the figure provides the required nests of peptides. Incorporation of a readily cleavable linkage allows the soluble peptide to be released as the synthesis is terminated.

as described above will identify them. Unfortunately, most epitopes on globular proteins recognized by antibody are discontinuous and this makes the job rather demanding, since one cannot predict which residues are likely to be brought together in space to form the epitope. To the extent that small linear sequences may contribute to a discontinuous epitope, the overlapping peptide strategy may provide some clues.

A potentially promising approach to this problem of mimicking the residues which constitute such epitopes (termed **mimotopes** by Geysen) is through the production of libraries of bacteriophages bearing all

possible random hexapeptides. These are produced by ligating degenerate oligonucleotide inserts (coding for hexapeptides) to a bacteriophage coat protein in a suitable vector; appropriate expression in *E. coli* can provide up to 10^9 different clones. The beauty of the system is that a bacteriophage expressing a given hexapeptide on its external coat protein also bears the sequence encoding the hexapeptide in its genome (cf. p. 124). Accordingly, sequential rounds of selection, in which the phages react with a biotinylated monoclonal antibody and are then panned on a streptavidin plate, should isolate those bearing the peptides which mimic the epitope recognized by the monoclonal; nucleotide sequencing will then give the peptide structure.

Even nonproteinaceous antigens can occasionally be mimicked using peptide libraries, one example being the use of a D-amino acid hexapeptide library to identify a mimotope for *N*-acetylglucosamine. Others have used a single-chain Fv (scFv) library to isolate an idiotypic mimic of a meningococcal carbohydrate.

MAKING ANTIBODIES TO ORDER

The monoclonal antibody revolution

First in rodents

A fantastic technological breakthrough was achieved by Köhler and Milstein who devised a technique for the production of 'immortal' clones of cells making single antibody specificities by fusing normal antibody-forming cells with an appropriate B-cell tumor line. These so-called 'hybridomas' are selected out in a tissue culture medium which fails to support growth of the parental cell types, and by successive dilutions or by plating out, single clones can be established (figure 6.20). These clones can be grown up in the ascitic form in mice when quite prodigious titers of monoclonal antibody can be attained, but bearing in mind the imperative to avoid using animals wherever feasible, propagation in large-scale culture is to be preferred. Remember that, even in a good antiserum, over 90% of the Ig molecules have little or no avidity for the antigen, and the 'specific antibodies' themselves represent a whole spectrum of molecules with different avidities directed against different determinants on the antigen. What a contrast is provided by the monoclonal antibodies, where all the molecules produced by a given hybridoma are identical: they have the same Ig class and allotype, the same variable region, structure, idiotype, affinity and specificity for a given epitope.

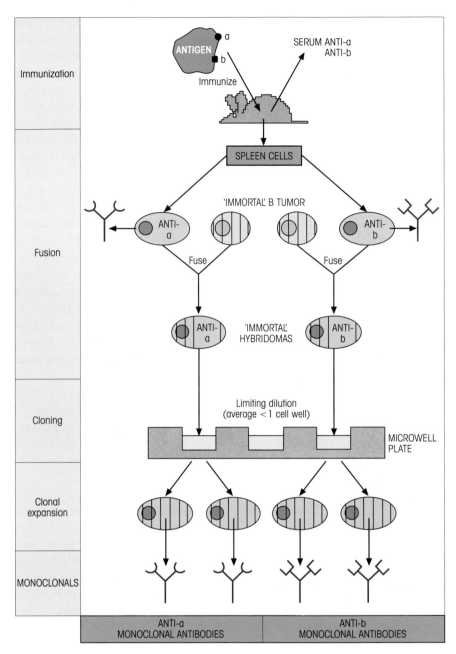

Figure 6.20. Production of monoclonal antibodies. Mice immunized with an antigen bearing (shall we say) two epitopes, a and b, develop spleen cells making anti-a and anti-b which appear as antibodies in the serum. The spleen is removed and the individual cells are fused in polyethylene glycol with constantly dividing (i.e. 'immortal') B-tumor cells selected for a purine enzyme deficiency and usually for their inability to secrete Ig. The resulting cells are distributed into microwell plates in HAT (hypoxanthine, aminopterin, thymidine) medium which kills off the fusion partners. They are seeded at such a dilution that on average each well will contain less than one hybridoma cell. Each hybridoma—the fusion product of a single antibody-forming cell and a tumor cell—will have the ability of the former to secrete a single species of antibody and the immortality of the latter enabling it to proliferate continuously. Thus, clonal progeny can provide an unending supply of antibody with a single specificity—the monoclonal antibody. In this example, we considered the production of hybridomas with specificity for just two epitopes, but the same technique enables monoclonal antibodies to be raised against complex mixtures of multiepitopic antigens. Fusions using rat cells instead of mouse may have certain advantages in giving a higher proportion of stable hybridomas, and monoclonals which are better at fixing human complement, a useful attribute in the context of therapeutic applications to humans involving cell depletion.

Naturally, for use in the human, the ideal solution is the production of purely human monoclonals. Human myeloma fusion partners have not found wide acceptance since they tend to have low fusion efficiencies, poor growth and secretion of the myeloma Ig which dilutes the desired monoclonal. A nonsecreting heterohybridoma obtained by fusing a mouse myeloma with human B-cells can be used as a productive fusion partner for antibody-producing human B-cells. Other groups have turned to the well-characterized murine fusion partners, and the heterohybridomas so formed grow well, clone easily and are productive. There is some instability from chromosome loss and it appears that antibody production is maintained by translocation of human *Ig* genes to mouse chromosomes. Fusion frequency is even better if Epstein–Barr virus (EBV)-transformed lines are used instead of B-cells.

Whereas the large amount of nonspecific, relative to antigen-specific, Ig in an antiserum means that background binding to antigen in any given immunological test may be uncomfortably high, the problem is greatly reduced with a monoclonal antibody preparation, since all the Ig is antibody, thus giving a much superior 'signal:noise' ratio. By being directed towards single epitopes on the antigen, monoclonal antibodies frequently show high specificity in terms of their low cross-reactivity with other antigens. Occasionally, however, one sees quite unexpected binding to molecules which react poorly, if at all, with a specific antiserum directed to the original antigen. The reason for this has already been discussed (see p. 89). Suffice it to say here that the problem can be circumvented by using a group of overlapping monoclonals reacting with the same determinant or a combination of monoclonals to more than one determinant on the same antigen.

An outstanding advantage of the monoclonal antibody as a reagent is that it provides a single standard material for all laboratories throughout the world to use in an unending supply if the immortality and purity of the cell line are nurtured; antisera raised in different animals, on the other hand, may be as different from each other as chalk and cheese. The monoclonal approach again shows a clean pair of heels relative to conventional strategies in the production of antibodies specific for individual components in a complex mixture of antigens. The uses of monoclonal antibodies are truly legion and include: immunoassay, diagnosis of malignancies, tissue typing, serotyping of microorganisms, the separation of individual cell types with specific surface markers (e.g. lymphocyte subpopulations), therapeutic neutralization of inflammatory cytokines and 'magic bullet' therapy with cytotoxic agents coupled to antitumor-specific antibody—these and many other areas have been transformed by hybridoma technology.

Catalytic antibodies

An especially interesting development with tremendous potential is the recognition that a monoclonal antibody to a stable analog of the transition state of a given reaction can act as an enzyme ('abzyme') in catalysing that reaction. The possibility of generating enzymes to order promises a very attractive future, and some exceedingly adroit chemical maneuvers have already extended the range of reactions which can be catalysed in this way. A recent demonstration of sequence-specific peptide cleavage with an antibody which incorporates a metal complex cofactor has raised the pulse rate of the *cognoscenti*, since this is an energetically difficult reaction which has an enormous range of applications. Another innovative approach is to immunize with an antigen which is so highly reactive that a chemical reaction occurs in the antibody combining site. This recruits antibodies which are not only complementary to the active chemical, but are also likely to have some enzymic power over the immunogen–substrate complex. Thus, using this strategy, an antibody with exceptionally broad substrate specificity for efficient catalysis of aldol and retro-aldol reactions was obtained. A key feature of this antibody is a reactive lysine buried within a hydrophobic pocket in the binding site. The antibody remains catalytically active for several weeks following i.v. injection into mice and has therapeutic potential for a version of antibody-directed enzyme prodrug therapy (ADEPT, see p. 392), here with the enzyme component being a catalytic antibody.

Large combinatorial antibody libraries created by random association between pools of heavy and light chains and expressed on bacteriophages (see below) can be screened for catalytic antibodies by using the substrate in a solid-phase state. Cleavage by the catalytic antibody leaves a solid-phase product which can now be identified by a double antibody system using antibodies specific for the product as distinct from the substrate.

An area of great interest is the presence of catalytic autoantibodies in certain groups of patients, with hydrolytic antibodies against vasoactive intestinal peptide, DNA and thyroglobulin having been described. Catalytic antibodies capable of factor VIII hydrolysis have also recently been discovered in hemophiliacs given this clotting factor, the antibodies preventing the coagulation function of the factor VIII.

Human monoclonals can be made

Mouse monoclonals injected into human subjects for therapeutic purposes are frightfully immunogenic and the human anti-mouse antibodies (HAMA in the trade) so formed are a wretched nuisance, accelerating clearance of the monoclonal from the blood and possibly causing hypersensitivity reactions; they also prevent the mouse antibody from reaching its target and, in some cases, block its binding to antigen. In some circumstances it is conceivable that a mouse monoclonal taken up by a tumor cell could be processed and become the MHC-linked target of cytotoxic T-cells or help to boost the response to a weakly immunogenic antigen on the tumor cell surface. In general, however, logic points to removal of the xenogeneic (foreign) portions of the monoclonal antibody and their replacement by human Ig structures using recombinant DNA technology. Chimeric constructs, in which the V_H and V_L mouse domains are spliced onto human C_H and C_L genes (figure 6.21a), are far less immunogenic in humans.

A more refined approach is to graft the six complementarity determining regions (CDRs) of a high affinity rodent monoclonal onto a completely human Ig framework without loss of specific reactivity (figure 6.21b). This is not a trivial exercise, however, and the objective of fusing human B-cells to make hybridomas is still appealing, taking into account not only the gross reduction in immunogenicity, but also the fact that, within a species, antibodies can be made to subtle differences such as major histocompatibility complex (MHC) polymorphic molecules and tumor-associated antigens on other individuals. In contrast, xenogeneic responses are more directed to immunodominant structures common to most subjects, making the production of variant-specific antibodies more difficult. Notwithstanding the difficulties in finding good fusion partners, large numbers of human monoclonals have been established. A further restriction arises because the peripheral blood B-cells, which are the only B-cells readily available in the human, are not normally regarded as a good source of antibody-forming cells.

Immortalized Epstein–Barr virus-transformed B-cell lines have also been used as a source of human monoclonal antibodies. Although these often produce relatively low affinity IgM antibodies, some useful higher affinity IgG antibodies can occasionally be obtained. The cell lines frequently lose their ability to secrete antibody if cultured for long periods of time, although they can sometimes be rescued by fusion with a myeloma cell line to produce hybridomas, or the genes can be isolated and used to produce a recombinant antibody.

A radically different approach involves the production of transgenic xenomouse strains in which megabase-sized unrearranged human Ig H and κ light chain loci have been introduced into mice whose endogenous murine Ig genes have been inactivated. Immunization of these mice yields high affinity (10^{-10}–10^{-11} M) human antibodies which can then be isolated using hybridoma or recombinant approaches. Potent anti-inflammatory (anti-IL-8) and anti-tumor (anti-epidermal growth factor receptor) therapeutic agents have already been obtained using such mice.

There is still a snag in that even human antibodies can provoke anti-idiotype responses; these may have to be circumvented by using engineered antibodies bearing different idiotypes for subsequent injections. Even more desirable would be if the prospective recipients could be first made tolerant to the idiotype, perhaps by coadministering the therapeutic antibody together with a nondepleting anti-CD4.

Many human monoclonals are awaiting the go-ahead for clinical use; one can cite IgG anti-RhD for the prevention of rhesus disease of the newborn (see p. 334), and highly potent monoclonals for protection against varicella zoster, cytomegalovirus, group B streptococci and lipopolysaccharide endotoxins of Gram-negative bacteria.

Engineering antibodies

There are other ways around the problems associated with the production of human monoclonals which exploit the wiles of modern molecular biology. Reference has already been made to the 'humanizing' of rodent antibodies (figure 6.21), but an important new strategy based upon bacteriophage expression and **selection** has achieved a prominent position. In essence, mRNA from primed human B-cells is converted to cDNA and the antibody genes, or fragments therefrom, expanded by the polymerase chain reaction (PCR). Single constructs are then made in which the light and heavy chain genes are allowed to combine randomly in tandem with the gene encoding bacteriophage coat protein III (pIII) (figure 6.22). This **combinatorial library** containing most random pairings of heavy and light chain genes encodes a huge repertoire of antibodies (or their fragments) expressed as fusion proteins with pIII on the bacteriophage surface. The extremely high number of phages produced by *E. coli* infection can now be panned on solid-phase antigen to select those bearing the highest affinity antibodies attached to their

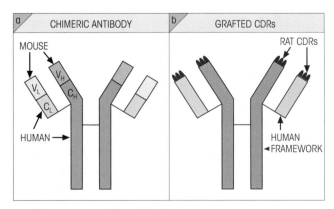

Figure 6.21. Genetically engineering rodent antibody specificities into the human. (a) Chimeric antibody with mouse variable regions fused to human Ig constant regions. (b) 'Humanized' rat monoclonal in which gene segments coding for all six CDRs are grafted onto a human Ig framework.

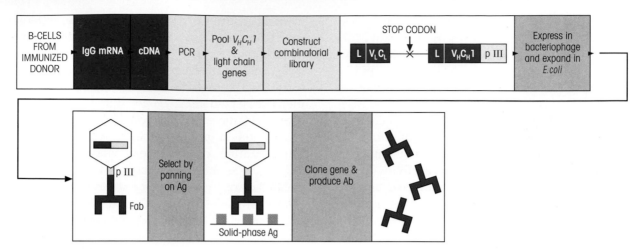

Figure 6.22. Selection of antibody genes from a combinatorial library. B-cells from an immunized donor (in one important experiment, human memory peripheral blood cells were boosted with tetanus toxoid antigen after transfer to SCID mice; Duchosal M.A. *et al.* (1992) *Nature* **355**, 258) are used for the extraction of IgG mRNA and the light chain ($V_L C_L$) and $V_H C_H 1$ genes (encoding Fab) randomly combined in constructs fused to the bacteriophage pIII coat protein gene as shown. These were incorporated into phagemids such as pHEN1 and expanded in *E. coli*. After infection with helper phage, the recombinant phages bearing the highest affinity were selected by rounds of panning on solid-phase antigen so that the genes encoding the Fabs could be cloned. L = bacterial leader sequence.

surface (figure 6.22). Because the genes which encode these highest affinity antibodies are already present within the selected phage, they can readily be cloned and the antibody expressed in bulk. It should be recognized that this **selection** procedure has an enormous advantage over techniques which employ **screening** because the number of phages which can be examined is several logs higher.

Combinatorial libraries have also been established using mRNA from **unimmunized** human donors. V_H, V_κ and V_λ genes are expanded by PCR and randomly recombined to form single-chain Fv (scFv) constructs (figure 6.23a) fused to phage pIII. Soluble fragments binding to a variety of antigens have been obtained. Of special interest are those which are autoantibodies to molecules with therapeutic potential such as CD4 and tumor necrosis factor-α (TNFα); lymphocytes expressing such autoantibodies could not be obtained by normal immunization since they would probably be tolerized, but the random recombination of V_H and V_L can produce entirely new specificities under conditions *in vitro* where tolerance mechanisms do not operate.

Although a 'test-tube' operation, this approach to the generation of specific antibodies does resemble the affinity maturation of the immune response *in vivo* (see p. 195) in the sense that antigen is the determining factor in selecting out the highest affinity responders.

In order to increase the affinities of antibodies pro-

duced by these techniques, antigen can be used to select higher affinity mutants produced by random mutagenesis or even more effectively by site-directed replacements at mutational hotspots (figure 6.23b), again mimicking the natural immune response which involves random mutation and antigen selection (see p. 192). Affinity has also been improved by gene 'shuffling' in which a V_H gene encoding a reasonable affinity antibody is randomly combined with a pool of V_L genes and subjected to antigen selection. The process can be further extended by mixing the V_L from this combination with a pool of V_H genes. It has also proved possible to shuffle individual CDRs between variable regions of moderate affinity antibodies obtained by panning on antigen, thereby creating antibodies of high affinity from relatively small libraries.

Other novel antibodies have been created. In one construct, two scFv fragments associate to form an antibody with two different specificities (figure 6.23c). Another consists of a single heavy chain variable region domain (DAB) whose affinity can be surprisingly high—of the order of 20nM. If it were possible to overcome the 'stickiness' of these miniantibodies, their small size could be exploited for tissue penetration. The design of potential 'magic bullets' for immunotherapy can be based on fusion of a toxin (e.g. ricin) to an antibody Fab (figure 6.23d).

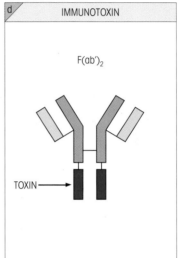

Figure 6.23. Other engineered antibodies. (a) A single gene encoding V_H and V_L joined by a sequence of suitable length gives rise to a single-chain Fv (scFv) antigen-binding fragment. (b) By site-specific mutagenesis of residues in or adjacent to the complementarity determining region (CDR), it is possible to increase the affinity of the antibody. (c) Two scFv constructs expressed simultaneously will associate to form a 'diabody' with two specificities. These bispecific antibodies have a number of uses. Note that such a bispecific antibody directed to two different epitopes on the same antigen will have a much higher affinity due to the 'bonus effect' of cooperation between the two binding sites (cf. p. 90). (d) Potential 'magic bullets' can be constructed by fusing the gene for a toxin (e.g. ricin) to the Fab.

Fields of antibodies

Not only can the genes for a monoclonal antibody be expressed in bulk in the milk of lactating animals but plants can also be exploited for this purpose. So-called '**plantibodies**' have been expressed in bananas, potatoes and tobacco plants. One can imagine a high-tech farmer drawing the attention of a bemused visitor to one field growing anti-tetanus toxoid, another anti-meningococcal polysaccharide, and so on. Multifunctional plants might be quite profitable with, say, the root being harvested as a food crop and the leaves expressing some desirable gene product. At this rate there may not be much left for science fiction authors to write about!

Drugs can be based on the CDRs of minibodies

Millions of **minibodies** composed of a segment of the V_H region containing three β-strands and the H1 and H2 hypervariable loops were generated by randomization of the CDRs and expressed on the bacteriophage pIII coat protein. By panning the library on functionally important ligand-binding sites, such as hormone receptors, useful lead candidates for drug design programs can be identified and their affinity improved by loop optimization, loop shuffling and further selection.

PURIFICATION OF ANTIGENS AND ANTIBODIES BY AFFINITY CHROMATOGRAPHY

The principle is simple and *very* widely applied. Antigen or antibody is bound through its free amino groups to cyanogen bromide-activated Sepharose particles. Insolubilized antibody, for example, can be used to pull the corresponding antigen out of solution, in

ACTIVATED SEPHAROSE	MONOCLONAL ANTIBODY	AFFINITY ABSORBENT	ANTIGEN MIXTURE			PURIFIED ANTIGEN
Add	Conjugate	Add	Absorb antigen	Wash	Elute	

Figure 6.24. Affinity chromatography. A column is filled with Sepharose-linked antibody. The antigen mixture is poured down the column. Only the antigen binds and is released by a change in pH, for example. Conversely, an antigen-linked affinity column can be used to purify antibody.

which it is present as one component of a complex mixture, by absorption to its surface. The uninteresting garbage is washed away and the required ligand released from the affinity absorbent by disruption of the antigen–antibody bonds by changing the pH or adding chaotropic ions such as thiocyanate (figure 6.24). Likewise, an antigen immunosorbent can be used to absorb out an antibody from a mixture whence it can be purified by elution.

NEUTRALIZATION OF BIOLOGICAL ACTIVITY

To detect antibody

A number of biological reactions can be inhibited by addition of specific antibody. Thus the agglutination of red cells by interaction of influenza virus with receptors on the erythrocyte surface can be blocked by antiviral antibodies and this forms the basis for their serological detection. A test for antibodies to *Salmonella* H antigen present on the flagella depends upon their ability to inhibit the motility of the bacteria *in vitro*. Likewise, *Mycoplasma* antibodies can be demonstrated by their inhibitory effect on the metabolism of the organisms in culture.

Using antibody as an inhibitor

The successful treatment of cases of drug overdose with the Fab fragment of specific antibodies has been described and may become a practical proposition if a range of hybridomas can be assembled. Conjugates of cocaine with keyhole limpet hemocyanin can provoke neutralizing antibodies. Antibodies to hormones such as insulin and thyroid-stimulating hormone (TSH), or to cytokines, can be used to probe the specificity of biological reactions *in vitro*. For example, the specificity of the insulin-like activity of a serum sample on rat epididymal fat pad can be checked by the neutralizing effect of an antiserum. Such antibodies can be effective *in vivo*, and anti-TNF treatment of patients with rheumatoid arthritis has confirmed the role of this cytokine in the disease process. Likewise, as part of the worldwide effort to prevent disastrous overpopulation, attempts are in progress to immunize against chorionic gonadotropin using fragments of the β chain coupled to appropriate carriers, since this hormone is needed to sustain the implanted ovum.

In a totally different context, antibodies raised against myelin-associated neurite growth inhibitory proteins revealed their importance in preventing nerve repair, in that treatment with these antibodies permitted the regeneration of corticospinal axons after a spinal cord lesion had been induced in adult rats. This quite remarkable finding significantly advances our understanding of the processes involved in regeneration and gives ground for cautious optimism concerning the development of treatment for spinal cord damage, although for various reasons this may not ultimately be based on antibody therapy.

SUMMARY

Estimation of antibody

- The antibody content of a polyclonal antiserum is defined entirely in operational terms by the nature of the assay employed.
- Antibody in solution can be assayed by the formation of frank precipitates which can be enhanced by countercurrent electrophoresis in gels.
- Nonprecipitating antibodies can be measured by laser nephelometry or by salt or anti-Ig coprecipitation with radioactive antigen.
- Affinity is measured by a variety of methods including surface plasmon resonance which gives a measure of both the on- and off-rates.
- Antibodies can also be detected by macroscopic agglutination of antigen-coated particles, and by one of the most important methods, ELISA, a two-stage procedure in which antibody bound to solid-phase antigen is detected by an enzyme-linked anti-Ig.

Identification and measurement of antigen

- Antigens can be separated and their mobility in an electric field determined by electrophoresis and immunofixation.
- Antigens can be quantified by their reaction in gels with antibody using single radial immunodiffusion.
- Higher concentrations of antigens are frequently estimated by nephelometry.
- Exceedingly low concentrations of antigens can be measured by immunoassay techniques which depend upon the relationship between Ag concentration and fractional occupancy of the binding antibody. Occupied sites are measured with a high specific activity second antibody directed to a different epitope; alternatively, unoccupied sites can be estimated by labeled Ag. Multiple assays on arrays of antibody microspots are being developed.
- Overlapping nests of peptides derived from the linear sequence of a protein can map T-cell epitopes and the linear elements of B-cell epitopes. Bacteriophages encoding all possible hexapeptides on their surface have provided some limited success in identifying discontinuous B-cell determinants.

Detection of immune complexes

- Serum complexes can be determined by precipitation with polyethylene glycol, reaction with C1q or bovine conglutinin, changes in C3 and C3c and binding to rheumatoid factors.

Making antibodies to order

- Immortal hybridoma cell lines making monoclonal antibodies provide powerful immunological reagents and insights into the immune response. Applications include enumeration of lymphocyte subpopulations, cell depletion, immunoassay, cancer diagnosis and imaging, purification of antigen from complex mixtures, and recently the use of monoclonals as artificial enzymes (catalytic antibodies).
- Genetically engineered human antibody fragments can be derived by expanding the V_H and V_L genes from unimmunized, but preferably immunized, donors and expressing them as completely randomized combinatorial libraries on the surface of bacteriophage. Phages bearing the highest affinity antibodies are selected by panning on antigens and the antibody genes can then be cloned from the isolated viruses.
- Single-chain Fv (scFv) fragments encoded by linked V_H and V_L genes and even single heavy chain domains can be created.
- The HAMA response against mouse monoclonal antibodies can be reduced by producing chimeric antibodies with mouse variable regions and human constant regions or, better still, using humanized antibodies in which all the mouse sequences except for the CDRs are replaced by human sequences.
- Transgenic mice bearing human *Ig* genes can be immunized. The mice produce high affinity fully human antibodies.
- Recombinant antibodies can be expressed on a large scale in plants.
- Combinatorial libraries of diabodies containing the H1 and H2 V_H CDR may be used to develop new drugs.

Affinity chromatography

- Insoluble immunoabsorbents prepared by coupling antibody to Sepharose can be used to affinity-purify antigens from complex mixtures and reciprocally to purify antibodies.

Neutralization of biological activity

- Antibodies can be detected by inhibition of biological functions such as viral infectivity or bacterial growth.
- Inhibition of biological function by known antibodies helps to define the role of the antigen, be it a hormone or cytokine for example, in complex responses *in vivo* and *in vitro*.

See the accompanying website (**www.roitt.com**) for multiple choice questions.

FURTHER READING

Ausubel F.M., Brent R., Kingston R.E., Moore D.D., Seidman J.G., Smith J.A. & Struhl K. (eds) (1987; continually updated) *Current Protocols in Molecular Biology, 1–2*. Greene Publishing Associates & Wiley-Interscience, New York.

Chowdhury P.S. & Pastan I. (1999) Improving antibody affinity by mimicking somatic hypermutation *in vitro*. *Nature Biotechnology* **17**, 568.

Coligan J.E., Kruisbeek A.M., Margulies D.H., Shevach E.M. & Strober W. (eds) (1991; continually updated) *Current Protocols in Immunology, 1–2*. Greene Publishing Associates & Wiley-Interscience, New York.

Delves P.J. (1995) *Antibody Applications*. J. Wiley & Sons, Chichester.

Delves P.J. (1997) *Antibody Production*. J. Wiley & Sons, Chichester.

Fishwild D.M. *et al.* (1996) High-avidity human IgGκ monoclonal antibodies from a novel strain of minilocus transgenic mice. *Nature Biotechnology* **14**, 845.

Friguet B., Chafotte A.F., Djavadi-Ohaniance L. & Goldberg M.E.J. (1985) Measurements of the true affinity constant in solution of antigen–antibody complexes by enzyme-linked immunosorbent assay. *Journal of Immunological Methods* **77**, 305.

Green L.L. (1999) Antibody engineering via genetic engineering of the mouse: xenomouse strains are a vehicle for the facile generation of therapeutic human monoclonal antibodies. *Journal of Immunological Methods* **231**, 11.

Lacroix-Desmazes S. *et al.* (1999) Catalytic activity of antibodies against factor VIII in patients with hemophilia A. *Nature Medicine* **5**, 1044.

Malik V.S. & Lillehoj E.P. (1994) *Antibody Techniques*. Academic Press, London. (Laboratory manual of pertinent techniques for production and use of monoclonal antibodies for the nonimmunologist.)

McGuinness B.T. *et al.* (1996) Phage diabody repertoires for selection of large numbers of bispecific antibody fragments. *Nature Biotechnology* **14**, 1149.

Mosier D.E. (ed.) (1996) Humanizing the mouse. *Seminars in Immunology* **8**, 185.

Pinilla C. *et al.* (1999) Exploring immunological specificity using synthetic peptide combinatorial libraries. *Current Opinion in Immunology* **11**, 193.

Ritter M.A. & Ladyman H.M. (1995) *Monoclonal Antibodies: Production, Engineering and Clinical Application*. Cambridge University Press, Cambridge. (An evaluation of different techniques available rather than a technical manual.)

Shabat D., Rader C., List B., Lerner R.A. & Barbas C.F., III (1999) Multiple event activation of a generic prodrug trigger by antibody catalysis. *Proceedings of the National Academy of Sciences of the United States of America* **96**, 6925.

Sikorski R.S. & Peters R. (1996) Antibodies on the web. *Nature Biotechnology* **14**, 775.

Vaughan T.J. *et al.* (1996) Human antibodies with subnanomolar affinities isolated from a large nonimmunized phage display library. *Nature Biotechnology* **14**, 309.

Watson J.D., Gilman M., Witkowski J. & Zoller M. (1992) *Recombinant DNA*, 2nd edn. Scientific American Books, New York.

Weir D.M. *et al.* (eds) (1996) *Handbook of Experimental Immunology: Volume 4*, 5th edn. Blackwell Scientific Publications, Oxford.

Zola H. (1999) *Monoclonal Antibodies*. Bios Scientific Publishers, Oxford.

Cellular techniques

INTRODUCTION

Techniques for probing the immunophenotype and function of cells of the immune system are becoming ever more sophisticated. In addition, it is possible to identify the function of individual genes by mutation and the creation of transgenic and 'knockout' animals.

ISOLATION OF LEUKOCYTE SUBPOPULATIONS

Bulk techniques

Separation based on physical parameters

Separation of cells on the basis of their differential **sedimentation rate**, which roughly correlates with **size**, can be carried out by centrifugation through a density gradient. Cells can be increased in mass by selectively binding particles such as red cells to their surface, the most notable example being the rosettes formed when sheep erythrocytes bind to the CD2 of human T-cells.

Buoyant density is another useful parameter. Centrifugation of whole blood over isotonic Ficoll–Hypaque (sodium metrizoate) of density 1.077 g/ml leaves the mononuclear cells (lymphocytes, monocytes and natural killer (NK) cells) floating in a band at the interface, while the erythrocytes and polymorphonuclear leukocytes, being denser, travel right down to the base of the tube. **Adherence** to plastic surfaces largely removes phagocytic cells, while passage down nylon-wool columns greatly enriches lymphocyte populations for T-cells at the expense of B-cells.

Separation exploiting biological parameters

Actively phagocytic cells which take up small iron particles can be manipulated by a magnet deployed externally. Lymphocytes which divide in response to a polyclonal activator (see p. 164), or specific antigen, can be eliminated by allowing them to incorporate 5-bromodeoxyuridine (BrdU); this renders them susceptible to the lethal effect of UV irradiation.

Selection by antibody

Several methods are available for the selection of cells specifically coated with antibody, some of which are illustrated in figure 7.1. Addition of complement or anti-Ig toxin conjugates will eliminate such populations. Magnetic beads coated with anti-Ig form clusters with antibody-coated cells which can be readily separated from uncoated cells. Another useful bulk selection technique is to pan antibody-coated cells on anti-Ig adsorbed to a surface. One variation on this theme used to isolate bone marrow stem cells with anti-CD34 is to coat the cells with biotinylated antibody and select with an avidin column or avidin magnetic beads.

Figure 7.1. Major methods for separating cells coated with a specific antibody.

Cocktails of antibodies coated onto beads are used in cell separation columns for the depletion of specific populations leading to, for example, enriched CD4⁺ CD45RA⁻ or CD4⁺ CD45RO⁻ lymphocytes.

Cell selection by the FACS

Cells coated with fluorescent antibody can be separated in the fluorescence-activated cell sorter (FACS) as described in Milestone 7.1 and figure 7.2 (see more in-depth discussion under 'Flow cytofluorimetry', p. 133).

Enrichment of antigen-specific populations

Selective expansion of antigen-specific T-cells by repeated stimulation with antigen and presenting cells in culture, usually alternated with interleukin-2 (IL-2) treatment, leads to an enrichment of heterogeneous T-cells specific for different epitopes on the antigen. Such **T-cell lines** can be distributed in microtiter wells at a high enough dilution such that **on average** there is less than one cell per well; pushing the cells to proliferate with antigen or anti-CD3 produces single T-cell clones which can be maintained with much obsessional care and attention, but my goodness they can be a pain! Potentially immortal **T-cell hybridomas**, similar in

principle to B-cell hybridomas, can be established by fusing cell lines with a T-tumor line and cloning.

Animals populated essentially by a single T-cell specificity can be produced by introducing the T-cell receptor α and β genes from a T-cell clone, as a transgene (see below); since the genes are already rearranged, their presence in every developing T-cell will switch off any other $V\beta$ gene recombinations.

No one has succeeded in cloning B-cells, except as hybridomas or Epstein–Barr virus-transformed cell lines, although, as with T-cells, transgenic animals expressing the same antibody in all their B-cells have been generated.

IMMUNOHISTOCHEMISTRY—LOCALIZATION OF ANTIGENS IN CELLS AND TISSUES

Immunofluorescence techniques

Because fluorescent dyes such as fluorescein and rhodamine can be coupled to antibodies without destroying their specificity, the conjugates can combine with antigen present in a tissue section and be visualized in the fluorescence microscope. In this way, the distribution of antigen throughout a tissue and within cells can be demonstrated. Looked at another way, the method can also be used for the detection of antibodies directed against antigens already known to be present in a given tissue section or cell preparation. There are two general ways in which the test is carried out.

Direct test with labeled antibody

The antibody to the tissue antigen is conjugated with the fluorochrome and applied directly (figure 7.3a). For example, suppose we wished to show the distribution of a thyroid autoantigen reacting with the autoantibodies present in the serum of a patient with Hashimoto's disease, a type of thyroid autoimmunity. We would isolate IgG from the patient's serum, conjugate it with fluorescein, and apply it to a section of human thyroid on a slide. When viewed in the fluorescence microscope we would see that the cytoplasm of the follicular epithelial cells was brightly stained (cf. figure 19.1a).

By using two antisera conjugated to dyes which emit fluorescence at different wavelengths, two different antigens can be identified simultaneously in the same preparation. In figure 2.6e, direct staining of fixed plasma cells with a mixture of rhodamine-labeled anti-IgG and fluorescein-conjugated anti-IgM craftily demonstrates that these two classes of antibody are produced by different cells. The technique of coupling

Milestone 7.1 — The Fluorescence-activated Cell Sorter (FACS)

The FACS was developed by the Herzenbergs and their colleagues to quantify the surface molecules on individual white cells by their reaction with fluorochrome-labeled monoclonal antibodies and to use the signals so generated to separate cells of defined phenotype from a heterogeneous mixture.

In this elegant but complex machine, the fluorescent cells are made to flow obediently in a single stream past a laser beam. Quantitative measurement of the fluorescent signal in a suitably placed photomultiplier tube relays a signal to the cell as it emerges in a single droplet; the cell

becomes charged and can be separated in an electric field (figure M7.1.1). Extra sophistication can be introduced by using additional lasers and fluorochromes, and both 90° and forward light scatter. This will be elaborated upon in the section on flow cytofluorimetry describing how this technique can be used for quantitative multi-parameter analysis of single-cell populations (cf. figure 7.6). Suffice to state that these latest FACS machines permit the isolation of cells with a complex phenotype from a heterogeneous population with a high degree of discrimination.

Figure M7.1.1. The principle of the FACS for flow cytofluorimetry of the fluorescence on stained cells (green rimmed circles) and physical separation from unstained cells. The charge signal can be activated to separate cells of high from low fluorescence and, using light scatter, of large from small size and dead from living.

biotin to the antiserum and then finally staining with fluorescent avidin is often employed.

Indirect test for antibody

In this double-layer technique, the unlabeled antibody is applied directly to the tissue substrate and visualized by treatment with a fluorochrome-conjugated anti-immunoglobulin serum (figure 7.3b). In this case, in order to find out whether or not the serum of a patient has antibodies to thyroid epithelial cells, we would first treat a thyroid section with the serum, wash well and then apply a fluorescein-labeled rabbit

anti-human immunoglobulin; if antibodies were present, there would be staining of the thyroid epithelial cells.

This technique has several advantages. In the first place the fluorescence is brighter than with the direct test since several fluorescent anti-immunoglobulins bind on to each of the antibody molecules present in the first layer (figure 7.3b). Second, even when many sera have to be screened for specific antibodies it is only necessary to prepare (or, more usually the case, purchase) a single labeled reagent, viz. the anti-immunoglobulin. Furthermore, the method has great flexibility. For example, by using conjugates of antisera

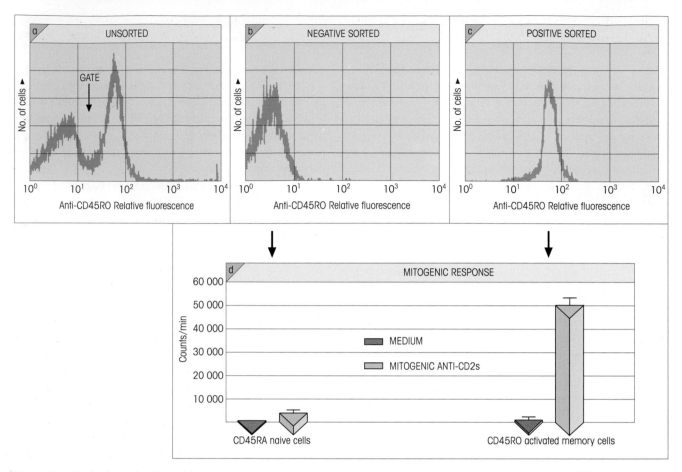

Figure 7.2. Separation of activated peripheral blood memory T-cells (CD45RO positive) from naive T-cells (CD45RO negative; but positive for the CD45RA isoform) in the FACS after staining the surface of the living cells in the cold with a fluorescent monoclonal antibody to the CD45RO (see p. 196). The unsorted cells showed two peaks (a); cells with fluorescence intensity lower than the arbitrary gate were separated from those with higher intensity giving (b) negative (CD45RA) and (c) positive (CD45RO) populations, which were each tested for their proliferative response to a mixture of two anti-CD2 monoclonals (OKT11 and GT2) in the presence of 10% antigen-presenting cells (d). ^{3}H-Thymidine was added after 3 days and the cells counted after 15 h. Clearly the memory cell population proliferated, whereas the naive population did not. (Data kindly provided by D. Wallace and R. Hicks.)

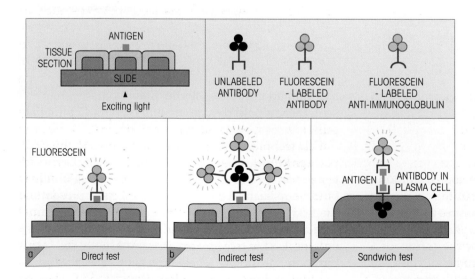

Figure 7.3. The basis of fluorescence antibody tests for identification of tissue antigens or their antibodies. ⬤ = fluorescein labeled.

to individual immunoglobulin heavy chains, the distribution of antibodies among the various classes and subclasses can be assessed at least semiquantitatively. One can also test for complement fixation on the tissue section by adding a mixture of the first antibody plus a source of complement, followed by a fluorescent anticomplement reagent as the second layer.

Further applications of the indirect test may be seen in Chapter 19.

High resolution with the confocal microscope

Fluorescent images at high magnification are usually difficult to resolve because of the flare from slightly out of focus planes above and below that of the object. All that is now past, with the advent of commercially available **scanning confocal microscopes** which focus the image of the laser source in a fine plane within the cell and collect the fluorescence emission in a photomultiplier tube (PMT) with a confocal aperture. Fluorescence from planes above and below the object plane fails to reach the PMT and so the sharpness of the image is unaffected. An X–Y scanning unit enables the whole of the specimen plane to be interrogated *quantitatively* and, with suitable optics, two different fluorochromes can be used simultaneously. The instrument software can compute three-dimensional fluorescent images from an automatic series of such X–Y scans accumulated in the Z axis (figure 7.4) and rotate them at the whim of the operator.

Flow cytofluorimetry

Cell surface antigens can be detected and localized by the use of labeled antibodies. Because antibodies cannot readily penetrate living cells except by endocytosis, treatment of cells with labeled antibody in the cold (to minimize endocytosis) leads to staining only of antigens on the surface (figure 7.2). Remember also a previous example of fluorescent staining of the surface of B-lymphocytes with anti-immunoglobulin (figure 2.6c).

It is possible to stain single cells with several different fluorochromes (figure 7.5) and analyse the cells in individual droplets as they flow past the monitoring section of a **flow cytometer**. This piece of equipment is essentially a FACS machine without the cell-sorting facility (figure 7.6). These instruments record quantitative data relating to the surface antigen content and physical nature of each individual cell, with multiple parameters being assessed per cell to give a phenotypic analysis on a single cell rather than a population average (figure 7.7). With the impressive number of monoclonal antibodies and of fluorochromes to hand, highly detailed analyses are now feasible, with a notable contribution to the diagnosis of leukemia (cf. p. 382).

We can also probe the cell *interior* in several ways. Permeabilization to allow penetration by fluorescent antibodies (preferably with small Fab or even single-chain Fv fragments) gives a readout of cytokines and other intracellular proteins. Cell cycle analysis can be achieved with DNA-binding dyes such as propidium iodide to measure DNA content and antibody detection of BrdU incorporation to visualize DNA synthesis. In addition, fluorescent probes for intracellular pH, thiol concentration, Ca^{2+}, Mg^{2+} and Na^+ have been developed.

A powerful analytical tool is the measurement of the intracellular expression of artificially introduced genes which comprise a coding sequence or regulatory region of interest fused to another gene for a molecule, such as green fluorescent protein (GFP), luciferase or LacZ (*Escherichia coli* β-galactosidase, detected via hydrolysis of the fluorogenic substrate fluorescein digalactoside). Depending on the construct used, the gene can be utilized as a marker for developmental and migration studies or as a reporter under the control of specified promoter or enhancer elements. As an example of the fancy flow cytofluorimetric analyses that can be carried out, transgenic replacement (cf. p. 143) of endogenous RAG-2 genes with a RAG-2–GFP fusion gene permitted the study of RAG-2 expression in individual lymphocytes whose phenotype was simultaneously defined by monoclonal antibody staining.

Other labeled antibody methods

In place of fluorescent markers, enzymes such as alkaline phosphatase (cf. figure 18.7) or peroxidase can be coupled to antibodies and then visualized by conventional histochemical methods at both light microscope (cf. figure 8.7f) and electron microscope level.

Colloidal gold bound to antibody is being widely used as an electron-dense immunolabel by electron microscopists. At least three different antibodies can be applied to the same section by labeling them with gold particles of different size (cf. figure 9.13). A new ultra-small probe consisting of Fab' fragments linked to undecagold clusters allows more accurate spatial localization of antigens and its small size enables it to mark sites which are inaccessible to the larger immunolabels. However, clear visualization requires a high-resolution scanning transmission electron microscope.

Figure 7.4. Construction of a three-dimensional fluorescent image with the confocal microscope. A spherical thyroid follicle in a thick razor-blade section of rat thyroid fixed in formalin was stained with a rhodamine–phalloidin conjugate which binds F-actin (similar results obtained with antibody conjugates). Although the sample was very thick, the microscope was focused on successive planes at 1 µm intervals from the top of the follicle (image no. 1) to halfway through (image no. 8), the total of the images representing a hemisphere. Note how the fluorescence in one plane does not interfere with that in another and that the composite photograph (image no. 9) of images 1–8 shows all the fluorescent staining in focus throughout the depth of the hemisphere. Clearly the antibody is staining hexagonal structures close to the apical (inner) surface of the follicular epithelial cells. Erythrocytes are visible near the top of the follicle. (Negatives kindly supplied by Dr Anna Smallcombe were taken by Bio-Rad staff on a Bio-Rad MRC-600 confocal imaging system using material provided by Professor V. Herzog and Fr. Brix of Bonn University.)

GENE EXPRESSION

Messenger RNA can be extracted from cells or tissues and then analysed in dot blots, by northern blotting or by PCR. The development of microarray technologies now permits the simultaneous measurement of expression of thousands of genes in a single experiment. Oligonucleotides or cDNA fragments are robotically spotted onto a gene chip and cDNA generated from, for example, T-cell mRNA is labeled and hybridized to the genes on the microarray. This provides a quantitative comparison of expression for every gene present on the chip. By accumulating such data it is possible to build up a complete picture of which genes are expressed in which cells (figure 7.8). One area in which this technology is being rapidly deployed is in the analysis of differences in gene expression between a tumor cell and its normal counterpart, thereby illuminating possible targets for therapeutic intervention.

Localization of mRNA to individual cells can be obtained by *in situ* hybridization of labeled oligonucleotide probes to either cell smears or to tissue sections.

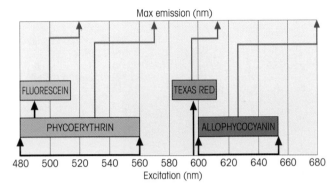

Figure 7.5. Fluorescent labels used in flow cytofluorimetry. The fluorescein longer wave emission overlaps with that of Texas Red and is corrected for in the software. The phycobiliproteins of red algae and cyanobacteria effect energy transfer of blue light to chlorophyll for photosynthesis; each molecule has many fluorescent groups giving a broad excitation range, but fluorescence is emitted within a narrow wavelength band with such high quantum efficiency as to obviate the need for a second amplifying antibody.

ASSESSMENT OF FUNCTIONAL ACTIVITY

The activity of phagocytic cells

The major tests employed to assess neutrophil function are summarized in table 7.1.

Lymphocyte responsiveness

When lymphocytes are stimulated by antigen or polyclonal activators *in vitro* they usually undergo mitosis (cf. figure 2.6b) and release cytokines. Mitosis is normally assessed by the incorporation of radiolabeled ^{3}H-thymidine or ^{125}I-UdR (5-iododeoxyuridine) into the DNA of the dividing cells.

Cytokines released into the culture medium can be measured by immunoassay or by a bioassay using a cell line dependent on a particular cytokine for its growth and survival. Individual cells synthesizing cytokines can be enumerated in the flow cytometer by permeabilizing and staining intracellularly with labeled antibody; alternatively the ELISPOT technique (see below) can be applied. As usual, molecular biology has a valuable, if more sophisticated, input since T-cells transfected with an IL-2 enhancer–*lacZ* construct will switch on *lacZ* β-galactosidase expression on activation of the IL-2 cytokine response (cf.

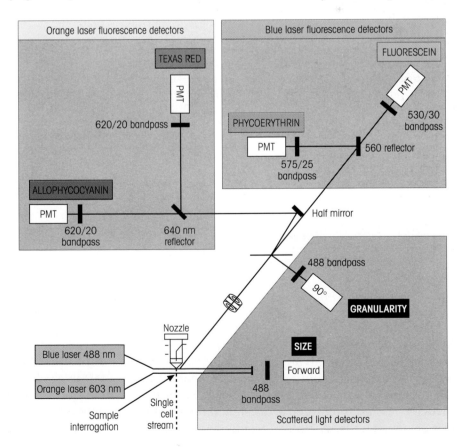

Figure 7.6. Six-parameter flow cytometry optical system for multicolor immunofluorescence analysis. Cell fluorescence excited by the blue laser is divided into green (fluorescein) and orange (phycoerythrin) signals, while fluorescence excited by the orange laser is reflected by a mirror and divided into near red (Texas Red) and far red (allophycocyanin) signals. Blue light scattered at small forward angles and at 90° is also measured in this system, providing information on cell size and internal granularity respectively. PMT, photomultiplier tube. (Based closely on Hardy R.R. (1998) In Delves P.J. & Roitt I.M. (eds) *Encyclopedia of Immunology*, 2nd edn, p. 946. Academic Press, London.) The recent use of three lasers and nine different fluorochromes pushes the system even further, providing 11 parameters!

Figure 7.7. Cytofluorimetric analysis of TCR Vβ6 usage by human peripheral blood lymphocytes. Cells stained with fluoresceinated anti-TCR Vβ6 and phycoerythrin-conjugated anti-CD3. Each dot represents an individual lymphocyte and the numbers refer to the percentage of lymphocytes lying within the four quadrants formed by the two gating levels arbitrarily used to segregate positive from negative values. Virtually no lymphocytes bearing the T-cell receptors belonging to the Vβ6 family lack CD3, while 4.6% (3.5 out of 77.0) of the mature T-cells express Vβ6. (Data kindly provided by D. Morrison.)

Table 7.1. Evaluation of neutrophil function.

Function	Test
Phagocytosis	Measure the uptake of particles such as latex or bacteria by counting or by chemiluminescence
Respiratory burst	Measure reduction of nitroblue tetrazolium
Intracellular killing	Microbicidal test using viable *Staphylococcus aureus*
Directional migration	Movement through filters up concentration gradient of chemotactic agent such as formyl.Met.Leu.Phe
Surface LFA-1 and CR3 upregulation	Ascertained with monoclonal antibody staining

Figure 7.8. Gene expression during lymphocyte development and activation. The data were generated from over 3.8 million measurements of gene expression made on 13 637 genes using 243 microarrays. Each experiment represents a different cell population. For example, experiment 1 utilized polyclonally activated fetal CD4+ thymic cells, whereas experiment 2 shows the same population prior to stimulation. Overexpressed or induced genes are colored red, underexpressed or repressed genes green. Certain gene expression signatures become apparent in the different cell populations, indicated on the right. For example, the T-cell gene expression signature includes CD2, TCR, TCR signaling molecules and many cytokines. (Reproduced with permission of the authors and the publishers from Alizadeh A.A. & Staudt L.M. (2000) *Current Opinion in Immunology* **12**, 219.)

p. 167) and this can be readily revealed with a fluorescent or chromogenic enzyme substrate.

The ability of cytotoxic T-cells to kill their cell targets extracellularly is usually evaluated by a chromium release assay. Target cells are labeled with ^{51}Cr and the release of radioactive protein into the medium over and above that seen in the controls is the index of cytotoxicity. The test is repeated at different ratios of effector to target cells. A similar technique is used to measure extracellular killing of antibody-coated or uncoated targets by NK cells. Now a word of caution regarding the interpretation of *in vitro* assays. Since one can manipulate the culture conditions within wide limits, it is possible to achieve a result that might not be attainable *in vivo*. Let us illustrate this point by reference to cytotoxicity for murine cells infected with lymphocytic choriomeningitis virus (LCMV) or vesicular stomatitis virus (VSV). The most sensitive *in vitro* technique proved to be chromium release from target cells after secondary stimulation of the lymphocytes. However, this needs 5 days, during which time a relatively small number of memory CD8 cytotoxic T-cell precursors can replicate and surpass the threshold required to produce a measurable assay. Nonetheless, a weak cytotoxicity assay under these conditions was not reflected by any of the *in vivo* assessments of antiviral function implying that they had no biological relevance.

Apoptosis

Programed cell death occurs frequently in the immune system in a number of different situations and a variety of approaches can be used to measure the apoptotic cells. Gel electrophoresis will detect the characteristic laddering pattern of the DNA fragments generated due to internucleosomal cleavage (see figure 1.19). An alternative way to detect this DNA fragmentation, known as the TUNEL (*T*dT-mediated d*U*TP (deoxyuridine triphosphate) *n*ick *e*nd *l*abeling) technique, utilizes the enzyme terminal deoxynucleotidyl transferase (TdT) to add labeled nucleotides to the 3' ends of the fragments. An earlier event in apoptosis is the loss of membrane symmetry resulting in the expression of phosphatidylserine on the cell surface—readily detected by flow cytometry using a labeled version of its ligand Annexin V. For sophisticates, more detailed analyses can be undertaken in which individual components of the apoptotic pathways, such as Bcl-2, Bcl-x$_L$, Bax, PARP (poly(ADP-ribose) polymerase) or specific procaspases and caspases, are measured in fluorimetric or colorimetric assays.

Precursor frequency

The magnitude of lymphocyte responses in culture is closely related to the number of antigen-specific lymphocytes capable of responding. Because of the clonality of the responses, it is possible to estimate the frequency of these antigen-specific precursors by **limiting dilution analysis**. In essence, the method depends upon the fact that, if one takes several replicate aliquots of a given cell suspension which would be expected to contain *on average* one precursor per aliquot, then Poisson distribution analysis shows that 37% of the aliquots will contain *no* precursor cells (through the randomness of the sampling). Thus, if aliquots are made from a series of dilutions of a cell suspension and incubated under conditions which allow the precursors to mature and be recognized through some amplification scheme, the dilution at which 37% of the aliquots give negative responses will be known to con-

tain an average of one precursor cell per aliquot, and one can therefore calculate the precursor frequency in the original cell suspension. An example is shown in some detail in figure 7.9.

It has been argued that limiting dilution analysis often underestimates the true precursor frequency. An accurate measure of the percentage of lymphocytes bearing a specific antigen receptor can be obtained by flow cytometry of cells stained with labeled antigen. In the case of B-cells this is fairly straightforward given that their antigen receptors recognize native antigen. However, it is only recently that technical finesse, in the form of peptide–MHC tetramers, has brought this technique to T-cells (figure 7.10). This approach overcomes the problem of the relatively weak intrinsic affinity of TCR for peptide–MHC by presenting a tagged peptide–MHC as a multivalent tetramer, thereby exploiting the bonus effect of multivalency (cf. p. 90). Peptide–MHC complexes are produced by permitting recombinant MHC molecules to refold with the appropriate synthetic peptide. The recombinant MHC molecules are biotinylated on a special carboxyterminal extension, which ensures that the biotin is incorporated at a distance from the site to which the TCR binds, and mixed with fluorescently labeled streptavidin, which not only binds biotin with a very high affinity but also has a valency of four with respect to the biotin—hence the formation of tetramers.

Numerous adaptations of this technology are appearing. For example, incubation at 37°C of tetramers bound to their cognate TCR leads to internalization; by tagging them with a toxin individual T-lymphocytes of a single specificity can be eliminated. Another approach is to use the FACS to directly sort stained cells into an ELISPOT microtiter plate in which cytokine secretion is measured, providing a functional analysis of the cells.

Enumeration of antibody-forming cells

The immunofluorescence sandwich test

This is a double-layer procedure designed to visualize specific intracellular antibody. If, for example, we wished to see how many cells in a preparation of lymphoid tissue were synthesizing antibody to *Pneumococcus* polysaccharide, we would first fix the cells with ethanol to prevent the antibody being washed away during the test, and then treat with a solution of the polysaccharide antigen. After washing, a fluorescein-labeled antibody to the polysaccharide would then be added to locate those cells which had specifically bound the antigen.

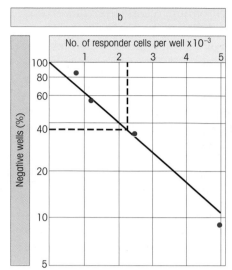

Figure 7.9. Limiting dilution analysis of cytotoxic T-cell precursor frequency in spleen cells from a BALB/c mouse stimulated with irradiated C57BL/6 spleen cells as antigen. BALB/c splenic responder cells were set up in 24 replicates at each concentration tested together with antigen and an excess of T-helper factors. The generation of cytotoxicity in each well was looked for by adding ^{51}Cr-labeled tumor cells (EL-4) of the C57BL/6 haplotype; cytotoxicity was then revealed by measuring the release of soluble ^{51}Cr-labeled intracellular material into the medium. (a) The points show the percentage of specific lysis of individual wells. The dashed line indicates three standard deviations above the medium release control,

and each point above that line is counted as positive for cytotoxicity. (b) The data replotted in terms of the percentage of negative wells at each concentration of responder cells over the range in which the data titrated (5×10^{-3}/well to 0.625×10^{-3}/well). The dashed line is drawn at 37% negative wells and this intersects the regression line to give a precursor (T_{cp}) frequency of 1 in 2327 responder cells. The regression line has an r^2 value of 1.00 in this experiment. (Reproduced with permission from Simpson E. & Chandler P. (1986) In Weir D.M. (ed.) *Handbook of Experimental Immunology*, figure 68.2. Blackwell Scientific Publications, Oxford.)

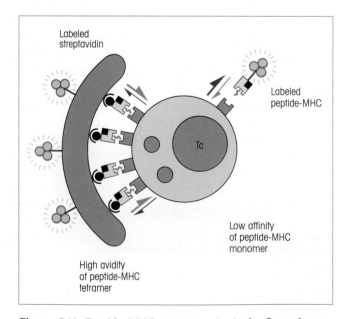

Figure 7.10. Peptide–MHC tetramer. A single fluorochrome-labeled peptide–MHC complex (top right) has only a low affinity for the TCR and therefore provides a very insensitive probe for its cognate receptor. However, by biotinylating (●) the MHC molecules and then mixing them with streptavidin, which has a valency of four with respect to biotin binding, a tetrameric complex is formed which has a much higher functional affinity (avidity) when used as a probe for the specific TCRs on the T-cell surface.

The name of the test derives from the fact that antigen is sandwiched between the antibody present in the cell substrate and that added as the second layer (figure 7.3c).

Plaque techniques

Antibody-secreting cells can be counted by diluting them in an environment in which the antibody formed by each individual cell produces a readily observable effect. In one technique, developed from the original method of Jerne and Nordin, the cells from an animal immunized with sheep erythrocytes are suspended together with an excess of sheep red cells and complement within a shallow chamber formed between two microscope slides. On incubation, the antibody-forming cells release their immunoglobulin which coats the surrounding erythrocytes. The complement will then cause lysis of the coated cells and a **plaque** clear of red cells will be seen around each antibody-forming cell (figure 7.11). Direct plaques obtained in this way largely reveal IgM producers since this antibody has a high hemolytic efficiency. To demonstrate IgG synthesizing cells it is necessary to increase the complement binding of the erythrocyte–IgG antibody complex by adding a rabbit anti-IgG serum; the 'indi-

Figure 7.11. Jerne plaque technique for enumerating antibody-forming cells (Cunningham modification). (a) The *direct* technique for cells synthesizing IgM hemolysin is shown. The *indirect* technique for visualizing cells producing IgG hemolysins requires the addition of anti-IgG to the system. The difference between the plaques obtained by direct and indirect methods gives the number of 'IgG' plaques. The *reverse plaque* assay enumerates total Ig-producing cells by capturing secreted Ig on red cells coated with anti-Ig. Multiple plaque assays can be carried out by a modification using microtiter plates. (b) Photograph of plaques which show as circular dark areas (some of which are arrowed) under dark-ground illumination. They vary in size depending upon the antibody affinity and the rate of secretion by the antibody-forming cell. (Courtesy of C. Shapland, P. Hutchings and Professor D. Male.)

rect plaques' thus developed can be used to enumerate cells making antibodies in different immunoglobulin subclasses, provided that the appropriate rabbit antisera are available. The method can be extended by coating an antigen such as *Pneumococcus* polysaccharide on to the red cell, or by coupling hapten groups to the erythrocyte surface.

In the **ELISPOT** modification, the antibody-forming cell suspension is incubated in microtiter wells containing filters coated with antigen. The secreted antibody is captured locally and is visualized, after removal of the cells, by treatment with enzyme-labeled anti-Ig and development of the color reaction with the substrate. The macroscopic spots can be readily enumerated (figure 7.12).

Analysis of functional activity by cellular reconstitution

Radiation chimeras

The entire populations of lymphocytes and polymorphs can be inactivated by appropriate doses of X-irradiation. Animals ablated in such a way may be reconstituted by injection of bone marrow hematopoietic stem cells which provide the precursors of all the formed elements of the blood (cf. figure 12.1). These chimeras of host plus hematopoietic grafted cells can be manipulated in many ways to analyse cellular function, such as the role of the thymus in the maturation of T-lymphocytes from bone marrow stem cells (figure 7.13).

Mice with severe combined immunodeficiency (SCID)

Mice with defects in the genes encoding the IL-2 receptor γ chain, the nucleotide salvage pathway enzymes adenosine deaminase or purine nucleoside phosphorylase, or the RAG enzymes, develop SCID due to a failure of B- and T-cells to differentiate. These special animals can be reconstituted with various human lymphoid tissues and their functions and responses analysed. Coimplantation of contiguous fragments of human fetal liver (hematopoietic stem cells) and thymus allows T-lymphopoiesis, production of B-cells and maintenance of colony-forming units of myeloid and erythroid lineages for 6–12 months. Adult peripheral blood cells injected into the peritoneal cavity of SCID mice treated with growth hormone can sustain the production of human B-cells and antibodies and can be used to generate human hybridomas making defined monoclonal antibodies. Immunotherapeutic antitumor responses can also be played with in these animals.

Cellular interactions in vitro

It is obvious that the methods outlined earlier for depletion, enrichment and isolation of individual cell populations enable the investigator to study cellular interactions through judicious recombinations. These interactions are usually more effective when the cells are operating within some sort of stromal network resembling the set-up of the tissues where their function is optimally expressed. For example, colonization of

Figure 7.12. ELISPOT (from ELISA spot) system for enumerating antibody-forming cells. The picture shows spots formed by hybridoma cells making autoantibodies to thyroglobulin revealed by alkaline phosphatase-linked anti-Ig (courtesy of P. Hutchings). Increasing numbers of hybridoma cells were added to the top two and bottom left-hand wells which show corresponding increases in the number of 'ELISPOTs'. The bottom right-hand well is a control using a hybridoma of irrelevant specificity.

murine fetal thymus rudiments in culture with T-cell precursors enables one to follow the pattern of proliferation, maturation, TCR rearrangement and positive and negative selection normally seen *in vivo* (cf.

Operation	Irradiation	Restitution	Induction of cell-mediated immunity
1 Sham thymectomy	(X)	Bone marrow	++
2 Thymectomy	(X)	Bone marrow	–
3 Thymectomy	(X)	Bone marrow + adult lymphocytes	++

Figure 7.13. Maturation of bone marrow stem cells under the influence of the thymus to become immunocompetent lymphocytes capable of cell-mediated immune reactions. X-irradiation (X) destroys the ability of host lymphocytes to mount a cellular immune response, but the stem cells in injected bone marrow can become immunocompetent and restore the response (1) unless the thymus is removed (2), in which case only already immunocompetent lymphocytes are effective (3). Incidentally, the bone marrow stem cells also restore the levels of other formed elements of the blood (red cells, platelets, neutrophils, monocytes) which otherwise fall dramatically after X-irradiation, and such therapy is crucial in cases where accidental or therapeutic exposure to X-rays or other antimitotic agents seriously damages the hematopoietic cells.

p. 225). An even more refined system involves the addition of selected lymphoid populations to disaggregated stromal cells derived from fetal thymic lobes depleted of endogenous lymphoid cells with deoxyguanosine. The cells can be spun into a pellet and cocultured in hanging drops; on transfer to normal organ culture conditions after a few hours, reaggregation to intact lobes takes place quite magically and the various differentiation and maturation processes then unfold.

Probing function with antibodies

Antibodies can be used to confirm the importance of cross-linking cell surface components for a number of functions. An excellent example is the induction of histamine release from mast cells by divalent $F(ab')_2$ anti-FcεRI but not by the univalent fragment. Similarly, divalent anti-FcγR triggers phagocytosis in macrophages, while a bispecific antibody to CD3 and CD4 brings the two molecules together on the T-cell surface and induces activation.

Spatially defined intracellular damage by chromophore-assisted laser inactivation can be carried out using antibodies. A neuronal growth cone in a living embryo, for example, can be permeabilized and loaded with anticalcineurin labeled with malachite green which absorbs light at 620 nm where most cellular constituents do not. A laser emitting light of this

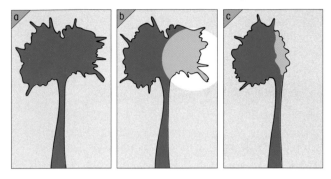

Figure 7.14. Microsurgery of a neuronal growth cone loaded with a malachite green-labeled antibody to calcineurin. The growth cone shows laser-induced retraction of membrane extensions: (a) before, (b) during and (c) after the laser flash. (Reproduced from a commentary by Muller B.K. & Bonhoeffer F. (1995) *Current Biology* **11**, 1255 on experiments by Jay D.G. and colleagues (1995) *Nature* **376**, 686, with permission.)

wavelength will irradiate the antibody–chromophore conjugate, so generating a pulse of highly reactive free radicals which cause inactivation in a small region of diameter around 15 Å. Figure 7.14 shows that the laser flash results in retraction of filopodial and lamellipodial membrane extensions. This in turn influences the direction of subsequent growth cone movement, so demonstrating the involvement of the calmodulin-dependent phosphatase, calcineurin, in growth cone steering. By operating at different embryonic stages the investigator can knock out functions in a temporally as well as spatially restricted fashion. This should prove to be a discriminating cellular microsurgical tool of considerable utility and applicability.

GENETIC ENGINEERING OF CELLS

Insertion and modification of genes in mammalian cells

Because gene transfer into mammalian cells is inefficient, it is customary to use immortal cell lines for such **transfections** and to include a selectable marker such as neomycin resistance. Genes can be introduced into cells as calcium phosphate precipitates or by electroporation, in which a brief electric pulse transiently creates holes in the cell membrane. Another approach is to incorporate the gene into liposomes which fuse with the cell membrane. Direct microinjection of DNA is also effective. Integration of the gene into the genome of a virus such as vaccinia provides an easy ride into the cell, although more stable long-term transfections are obtained with modified retroviral vectors. One of the latest fads is transfection by biolistics, the buzz word for biological ballistics. DNA coated on to gold

microparticles is literally fired from a high-pressure helium gun and penetrates the cells; even plant cells with their cellulose coats are easy meat for this technology. Skin and surgically exposed tissues can also be penetrated with ease.

Studying the effect of *adding* a gene, then, does not offer too many technological problems. How does one assess the impact of *removing* a gene? One versatile strategy to delete endogenous gene function is to target the gene's mRNA as distinct from the gene itself. Nucleotide sequences complementary to the mRNA of the target gene are introduced into the cell, usually in a form which allows them to replicate. The **antisense** molecules so produced base pair with the target mRNA and block translation into protein.

Introducing new genes into animals

Establishing 'designer mice' bearing new genes

Female mice are induced to superovulate and are then mated. The fertilized eggs are microinjected with the gene and surgically implanted in females. Between 5% and 40% of the implanted oocytes develop to term and, of these, 10–25% have copies of the injected gene, stably integrated into their chromosomes, detectable by PCR. These 'founder' transgenic animals are mated with nontransgenic mice and pure transgenic lines are eventually established (figure 7.15).

Expression of the transgene can be directed to particular tissues if the relevant promoter is included in the construct, for example the thyroglobulin promoter will confine expression to the thyroid. A different approach is to switch a gene on and off at will by incorporating an inducible promoter. Thus, the metallothionine promoter will enable expression of its linked gene only if zinc is added to the drinking water given to the mice. One needs to confirm that only the desired expression is obtained as, in some situations, promoters may misbehave leading to 'leaky' expression of the associated gene.

Transgenes introduced into embryonic stem cells

Embryonic stem (ES) cells can be obtained by culturing the inner cell mass of mouse blastocysts. After transfection with the appropriate gene, the transfected cells can be selected and reimplanted after injection into a new blastocyst. The resulting mice are chimeric, in that some cells carry the transgene and others do not. The same will be true of germ cells and, by breeding for germ-line transmission of the transgene, pure strains can be derived (figure 7.16).

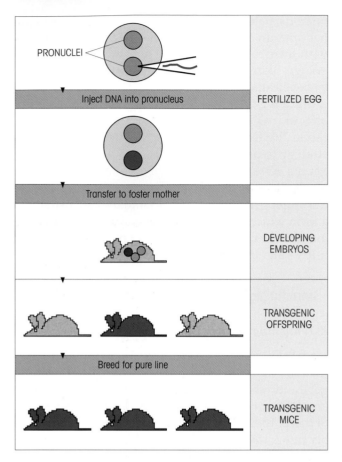

Figure 7.15. Production of pure strain transgenic mice by microinjection of fertilized egg, implantation into a foster mother and subsequent inbreeding.

Figure 7.16. Introduction of a transgene through transfection of embryonic stem cells. The transfected cells can be selected, e.g. for homologous recombinant 'knockouts', before reimplantation. LIF, leukemia inhibitory factor.

The advantage over microinjection is that the cells can be selected after transfection, and this is especially important if **homologous recombination** is required in order to generate '**knockout mice**' lacking the gene which has been targeted. In this case, a DNA sequence which will disrupt the reading frame of the endogenous gene is inserted into the ES cells. Because homologous recombination is a rare event compared to random integration, selectable markers are incorporated into the construct in order to transfer only those ES cells in which the endogenous gene has been deleted (figure 7.17). This is a truly powerful technology and the whole biological community has been suffused with boxing fever, knocking out genes right, left and center. Just a few examples of knockout mice of interest to immunologists are listed in table 7.2.

It is not a particularly rare finding to observe that knocking out a gene unexpectedly leads to developmental defects. Whilst this in itself can provide important information implicating the gene in the developmental biology of the animal, it can frustrate the original aim of the experiment. Indeed, a number of knockouts are nonviable due to embryonic lethality. Never fear, ingenuity once again triumphs, in this case by the harnessing of viral or yeast recombinase systems. Instead of using a nonfunctional gene to create the knockout mouse, the targeting construct contains the normal form of the gene but flanked with recognition sequences (*loxP* sites) for a recombinase enzyme called Cre. These mice are mated with transgenic mice containing the bacteriophage P1-derived *Cre* transgene linked to an inducible or tissue-specific promoter. The endogenous gene of interest will be deleted only

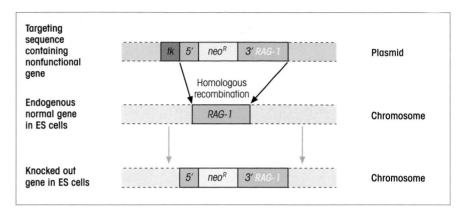

Figure 7.17. Gene disruption by homologous recombination with plasmid DNA containing a copy of the gene of interest (in this example *RAG-1*) into which a sequence specifying neomycin resistance (*neo^R*) has been inserted in such a way as to destroy the *RAG-1* reading frame between the 5′ and 3′ ends of the gene. Embryonic stem (ES) cells in which the targeting sequence has been incorporated into the chromosomal DNA by homologous recombination will be resistant to the neomycin analog G418. Stem cells in which nonhomologous recombination into chromosomal DNA has occurred would additionally incorporate the *thymidine kinase* (*tk*) gene which can be used to destroy such cells by culturing them in the presence of ganciclovir, leaving only ES cells in which homologous recombination has been achieved. These are then used to create a knockout mouse.

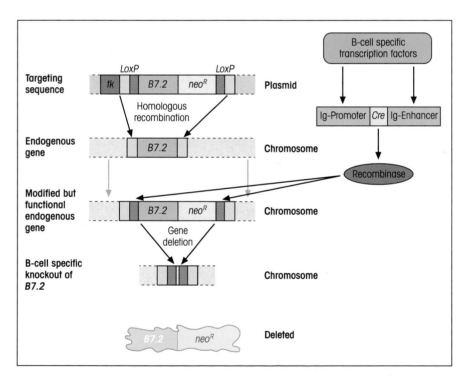

Figure 7.18. Conditional knockout. The endogenous gene that is under study (here *B7.2*) is homologously replaced in ES cells with an identical gene, as in figure 7.17, but here flanked by *loxP* sequences (brown boxes) and with the *neo^R* gene incorporated in a nondisruptive manner purely for selection purposes. Nonhomologous recombinants will contain the *tk* gene and are eliminated using ganciclovir. Transgenic animals are then generated from ES cells which are resistant to G418. If homozygous *B7.2–loxP* transgenics are mated with mice which contain a transgene for the Cre recombinase under the control of specific regulatory elements, only those cells in which the promoter is active will produce the Cre enzyme necessary to delete the sequence flanked by *loxP*. The example given would represent an experiment aimed at investigating the effect of specifically knocking out *B7.2* in B-cells whilst maintaining its expression in, for example, dendritic cells.

when and where Cre is expressed (figure 7.18). The Cre/*loxP* system can also be organized in such a way as to turn on expression of a gene by incorporating a stop sequence flanked by *loxP* sites.

Mice in which an endogenous gene is purposefully replaced by a functional gene, be it a modified version of the original gene or an entirely different gene, are referred to as **'knocked in mice'**. Hence, in the example above, knocking in a *loxP* flanked gene leads eventually to a knocked out gene in a selected cell type. Another

Table 7.2. Some gene 'knockouts' and their effects.

Knockout target	Phenotype of knockout mice
CD8 α-chain	Absence of cytotoxic T-cells
p59 ^{fynT}	Defective signalling in thymocytes but not peripheral T-cells
HOX 11	No spleen
IgE	No defects observed!
FcεRI α-chain	Resistant to cutaneous and systemic anaphylaxis
IgM μ-chain membrane exon	Absence of B-cells
IL-6	No bone loss when ovariectomized (implications for osteoporosis?)
IL-18	Susceptible to *Leishmania major*; shift from Th1 to Th2 response (decreased IFNγ and increased IL-4 production)
MHC class II Aβ	Decreased CD4 T-cells; inflammatory bowel disease
Perforin	Impaired CTL and NK cell function
TAP1	Lack CD8 cells
TNFR-1	Resistant to endotoxic shock; susceptible to *Listeria*

Modified from Brandon (1995) *Current Biology* **5**, 625.

example of a knocked in gene was seen on p. 133 with the replacement of endogenous *RAG-2* with a *RAG-2–GFP* fusion gene.

Gene therapy in humans. We seem to be catching up with science fiction and are in the early stages of being able to correct genetic misfortune by the introduction of 'good' genes. Effective gene delivery still poses major problems but there have been some recent successes. One form of severe combined immunodeficiency (SCID) is due to a mutation in the χc gene which encodes a subunit of the cytokine receptors for IL-2, -4, -7, -9 and -15. Correction of this defect in children has been achieved by *in vitro* transfer of the normal gene into CD34$^+$ bone marrow stem cells using a vector derived from a Moloney retrovirus, a convincing proof of principle for human gene therapy. Adenovirus vectors have also proved popular in past attempts at gene therapy but are increasingly being replaced by adeno-associated virus (AAV) which may be safer. Some success has been achieved using intramuscular injection of AAV-based vectors to transfer human blood clotting factor IX into patients with hemophilia B.

SUMMARY

Isolation of leukocyte subpopulations

• Cells can be separated on the basis of physical characteristics such as size, buoyant density and adhesiveness.

• Phagocytic cells can be separated by a magnet after taking up iron particles, and cells which divide in response to a specific stimulus, e.g. antigen, can be eliminated by ultraviolet light after incorporation of 5-bromodeoxyuridine.

• Antibody-coated cells can be eliminated by complement-mediated cytotoxicity or anti-Ig–ricin conjugates; they can be isolated by panning on solid-phase anti-Ig or by cluster formation with magnetic beads bearing anti-Ig on their surface.

• Smaller numbers of cells can be fractionated by coating with a fluorescent monoclonal antibody and separating them from nonfluorescent cells in the FACS.

• Antigen-specific T-cells can be enriched as lines or clones by driving them with antigen; fusion to appropriate T-cell tumor lines yields immortal antigen-specific T-cell hybridomas.

Immunohistochemical localization of antigens in cells and tissues

• Antigens can be localized if stained by fluorescent antibodies and viewed in a fluorescence microscope.

• Confocal microscopy scans a very thin plane at high magnification and provides quantitative data on extremely sharp images of the antigen-containing structures which can also be examined in three dimensions.

• Antibodies can either be labeled directly or visualized by a second antibody, a labeled anti-Ig.

• In a flow cytometer single cells in individual droplets are interrogated by one or more lasers and quantitative data using different fluorescent labels can be logged, giving a complex phenotypic analysis of each cell in a heterogeneous mixture. In addition, forward scatter of the laser light defines cell size and 90° scatter, cell granularity.

• Fluorescent antibodies or their fragments can also be used for staining intracellular antigens in permeabilized cells. Intracellular probes for pH, Ca^{2+}, Mg^{2+}, Na^+, thiols and DNA content are also available. Gene regulatory elements linked to a reporter gene such as *GFP* can also now be studied at the single-cell level by flow cytometry.

• Antibodies can be enzyme-labeled for histochemical definition of antigens at the light microscope level, and coupled with different-sized colloidal gold particles for ultrastructural visualization in the electron microscope.

(continued)

Gene expression

- mRNA expression can be localized by *in situ* hybridization using a complementary oligonucleotide probe.
- A complete picture of cellular gene expression is now attainable by hybridization to microarray chips.

Assessment of functional activity

- Neutrophil chemotaxis, phagocytosis, NADH (reduced nicotinamide adenine dinucleotide) oxidase activity and microbicidal potency can all be studied, almost on a routine basis.
- Lymphocyte responses to antigen are monitored by proliferation and/or cytokine release. Individual cells secreting cytokines can be identified by the ELISPOT technique in which the secreted product is captured by a solid-phase antibody and then stained with a second labeled antibody.
- Extracellular killing by cytotoxic T-cells, and NK cells, can be measured by the release of radioactive ^{51}Cr from prelabeled target cells.
- The precursor frequency of effector T-cells can be measured by staining the cells with peptide–MHC tetramers or by limiting dilution analysis.
- Antibody-forming cells can be enumerated, either by an immunofluorescence sandwich test or by plaque techniques in which the antibody secreted by the cells causes complement-mediated lysis of adjacent red cells, or is captured by solid-phase antigen in an ELISPOT assay.
- Functional activity can be assessed by cellular reconstitution experiments in which leukocyte sets and selected lymphoid tissue can be transplanted into unresponsive hosts such as X-irradiated recipients or SCID mice. Defined cell populations can also be separated and selectively recombined *in vitro*.
- Antibodies can be used to probe cellular function by cross-linking cell surface components or by selective destruction of particular intracellular sites by laser irradiation of chromophore-conjugated specific antibodies which localize to the target area by penetrating permeabilized cells.

Genetic engineering of cells

- Genes can be inserted into mammalian cells by transfection using calcium phosphate precipitates, electroporation, liposomes and microinjection.
- Genes can also be taken into a cell after incorporation into vaccinia or retroviruses.
- Endogenous gene function can be inhibited by antisense RNA or by homologous recombination with a disrupted gene.
- Transgenic mice bearing an entirely new gene introduced into the fertilized egg by microinjection of DNA can be established as inbred lines.
- Genes can be introduced into embryonic stem cells; these modified stem cells are injected back into a blastocyst and can develop into founder mice from which pure transgenic animals can be bred. One very important application of this technique involves the disruption of a targeted gene in the embryonic stem cell by homologous recombination, producing 'knockout' mice lacking a specific gene. Conditional knockouts employ recombinase systems such as Cre/*loxP* in order to control the deletion either temporally or in a tissue-specific manner.
- 'Knock in' mice have a specified endogenous gene homologously replaced with either a variant of that gene or an entirely different gene.
- Human gene therapy promises an exciting future. Delivery of genes by vectors based on retroviruses or adeno-related virus is under intensive investigation.

See the accompanying website (**www.roitt.com**) for multiple choice questions.

FURTHER READING

Ausubel F.M., Brent R., Kingston R.E., Moore D.D., Seidman J.G., Smith J.A. & Struhl K. (eds) (1987; continually updated) *Current Protocols in Molecular Biology, 1–2*. Greene Publishing Associates & Wiley-Interscience, New York.

Brandtzaeg P. (1998) The increasing power of immunohistochemistry and immunocytochemistry. *Journal of Immunological Methods* **216**, 49.

Carter L.L. & Swain S.L. (1997) Single cytokine analysis of cytokine production. *Current Opinion in Immunology* **9**, 177.

Cavazzana-Calvo S. *et al.* (2000) Gene therapy of human severe combined immunodeficiency (SCID)-XI disease. *Science* **288**, 669.

Coligan J.E., Kruisbeek A.M., Margulies D.H., Shevach E.M. & Strober W. (eds) (1991; continually updated) *Current Protocols in Immunology, 1–2*. Greene Publishing Associates & Wiley-Interscience, New York.

Cotter T.G. & Martin S.J. (eds) (1996) *Techniques in Apoptosis: A User's Guide*. Portland Press, London.

Lefkovits I. & Waldmann H. (1999) *Limiting Dilution Analysis of Cells of the Immune System*, 2nd edn. Oxford University Press, Oxford.

Monroe R.J. *et al.* (1999) RAG2:GFP knockin mice reveal novel aspects of RAG2 expression in primary and peripheral lymphoid tissues. *Immunity* **11**, 201.

Ogg G.S. & McMichael A.J. (1998) HLA–peptide tetrameric complexes. *Current Opinion in Immunology* **10**, 393.

Robinson J.P. & Babcock G.F. (eds) (1998) *Phagocyte Function: A Guide for Research and Clinical Evaluation*. Wiley-Liss, New York.

Staudt L.M. & Brown P.O. (2000) Genomic views of the immune system. *Annual Reviews of Immunology* **18**, 829.

Storch W.B. (2000) *Immunofluorescence in Clinical Immunology: A Primer and Atlas*. Birkhäuser Verlag AG, Basel.

Watson J.D., Gilman M., Witkowski J. & Zoller M. (1992) *Recombinant DNA*, 2nd edn. Scientific American Books, New York.

Weir D.M. *et al.* (eds) (1996) *Handbook of Experimental Immunology: Volume 4*, 5th edn. Blackwell Scientific Publications, Oxford.

The anatomy of the immune response

INTRODUCTION

In order to discuss the events which occur in the operation of the immune system as a whole, it is imperative to establish a nomenclature which identifies the surface markers on the cells involved since these are used for communication and are usually functional molecules reflecting the state of cellular differentiation. The nomenclature system is established as follows. Immunologists from the far corners of the world who have produced monoclonal antibodies directed to surface molecules on B- and T-cells, macrophages, neutrophils and natural killer (NK) cells, and so on, get together every so often to compare the specificities of their reagents in international workshops whose spirit of cooperation should be a lesson to most politicians. Where a cluster of monoclonals are found to react with the same polypeptide, they clearly represent a series of reagents defining a given marker and are labeled with a CD (**cluster of differentiation**) number. Currently, there are nearly 250 CD numbers assigned, with some of them having subdivisions, but those in table 8.1 are most relevant to our discussions. A complete list of CD markers is given in Appendix 1. It is important to appreciate that the expression level of cell surface molecules often changes as cells differentiate or become activated and that 'subpopulations' of cells exist which differentially express particular molecules. When expressed at a low level the 'presence' or 'absence' of a given CD antigen may be rather subjective, but be aware that low level expression does not necessarily imply biological irrelevance.

THE NEED FOR ORGANIZED LYMPHOID TISSUE

For an effective immune response, an intricate series of cellular events must occur. Antigen must bind and if necessary be processed by antigen-presenting cells, which must then make contact with and activate T- and B-cells; T-helpers must assist B-cells and cytotoxic T-cell precursors, and there have to be mechanisms which amplify the numbers of potential effector cells by proliferation and then bring about differentiation to generate the mediators of humoral and cellular immunity. In addition, memory cells for secondary responses must be formed and the whole response controlled so that it is adequate but not excessive and is appropriate to the type of infection being dealt with. By working hard, we can isolate component cells of the immune system and persuade them to carry out a number of responses to antigen in the test-tube, but compared with the efficacy of the overall development of immunity in the body, our efforts still leave much to be desired. *In vivo* the integration of the complex cellular interactions which form the basis of the immune response takes place within the organized architecture

Table 8.1. Some of the major clusters of differentiation (CD) markers on human cells.

CD	Expression	Functions
CD1	IDC, B subset	Presents glycolipid and other non-peptide antigens to T-cells
CD2	T, NK	Receptor for CD58 (LFA-3) costimulator. Binds sheep rbc
CD3	T	Transducing elements of T-cell receptor
CD4	T-helper, Mo, Mϕ	MHC class II. HIV receptor
CD5	T, B subset	Involved in antigen receptor signaling
CD8	T-cytotoxic	MHC class I receptor
CD14	G, Mo, Mϕ	LPS/LBP complex receptor
CD16	G, NK, B, Mϕ, IDC	FcγRIII (medium affinity IgG receptor)
CD19	B, FDC	Part of B-cell antigen receptor complex
CD20	B	Unknown, but able to provide intracellular signals
CD21	B, FDC	CR2. Receptor for C3d and Epstein–Barr virus. Part of B-cell antigen receptor complex
CD23	B, Mo, FDC	FcεRII (low affinity IgE receptor)
CD25	*T, *B, *Mo, *Mϕ	IL-2 receptor α chain
CD28	T, *B	Receptor for CD80/CD86 (B7.1 and B7.2) costimulators
CD32	Mo, Mϕ, IDC, FDC, G, NK, B,	FcγRII (low affinity IgG receptor)
CD34	Progenitors	Adhesion molecule. Stem cell marker
CD40	B, Mϕ, IDC, FDC	Receptor for CD40L costimulator
CD45RA	Resting/Naive T-cells, B, G, Mo, NK	Phosphatase, cell activation
CD45RO	Activated/Memory T-cells, Mo, DC	Phosphatase, cell activation
CD64	Mo, Mϕ, DC	FcγRI (high affinity IgG receptor)
CD79a/CD79b	B	Transducing elements of B-cell receptor
CD80	*B, *T, Mϕ, DC	B7.1 receptor for CD28 costimulator and for CTLA4 inhibitory signal
CD86	B, IDC, Mo	B7.2 receptor for CD28 costimulator and for CTLA4 inhibitory signal
CD95	Widespread	Fas receptor for FasL. Transmits apoptotic signals

*, activated; B, B-lymphocytes; FDC, follicular dendritic cells; G, granulocytes; IDC, interdigitating dendritic cells; Mast, mast cells; Mϕ, macrophages; Mo, monocytes; NK, natural killer cells; T, T-lymphocytes.

of peripheral, or secondary, lymphoid tissue which includes the lymph nodes, spleen and unencapsulated tissue lining the respiratory, gastrointestinal and genitourinary tracts.

These tissues become populated by cells of reticular origin and by macrophages and lymphocytes derived

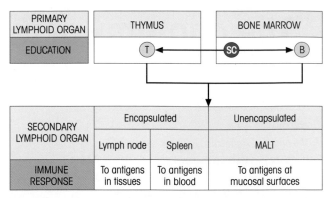

Figure 8.1. **The functional organization of lymphoid tissue.** Stem cells (SC) arising in the bone marrow differentiate into immunocompetent T- and B-cells in the primary lymphoid organs and then colonize the secondary lymphoid tissues where immune responses are organized. The mucosal-associated lymphoid tissue (MALT) produces antibodies for mucosal secretions.

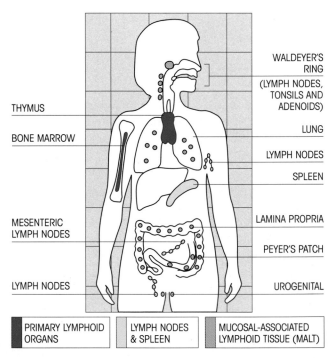

Figure 8.2. **The distribution of major lymphoid organs and tissues throughout the body.**

from bone marrow stem cells, the T-cells first differentiating into immunocompetent cells by a high-pressure training period in the thymus, the B-cells undergoing their education in the bone marrow itself (figure 8.1). In essence, the lymph nodes filter off and, if necessary, respond to foreign material draining body tissues, the spleen monitors the blood and the unencapsulated lymphoid tissue is strategically integrated into mucosal surfaces of the body as a forward defensive system based on IgA secretion.

The anatomical disposition of these lymphoid tissues is illustrated in figure 8.2. The lymphatics and associated lymph nodes form an impressive network, draining the viscera and the more superficial body structures before returning to the blood by way of the thoracic duct (figure 8.3).

Communication between these tissues and the rest of the body is maintained by a pool of recirculating lymphocytes which pass from the blood into the lymph nodes, spleen and other tissues and back to the blood by the major lymphatic channels such as the thoracic duct (figures 8.4 and 8.10).

LYMPHOCYTES TRAFFIC BETWEEN LYMPHOID TISSUES

This traffic of lymphocytes between the tissues, the bloodstream and the lymph nodes enables antigen-sensitive cells to seek the antigen and to be recruited to sites at which a response is occurring, while the dissemination of memory cells and their progeny enables a more widespread response to be organized throughout the lymphoid system. Thus, antigen-reactive cells are depleted from the circulating pool of lymphocytes within 24 hours of antigen first localizing in the lymph nodes or spleen; several days later, after proliferation at the site of antigen localization, a peak of activated cells appears in the thoracic duct. When antigen reaches a lymph node in a primed animal, there is a dramatic fall in the output of cells in the efferent lymphatics, a phenomenon described variously as 'cell shutdown' or 'lymphocyte trapping' and which is thought to result from the antigen-induced release of soluble factors from T-cells (cf. the cytokines, p. 179); this is followed by an output of activated blast cells which peaks at around 80 hours.

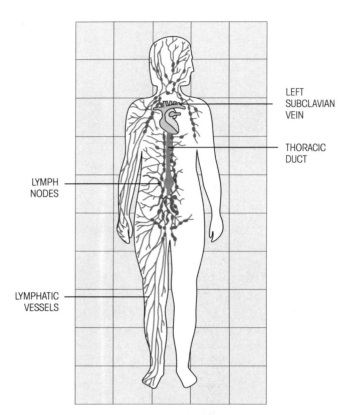

Figure 8.3. The network of lymph nodes and lymphatics. Lymph nodes occur at junctions of the draining lymphatics. The lymph finally collects in the thoracic duct and thence returns to the bloodstream via the left subclavian vein.

Lymphocytes home to their specific tissues

Naive lymphocytes enter a lymph node through the afferent lymphatics and by guided passage across the

Figure 8.4. Traffic and recirculation of lymphocytes through encapsulated lymphoid tissue and sites of inflammation. Blood-borne lymphocytes enter the tissues and lymph nodes passing through the high-walled endothelium of the postcapillary venules (HEV) and leave via the draining lymphatics. The efferent lymphatics, finally emerging from the last node in each chain, join to form the thoracic duct which returns the lymphocytes to the bloodstream. In the spleen, which lacks HEVs, lymphocytes enter the lymphoid area (white pulp) from the arterioles, pass to the sinusoids of the erythroid area (red pulp) and leave by the splenic vein. Traffic through the mucosal immune system is elaborated in figure 8.10.

(a)

(b)

(c)

Figure 8.5. Lymphocyte association with postcapillary venules. (a) High-walled endothelial cells (HEC) of postcapillary venules in rat cervical lymph nodes showing intimate association with lymphocytes (Ly). (b) Flattened capillary endothelial cell (EC) for comparison. (c) Lymphocytes adhering to HEC (scanning electron micrograph). ((a) and (b) Kindly provided by Dr Ann Ager and (c) by Dr W. van Ewijk.)

specialized **high-walled endothelium of the postcapillary venules (HEVs)** (figure 8.5). Comparable HEVs offer the transit of cells concerned in mucosal immunity to Peyer's patches. In other cases involving migration into normal and inflamed tissues, the lymphocytes bind to and cross nonspecialized flatter endothelia. Lymphoblasts and memory cell populations display tissue-restricted migration to extralymphoid sites such as skin or mucosal epithelium, while lymphocytes, as well as neutrophils and monocytes, target and migrate into sites of inflammation in response to locally produced mediators.

This highly organized traffic is orchestrated by directing the relevant lymphocytes to different parts of the lymphoid system and the various other tissues by a series of **homing receptors** which include members of the **integrin** superfamily (table 8.2) and also a member of the selectin family, L-selectin. Integrins can bind to extracellular matrix, plasma proteins and to other cell surface molecules, and they are widely involved in embryogenesis, cell growth, differentiation, adhesion, motility, programed cell death and tissue maintenance. Within the immune system their complementary ligands include cell surface **vascular addressins** present on the appropriate blood vessel endothelium (figure 8.6). These act as selective gateways which allow partic-

ular populations of lymphocytes access to the appropriate tissue (table 8.3). Chemokines such as SLC (*secondary lymphoid tissue chemokine*), presented by vascular endothelium, play a key role in triggering lymphocyte arrest, the chemokine receptors on the lymphocyte being involved in the functional upregulation of integrins. With respect to lymphocytes and dendritic cells which are destined for the skin, E-selectin on the endothelium recognizes cutaneous leukocyte antigen (CLA) on these cells.

Transmigration occurs in three stages

Step 1: Tethering and rolling

In order for the lymphocyte to become attached to the endothelial cell, it has to overcome the shear forces created by the blood flow. This is effected by a force of attraction between the homing receptors and their ligands on the vessel wall which operates through microvilli on the leukocyte surface (figure 8.6). After this tethering process, the lymphocyte rolls along the endothelial cell, with the integrins VLA-4 or LPAM-1 on the lymphocyte binding to their ligands on the endothelium.

Step 2: LFA-1 activation and cell flattening

This process leads to activation and recruitment of LFA-1 to the nonvillous surface of the lymphocyte. This integrin binds very strongly to ICAM-1 and -2 on the endothelial cell, the intimate contact causing the lymphocyte to flatten.

Table 8.2. The integrin superfamily. In general, the integrins are concerned with intercellular adhesion and adhesion to extracellular matrix components. Many of them are also involved in cell signal transduction. They are heterodimers with unique but related α chains which can be grouped into subsets, each of which has a common β chain. The VLA subfamily took its name from VLA-1 and -2 which appeared as very late antigens (VLA) on T-cells, 2–4 weeks after *in vitro* activation. However, VLA-3, -4 and -5 belong to the same family but are not 'very late' and are found to different extents on lymphocytes, monocytes, platelets and probably hematopoietic progenitors. A structure called the I (inserted) domain is present in many integrin subunits and contains the *m*etal *i*on-*d*ependent *a*dhesion *s*ite (MIDAS) which, in the presence of Mg^{2+}, is involved in binding the Arg.Gly.Asp. (RGD) motif on many of the ligands essential for cell adhesion.

Integrin	Subunits	*CD group	Expression	Ligand
		VLA proteins		
VLA-1	$\alpha_1\beta_1$	CD49a/CD29	Widespread	LM, CO
VLA-2	$\alpha_2\beta_1$	CD49b/CD29	Widespread	LM, CO
VLA-3	$\alpha_3\beta_1$	CD49c/CD29	Widespread	FN, LM, CO, EN
VLA-4	$\alpha_4\beta_1$	CD49d/CD29	Widespread	FN, VCAM-1
VLA-5	$\alpha_5\beta_1$	CD49e/CD29	Widespread	FN
VLA-6	$\alpha_6\beta_1$	CD49f/CD29	Widespread	LM
		Leukocyte integrins		
LFA-1	$\alpha_L\beta_2$	CD11a/CD18	Leukocytes	ICAM-1,-2,-3
CR3 (Mac-1)	$\alpha_M\beta_2$	CD11b/CD18	N, Mo, LGL	ICAM-1, C3bi, FG, FX
p150,95	$\alpha_X\beta_2$	CD11c/CD18	M, Mo, N	C3bi, LPS
	$\alpha_D\beta_2$	CD11d/CD18	Tissue M	ICAM-3
LPAM-1	$\alpha_4\beta_7$	CD49d/ND	Lymphocytes	MAdCAM-1, VCAM-1, FN
	$\alpha_E\beta_7$	CD103/ND	Intraepithelial T-cells	E-cadherin
		Cytoadhesins		
GPIIb/IIIa	$\alpha_{IIb}\beta_3$	CD41/CD61	Megakaryocytes, platelets	FN,VN,FG, VWF, THR
VN receptor	$\alpha_V\beta_3$	CD51/CD61	Widespread	VN,FN,FG, VWF, THR, TN

CO, collagen; CR3, complement receptor 3; EN, entactin; FG, fibrinogen; FN, fibronectin; FX, factor X; GPIIb/IIIa, integrin glycoproteins IIb and IIIa; ICAM, intercellular adhesion molecule; LFA, lymphocyte function-associated molecule; LGL, large granular lymphocyte; LM, laminin; LPAM, lymphocyte Peyer's patch adhesion molecule; M, macrophage; MAdCAM, mucosal addressin cell adhesion molecule; Mo, monocyte; N, neutrophil; THR, thrombospondin; TN, tenascin; VCAM, vascular cell adhesion molecule; VLA, very late antigen (although they are not all expressed late!); VN, vitronectin; VWF, von Willebrand factor. *CD markers are explained on p. 147. ND, no CD designation yet assigned.

Step 3: Diapedesis

The flattened lymphocyte now uses the LFA-1–ICAM interaction and the immunoglobulin superfamily member PECAM-1 (*p*latelet *e*ndothelial *c*ell *a*dhesion *m*olecule, CD31; not only present on platelets, see Appendix 1), to elbow its way between the endothelial cells and into the tissue in response to a chemotactic signal.

A closer look at the interacting receptors and their ligands

The ligands for selectins tend to be mucinous molecules covered with dense patches of O-linked sugars. The selectins generally terminate in a lectin domain (hence 'selectin'), as might be expected given the nature of the ligands.

P- and E-selectins allow memory T-cells expressing high levels of VLA-4 to localize at sites of inflammation where subsequent interaction with the upregulated vascular cell adhesion molecule (VCAM-1) on the inflamed endothelium, and with various cytokine and chemokine inflammatory mediators presented on the surface of extracellular matrix proteoglycans, leads to lymphocyte transmigration. Secretion of heparanase by the stimulated T-cell could break down elements of the extracellular matrix, thereby facilitating movement towards the sounds of inflammatory gunfire.

Homing previously activated and memory lymphocytes to sites of inflammation provoked by infectious agents makes a great deal of sense. The same may be said for the mechanisms which enable lymphocytes bearing receptors for mucosal-associated lymphoid tissue (MALT) to circulate within and between the collections of lymphoid tissue guarding the external body surfaces (see figure 8.10). In this way, lymphocytes, such as those programed to support the synthesis of IgA destined for secretion, will not waste time cooling their heels in encapsulated peripheral lymph nodes which play no role in mucosal protection.

ENCAPSULATED LYMPH NODES

The encapsulated tissue of the lymph node contains a meshwork of reticular cells and their fibers organized into sinuses. These act as a filter for lymph draining the body tissues, and possibly bearing foreign antigens, which enters the subcapsular sinus by the afferent vessels and diffuses past the lymphocytes in the cortex to reach the macrophages of the medullary sinuses (figure 8.7) and thence the efferent lymphatics (figures 8.4 and 8.7). What is so striking about the organization of the lymph node is that the T- and B-lymphocytes are very largely separated into different anatomical compartments.

B-cell areas

The follicular aggregations of B-lymphocytes are a prominent feature of the outer cortex. In the unstimulated node they are present as spherical collections of cells termed **primary follicles** (figure 8.7i), but after

Figure 8.6. Homing and transmigration of lymphocytes. Fast-moving lymphocytes are tethered (Step 1) to the vessel walls of the tissue they are being guided to enter through an interaction between specific homing receptors, such as L-selectin (•) or LPAM-1 (•) located on the microvilli of the lymphocyte, and their ligands, for example GlyCAM-1 or MAdCAM-1, on the endothelium of the vessel wall. After rolling along the surface of the endothelial cells (Step 2), activation of the lymphocyte LFA-1 integrin (cf. table 8.2) occurs (Step 3, •). Note that, because this integrin is absent from the microvilli, firm binding occurs by the body of the lymphocyte to its ligands, ICAM-1/2, on the endothelium. This process results in cell flattening (Step 4) and migration of the lymphocyte between adjacent endothelial cells, a process referred to as diapedesis (Step 5).

Table 8.3. Ligand–receptor interactions determining the homing of defined lymphocyte populations.

Homing	*Ligand on endothelium	Receptor on lymphocyte	Result of interaction				
			Tethering	Rolling	LFA-1 activation	Flattening	Diapedesis
Naive and memory T-cells into a lymph node	GlyCAM-1 VCAM-1 SLC ICAM-1/2	L-selectin VLA-4 CCR7 LFA-1					
Naive T-cells into Peyer's patches	MAdCAM-1 MAdCAM-1 SLC ICAM-1/2	L-selectin LPAM-1 CCR7 LFA-1					
LPAM-1ʰⁱ lymphoblasts and memory T-cells into Peyer's patch and lamina propria	MAdCAM-1 ICAM-1/2	LPAM-1 LFA-1					
LPAM-1ʰⁱ memory T-cells into site of inflammation	P-selectin E-selectin VCAM-1 ICAM-1/2	PSGL-1 and ESL-1 ESL-1 VLA-4 LFA-1					

*In lymph node and Peyer's patches the molecules are present on the specialized HEV.
CCR7, CC subgroup chemokine receptor-7; ESL, E-selectin ligand; GlyCAM, glycosylation-dependent cell adhesion molecule; PSGL, P-selectin glycoprotein ligand; SLC, secondary lymphoid tissue chemokine.

antigenic challenge they form **secondary follicles** (figure 8.7f) which consist of a corona or mantle of concentrically packed, resting, small B-lymphocytes possessing both IgM and IgD on their surface surrounding a pale-staining **germinal center** (figure 8.7b). This contains large, usually proliferating, B-blasts, a minority of T-cells, scattered conventional reticular macrophages containing 'tingible bodies' of phagocytosed lymphocytes, and a tight network of specialized **follicular dendritic cells** (FDCs) with elongated cytoplasmic processes and few, if any, lysosomes. Germinal centers are greatly enlarged in secondary antibody

Figure 8.7. Lymph node. (a) Diagrammatic representation of section through a whole node. (b) Diagram showing differentiation of B-cells during passage through different regions of an active germinal center. FDC, follicular dendritic cell; Mφ, macrophage; ×, apoptotic B-cell. (c) Human lymph node, low-power view. (d) Medulla stained with methyl green (DNA)/pyronin (RNA) to show the basophilic (pink) cytoplasm of the plasma cells with their abundant ribosomes. (e) Medullary sinus of lymph node draining site of lithium carmine injection showing macrophages which have phagocytosed the colloidal dye (one is arrowed). (f) Secondary lymphoid follicle showing germinal center surrounded by a mantle of small B-lymphocytes stained by anti-human IgD labeled with horseradish peroxidase (brown color). There are few IgD-positive cells in the center but both areas contain IgM-positive B-lymphocytes. (g) Node from mouse immu-

nized with the thymus-independent antigen, *Pneumococcus* polysaccharide SIII, revealing prominent stimulation of secondary follicles with germinal centers. (h) Methyl green/pyronin stain of lymph node draining site of skin painted with the contact sensitizer oxazolone, highlighting the generalized expansion and activation of the paracortical T-cells, the T-blasts being strongly basophilic. (i) The. same study in a neonatally thymectomized mouse shows a lonely primary nodule (follicle) with complete lack of cellular response in the paracortical area. GC, germinal center; LM, lymphocyte mantle of secondary follicle; MC, medullary cords; MS, medullary sinus; PA, paracortical area; PC, plasma cell; PF, primary follicle; SF, secondary follicle; SM, sinusoidal macrophage; SS, subcapsular sinus. ((c) Photographed by Professor P.M. Lydyard; (d–f) by Dr K.A. MacLennan; (g–i) courtesy of Dr M. de Sousa and Professor D.M.V. Parrott.)

responses during which they constitute sites of B-cell maturation and the generation of B-cell memory.

In the absence of antigen drive, the primary follicles are composed of a mesh of FDCs whose spaces are filled with recirculating, but resting, small B-lymphocytes. On priming with a single dose of a T-dependent antigen (i.e. antigen for which the B-cells require cooperation from T-helper cells; cf. p. 171), the FDC network can be colonized by as few as three primary B-blasts which undergo exponential growth, producing around 10^4 so-called centroblasts and displacing the original resting B-cells which now form the follicular mantle. These highly mitotic centroblasts, with no surface IgD (sIgD) and very little sIgM, then differentiate into light zone centrocytes which are noncycling and begin to upregulate their expression of sIg. At this stage there is very extensive apoptotic cell death, giving rise to DNA fragments which are visible as 'tingible bodies' within the macrophages, the final resting place of the dead cells. The survivors undergo their final training in the apical light zone. A proportion of those which are shunted down the **memory** cell pathway take up residence in the mantle zone population, the remainder joining the recirculating B-cell pool. Other cells differentiate into plasmablasts with a well-defined endoplasmic reticulum, prominent Golgi apparatus and cytoplasmic Ig; these migrate to become plasma cells in the medullary cords which project between the medullary sinuses (figure 8.7d). This maturation of antibody-forming cells at a site distant from that at which antigen triggering has occurred is also seen in the spleen, where plasma cells are found predominantly in the marginal zone. One's guess is that this movement of cells acts to prevent the generation of high local concentrations of antibody within the germinal center, so avoiding neutralization of the antigen on the FDCs and premature shutting off of the immune response.

The remainder of the outer cortex is also essentially a B-cell area with scattered T-cells.

T-cell areas

T-cells are mainly confined to a region referred to as the paracortical (or thymus-dependent) area (figure 8.7a); in nodes taken from children with selective T-cell deficiency (figure 15.5), or from neonatally thymectomized mice (figure 8.7i), the paracortical region is seen to be virtually devoid of lymphocytes. Furthermore, when a T-cell-mediated response is elicited in a normal animal, say by a skin graft or by painting chemicals such as picryl chloride on the skin to induce contact hypersensitivity, there is a marked prolifera-

tion of cells in the thymus-dependent area and typical lymphoblasts are evident (figure 8.7h). In contrast, stimulation of antibody formation by the thymus-independent antigen, *Pneumococcus* polysaccharide SIII, leads to proliferation in the cortical lymphoid follicles with the development of germinal centers, while the paracortical region remains inactive, reflecting the inability to develop cellular hypersensitivity to the polysaccharide (figure 8.7g). As expected, nodes taken from children with congenital hypogammaglobulinemia associated with failure of B-cell development conspicuously lack primary and secondary follicles.

SPLEEN

On a fresh section of spleen, the lymphoid tissue forming the white pulp is seen as circular or elongated gray areas (figure 8.8b) within the erythrocyte-filled red pulp which consists of splenic cords lined with macrophages and venous sinusoids. As in the lymph node, T- and B-cell areas are segregated (figure 8.8a). The spleen is a very effective blood filter removing effete red and white cells and responding actively to blood-borne antigens, the more so if they are particulate. Plasmablasts and mature plasma cells are present in the marginal zone extending into the red pulp (figure 8.8c).

MUCOSAL-ASSOCIATED LYMPHOID TISSUE (MALT)

The respiratory, gastrointestinal and genitourinary tracts are guarded immunologically by subepithelial accumulations of lymphoid tissue which are not constrained by a connective tissue capsule (figure 8.9). These may occur as diffuse collections of lymphocytes, plasma cells and phagocytes throughout the lung and the lamina propria of the intestinal wall (figure 8.9a and b), or as more clearly organized tissue with well-formed follicles. In humans, the latter includes the lingual, palatine and pharyngeal tonsils (figure 8.9c), the Peyer's patches of the small intestine (figure 8.9d) and the appendix. MALT forms an interconnected secretory system within which cells committed to IgA or IgE synthesis may circulate (figure 8.10).

In the gut, antigen enters the Peyer's patches (figure 8.9d) across specialized epithelial cells (cf. figure 8.15) and stimulates the antigen-sensitive lymphocytes. After activation these drain into the lymph and, after a journey through the mesenteric lymph nodes and the thoracic duct, they pass from the bloodstream into the

(a)

(b)

(c)

(d)

Figure 8.8. Spleen. (a) Diagrammatic representation. (b) Low-power view showing lymphoid white pulp (WP) and red pulp (RP). (c) High-power view of germinal center (GC) and lymphocyte mantle (M) surrounded by marginal zone (MZ) and red pulp (RP). Adjacent to the follicle, an arteriole (A) is surrounded by the peri-arteriolar lymphoid sheath (PALS) predominantly consisting of T-cells. Note that the marginal zone is only present above the secondary follicle. (d) Localization of the thymus-independent antigen, ficoll, on the marginal zone macrophages. The ficoll is visualized by labeling with the red fluorescent dye tetramethyl-rhodamine. ((b) Photographed by Professor P.M. Lydyard; (c) by Professor I.C.M. MacLennan; (d) kindly provided by Professor J.H. Humphrey.)

lamina propria (figure 8.10) where they become IgA-forming cells which, because they are now broadly distributed, protect a wide area of the bowel with protective antibody. The cells also appear in the lymphoid tissue of the lung and in other mucosal sites guided by the interactions of specific homing receptors with appropriate HEV addressins as discussed earlier. Similarly, intranasal immunization is particularly effective at generating antibody production in the genitourinary tract.

Intestinal lymphocytes

The intestinal **lamina propria** is home to a predominantly activated T-cell population rich in the LPAM-1 integrin (table 8.2), the ligand for MAdCAM-1 on the lamina propria postcapillary venules (figure 8.11). These T-cells bear a phenotype roughly comparable to that of peripheral blood lymphocytes: viz. > 95% T-cell receptor (TCR) αβ and a CD4:CD8 ratio of 7:3. Within the lamina propria there is also a generous sprinkling of activated B-blasts and plasma cells secreting IgA for transport by the poly-Ig receptor to the intestinal lumen (cf. p. 53).

Intestinal **intraepithelial lymphocytes** (IELs) are quite a different kettle of fish. They are also mostly T-cells, 10–40% of which have a γδ TCR. Of those bearing an αβ TCR, most are CD8 positive and can be divided into two populations. One-third of them possess the conventional form of CD8, which is a heterodimer

Figure 8.9. The IgA secretory immune system (MALT). (a) Section of lung showing a diffuse accumulation of lymphocytes (Ly) in the bronchial wall. (b) Section of human jejunum showing lymphoid cells (Ly), stained green by a fluorescent antileukocyte monoclonal antibody, in the mucosal epithelium (ME) and in the lamina propria (LP). A red fluorescent anti-IgA conjugate stains the cytoplasm of plasma cells (PC) in the lamina propria and detects IgA in the surface mucus; altogether a super picture! (c) Low-power view of human tonsil showing the MALT with numerous secondary follicles (SF) containing germinal centers. (d) Peyer's patches (PP) in mouse ileum. The T-cell areas are stained brown by a peroxidase-labeled monoclonal antibody to Thy 1. ((a) Kindly provided by Professor P. Lydyard; (b) by Professor G. Jannosy; (c) by Mr C. Symes; and (d) by Dr E. Andrew.)

composed of a CD8 α chain and a CD8 β chain. However, two-thirds of them instead express a CD8 αα homodimer which is almost exclusively found only on IELs. Whilst the CD8 αβ IELs are restricted by classical MHC class I molecules, the CD8 αα IELs appear to recognize nonclassical MHC molecules (cf. p. 77) perhaps including TL and Qa1 but not, apparently, CD1. The antigen specificity of most IELs is unknown. Intraepithelial lymphocytes and intraepithelial dendritic cells express high levels of the $\alpha_E\beta_7$ integrin which binds E-cadherin on intestinal epithelial cells.

The relatively high proportion of TCR γδ cells is also unusual and most of these also express the CD8 αα characteristic of IELs. Since a number of cloned γδ T-cells have been found to have specificity for heat-shock proteins, which are widely distributed in nature and usually highly immunogenic, it has been postulated that they act as a relatively primitive first line of defense at the outer surfaces of the body.

Reflect for a moment on the fact that roughly 10^{14} bacteria reside in the intestinal lumen of the normal adult human. That is a pretty impressive number of 'noughts' to swallow. Yet combined with the barrier of mucins produced by goblet cells and the protective zone of secreted IgA antibodies, these collections of intestinal lymphocytes represent a crucial line of defense.

It is not only the intestine that has a localized

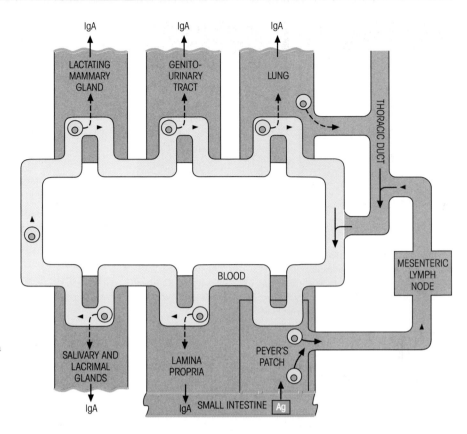

Figure 8.10. Circulation of lymphocytes within the mucosal-associated lymphoid system. Antigen-stimulated cells move from Peyer's patches to colonize the lamina propria and the other mucosal surfaces (～～～～), forming what has been described as a common mucosal immune system.

Figure 8.11. Selective expression of the mucosal vascular addressin MAdCAM-1 on endothelium involved in lymphocyte homing to gastrointestinal sites. Immunohistologic staining reveals the presence of MAdCAM-1 (a) on postcapillary venules in the small intestinal lamina propria and (b) on HEV in Peyer's patches, but its absence from (c) HEV in peripheral lymph nodes. (Reproduced with permission from Butcher E.C. *et al.* (1999) *Advances in Immunology* **72**, 209.) At least some component of intestinal trafficking appears to operate as a subcomponent of a common mucosal immune system (cf. figure 8.10), MAdCAM-1 being largely absent from the genitourinary tract, lung, salivary and lacrimal gland, although it is present on vascular endothelium in the mammary gland.

immune system composed mostly of resident T-lymphocytes; similar set-ups appear to apply to the skin and to the liver. Nonclassical MHC antigens seem to play an important role in these specialized locales, with the MHC class I chain-related (MIC) family members MICA and MICB (cf. p. 78) implicated in the activation of human γδ TCR IELs, and CD1 in antigen presentation to liver NK T-cells (cf. p. 102).

BONE MARROW CAN BE A MAJOR SITE OF ANTIBODY SYNTHESIS

A few days after a secondary response, activated memory B-cells migrate to the bone marrow where they mature into plasma cells (figure 8.12). The bone marrow is a major source of serum Ig, contributing up to 80% of the total Ig-secreting cells in the 100-week-

Figure 8.12. Plasma cells in human bone marrow. Cytospin preparation stained with rhodamine (orange) for IgA heavy chain and fluorescein (green) for lambda light chain. One cell is IgA.λ, another IgA.non-λ and the third is non-IgA.λ positive. (Photograph kindly supplied by Drs Benner, Hijmans and Haaijman.)

old mouse. The peripheral lymphoid tissue responds rapidly to antigen, but only for a relatively short time, whereas bone marrow starts slowly and gives a long-lasting massive production of antibody to antigens which repeatedly challenge the host.

THE ENJOYMENT OF PRIVILEGED SITES

Certain selected parts of the body, for example brain, anterior chamber of the eye and testis, have been designated **privileged immunological sites**, in the sense that antigens located within them do not provoke reactions against themselves. It has long been known, for example, that foreign corneal grafts can take up long-term residence, and a number of viruses have been expanded by repeated passage through animal brain.

Generally speaking, privileged sites are protected by rather strong blood–tissue barriers and low permeability to hydrophilic compounds and carrier-mediated transport systems. Functionally insignificant levels of complement reduce the threat of acute inflammatory reactions and unusually high concentrations of immunomodulators, such as IL-10 and transforming growth factor-β (TGFβ; cf. p. 179), endow macrophages with an immunosuppressive capacity. Immune privilege may also be maintained by Fas (CD95)-induced apoptosis of autoaggressive cells. Lesley Brent put it rather well: 'It may be supposed that it is beneficial to the organism not to turn the anterior chamber or the cornea of the eye, or the brain, into an inflammatory battle-field, for the immunological response is sometimes more damaging than the antigen insult that provoked it.'

However, inflammatory reactions at the blood–tissue barrier can open the gates to invasion by immunological marauders—witness the inability of corneal grafts to take in the face of a local pre-existing inflammation.

THE HANDLING OF ANTIGEN

Where does antigen go when it enters the body? If it penetrates the tissues, it will tend to finish up in the draining lymph nodes. Antigens which are encountered in the upper respiratory tract or intestine are trapped by local MALT, whereas antigens in the blood provoke a reaction in the spleen. Macrophages in the liver will filter blood-borne antigens and degrade them without producing an immune response since they are not strategically placed with respect to lymphoid tissue.

Macrophages are general antigen-presenting cells

'Classically', it has always been recognized that antigens draining into lymphoid tissue are taken up by macrophages. The antigens are then partially, if not completely, broken down in the lysosomes; some may escape from the cell in a soluble form to be taken up by other antigen-presenting cells and a fraction may reappear at the surface, either as a large fragment or as a processed peptide associated with class II major histocompatibility molecules. Although resting, resident macrophages do not express MHC class II, antigens are usually encountered in the context of a microbial infectious agent which can induce the expression of class II by its adjuvant-like properties involving molecules such as bacterial lipopolysaccharide (LPS). The antigen-presenting cell must bear antigen on its surface for effective activation of lymphocytes and there is ample evidence that antigen-pulsed macrophages can stimulate specific T- and B-cells both *in vitro* and when injected back *in vivo*. Some antigens, such as polymeric carbohydrates like ficoll, cannot be degraded because the macrophages lack the enzymes required; in these instances, specialized macrophages in the marginal zone of the spleen (see figure 8.8d), or the lymph node subcapsular sinus, trap and present the antigen to B-cells directly, apparently without any processing or intervention from T-cells.

Interdigitating dendritic cells present antigen to T-lymphocytes

Notwithstanding this impressive account of the mighty macrophage in antigen presentation, there is one function where it is seemingly deficient, namely the priming of naive lymphocytes. Animals which have been depleted of macrophages, by selective uptake of liposomes containing the drug dichlorome-thylene diphosphonate, are as good as their controls with intact macrophages in responding to T-dependent antigens. We must conclude that cells other than macrophages prime T-helper cells, and it is now generally accepted that these are the interdigitating dendritic cells (IDCs). These cells, which are of bone marrow origin, have the awesome capacity to process four times their own volume of extracellular fluid in 1 hour, thereby facilitating antigen capture and processing in their abundant intracellular MHC class II-rich compartments (MIIC; cf. p. 95).

The IDCs are the *crème de la crème* of the antigen-presenting cells and, if pulsed with antigen before injection into animals, usually produce stunning immune responses. In this connection, it is relevant to note that large numbers of these dendritic cells can be generated from peripheral blood by cultivation with granulocyte–macrophage colony-stimulating factor (GM-CSF) (cf. p. 179) to promote proliferation and IL-4 to suppress macrophage overgrowth; this means that it is perfectly feasible to contemplate their use for immunotherapy, e.g. pulsing autologous dendritic cells with the patient's tumor antigens and then rein-jecting them to evoke an immune response.

Immature dendritic cells in the blood that are destined to become skin Langerhans' cells express cutaneous leukocyte antigen (CLA), directing their homing to skin via interaction with E-selectin on the relevant vascular endothelial cells just as occurs for cutaneous T-cells. The Langerhans' cells, and dendritic cells in other tissues, act as antigen sampling agents. They are only moderately phagocytic but display extremely active endocytosis. Receptors involved in antigen capture, including the mannose receptor and the immunoglobulin receptors FcγRII, FcεRI and FcεRII, are expressed at high levels. Unlike macrophages, however, they do not express appreciable amounts of the high affinity FcγRI. The expression of cell surface MHC class II, and of adhesion and co-stimulatory molecules, is low at this early stage of the dendritic cells' life. However, as they differentiate into fully fledged antigen-presenting cells, they decrease their phagocytic and endocytic activity, show reduced levels of molecules involved in antigen capture, but dramatically increase their MHC class II and CD1. Costimulatory molecules such as B7.1, B7.2 and CD40 are also upregulated at this stage, as are ICAM-1 and ICAM-2 which are thought to contribute to both the migratory and antigen-presenting properties of these

cells. Their expression of CD4 and the chemokine receptors CCR5 and CXCR4 (cf. table 10.3) means that they are attracted to and migrate into T-cell areas and incidently become susceptible to infection by HIV (see p. 314).

There is evidence for different populations of IDCs, although this is still a somewhat shaky area. Two separate developmental pathways have been described, one which involves CD1a$^+$ CD14$^-$ cells with features of Langerhans' cells, and the other involving CD1a$^-$ CD14$^+$ cells that can differentiate into dermal dendritic cells that lack Langerhans' cell markers, such as Birbeck granules. Another subdivision that has been described involves the ability of murine CD8 α$^-$ myeloid lineage dendritic cells to induce a Th2-type response, whilst CD8 α$^+$ lymphoid lineage dendritic cells activate Th1 differentiation (cf. p. 181). Recent data suggest a rather more complex situation, with dendritic cells arising from several different types of progenitor cells and the potential for functionally different types of dendritic cells to arise from the same progenitor, their function depending upon their maturation stage and the local cytokine environment.

What is clear is that, in addition to their antigen-presenting function, dendritic cells are important producers of chemokines. Lymph node IDCs that have matured from Langerhans' cells secrete T-cell-attracting chemokines, such as MDC (*m*acrophage-*d*erived *c*hemokine) and TARC (*t*hymus- and *a*ctivation-*r*egulated *c*hemokine), with production localized to regions of the T-cell zone proximal to lymphoid follicles. MDC and perhaps TARC attract T-cells that are already to some extent activated. An apparently separate dendritic cell population constitutively expresses ELC (*E*BI-1 *l*igand *c*hemokine) and SLC (*s*econdary *l*ymphoid tissue *c*hemokine) in the T-cell zone and attracts naive T-cells. Thus a first phase of recruitment may occur involving naive T-cells, followed by a second wave of activated cells, thereby enhancing the possibility of encounter between antigen-bearing dendritic cells and their cognate antigen-specific T-cells. Once these cells get together, there are a number of receptor–ligand interactions involved in dendritic cell activation of T-cells aside from MHC–peptide recognition by the TCR. These include B7–CD28, CD40–CD40L, OX40L–OX40 (CD134) and TRANCE (*T*NF-*r*elated *a*ctivation-induced *c*ytokine)–TRANCE receptor recognition events. In addition to the T-cell zone, IDCs are also present in germinal centers, although not as prominently as the follicular dendritic cells to be discussed below. These germinal center IDCs may play a role in B-cell expansion and differentiation via their production of cytokines.

It is worth noting that, unlike macrophages, which in a sense are 'brutal microbe crunchers', the dendritic cells are not strongly phagocytic and they do need help from the macrophages in the preprocessing of particulate antigens, since these responses are completely abolished in macrophage-depleted animals.

To summarize, the scenario for T-cell priming appears to be as follows. Peripheral immature dendritic cells such as the Langerhans' cells (cf. figure 2.6f), which bind to skin keratinocytes through surface expression of E-cadherin, can pick up and process antigen. As maturation proceeds, they lose their E-cadherin and produce collagenase, presumably to facilitate their crossing of the basement membrane. They then travel as 'veiled' cells in the lymph (figure 8.13b) before settling down as IDCs in the paracortical T-cell zone of the draining lymph node (figure 8.13a). There, maturation is completed (figure 8.14), the IDC delivers the antigen with costimulatory signals for potent stimulation of naive and subsequently of activated, specific T-cells, which take advantage of the large surface area to bind to the MHC–peptide complex on the IDC membrane.

We will meet IDCs again in Chapter 12 when we discuss their central role within the thymus where they present self-peptides to developing autoreactive T-cells and trigger their apoptotic execution (known more gently as 'clonal deletion'; cf. p. 231).

Follicular dendritic cells stimulate B-cells in germinal centers

Another type of cell with dendritic morphology, but this time of mesenchymal origin, exists within lymphoid tissues and is referred to as the **follicular dendritic cell** (FDC). These are nonphagocytic and lack lysosomes but have very elongated processes which can make contact with numerous lymphocytes present within the germinal centers of secondary follicles. Their possession of FcγRII, FcεRII and complement receptors enables them to trap complexed antigen very efficiently and hold it in its native form on their surface for extended periods, in keeping with the memory function of secondary follicles. This would explain the fact that secondary antibody responses can be boosted by quite small amounts of immunogen which become bound by circulating antibody and then fix C3. Evidence for this notion may be derived from animals effectively depleted of complement by injection of cobra venom factor which contains the reptilian equivalent of C3b. This fires the alternative complement pathway by forming a complex with factor B but, because of its insensitivity to the mammalian C3 inactivator, it persists long enough to discharge the feedback loop to exhaustion and deplete C3 completely. Such mice can neither localize antigen–antibody complexes on their

(a)

(b)

Figure 8.13. Dendritic antigen-presenting cell. (a) Interdigitating dendritic cell (IDC) in the thymus-dependent area of the rat lymph node. This is thought to be an antigen-presenting cell derived from the Langerhans' cell in the skin and dendritic cells in other tissues, which travels to the node in the afferent lymph as a 'veiled' cell bearing antigen on its profuse surface processes. Intimate contacts are made with the surface membranes (arrows) of the surrounding T-lymphocytes (TL). The cytoplasm of the IDC contains relatively few organelles and does not show Birbeck granules (racket-shaped cytoplasmic organelles, characteristic of the Langerhans' cell), although some IDCs in lymph nodes do possess these granules, perhaps after antigenic stimulation (×2000). (b) Scanning electron micrograph of a veiled cell. In contrast with these dendritic cells which present antigen to T-cells, the follicular dendritic cells in germinal centers stimulate B-cells. ((a) Reproduced with permission of the authors and publishers from Kamperdijk E.W.A., Hoefsmit E.Ch.H., Drexhage H.A. & Balfour B.H. (1980) In Van Furth R. (ed.) *Mononuclear Phagocytes*, 3rd edn. Rijhoff Publishers, The Hague. (b) Courtesy of Dr G.G. MacPherson.)

Figure 8.14. Migration and maturation of interdigitating dendritic cells. The precursors of the IDCs are derived from bone marrow stem cells. They travel via the blood to nonlymphoid tissues. These immature IDCs, e.g. Langerhans' cells in skin, are specialized for antigen uptake. Subsequently they travel via the afferent lymphatics as veiled cells (cf. figure 8.13b) to take up residence within secondary lymphoid tissues (cf. figure 8.13a) where they express high levels of MHC class II and costimulatory molecules such as B7. These cells are highly specialized for the activation of naive T-cells.

Figure 8.15. M-cell within Peyer's patch epithelium. (a) Scanning electron micrograph of the surface of the Peyer's patch epithelium. The antigen-sampling M-cell in the center is surrounded by absorptive enterocytes covered by closely packed, regular microvilli. Note the irregular and short microfolds of the M-cell. (Reproduced with permission of the authors and publishers from Kato T. & Owen R.L. (1999) In Ogra R. *et al.* (eds) *Mucosal Immunology*, 2nd edn. Academic Press, San Diego.) (b) After uptake and transcellular transport by the M-cell (M), antigen is processed by macrophages and thence by IDCs which present antigen to T-cells in Peyer's patches and mesenteric lymph nodes. E, enterocyte; L, lymphocyte; Mφ, macrophage. (c) Electron photomicrograph of an M-cell (M in nucleus) with adjacent lymphocyte (L in nucleus). Note the flanking epithelial cells are both absorptive enterocytes with a typical brush border. In some cases, proteases on the surface of the M-cells modify the pathogen so that it can adhere and be taken up. Pathogenic *Salmonella* can invade and destroy M-cells, making a hole through which other bacteria can invade the underlying tissue. (Lead citrate and uranyl acetate, ×1600.) ((b) Based on Sminia T. & Kraal G. (1998) In Delves P.J. & Roitt I.M. (eds) *Encyclopedia of Immunology*, 2nd edn, p. 188. Academic Press, London.)

follicular dendritic cells, nor generate memory B-cells in response to T-dependent antigens (see p. 171).

Classically, a secondary response would be initiated at the T-helper level by antigen, alone or as a complex, being taken up by IDCs and macrophages. However, the capture of immune complexes on the surface of FDCs opens up an alternative pathway. One to three days after secondary challenge, the filamentous dendrites on the follicular cells, to which the immune complexes are bound, form into beads which break off as structures called 'iccosomes' (*i*mmune *c*omplex-*co*ated bodies). These bind to germinal center B-cells which then endocytose and process the antigen for presentation by the B-cell MHC class II, and subsequent stimulation of T-helper cells to kick off the secondary response.

M-cells provide the gateway to the mucosal lymphoid system

The mucosal surface is in the front line facing an unfriendly sea of microbes and, generally, antigens are excluded by the epithelium with its tight junctions and mucous layer. Gut lymphoid tissue is separated from the lumen by a layer of columnar epithelium interspersed with microfold (M)-cells (figure 8.15a); specialized antigen-transporting cells with short, irregular microvillae, strong nonspecific esterase activity and no MHC class II. They overlay intraepithelial lymphocytes and macrophages (figure 8.15b and c). Foreign material, including bacteria, is taken up by M-cells and passed on to the underlying antigen-presenting cells which, in turn, migrate to the local lymphoid tissue to activate the appropriate lymphocytes.

SUMMARY

The surface markers of cells in the immune system
• Individual surface molecules are assigned a *cluster of differentiation* (CD) number defined by a cluster of monoclonal antibodies reacting with that molecule.

Organized lymphoid tissue
• The complexity of immune responses is catered for by a sophisticated structure.
• Lymph nodes filter and screen lymph flowing from the body tissues while spleen filters the blood.
• B- and T-cell areas are separated.
• B-cell structures appear in the lymph node cortex as primary follicles which become secondary follicles with germinal centers after antigen stimulation.
• Germinal centers with their meshwork of follicular dendritic cells expand B-cell blasts produced by secondary antigen challenge and direct their differentiation into memory cells and antibody-forming plasma cells.

Mucosal-associated lymphoid tissue
• Lymphoid tissue guarding the gastrointestinal tract is unencapsulated and somewhat structured (tonsils, Peyer's patches, appendix), or present as diffuse cellular collections in the lamina propria. Intraepithelial lymphocytes are mostly T-cells and include some novel subsets, e.g. CD8 αα-bearing cells which use nonclassical MHC molecules as restriction elements for antigen presentation.
• Together with the subepithelial accumulations of cells lining the mucosal surfaces of the respiratory and genitourinary tracts, this lymphoid tissue forms the 'secretory immune system' which bathes the surface with protective IgA antibodies.

Other sites
• Bone marrow is a major site of antibody production.
• The brain, anterior chamber of the eye and testis are privileged sites in which antigens can be safely sequestered.

Lymphocyte traffic
• Lymphocyte recirculation between the blood and lymphoid tissues is guided by specialized homing receptors on the surface of the high-walled endothelium of the postcapillary venules.
• Lymphocytes are tethered and then roll along the surface of the selected endothelial cells through interactions between selectins and integrins and their respective ligands. Flattening of the lymphocyte and transmigration across the endothelial cell follow LFA-1 activation.
• Entry of memory T-cells into sites of inflammation is facilitated by upregulation of integrin molecules (VLA-4 and LFA-1) on the lymphocyte and corresponding binding ligands on the vascular endothelium (VCAM-1 and ICAM-1/2 respectively).

The handling of antigen
• Macrophages are general antigen-presenting cells for primed lymphocytes but cannot stimulate naive T-cells.
• This is effected by dendritic cells of hematopoietic origin which process antigen, migrate to the draining lymph node and settle down as interdigitating dendritic cells. They can present antigen-derived peptides to naive T-cells, thereby powerfully initiating primary T-cell responses.
• Follicular dendritic cells in germinal centers bind immune complexes to their surface through Ig and C3b receptors. The complexes are long-lived and provide a sustained source of antigenic stimulation for B-cells.
• Specialized antigen-transporting M-cells provide the gateway for antigens to the mucosal lymphoid tissue.

See the accompanying website (**www.roitt.com**) for multiple choice questions.

FURTHER READING

Barclay A.N. *et al.* (1997) *The Leucocyte Antigen Factsbook*, 2nd edn. Academic Press, London.

Bell D., Young J.W. & Bancherau J. (1999) Dendritic cells. *Advances in Immunology* **72**, 255.

Butcher E.C. *et al.* (1999) Lymphocyte trafficking and regional immunity. *Advances in Immunology* **72**, 209.

Caligaris-Cappio F. (1998) Germinal centers. In Delves P.J. & Roitt I.M. (eds) *Encyclopedia of Immunology*, 2nd edn, p. 992. Academic Press, London.

Cyster J.G. (1999) Chemokines and cell migration in secondary lymphoid organs. *Science* **286**, 2098.

Grabbe S., Kämpgen, E. & Schuler G. (2000) Dendritic cells: multi-lineal and multi-functional. *Immunology Today* **21**, 431.

Pringault E. (ed.) (1999) M cell development and function in physiology and disease. *Seminars in Immunology* **11**, 155.

Shaw S., Turni L.A. & Katz K.S. (eds) *Protein Reviews on the Web (PROW)*. http://www.ncbi.nlm.nih.gov/prow.

Shimizu Y., Rose D.M. & Ginsberg M.H. (1999) Integrins in the immune system. *Advances in Immunology* **72**, 325.

CHAPTER 9

Lymphocyte activation

INTRODUCTION

The differences which distinguish immunocompetent T- and B-cells are sharply demarcated at the cell surface (table 9.1). The most clear-cut discrimination is established by reagents which recognize components of the antigen receptors, anti-CD3 for T-cells and anti-immunoglobulin for B-cells, and in laboratory practice these are the markers most often used to enumerate the two lymphocyte populations. The surface expression of receptors for Ig and complement also distinguishes T- and B-cells, while the adventitious formation of rosettes through the binding of sheep erythrocytes to CD2 is sometimes used for the detection and separation of T-cells.

Differences in the CD markers determined by monoclonal antibodies reflect disparate functional properties and in particular define specialized T-cell subsets. CD4 is a marker of T-helper cell populations which promote activation and maturation of B-cells and cytotoxic T-cells, and control antigen-specific chronic inflammatory reactions through stimulation of macrophages. CD4 molecules form links with class II *m*ajor *h*istocompatibility *c*omplex (MHC) on the cell presenting antigen. Similarly, the CD8 molecules on cytotoxic T-cells associate with MHC class I (figure 9.1).

Attention should also be drawn to the 'nonspecific mitogens' which activate populations and sometimes subpopulations of T- or B-cells in a way which is unrelated to the antigen specificity of the lymphocyte receptors. They react with constant, as distinct from highly variable, structures on the cell surface. For this reason, they are often termed polyclonal B- or T-cell activators (table 9.1). We have already drawn attention in Chapter 5 to the ability of superantigens such as staphylococcal enterotoxins to act as polyclonal activators by stimulating all T-cells bearing certain T-cell receptor (TCR) Vβ families irrespective of their specificity for antigen.

T-LYMPHOCYTES AND ANTIGEN-PRESENTING CELLS INTERACT THROUGH SEVERAL PAIRS OF ACCESSORY MOLECULES

The affinity of an individual TCR for its specific MHC–antigen peptide complex is relatively low (figure 9.2) and a sufficiently stable association with the antigen-presenting cell (APC) can only be achieved by the interaction of complementary pairs of accessory

Figure 9.1. Helper and cytotoxic T-cell subsets are restricted by MHC class. CD4 on helper T-cells contacts MHC class II; CD8 on cytotoxic T-cells associates with class I.

Table 9.1. Comparison of human T- and B-cells.

	T-cells	B-cells
% in peripheral blood	65–80	8–15
ANTIGEN RECOGNITION	Processed	Native
CELL SURFACE MOLECULES		
Antigen receptor	TCR/CD3	Surface Ig
MHC class I	+	+
MHC class II	only after activation	+
CD2	+	–
CD4	MHC class II-restricted (helper)	–
CD5	+	only on B1a minor subset
CD8	MHC class I-restricted (cytotoxic)	–
CD19	–	+
CD20	–	+
CD21 (CR2: C3d and EBV receptor	–	+
CD23 (FcεRII)	–	+
CD32 (FcγRII)	–	+
POLYCLONAL ACTIVATION	Anti-CD3 Phytohemagglutinin Pokeweed mitogen *S.aureus enterotoxin	Anti-Ig Epstein-Barr virus Pokeweed mitogen S.aureus Cowan I strain

*Staphylococcal superantigen, polyclonal response restricted to certain TCR Vβ families.

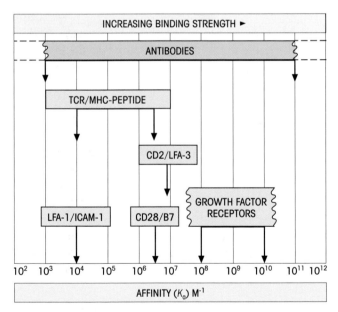

Figure 9.2. The relative affinities of molecular pairs involved in interactions between T-lymphocytes and cells presenting antigen. The ranges of affinities for growth factors and their receptors, and of antibodies, are shown for comparison. (Based on Davies M.M. & Chien Y.-H. (1993) *Current Opinion in Immunology* **5**, 45.)

molecules such as LFA-1/ICAM-1, CD2/LFA-3, and so on (figure 9.3). However, these molecular couplings are not necessarily concerned just with intercellular adhesion.

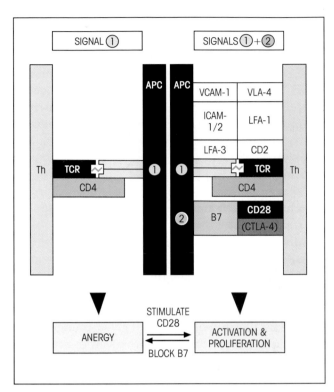

Figure 9.3. Activation of resting T-cells. Interaction of costimulatory molecules leads to activation of resting T-lymphocyte by antigen-presenting cell (APC) on engagement of the T-cell receptor (TCR) with its antigen–MHC complex. Engagement of the TCR signal 1 without accompanying costimulatory signal 2 leads to anergy. Note, a cytotoxic rather than a helper T-cell would, of course, involve coupling of CD8 to MHC I. Engagement of CTLA-4 with B7 downregulates signal 1. ICAM-1/2, intercellular adhesion molecule-1/2; LFA-1/2, lymphocyte function-associated molecule-1/2; VCAM-1, vascular cell adhesion molecule-1; VLA-4, very late antigen-4. (Based on Liu Y. & Linsley P.S. (1992) *Current Opinion in Immunology* **4**, 265.)

THE ACTIVATION OF T-CELLS REQUIRES TWO SIGNALS

Antibodies to the TCR, either anti-idiotype or anti-CD3, when insolubilized by coupling to Sepharose, will not fully activate resting helper T-cells on their own. Upon addition of interleukin-1 (IL-1), however, RNA and protein synthesis is induced, the cell enlarges to a blast-like appearance, interleukin-2 (IL-2) synthesis begins and the cell moves from G0 into the G1 phase of the mitotic cycle. Thus, two signals are required for the activation of a resting helper T-cell (figure 9.3). Antigen in association with MHC class II on the surface of APCs is clearly capable of fulfilling these requirements. Complex formation between the TCR, antigen and MHC provides signal 1, through the receptor–CD3 complex, and this is greatly enhanced by the coupling of CD4 with the MHC. The T-cell is now exposed to a costimulatory signal 2 from the APC. Although this could be IL-1, it would appear that the most potent costimulator is B7 on the APC binding to CD28. Thus activation of resting T-cells can be blocked by anti-B7; surprisingly, this renders the T-cell **anergic**, i.e. unresponsive to any further stimulation by antigen. As we shall see in later chapters, the principle that two signals activate, but one may induce anergy in, an antigen-specific cell provides a potential for targeted immunosuppressive therapy. Unlike resting T-lymphocytes, **activated T-cells proliferate in response to a** *single* **signal**.

Adhesion molecules such as ICAM-1, VCAM-1 and LFA-3 are not themselves costimulatory but augment the effect of other signals (figure 9.3); an important distinction. Early signaling events involve the aggregation of **lipid rafts** composed of membrane subdomains enriched in cholesterol and glycosphingolipids. The cell membrane molecules involved in activation become concentrated within these structures.

PROTEIN TYROSINE PHOSPHORYLATION IS AN EARLY EVENT IN T-CELL SIGNALING

If a **protein tyrosine kinase (PTK)** phosphorylates and thereby activates a kinase precursor, which in turn switches on a second kinase precursor and so on, one has the basis for an enzymic phosphorylation cascade which could amplify an initial signal, just as the proteolytic enzyme cascade amplifies the triggering event of the complement system (cf. p. 10). As we shall see shortly, these signaling cascades can become quite extensive! (figure 9.4); but take it one step at a time and you'll be O.K.

The initial signal for T-cell activation through the TCR is greatly enhanced by cross-linking the TCR with CD4 which brings the CD4-associated PTK, **Lck**, close to the CD3-associated **ζ chains**. *I*mmunoreceptor *t*yrosine-based *a*ctivation *m*otifs (ITAMs) on the ζ chains become phosphorylated and bind to the SH2 domains of **ZAP-70**, which now becomes an active PTK (figure 9.5) capable of initiating a series of downstream biochemical events. The key role of these tyrosine kinases is underlined by the ability of the PTK inhibitor herbimycin-A to block proximal TCR-mediated signaling events such as phosphatidylinositol turnover as well as later manifestations like IL-2 production. Receptor proximal events are coupled to

Figure 9.4. Signaling pathways can become quite complex. (Reproduced with permission from Zolnierowicz S. & Bollen M. (2000) *EMBO Journal* **19**, 483.)

Figure 9.5. Signals through the TCR/CD3/CD4/8 complex initiate a protein tyrosine kinase (PTK) cascade. The PTK Lck (p56^{lck}) phosphorylates the tyrosine within the ITAM sequences of CD3-associated ζ chains. These bind the ζ-associated protein (ZAP-70) through its SH2 (Src homology-2) domains and this in turn acquires PTK activity for downstream phosphorylation of later components in the chain. In contrast to the three ITAMs on each ζ chain, the CD3 γ, δ and ε chains each bear a single ITAM.

downstream signaling cascades by nonenzymic **adaptor proteins** which link together the enzymes necessary for signal transduction.

DOWNSTREAM EVENTS FOLLOWING TCR SIGNALING

Ras function

Following TCR signaling, there is an early increase in the level of active Ras–GTP (guanosine triphosphate) complexes which regulate pivotal *mitogen-activated protein kinases* (**MAPK**), such as JNK or ERK, through sequential kinase cascades. Thus, in one of the phosphorylation amplifying cascades, MEK (*MAP-ERK kinase*) acts as a MAP kinase kinase and Raf as a MAP kinase kinase kinase or MAPKKK (figure 9.6)! As illustrated in figure 9.7, this is just one of a number of

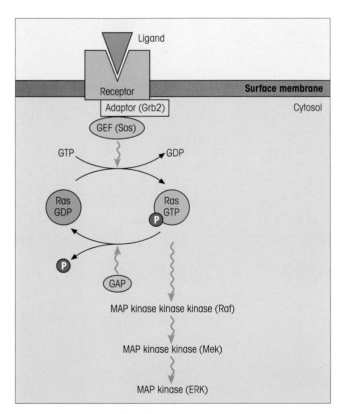

Figure 9.6. Regulation of Ras activity controls kinase amplification cascades. A number of cell surface receptors signal through Ras-regulated pathways. Ras cycles between inactive Ras–GDP and active Ras–GTP, regulated by guanine nucleotide exchange factors (GEFs) which promote the conversion of Ras–GDP to Ras–GTP, and by GTPase-activating proteins (GAPs) which increase the intrinsic GTPase activity of Ras. Upon ligand binding to receptor, receptor tyrosine kinases recruit adaptor proteins, e.g. Grb2, and GEF proteins, such as Sos ('son of sevenless'), to the plasma membrane. These events generate Ras–GTP which activates Raf. (Modified with permission from Olson M.F. & Marais R. (2000) *Seminars in Immunology* **12**, 63.)

different pathways involved in T-cell activation. The MAP kinases themselves may also be influenced by CD28 operating through phosphatidylinositol 3-kinase (PI3K). It should be stressed that the details of these various pathways are not yet inscribed in tablets of stone.

The phosphatidylinositol pathway

Within 15 seconds of TCR stimulation, the $\gamma 1$ isoform of **phospholipase C** (PLCγ1), an enzyme which (like the $\gamma 2$ isoform) activates the phosphatidylinositol pathway, is phosphorylated and its catalytic activity increased. This early increase in phospholipase C activity accelerates the hydrolysis of phosphatidylinositol 4,5-biphosphate (PIP$_2$) to diacylglycerol (DAG) and inositol 1,4,5-triphosphate (IP$_3$) (figure 9.7). The triphosphate binds to specific receptors on specialized calcium storage vesicles and triggers the release of Ca^{2+} into the cytosol; this is supplemented by an influx from the external milieu. The **raised Ca^{2+}** level has at least two consequences. First, it synergizes with diacylglycerol to activate **protein kinase C** (PKC); second, it acts together with **calmodulin** to increase the activity of **calcineurin**.

Control of IL-2 gene transcription

Transcription of IL-2 is one of the key elements in preventing the signaled T-cell from lapsing into anergy and is controlled by multiple receptors for transcriptional factors in the promoter region (figure 9.7). The MAP kinase JNK phosphorylates Jun, which then binds as a binary complex with Fos to the **AP-1** site, deletion of which abrogates 90% of IL-2 enhancer activity.

Under the influence of calcineurin, the cytoplasmic component of the *nuclear factor of activated T*-cells (**NFAT$_c$**) becomes activated and translocates to the nucleus where it forms a binary complex with NFAT$_n$, its partner which is constitutively expressed in the nucleus. The NFAT complex binds to two different IL-2 regulatory sites (figure 9.7). Note here that the calcineurin effect is blocked by the anti-T-cell drugs cyclosporin and FK506 (see Chapter 17). PKC- and calcineurin-dependent pathways synergize in activating the multisubunit IκB kinase (IKK), which phosphorylates the inhibitor IκB thereby targeting it for ubiquitination and subsequent degradation by the proteasome. Loss of IκB from the IκB–NFκB complex exposes the nuclear localization signal on the NFκB transcription factor which then swiftly enters the nucleus. In addition, the ubiquitous transcription

factor **Oct-1** interacts with specific octamer-binding sequence motifs.

We have concentrated on IL-2 transcription as an early and central consequence of T-cell activation, but more than 70 genes are newly expressed within 4 hours of T-cell activation, leading to proliferation and the synthesis of several cytokines and their receptors (see Chapter 10).

Further thoughts on T-cell triggering

A serial TCR engagement model for T-cell activation

We have already commented that the major docking forces which conjugate the APC and its T-lymphocyte counterpart must come from the complementary accessory molecules such as ICAM-1/LFA-1 and LFA-

Figure 9.7. T-cell signaling leads to activation. The signals through the MHC–antigen complex (signal 1) and costimulator B7 (signal 2) initiate a protein kinase cascade and a rise in intracellular calcium, thereby activating transcription factors which control entry in the cell cycle from G0 and regulate the expression of IL-2 and many other cytokines. Itk is a member of the Tec family of kinases which associates with a multimeric complex containing a number of adaptor proteins involved in PLCγ1 activation and thereby stimulates the IP$_3$ and DAG pathways. Upon activation by calcineurin, NFAT$_c$ translocates from the cytoplasm to the nucleus and complexes with the nuclear component NFAT$_n$. The complex then binds to the NFAT transcription sites. The IκB kinase (IKK) mediates the release of NFκB from its inhibitor IκB, whence it translocates to the nucleus and binds to a specific regulatory site. The Ras pathway activates the Raf, MEK, ERK and Elk kinases, finally activating the transcription factor Fos. Ras also activates Rac, which then phosphorylates JNKK, the kinase which activates JNK, and finally the transcription factor Jun which, complexed with Fos, binds to the AP-1 transcription site. B7 can incite a negative signal through CTLA-4. Note that the adaptor protein SLAP, also called Fyb, can play an inhibitory role in signaling by abrogating the function of SLP-76. The scheme presented omits several molecules which are thought to play important additional roles in signal transduction. As well as Lyk, other Src family PTKs, such as Fyn and Lyn, can phosphorylate ITAM motifs associated with a number of receptors including TCR, BCR and FcR. Transmembrane adaptors not shown include SIT (*SHP-2 interacting transmembrane adaptor*) and TRIM (*T-cell receptor interacting molecule*): the latter may act through the Grb2 adaptor as a positive regulator, whereas SIT may be a negative regulator. Abbreviations: DAG, diacylglycerol; ERK, *extracellular signal regulated kinase*; IP$_3$, inositol triphosphate; JNK, *Jun N-terminal kinase*; LAT, *linker for activated T-cells*; NFκB, *nuclear factor κβ*; NFAT, *nuclear factor of activated T-cells*; OCT-1, octamer-binding factor; Pak, *p21-activated kinase*; PI3K, phosphatidylinositol 3-kinase; PIP$_2$, phosphatidylinositol diphosphate; PKC, protein kinase C; PLC, phospholipase C; SH2, *Src-homology domain 2*; SLAP, *SLP-76-associated phosphoprotein*; SLP-76, *SH2-domain containing leukocyte-specific 76 kDa phosphoprotein*; ZAP-70, *ζ chain-associated protein kinase*. ⟿, Positive signal transduction; – – ➤, negative signal transduction; ▢, adaptor proteins; ▪, guanine nucleotide exchange factors; ▪, kinases; ▢, transcription factors; ▪, other molecules.

3/CD2, rather than through the relatively low affinity TCR–MHC plus peptide links (figure 9.3). Nonetheless, cognate antigen recognition by the TCR remains a *sine qua non* for T-cell activation. Fine, but how can as few as 100 MHC–peptide complexes on an APC, through their low affinity complexing with TCRs, effect the Herculean task of sustaining a raised intracellular calcium flux for the 60 minutes required for full cell activation? Any fall in calcium flux, as may be occasioned by adding an antibody to the MHC, and NFAT$_c$ dutifully returns from the nucleus to its cytoplasmic location, so aborting the activation process.

Surprisingly, Valitutti and Lanzavecchia have shown that as few as 100 MHC–peptide complexes on an APC can downregulate 18000 TCRs on its cognate T-lymphocyte partner. They suggest that each MHC–peptide complex can *serially* engage up to 200 TCRs. In their model, conjugation of an MHC–peptide dimer with two TCRs (cf. p. 100) activates signal transduction, phosphorylation of the CD3-associated ζ chains with subsequent downstream events, and then downregulation of those TCRs. Intermediate affinity binding favors dissociation of the MHC–peptide, freeing it to engage and trigger another TCR, so sustaining the required intracellular activation events. The model for **agonist** action would also explain why peptides giving interactions of lower or higher affinity than the optimum could behave as **antagonists** (figure 9.8). The important phenomenon of modified peptides behaving as **partial agonists**, with differential effects on the outcome of T-cell activation, is addressed in the legend to figure 9.8.

The immunological synapse

Experiments using peptide–MHC and ICAM-1 molecules labeled with different fluorochromes and inserted into a planar lipid bilayer on a glass support have provided evidence for the idea that T-cell activation occurs in the context of an **immunological synapse.** A clustered area of integrins acts as an anchor to permit optimal interaction between the opposing cell surfaces. Initially unstable TCR–MHC interactions occur in a broad outer ring surrounding the integrins. The peptide–MHC molecules then move towards the center of the synapse, changing places with the adhesion molecules which now form the outer ring (figure 9.9). It has been suggested that the generation of the immunological synapse only occurs after a certain initial threshold level of TCR triggering has been achieved, its formation being dependent upon cytoskeletal reorganization and leading to potentiation of the signal.

Affinity of MHC/peptide–TCR interaction	Duration, frequency and quality of complex formation	No. of successful complexes formed in given time	Outcome
Low		V. low	**Antagonist**
Intermediate		High	**Agonist**
High		Too low	**Antagonist**

APC–T-cell interaction time

Figure 9.8. Serial triggering model of TCR activation (Valitutti S. & Lanzavecchia A. (1995) *The Immunologist* **3**, 122). Intermediate affinity complexes between MHC–peptide and TCR survive long enough for a successful activation signal to be transduced by the TCR, and the MHC–peptide dissociates and fruitfully engages another TCR. A sustained high rate of formation of successful complexes is required for full T-cell activation. Low affinity complexes have a short half-life which either has no effect on the TCR or produces inactivation, perhaps through partial phosphorylation of ζ chains (◓, successful TCR activation; ●, TCR inactivation; ▬, no effect: the length of the horizontal bar indicates the lifetime of that complex). Being of low affinity, they recycle rapidly and engage and inactivate a large number of TCRs. High affinity complexes have such a long lifetime before dissociation that insufficient numbers of successful triggering events occur. Thus modified peptide ligands of either low or high affinity can act as antagonists by denying the agonist access to adequate numbers of vacant TCRs. Some modified peptides act as partial agonists in that they produce differential effects on the outcomes of T-cell activation. For example, a single residue change in a hemoglobin peptide reduced IL-4 secretion 10-fold but completely knocked out T-cell proliferation. The mechanism presumably involves incomplete or inadequately transduced phosphorylation events occurring through a truncated half-life of TCR engagement, allosteric effects on the MHC–TCR partners, or orientational misalignment of the peptide within the complex. Reproduced with permission of Hogrefe & Huber Publishers.

Damping T-cell enthusiasm

We have frequently reiterated the premise that no self-respecting organism would permit the operation of an expanding enterprise such as a proliferating T-cell population without some sensible controlling mechanisms.

Whereas CD28 is constitutively expressed on T-cells, CTLA-4 is not found on the resting cell but is rapidly upregulated following activation. It has a 10–20-fold higher affinity for both B7.1 and B7.2 and, in contrast to costimulatory signals generated through CD28, B7 engagement of CTLA-4 downregulates T-cell activation (figure 9.7), although the mechanism by which it does so is unknown.

A number of adaptor molecules have been identified which may be involved in reigning in T-cell activation. These include SLAP, SIT and members of the Cbl family. Cbl-b appears to influence the CD28 dependence of IL-2 production during T-cell activation, perhaps via an effect on the guanine nucleotide exchange

Figure 9.9. The immunological synapse. (a) The formation of the immunological synapse. T-cells were brought into contact with planar lipid bilayers and the positions of engaged MHC–peptide (green) and engaged ICAM-1 (red) at the indicated times after initial contact are shown (reproduced with permission from Grakoui A., Dustin M.L. *et al.* (1999) *Science* **285**, 221. © American Association for the Advancement of Science.). (b) Diagrammatic representation of the resolved synapse in which the adhesion molecule pairs CD2/LFA-3 and LFA-1/ICAM-1, which were originally in the center, have moved to the outside and now encircle the antigen recognition and signaling interaction between TCR and MHC–peptide and the costimulatory interaction between CD28 and B7. The CD43 molecule has been reported to bind to three different ligands, ICAM-1, galectin-1 and MHC class I, and upon ligation is able to induce IL-2 mRNA, CD69 and CD154 (CD40L) expression and activate the DNA-binding activity of the AP-1, NFκB and NFAT transcription factors.

factor Vav. Another member of the Cbl family, Cbl-c, is a negative regulator of Syk and ZAP-70, and may thereby alter the triggering threshold of the antigen receptors on both T- and B-cells.

Tempting though it might be, phosphatases should not automatically be equated with downregulation of a phosphorylation cascade. The observation that

T-cell mutants lacking CD45 do not possess signal transduction capacity was at first sight deemed to be strange because CD45 has phosphatase activity and was thought thereby to downregulate signaling. However, the Lck kinase in the CD45-deficient cells is phosphorylated on tyrosine-505 which is a negative regulatory site for kinase activity; hence dephosphorylation by CD45 activates the Lck enzyme and the paradox is resolved.

B-CELLS RESPOND TO THREE DIFFERENT TYPES OF ANTIGEN

1 Type 1 thymus-independent antigens

Certain antigens, such as bacterial lipopolysaccharides, at a high enough concentration, have the ability to activate a substantial proportion of the B-cell pool polyclonally, i.e. without reference to the antigen specificity of the surface receptor hypervariable regions. They do this through binding to a surface molecule which bypasses the early part of the biochemical pathway mediated by the specific antigen receptor. At concentrations which are too low to cause polyclonal activation through unaided binding to these mitogenic bypass molecules, the B-cell population with Ig receptors specific for these antigens will selectively and passively focus them on their surface, where the resulting high local concentration will suffice to drive the activation process (figure 9.10a).

2 Type 2 thymus-independent antigens

Certain linear antigens which are not readily degraded in the body and which have an appropriately spaced, highly repeating determinant—*Pneumococcus* polysaccharide, ficoll, D-amino acid polymers and poly-

vinylpyrrolidone, for example—are also thymus-independent in their ability to stimulate B-cells directly without the need for T-cell involvement. They persist for long periods on the surface of specialized macrophages located at the subcapsular sinus of the lymph nodes and the splenic marginal zone, and can bind to antigen-specific B-cells with great avidity through their multivalent attachment to the complementary Ig receptors which they cross-link (figure 9.10b).

In general, the thymus-independent antigens give rise to predominantly low affinity IgM responses, some IgG3 in the mouse, and relatively poor, if any, memory. Neonatal B-cells do not respond well to type 2 antigens and this has important consequences for the efficacy of carbohydrate vaccines in young children.

3 Thymus-dependent antigens

The need for collaboration with T-helper cells

Many antigens are thymus-dependent in that they provoke little or no antibody response in animals which have been thymectomized at birth and have few T-cells (Milestone 9.1). Such antigens cannot fulfil the molecular requirements for direct stimulation; they may be univalent with respect to the specificity of each determinant; they may be readily degraded by phagocytic cells; and they may lack mitogenicity. If they bind to B-cell receptors, they will sit on the surface just like a hapten and do nothing to trigger the B-cell (figure 9.11). Cast your mind back to the definition of a hapten—a small molecule like dinitrophenyl (DNP) which binds to preformed antibody (e.g. the surface receptor of a specific B-cell) but fails to stimulate antibody production (i.e. stimulate the B-cell). Remember also that haptens become immunogenic when coupled to an

Figure 9.10. B-cell recognition of (a) type 1 and (b) type 2 thymus-independent antigens. The complex gives a sustained signal to the B-cell because of the long half-life of this type of molecule. ⌇➔, activation signal; ⌇, surface Ig receptor; – – –, cross-linking of receptors.

Milestone 9.1 — T–B Collaboration for Antibody Production

In the 1960s, as the mysteries of the thymus were slowly unraveled, our erstwhile colleagues pushing back the frontiers of knowledge discovered that neonatal thymectomy in the mouse abrogated not only the cellular rejection of skin grafts, but also the antibody response to some but not all antigens (figure M9.1.1). Subsequent investigations showed that both thymocytes and bone marrow cells were needed for optimal antibody responses to such **thymus-dependent antigens** (figure M9.1.2). By carrying out these transfers with cells from animals bearing a recognizable chromosome marker (T6), it became evident that the antibody-forming cells were derived from the bone marrow inoculum, hence the nomenclature 'T' for *Thymus*-derived lymphocytes and 'B' for antibody-forming cell precursors originating in the *Bone* marrow. This convenient nomenclature has stuck even though bone marrow contains embryonic T-cell precursors since the immuno-competent T- and B-cells differentiate in the thymus and bone marrow respectively (see Chapter 12).

Figure M9.1.1. The antibody response to some antigens is thymus-dependent and, to others, thymus-independent. The response to tetanus toxoid in neonatally thymectomized animals could be restored by the injection of thymocytes.

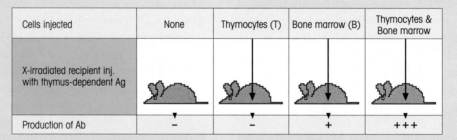

Cells injected	None	Thymocytes (T)	Bone marrow (B)	Thymocytes & Bone marrow
X-irradiated recipient inj. with thymus-dependent Ag				
Production of Ab	–	–	+	+++

Figure M9.1.2. The antibody response to a thymus-dependent antigen requires two different cell populations. Different populations of cells from a normal mouse histocompatible with the recipient (i.e. of the same H-2 haplotype) were injected into recipients which had been X-irradiated to destroy their own lymphocyte responses. They were then primed with a thymus-dependent antigen such as sheep red blood cells (i.e. an antigen which fails to give a response in neonatally thymectomized mice; figure M9.1.1) and examined for the production of antibody after 2 weeks. The small amount of antibody synthesized by animals receiving bone marrow alone is due to the presence of thymocyte precursors in the cell inoculum which differentiate in the intact thymus gland of the recipient.

appropriate carrier protein (see p. 80). Building on the knowledge that both T- and B-cells are necessary for antibody responses to thymus-dependent antigens (Milestone 9.1), we now know that the carrier functions to stimulate T-helper cells which cooperate with B-cells to enable them to respond to the hapten by providing accessory signals (figure 9.11). It should also be evident from figure 9.11 that, while one determinant on a typical protein antigen is behaving as a hapten in binding to the B-cell, the other determinants subserve a carrier function in recruiting T-helper cells.

Antigen processing by B-cells

The need for **physical linkage of hapten and carrier** strongly suggests that T-helpers must recognize the carrier determinants on the responding B-cell in order to provide the relevant accessory stimulatory signals. However, since T-cells only recognize processed membrane-bound antigen in association with MHC molecules, the T-helpers cannot recognize native antigen bound simply to the Ig receptors of the B-cell as naively depicted in figure 9.11. All is not lost, however, since **primed B-cells can present antigen to T-helper cells**—in fact, they work at much lower antigen concentrations than conventional presenting cells because they can focus antigen through their surface receptors. Antigen bound to surface Ig is internalized in endosomes which then fuse with vesicles containing MHC class II molecules with their invariant chain. Processing of the protein antigen then occurs as described in Chapter 5 (see figure 5.18) and the resulting antigenic peptide is recycled to the surface in association with the class II molecules where it is available for recognition by specific T-helpers (figures 9.12 and 9.13). The need for the physical union of hapten and carrier is now revealed; the hapten leads the carrier to be processed into the cell which is programed to make

antihapten antibody and, following stimulus by the T-helper-recognizing processed carrier, it will carry out its program and ultimately produce antibodies which react with the hapten (is there no end to the wiliness of nature?!).

THE NATURE OF B-CELL ACTIVATION

B-cells are stimulated by cross-linking surface Ig

Cross-linking of the B-cell receptor (BCR), for example by anti-IgM conjugated to insoluble Sepharose particles or by polymeric type 2 thymus-independent antigens with repeating determinants, induces the early activation events. Coligation of the pan-B-cell marker CD19 with surface Ig (sIg) reduces the threshold for cell activation 100-fold. *In vivo* this could be brought about by bridging the Ig and CR2 complement receptors on the B-cell surface by antigen–C3d complexes bound to the surface of APCs, since CD19 and CR2 (CD21) molecules enjoy mutual association.

Within 1 minute of surface Ig ligation, Src family kinases rapidly phosphorylate the Syk kinase, Bruton's tyrosine kinase (Btk) and the ITAMs on the sIg receptor chains Ig-α and Ig-β. Syk binds to the Ig-α and Ig-β ITAMs, analogously to ZAP-70 binding to the ITAMs on the TCR-associated ζ chains. CD19 also becomes phosphorylated, possibly by Lyn, thereby creating binding sites for the SH2 domains of phosphatidylinositol 3-kinase and the guanine nucleotide exchange factor Vav. Although B-cells lack the LAT and SLP-76 adaptors of T-cells (cf. figure 9.7), they possess a homolog of SLP-76 variously referred to as SLP-65, BLNK

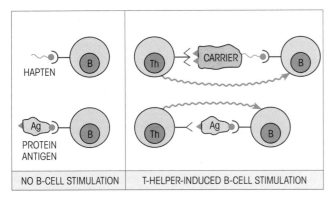

Figure 9.11. T-helper cells cooperate through protein carrier determinants to help B-cells respond to hapten or equivalent determinants on antigens by providing accessory signals. (For simplicity we are ignoring the MHC component and epitope processing in T-cell recognition, but we won't forget it.)

Figure 9.12. B-cell handling of a thymus-dependent antigen. Antigen captured by the surface Ig receptor is internalized within an endosome, processed and expressed on the surface with MHC class II (cf. figure 5.18). Costimulatory signals through the CD40–CD40L (CD154) interaction are required for the activation of the resting cell by the T-helper. sIg cross-linking by antigen on the surface of an antigen-presenting cell is likely during secondary responses within the germinal centers when complement-containing complexes on follicular dendritic cells interact with B-lymphoblasts. ⌇⌇⌇, activation signal; ⋎⋎⋎, cross-linking of receptors.

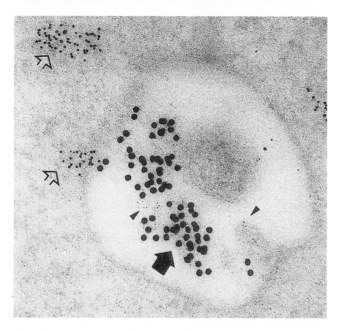

Figure 9.13. Demonstration that endocytosed B-cell surface Ig receptors enter cytoplasmic vesicles geared for antigen processing. Surface IgG was cross-linked with goat anti-human Ig and rabbit anti-goat Ig conjugated to 15-nm gold beads (large, dark arrow). After 2 minutes, the cell sections were prepared and stained with anti-HLA-DR invariant chain (2 nm gold; arrowheads) and an antibody to a cathepsin protease (5 nm gold; open arrows). Thus the internalized IgG is exposed to proteolysis in a vesicle containing class II molecules. The presence of invariant chain shows that the class II molecules derive from the endoplasmic reticulum and Golgi, not from the cell surface. Note the clever use of different-sized gold particles to distinguish the antibodies used for localizing the various intravesicular proteins, etc. (Photograph reproduced with permission from the authors and the publishers from Guagliardi L.E. *et al.* (1990) *Nature* **343**, 133. Copyright © 1990 Macmillan Magazines Ltd.)

(B-cell linker protein) or BASH (B-cell adaptor containing SH2 domain). SLP-65 is phosphorylated by Syk and forms a multimeric complex incorporating Vav, Btk and phospholipase Cγ2 (PLCγ2), the latter kicking off the PIP$_2$ pathway. Just as in the T-cell, this generates inositol triphosphate and diacylglycerol with a subsequent rise in intracellular calcium and activation of protein kinase C (cf. figure 9.7). The enhancer-binding protein NFκB is released from its inhibitor IκB on activation of protein kinase C and moves into the nucleus, where its appearance is associated with κ light chain gene transcription. The SLP-65 adaptor also links B-cell signaling into activation of the ERK and JNK pathways.

The BCR cross-linking model seems appropriate for an understanding of stimulation by type 2 thymus-independent antigens, since their repeating determinants ensure strong binding to, and cross-linking of, multiple Ig receptors on the B-cell surface to form aggregates which persist owing to the long half-life of the antigen and sustain the high intracellular calcium needed for activation. On the other hand, type 1 T-independent antigens, like the T-cell polyclonal activators, probably bypass the specific receptor and act directly on downstream molecules such as diacylglycerol and protein kinase C since Ig-α and Ig-β are not phosphorylated.

T-helper cells activate resting B-cells

T-dependent antigens pose a different problem, since they are usually univalent with respect to B-cell receptors, i.e. each epitope appears once on a monomeric protein, and as a result they cannot cross-link the surface Ig. However, we have discussed in some detail how antigen captured by a B-cell receptor can be internalized and processed for surface presentation as a peptide complexed with class II MHC (cf. figure 9.12). This can now be recognized by the TCR of a carrier-specific T-helper cell and, with the assistance of costimulatory signals arising from the interaction of **CD40 with its ligand CD40L** (cf. figure 9.12), B-cell activation is ensured.

In effect, the B-lymphocyte is acting as an antigen-presenting cell and, as mentioned above, it is very efficient because of its ability to concentrate the antigen by focusing onto its surface Ig. Nonetheless, although a preactivated T-helper can mutually interact with and stimulate a resting B-cell, a *resting* T-cell can only be triggered by a B-cell that has acquired the B7 costimulator and this is only present on activated, not resting, B-cells.

Presumably the immune complexes on follicular dendritic cells in germinal centers of secondary follicles can be taken up by the B-cells for presentation to T-helpers, but, additionally, the complexes could cross-link the sIg of the B-cell blasts and drive their proliferation in a T-independent manner. This would be enhanced by the presence of C3 in the complexes since the B-cell complement receptor (CR2) is comitogenic.

SUMMARY

Immunocompetent T- and B-cells differ in many respects

• The antigen-specific receptors, TCR/CD3 on T-cells and surface Ig on B-cells, provide a clear distinction between these two cell types.

• T- and B-cells differ in their receptors for C3d, IgG and certain viruses.

• There are distinct polyclonal activators of T-cells (PHA, anti-CD3) and of B-cells (anti-Ig, Epstein–Barr virus).

T-lymphocytes and antigen-presenting cells interact through pairs of accessory molecules

• The docking of T-cells and APCs depends upon strong mutual interactions between complementary molecular pairs on their surfaces: MHC II–CD4, MHC I–CD8, VCAM-1–VLA-4, ICAM-1–LFA-1, LFA-3–CD2, B7–CD28 (and CTLA-4).

Activation of T-cells requires two signals

• Two signals activate T-cells, but one alone produces unresponsiveness (anergy).

• One signal is provided by the low affinity cognate TCR–MHC plus peptide interaction.

• The second costimulatory signal is mediated through ligation of CD28 by B7.

Protein tyrosine phosphorylation is an early event in T-cell signaling

• The TCR signal is transduced and amplified through a protein tyrosine kinase (PTK) enzymic cascade.

• CD4/TCR colocation leads to phosphorylation of ITAM sequences on CD3-associated ζ chains by the CD4-associated Lck PTK. The phosphorylated ITAMs bind and then activate the ZAP-70 kinase.

Downstream events following TCR signaling

• Nonenzymic adaptor proteins form multimeric complexes with kinases and guanine nucleotide exchange factors (GEFs).

• Hydrolysis of phosphatidylinositol diphosphate by phospholipase Cγ1 or Cγ2 produces inositol triphosphate (IP$_3$) and diacylglycerol (DAG).

• IP$_3$ mobilizes intracellular calcium.

• DAG and increased calcium activate protein kinase C.

• The raised calcium together with calmodulin also stimulates calcineurin activity.

• Activation of Ras by the guanine nucleotide exchange factor Sos sets off a kinase cascade operating through Raf,

the MAP kinase kinase MEK and the MAP kinase ERK. CD28 through PI3 kinase can also influence MAP kinase.

• The transcription factors Fos and Jun, NFAT and NFκB are activated by MAP kinase, calcineurin and PKC, respectively, and bind to regulatory sites in the IL-2 promoter region.

• A small number of MHC–peptide complexes can serially trigger a much larger number of TCRs thereby providing the sustained signal required for activation.

• Initial binding of integrins facilitates the formation of an immunological synapse, the core of which exchanges integrins for TCR interacting with MHC–peptide.

• B7 delivers a negative signal through CTLA-4, and Cbl family adaptor molecules are also involved in negative signaling pathways.

• The phosphatase domains on CD45 are required to remove phosphates at inhibitory sites on kinases.

B-cells respond to three different types of antigen

• Type 1 thymus-independent antigens are polyclonal activators focused onto the specific B-cells by sIg receptors.

• Type 2 thymus-independent antigens are polymeric molecules which cross-link many sIg receptors and, because of their long half-lives, provide a persistent signal to the B-cell.

• Thymus-dependent antigens require the cooperation of helper T-cells to stimulate antibody production by B-cells.

• Antigen captured by specific sIg receptors is taken into the B-cell, processed and expressed on the surface as a peptide in association with MHC II.

• This complex is recognized by the T-helper cell which activates the resting B-cell.

• The ability of protein carriers to enable the antibody response to haptens is explained by T–B collaboration, with T-cells recognizing the carrier and B-cells the hapten.

The nature of B-cell activation

• Cross-linking of surface Ig receptors (e.g. by type 2 thymus-independent antigens) activates B-cells.

• T-helper cells activate resting B-cells through TCR recognition of MHC II–carrier peptide complexes and costimulation through CD40L–CD40 interactions (analogous to the B7–CD28 second signal for T-cell activation).

See the accompanying website (**www.roitt.com**) for multiple choice questions.

FURTHER READING

Acuto O. & Cantrell D. (2000) T cell activation and the cytoskeleton. *Annual Reviews in Immunology* **18**, 165.

Bromley S.K., Burack W.R., Johnson K.G. *et al.* (2001) The immunological synapse. *Annual Review of Immunology* **19**, 375.

Grakoui A. *et al.* (1999) The immunological synapse: a molecular machine controlling T cell activation. *Science* **285**, 221.

Jenkins M.K., Khoruts A., Ingulli E. *et al.* (2001) In vivo activation of antigen-specific CD4 T cells. *Annual Review of Immunology* **19**, 23.

Michel G. (ed.) (1999) *Biochemical Pathways: An Atlas of Biochemistry and Molecular Biology.* John Wiley & Sons, New York.

Myung P.S., Boerthe N.J. & Koretzky G.A. (2000) Adaptor proteins in lymphocyte antigen-receptor signaling. *Current Opinion in Immunology* **12**, 256.

Olson M.F. & Marais R. (2000) Ras protein signalling. *Seminars in Immunology* **12**, 63.

Oosterwegel A. *et al.* (1999) CTLA-4 and T cell activation. *Current Opinion in Immunology* **11**, 294.

Schraven B. *et al.* (1999) Integration of receptor-mediated signals in T cells by transmembrane adaptor proteins. *Immunology Today* **20**, 431.

The production of effectors

INTRODUCTION

We have dwelt upon the early events in lymphocyte activation consequent upon the engagement of the T-cell receptor (TCR) and the provision of an appropriate costimulatory signal. A complex series of tyrosine and serine/threonine phosphorylation reactions produces the factors which push the cell into the mitotic cycle and drive clonal proliferation and the differentiation to effectors. A succession of genes are upregulated by T-cell activation. Within the first half hour, nuclear transcription factors such as Fos/Jun and NFAT, which regulate interleukin-2 (IL-2) expression and the cellular protooncogene c-*myc*, are expressed, but the next few hours see the synthesis of a range of **soluble cytokines and their receptors**. Much later we see molecules like the transferrin receptor related to cell division and very late antigens such as the adhesion molecule VLA-1.

CYTOKINES ACT AS INTERCELLULAR MESSENGERS

In contrast with the initial activation of T-cells and T-dependent B-cells, which involves intimate contact with the antigen-presenting cells (APCs), subsequent proliferation and maturation of the response are orchestrated by soluble mediators generically termed cytokines (figure 10.1). With the realization that a given cytokine can be produced by many different cell types, terms such as lymphokine or monokine have become somewhat obsolete (table 10.1).

Cytokine action is transient and usually short range

These low molecular weight secreted proteins, usually 15–25 kDa, mediate cell growth, inflammation, immunity, differentiation, migration and repair. Because they regulate the amplitude and duration of the immune–inflammatory responses, they must be produced in a transient manner tightly regulated by the presence of foreign material, and it is relevant that the AU-rich sequences in the 3' untranslated regions of the mRNA of many cytokines are correlated directly with rapid degradation and therefore short half-life. Unlike endocrine hormones, the majority of cytokines normally act locally in a paracrine or even autocrine fashion. Thus cytokines derived from lymphocytes rarely persist in the circulation, but nonlymphoid cells can be triggered by bacterial products to release cytokines which may be detected in the bloodstream, often to the detriment of the host. Certain cytokines,

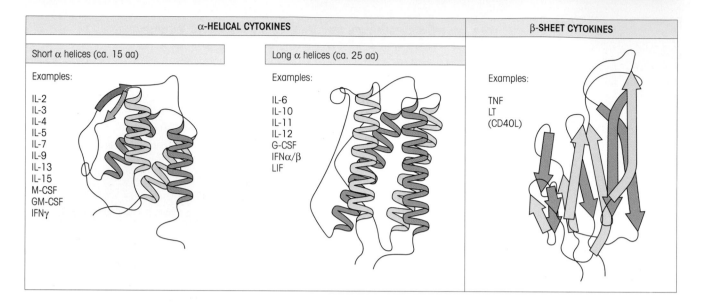

| α-HELICAL CYTOKINES | | β-SHEET CYTOKINES |

Short α helices (ca. 15 aa)

Examples:

IL-2
IL-3
IL-4
IL-5
IL-7
IL-9
IL-13
IL-15
M-CSF
GM-CSF
IFNγ

Long α helices (ca. 25 aa)

Examples:

IL-6
IL-10
IL-11
IL-12
G-CSF
IFNα/β
LIF

β-SHEET CYTOKINES

Examples:

TNF
LT
(CD40L)

Figure 10.1. Cytokine structures. Cytokines can be divided into a number of different structural groups. Illustrated here are three of the main types of structure and some named examples of each type: (a) four short (~15 amino acids) α-helices, (b) four long (~25 amino acids) α-helices and (c) a β-sheet structure. (Reproduced with permission from Michal G. (ed.) (1999) *Biochemical Pathways: An Atlas of Biochemistry and Molecular Biology.* John Wiley & Sons, New York.)

including IL-1 and tumor necrosis factor (TNF), also exist in membrane forms which can exert their stimulatory effects without becoming soluble.

Cytokines act through cell surface receptors

Cytokines are highly potent, often acting at femtomolar (10^{-15} M) concentrations, combining with small numbers of high affinity cell surface receptors to produce changes in the pattern of RNA and protein synthesis. A common feature in the triggering of the cytokine receptors is the ligand-induced association of receptor subunits which allows signal transduction through the interplay of their juxtaposed cytoplasmic domains. There are six major cytokine receptor structural families (figure 10.2).

Hematopoietin receptors

These are the largest family, sometimes referred to simply as the cytokine receptor superfamily. These receptors generally consist of one or two polypeptide chains responsible for cytokine binding and an additional shared (common or 'c') chain involved in signal transduction. The γc (CD132) chain is used by the IL-2

receptor (figure 10.2a) and IL-4, IL-7, IL-9, IL-13 and IL-15 receptors, a βc (CDw131) chain by IL-3, IL-5 and granulocyte–macrophage colony-stimulating factor (GM-CSF) receptors, and gp130 (CD130) shared chain by the IL-6, IL-11, IL-12, oncostatin M, ciliary neurotrophic factor and leukemia inhibitory factor (LIF) receptors.

Interferon receptors

These also consist of two polypeptide chains and, in addition to the IFNα, IFNβ and IFNγ receptors (figure 10.2b), this family includes the IL-10 receptor.

TNF receptors

The receptor polypeptides are cysteine rich and trimerize following cytokine binding. They include the tumor necrosis factor (TNF) receptor (figure 10.2c), lymphotoxin (LT) and nerve growth factor (NGF) receptors, and the cell surface-associated molecules CD40 and CD95 (Fas).

IgSF cytokine receptors

Immunoglobulin superfamily members are broadly utilized in many aspects of cell biology (cf. p. 245) and include the IL-1 receptor (figure 10.2d), and the macrophage colony-stimulating factor (M-CSF) and stem cell factor (SCF/c-kit) receptors.

Chemokine receptors

As we shall discover shortly, these comprise a family of approximately 20 different G-protein-coupled,

Table 10.1. Cytokines: their origin and function.

CYTOKINE	SOURCE	EFFECTOR FUNCTION
INTERLEUKINS		
IL-1α, IL-1β	Mono, Mφ, DC, NK, B, Endo	Costimulates T activation by enhancing production of cytokines including IL-2 and its receptor; enhances B proliferation and maturation; NK cytotoxicity; induces IL-1,-6,-8, TNF, GM-CSF and PGE$_2$ by Mφ; proinflammatory by inducing chemokines and ICAM-1 and VCAM-1 on endothelium; induces fever, APP, bone resorption by osteoclasts
IL-2	Th1	Induces proliferation of activated T- and B-cells; enhances NK cytotoxicity and killing of tumor cells and bacteria by monocytes and Mφ
IL-3	T, NK, MC	Growth and differentiation of hematopoietic precursors; MC growth
IL-4	Th2, Tc2, NK, NK-T, γδ T, MC	Induces Th2 cells; stimulates proliferation of activated B, T, MC; upregulates MHC class II on B and Mφ, and CD23 on B; downregulates IL-12 production and thereby inhibits Th1 differentiation; increases Mφ phagocytosis; induces switch to IgG1 and IgE
IL-5	Th2, MC	Induces proliferation of eosino and activated B; induces switch to IgA
IL-6	Th2, Mono, Mφ, DC, BM stroma	Differentiation of myeloid stem cells and of B into plasma cells; induces APP; enhances T proliferation
IL-7	BM and thymic stroma	Induces differentiation of lymphoid stem cells into progenitor T and B; activates mature T
IL-8	Mono, Mφ, Endo	Mediates chemotaxis and activation of neutrophils
IL-9	Th	Induces proliferation of thymocytes; enhances MC growth; synergizes with IL-4 in switch to IgG1 and IgE
IL-10	Th (Th2 in mouse), Tc, B, Mono, Mφ	Inhibits IFNγ secretion by mouse, and IL-2 by human, Th1 cells; downregulates MHC class II and cytokine (including IL-12) production by mono, Mφ and DC, thereby inhibiting Th1 differentiation; inhibits T proliferation; enhances B differentiation
IL-11	BM stroma	Promotes differentiation of pro-B and megakaryocytes; induces APP
IL-12	Mono, Mφ, DC, B	Critical cytokine for Th1 differentiation; induces proliferation and IFNγ production by Th1, CD8$^+$ and γδ T and NK; enhances NK and CD8$^+$ T cytotoxicity
IL-13	Th2, MC	Inhibits activation and cytokine secretion by Mφ; co-activates B proliferation; upregulates MHC class II and CD23 on B and mono; induces switch to IgG1 and IgE; induces VCAM-1 on endo
IL-15	T, NK, Mono, Mφ, DC, B	Induces proliferation of T-, NK and activated B and cytokine production and cytotoxicity in NK and CD8$^+$ T; chemotactic for T; stimulates growth of intestinal epithelium
IL-16	Th, Tc	Chemoattractant for CD4 T, mono and eosino; induces MHC class II
IL-17	T	Proinflammatory; stimulates production of cytokines including TNF, IL-1β,-6,-8, G-CSF
IL-18	Mφ, DC	Induces IFNγ production by T; enhances NK cytotoxicity
IL-19	Mono	Modulation of Th1 activity
IL-20	Keratinocytes?	Regulation of inflammatory responses to skin?
IL-21	Th	Regulation of hematopoiesis; NK differentiation; B activation; T costimulation
IL-22	T	Inhibits IL-4 production by Th2
IL-23	DC	Induces proliferation and IFNγ production by Th1; induces proliferation of memory cells
COLONY STIMULATING FACTORS		
GM-CSF	Th, Mφ, Fibro, MC, Endo	Stimulates growth of progenitors of mono, neutro, eosino and baso; activates Mφ
G-CSF	Fibro, Endo	Stimulates growth of neutro progenitors
M-CSF	Fibro, Endo, Epith	Stimulates growth of mono progenitors
SLF	BM stroma	Stimulates stem cell division (c-*kit* ligand)
TUMOR NECROSIS FACTORS		
TNF (TNFα)	Th, Mono, Mφ, DC, MC, NK, B	Tumor cytotoxicity; cachexia (weight loss); induces cytokine secretion; induces E-selectin on endo; activates Mφ; antiviral
Lymphotoxin (TNFβ)	Th1 Tc	Tumor cytotoxicity; enhances phagocytosis by neutro and Mφ; involved in lymphoid organ development; antiviral
INTERFERONS		
IFNα	Leukocytes	Inhibits viral replication; enhances MHC class I
IFNβ	Fibroblasts	Inhibits viral replication; enhances MHC class I
IFNγ	Th1, Tc1, NK	Inhibits viral replication; Enhances MHC class I and II; activates Mφ; induces switch to IgG2a; antagonizes several IL-4 actions; inhibits proliferation of Th2
OTHERS		
TGFβ	Th3, B, Mφ, MC	Proinflammatory by, e.g., chemoattraction of mono and Mφ but also anti-inflammatory by, e.g. inhibiting lymphocyte proliferation; induces switch to IgA; promotes tissue repair
LIF	Thymic epith, BM stroma	Induces APP
Eta-1	T	Stimulates IL-12 production and inhibits IL-10 production by Mφ
Oncostatin M	T, Mφ	Induces APP

APP, acute phase proteins; B, B-cell; baso, basophil; BM, bone marrow; Endo, endothelium; eosino, eosinophil; Epith, epithelium; Fibro, fibroblast; GM-CSF, granulocyte–macrophage colony-stimulating factor; IL, interleukin; LIF, leukemia inhibitory factor; Mφ, macrophage; MC, mast cell; Mono, monocyte; neutro, neutrophil; NK, natural killer; SLF, steel locus factor; T, T-cell; TGFβ, transforming growth factor-β. Note that there is not an interleukin-14. This designation was given to an activity that, upon further investigation, could not be unambiguously assigned to a single cytokine. IL-8 is a member of the chemokine family. These cytokines are listed separately in table 10.3.

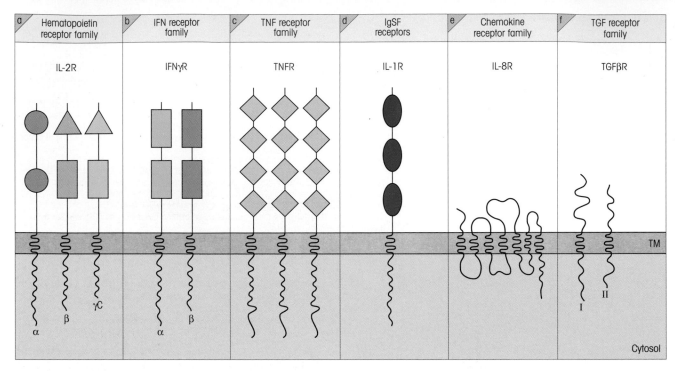

Figure 10.2. Cytokine receptor families. One example is shown for each family. (a) The **hematopoietin receptors** operate through a common subunit (γc, βc or gp130, depending on the subfamily) which transduces the signal to the interior of the cell. In essence, binding of the cytokine to its receptor must initiate the signaling process by mediating hetero- or homodimer formation involving the common subunit. In some cases the cytokine is active when bound to the receptor either in soluble or membrane-bound form (e.g. IL-6). The IL-2 receptor is interesting with respect to its ligand binding. The α chain (CD25, reacting with the Tac monoclonal) of the receptor possesses two complement control protein structural domains and binds IL-2 with a low affinity; the β chain (CD122) has a membrane proximal fibronectin type III structural domain and a membrane distal cytokine receptor structural domain, and associates with the common γ chain (CD132) which has a similar structural organization. The β chain binds IL-2 with intermediate affinity. IL-2 binds to and dissociates from the α chain very rapidly but the same processes involving the β chain occur at two or three orders of magnitude more slowly. When the α, β and γ chains form a single recep-

tor, the α chain binds the IL-2 rapidly and facilitates its binding to a separate site on the β chain from which it can only dissociate slowly. Since the final affinity (K_d) is based on the ratio of dissociation to association rate constants, then $K_d = 10^{-4}\,\text{sec}^{-1}/10^7\,\text{M}^{-1}\,\text{sec}^{-1} = 10^{-11}\,\text{M}$, which is a very high affinity. The γ chain does not itself bind IL-2 but contributes towards signal transduction. (b) The **interferon receptor** family consists of heterodimeric molecules each of which bears two fibronectin type III domains. (c) The receptors for **TNF** and related molecules consist of a single polypeptide with four TNFR domains. The receptor trimerizes upon ligand binding and, in common with a number of other receptors, is also found in a soluble form which, when released from a cell following activation, can act as an antagonist. (d) Another group of receptors contains varying numbers of **Ig superfamily domains**, whereas (e) **chemokine receptors** are members of the G-protein-coupled receptor superfamily and have seven hydrophobic transmembrane domains. (f) The final family illustrated are the **TGF receptors** which require association between two molecules, referred to as TGFR type I and TGFR type II, for signaling to occur.

seven transmembrane segment, receptors (figure 10.2e).

TGF receptors

Receptors for transforming growth factors such as the TGFβ receptor (figure 10.2f) possess cytoplasmic portions with serine/threonine kinase activity.

Signal transduction through cytokine receptors

The ligand-induced homo- or heterodimerization of cytokine receptor subunits represents a common theme for signaling by cytokines. The two major routes that are utilized are the Janus kinase (JAK)–STAT

and the Ras–MAP kinase pathways. Members of the cytokine receptor superfamily (hematopoietin receptors) lack catalytic domains and therefore associate with JAKs including JAK1, JAK2, JAK3 and Tyk2. Upon cytokine-induced receptor dimerization, the JAKs reciprocally phosphorylate, and thereby activate, each other. Once activated, they can phosphorylate the cytoplasmic domains of the receptors to create binding sites for SH2-containing signaling proteins. These include one or more of the group of transcription factors termed **STATs** (*s*ignal *t*ransducers and *a*ctivators of *t*ranscription), which also become phosphorylated by the workaholic JAKs, an event which causes the STATs to dissociate from the receptor and dimerize. The dimerized STATs then translocate to the nucleus

Figure 10.3. Cytokine receptor-mediated pathways for gene transcription. Cytokine-induced receptor oligomerization activates the associated JAK kinases. These phosphorylate the STAT DNA-binding transcription factors which dimerize and translocate to the nucleus. Cytokine receptors can also activate src family kinases which, via adaptor proteins such as Shc, Grb2 and SHP-2, could generate transcription factors via the two routes shown. MAPK, mitogen-activated protein kinases (see figure 9.7); MEK, kinase activator of MAPK; PI-3 kinase, phosphatidylinositol 3-kinase.

where they play an important role in pushing the cell through the mitotic cycle (figure 10.3). JAKs may also act through src family kinases to generate other transcription factors via the Ras–MAP kinase route (figure 10.3). Some cytokines also activate phosphatidylinositol 3-kinase (PI3K) and phospholipase C (PLCγ).

Downregulation of cytokine receptor-mediated signals involves members of the SOC (*s*uppressor *o*f *c*ytokine *s*ignaling) and CIS (*c*ytokine-*i*nducible *s*rc homology domain 2 [SH2]-containing) families. Although their mode of action is still being evaluated, some of these molecules may function by directly blocking phosphorylation motifs on the receptor, or possibly by acting as scavengers of tyrosine phosphorylated proteins, targeting them for ubiquitin/proteasome (cf. p. 94) degradation.

Cytokines often have multiple effects

In general, cytokines are **pleiotropic**, i.e. exhibit multiple effects on a variety of cell types (table 10.1),

and there is considerable overlap and *redundancy* between them with respect to individual functions, partially accounted for by the sharing of receptor components and the utilization of common transcription factors. For example, many of the biological activities of IL-4 overlap with those of IL-13. However, it should be pointed out that virtually all cytokines have at least some unique properties.

Their roles in the generation of T- and B-cell effectors, and in the regulation of chronic inflammatory reactions (figure 10.4a and b), will be discussed at length later in this chapter. We should note here the important role of cytokines in the control of hematopoiesis (figure 10.4c). The differentiation of stem cells to become the formed elements of blood within the environment of the bone marrow is carefully nurtured through the production of cytokines by the stromal cells. These include GM-CSF, G-CSF (granulocyte colony-stimulating factor), M-CSF, IL-6 and -7 and LIF (see table 10.1), and many of them are also derived from T-cells and macrophages. It is not surprising therefore that, during a period of chronic inflammation, the cytokines that are produced recruit new precursors into the hematopoietic differentiation pathway—a useful exercise in the circumstances. One of the cytokines, IL-3, should be highlighted for its exceptional ability to support the early cells in this pathway, particularly in synergy with IL-6 and G-CSF.

Network interactions

The complex and integrated relationships between the different cytokines are mediated through cellular events. The genes for IL-3, -4 and -5 and GM-CSF are all tightly linked on chromosome 5 in a region containing genes for M-CSF and its receptor and several other growth factors and receptors. Interaction may occur through a cascade in which one cytokine induces the production of another, through transmodulation of the receptor for another cytokine and through synergism or antagonism of two cytokines acting on the same cell (figure 10.5). The means by which target cells integrate and interpret the complex patterns of stimuli induced by these multiple soluble factors is only slowly unfolding.

DIFFERENT T-CELL SUBSETS CAN MAKE DIFFERENT CYTOKINE PATTERNS

The bipolar Th1/Th2 concept

Helper T-cell clones can be divided into two main types with distinct cytokine secretion phenotypes

Figure 10.4. Cytokine action. A general but not entirely comprehensive guide to indicate the scope of cytokine interactions (e.g. for reasons of simplicity we have omitted the inhibitory effects of IL-10 on monocytes and the activation of NK cells by IL-12). EOSINϕ, eosinophil; LAK, lymphokine-activated killer; Mϕ, macrophage; NK, natural killer cell; PMN, polymorphonuclear neutrophil.

Table 10.2. Cytokine patterns of helper T-cell clones. Interleukin-10 is not listed in the table. Although classed as a Th2 cytokine in the mouse, it is produced by both Th1 and Th2 cells in the human.

CYTOKINE PATTERNS OF T-CELL CLONES		
	Th1	Th2
IFNγ	++	Negative
IL-2	++	Negative
Lymphotoxin (TNFβ)	++	Negative
TNF (TNFα)	++	
GM-CSF	++	
IL-3	++	++
IL-4	Negative	++
IL-5	Negative	++
IL-6	Negative	++
IL-13	Negative	++

██ ++   ░░ +   ☐ Negative

Th1/2, T-helper 1/2.

(table 10.2). This makes biological sense in that Th1 cells producing cytokines such as IFNγ would be especially effective against intracellular infections with viruses and organisms which grow in macrophages, whereas Th2 cells are very good helpers for B-cells and would seem to be adapted for defense against parasites which are vulnerable to IL-4-switched IgE, IL-5-induced eosinophilia and IL-3/4-stimulated mast cell proliferation. Thus, studies on the infection of mice with the pathogenic protozoan *Leishmania major* demonstrated that intravenous or intraperitoneal injection of killed promastigotes leads to protection against challenge with live parasites associated with high expression of IFNγ mRNA and low levels of IL-4 mRNA; the reciprocal finding of low IFNγ and high IL-4 expression was made after subcutaneous immunization which failed to provide protection. Furthermore, nonvaccinated mice infected with live organisms could be saved by injection of IFNγ and anti-IL-4. These results are consistent with the preferential expansion of a population of protective IFNγ-secreting Th1 cells by intraperitoneal or intravenous immunization, and of nonprotective Th2 cells producing IL-4 in the subcutaneously injected animals. The ability of IFNγ, the characteristic Th1 cytokine, to inhibit the proliferation of Th2 clones, and of Th2-derived IL-4 and -10 to block both proliferation and cytokine release by Th1 cells, would seem to put the issue beyond reasonable doubt (figure 10.6).

The original Mosmann–Coffman classification into Th1 and Th2 subsets was predicated on data obtained

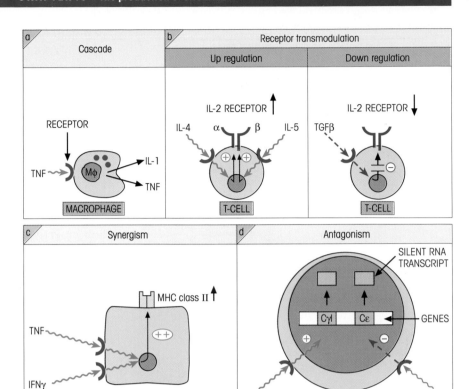

Figure 10.5. Network interactions of cytokines. (a) Cascade: in this example TNF induces secretion of IL-1 and of itself (autocrine) in the macrophage. (Note that all diagrams in this figure are simplified in that the effects on the nucleus are due to messengers resulting from the combination of cytokine with its surface receptor.) (b) Receptor transmodulation showing upregulation of each chain forming the high affinity IL-2 receptor in an activated T-cell by individual cytokines and downregulation by TGFβ. (c) Synergy of TNF and IFNγ in upregulation of surface MHC class II molecules on cultured pancreatic insulin-secreting cells. (d) Antagonism of IL-4 and IFNγ on transcription of silent ('sterile') mRNA relating to isotype switch (cf. figure 10.17).

with clones which had been maintained in culture for long periods and might have been artifacts of conditions *in vitro*. The use of cytokine-specific monoclonal antibodies for intracellular fluorescent staining, and of ELISPOT assays (cf. p. 140) for the detection of the secreted molecules, has demonstrated that the Th1/Th2 dichotomy is also apparent in freshly sampled cells and thus also applies *in vivo*. Nonetheless, it is perhaps best not to be too rigidly constrained in one's thinking by the Th1/Th2 paradigm, but rather to look upon T-cells as potentially producing a whole spectrum of cytokine profiles (Th0, figure 10.6), with possible skewing of the responses towards the extreme Th1 and Th2 patterns depending on the nature of the antigen stimulus. Thus, other subsets may also exist, in particular the transforming growth factor-β (TGFβ) and IL-10-producing Th3/Tr1 (T-regulatory 1) cells, which are of interest because these cytokines can mediate immunosuppressive effects and may be involved in the induction of mucosally induced tolerance (cf. p. 444).

Interactions with cells of the innate immune system biases the Th1/Th2 response

Antigen-presenting cells, and in particular dendritic cells, appear to be pivotal in driving differentiation towards a Th1 or Th2 phenotype. IL-12 seems to be par-

ticularly important for the production of Th1 cells and IL-4 for the production of Th2 cells. Invasion of phagocytic cells by intracellular pathogens induces copious secretion of IL-12, which in turn stimulates IFNγ production by NK cells. These two cytokines selectively drive differentiation of Th1 development and inhibit Th2 responses (figure 10.6). However, IL-4 effects appear to be dominant over IL-12 and therefore the amounts of IL-4 relative to the amounts of IL-12 and IFNγ will be of paramount importance in determining the differentiation of Th0 cells into Th1 or Th2 (figure 10.7). IL-4 downregulates the expression of the IL-12R $β_2$ subunit necessary for responsiveness to IL-12, further polarizing the Th2 dominance.

A special cell population, the NK-T cells bearing the NK1.1$^+$ marker, rapidly releases an IL-4-dominated pattern of cytokines on stimulation. These cells have many unusual features. They may be CD4$^-$8$^-$ or CD4$^+$8$^-$ and express low levels of T-cell αβ receptors with an invariant α chain and very restricted β, many of these receptors recognizing the nonclassical MHC-like CD1 molecule. Their morphology and granule content are intermediate between T-cells and NK cells. Although they express TCRαβ, there is an inclination to classify them on the fringe of the 'innate' immune system with regard to their primitive characteristics and possession of the lectin-like NK1.1 receptor which

Figure 10.6. The generation of Th1 and Th2 CD4 subsets. It is envisaged that, following the initial stimulation of T-cells, a range of cells producing a spectrum of cytokine patterns emerges. Under different conditions, the resulting population can be biased towards two extremes. IL-12, possibly produced through an 'innate'-type effect of an intracellular infection on macrophages, encourages the development of Th1 cells which produce the cytokines characteristic of *cell-mediated immunity*. IL-4, possibly produced by interaction of microorganisms with the lectin-like NK1.1⁺ receptor on NK-T cells, skews the development to the production of Th2 cells whose cytokines assist the progression of B-cells to antibody secretion and the provision of *humoral immunity*. Cytokines produced by polarized Th1 and Th2 subpopulations are mutually inhibitory. LT, lymphotoxin (TNFβ); Thp, T-helper precursor; Th0, early helper cell producing a spectrum of cytokines; other abbreviations as in table 10.1.

may be involved in the recognition of microbial carbohydrates.

Whilst there is a certain amount of evidence indicating the existence of subpopulations of dendritic cells specialized for the stimulation of either Th1 or Th2

populations, this is an area that is still under intensive investigation. However, it should be obvious from the above discussion that the cytokines produced in the immediate vicinity of the T-cell will be important. To give one recent example, Cantor and colleagues homologously deleted the gene for the cytokine Eta-1 (osteopontin) in mice and found that these animals had severely impaired immunity to infection with herpes simplex virus and to the intracellular bacterium *Listeria monocytogenes*. This was due to a deficient Th1 immunity caused by reduced IL-12 and IFNγ and enhanced IL-10 production. It appears that Eta-1 production by activated T-cells stimulates IL-12 production by macrophage lineage cells and downregulates IL-10 production. Interestingly, both serine phosphorylated and nonphosphorylated forms of Eta-1 are secreted by T-cells, and the IL-12 effect is phosphorylation-dependent whereas the IL-10 effect is not, indicating that phosphorylation can regulate the activity of secreted proteins.

Cytotoxic T-cells can also be subdivided into Tc1/Tc2

Clones of human cytotoxic T-cells obtained by limiting dilution also characteristically secrete particular cytokines. Thus, Tc1 cells secrete IFNγ but not IL-4, whilst Tc2 cells secrete IL-4 but not IFNγ. These clones show no differences in their cytolytic function but, when cocultured with CD4⁺ T-cells, Tc1 clones induce Th1 cells, whilst Tc2 clones induce Th2 cells.

ACTIVATED T-CELLS PROLIFERATE IN RESPONSE TO CYTOKINES

In so far as T-cells are concerned, amplification following activation is critically dependent upon IL-2 (figure 10.8). This cytokine is a single peptide of molecular weight 15.5 kDa which acts only on cells which express high affinity IL-2 receptors (figure 10.2). These receptors are not present on resting cells, but are synthesized within a few hours after activation.

Separation of an activated T-cell population into those with high and low affinity IL-2 receptors showed clearly that an adequate number of high affinity receptors were mandatory for the mitogenic action of IL-2. The numbers of these receptors on the cell increase under the action of antigen and of IL-2 and, as antigen is cleared, so the receptor numbers decline and, with that, the responsiveness to IL-2. It should be appreciated that, although IL-2 is an immunologically nonspecific T-cell growth factor, it only functions appropriately in specific responses because unstimulated T-cells do not express IL-2 receptors.

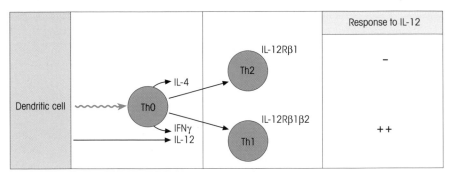

Figure 10.7. Polarization of T-helper responses is driven by dendritic cells. Initial activation of the Th0 cell is dependent upon presentation of peptide–MHC to the TCR, together with costimulatory signals such as that provided by CD80 and CD86 (B7.1 and B7.2 respectively) on the dendritic cell. Subsequently, the T-cells are driven towards a Th2 phenotype by the presence of IL-4 or a Th1 phenotype by the presence of IL-12 and IFNγ. The Th0 cells express both the β$_1$ and β$_2$ chains of the IL-12 receptor, but IL-4 causes loss of expression of the β$_2$ chain. Whilst IL-12 is predominantly a product of the macrophage/dendritic cell lineage, IL-4 is produced by a number of cell types including mast cells, γδ T-cells, NK-T cells, Th0 and Th2 cells.

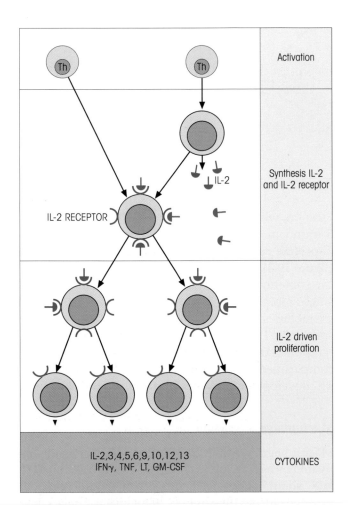

Figure 10.8. Activated T-blasts expressing surface receptors for IL-2 proliferate in response to IL-2 produced by itself or by another T-cell subset. Expansion is controlled through downregulation of the IL-2 receptor by IL-2 itself. The expanded population secretes a wide variety of biologically active cytokines of which IL-4 also enhances T-cell proliferation.

The T-cell blasts also produce an impressive array of other cytokines, and the proliferative effect of IL-2 is reinforced by the action of IL-4 and, to some extent, IL-6, which react with corresponding receptors on the dividing T-cells. We must not lose sight of the importance of control mechanisms, and obvious candidates to subsume this role are TGFβ, which blocks IL-2-induced proliferation (figure 10.5b) and the production of TNF (TNFα) and lymphotoxin (TNFβ), and the cytokines IFNγ, IL-4 and IL-12, which mediate the mutual antagonism of Th1 and Th2 subsets.

T-CELL EFFECTORS IN CELL-MEDIATED IMMUNITY

Cytokines mediate chronic inflammatory responses

In addition to their role in the adaptive response, T-cell cytokines are responsible for generating antigen-specific chronic inflammatory reactions which deal with intracellular parasites (figure 10.4b and 10.9), although there is a different emphasis on the pattern of factors involved (cf. p. 274).

Early events

The initiating event is probably a local inflammatory response to tissue injury caused by the infectious agent which would upregulate the synthesis of adhesion molecules such as VCAM-1 (vascular cell adhesion molecule) and ICAM-1 on adjacent vascular endothelial cells. These would permit entry of memory T-cells to the infected site through their VLA-4 and LFA-1 homing receptors (cf. p. 152). Contact with processed

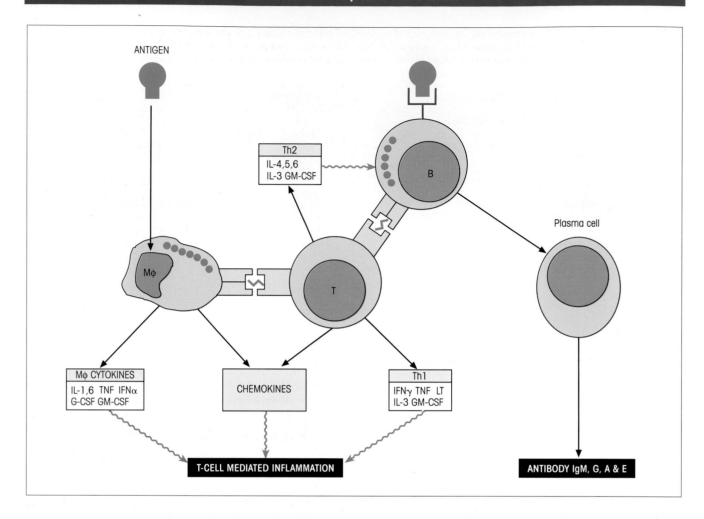

Figure 10.9. Cytokines controlling the antibody and T-cell-mediated inflammatory responses. Abbreviations as in table 10.1.

antigen derived from the intracellular parasite will activate the specific T-cell and induce the release of secreted cytokines. TNF will further enhance the expression of endothelial accessory molecules and increase the chances of other memory cells in the circulation homing in to meet the antigen provoking inflammation.

Chemotaxis

The recruitment of T-cells and macrophages to the inflammatory site (figure 10.9) is greatly enhanced by the action of chemotactic cytokines termed **chemokines** (*chemo*attractant cyto*kine*). These can be potentially produced by a variety of cell types and are divided into four families based on the disposition of the first (N-terminal) two of the four canonical cysteine residues (table 10.3). CXC chemokines have one amino acid and CX3C have three amino acids between the two cysteines. CC chemokines have adjacent cysteines at this

location, whereas C chemokines lack cysteines 1 and 3 found in other chemokines. Chemokines bind to G-protein-coupled seven transmembrane receptors (figure 10.2). Despite the fact that a single chemokine can sometimes bind to more than one receptor, and a single receptor can bind several chemokines, many chemokines exhibit a strong tissue and receptor specificity. They play important roles in inflammation, lymphoid organ development, cell trafficking, cell compartmentalization within lymphoid tissues, Th1/Th2 development, angiogenesis and wound healing.

Macrophage activation

Macrophages with intracellular organisms are activated by agents such as IFNγ, GM-CSF, IL-2 and TNF and should become endowed with microbicidal powers. During this process, some macrophages may die (probably helped along by cytotoxic T-cells) and release living parasites, but these will be dealt with by fresh macrophages brought to the site by chemotaxis and newly activated by local cytokines so that they have passed the stage of differentiation at which the

Table 10.3. Chemokines and their receptors. The chemokines are grouped according to the arrangement of their cysteines (see text). The letter L designates ligand (i.e. the individual chemokine), whereas the letter R designates receptors. Names in parentheses refer to the murine homologs of the human chemokine where the names of these differ, or the murine chemokine alone if no human equivalent has been described.

FAMILY	CHEMOKINE	ALTERNATIVE NAMES	CHEMOTAXIS	RECEPTORS
CXC	CXCL1	GROα/MGSAα	Neutro	CXCR2>CXCR1
	CXCL2	GROβ/MGSAβ	Neutro	CXCR2
	CXCL3	GROγ/MGSAγ	Neutro	CXCR2
	CXCL4	PF4	Eosino,Baso	?
	CXCL5	ENA-78	Neutro	CXCR2
	CXCL6	GCP-2/(CKα-3)	Neutro	CXCR1, CXCR2
	CXCL7	NAP-2	Neutro	CXCR2
	CXCL8	IL-8	Neutro	CXCR1, CXCR2
	CXCL9	Mig	T, NK	CXCR3
	CXCL10	IP-10	T, NK	CXCR3
	CXCL11	I-TAC	T, NK	CXCR3
	CXCL12	SDF-1α/β	T, B, DC, Mono	CXCR4
	CXCL13	BLC/BCA-1	B	CXCR5
	CXCL14	BRAC/Bolekine	?	?
	CXCL15	Lungkine	Neutro	?
C	XCL1	Lymphotactin/SCM-1α/ATAC	T	XCR1
	XCL2	SCM-1β	T	XCR1
CX3C	CX3CL1	Fractalkine/Neurotactin	T, NK, Mono	CX3CR1
CC	CCL1	I-309/(TCA-3/P500)	Mono	CCR8
	CCL2	MCP-1/MCAF	T, NK, DC, Mono, Baso	CCR2
	CCL3	MIP-1α/LD78α	T, NK, DC, Mono, Eosino	CCR1, CCR5
	CCL4	MIP-1β	T, NK, DC, Mono	CCR5
	CCL5	RANTES	T, NK, DC, Mono, Eosino, Baso	CCR1, CCR3, CCR5
	(CCL6)	(C10/MRP-1)	?	?
	CCL7	MCP-3	T, NK, DC, Mono, Eosino, Baso	CCR1,CCR2, CCR3
	CCL8	MCP-2	T, NK, DC, Mono, Baso	CCR3
	(CCL9/10)	(MRP-2/CCF18/MIP-1γ)	?	?
	CCL11	Eotaxin-1	T, DC, Eosino, Baso	CCR3
	(CCL12)	(MCP-5)	T, NK, DC, Mono, Baso	CCR2
	CCL13	MCP-4	T, NK, DC, Mono, Eosino, Baso	CCR2, CCR3
	CCL14	HCC-1/HCC-3	T, Mono, Eosino	CCR1
	CCL15	HCC-2/Leukotactin-1/MIP-1δ	T	CCR1, CCR3
	CCL16	HCC-4/LEC/(LCC-1)	T	CCR1
	CCL17	TARC	T, DC, Mono	CCR4
	CCL18	DCCK1/PARC/AMAC-1	T	?
	CCL19	MIP-3β/ELC/Exodus-3	T, B, DC	CCR7
	CCL20	MIP-3α/LARC/Exodus-1	DC	CCR6
	CCL21	6Ckine/SLC/Exodus-2/(TCA-4)	T, DC	CCR7
	CCL22	MDC/STCP-1/ABCD-1	T, DC, Mono	CCR4
	CCL23	MPIF-1	T	CCR1
	CCL24	MPIF-2/Eotaxin-2	T, DC, Eosino, Baso	CCR3
	CCL25	TECK	T, DC, Mono	CCR9
	CCL26	SCYA26/Eotaxin-3	T	CCR3
	CCL27	CTACK/ALP/ESkine	T	CCR10

B, B-cell; Baso, basophil; DC, dendritic cell; Eosino, eosinophil; Mono, monocyte; Neutro, neutrophil; NK, natural killer; T, T-cell.

intracellular parasites can subvert their killing mechanisms (cf. p. 263).

Combating viral infection

Virally infected cells require a different strategy and one strand of that strategy exploits the innate interferon mechanism to deny the virus access to the cell's replicative machinery. IFNγ, TNF and lymphotoxin all induce 2'–5' (A) synthetase, a protein which is involved in viral protection. TNF has another string to its bow in its ability to kill certain cells, since death of an infected cell before viral replication has occurred is obviously beneficial to the host. Its cytotoxic potential was first recognized using tumor cells as targets (hence the name), and IFNγ and lymphotoxin can act synergistically, with IFNγ setting up the cell for destruction by inducing the formation of TNF receptors.

Killer T-cells

The generation of cytotoxic T-cells

Cytotoxic T-cells (Tc), also referred to as cytotoxic T-lymphocytes (CTLs), represent the other major arm of the cell-mediated immune response and are of strategic importance in the killing of virally infected cells and possibly in contributing to the postulated surveillance mechanisms against cancer cells.

The cytotoxic cell precursors recognize antigen on the surface of cells in association with class I major histocompatibility complex (MHC) molecules and, like B-cells, they usually require help from T-cells. The mechanism by which help is proffered may, however, be quite different. As explained earlier (see p. 173), effective T–B collaboration is usually 'cognate' in that the collaborating cells recognize two epitopes which are physically linked (usually on the same molecule). If we may remind the reader without causing offense, the reason for this is that the surface Ig receptors on the B-cell capture native antigen, process it internally and present it to the Th as a peptide in association with MHC class II. Although it has been shown that linked epitopes on the antigen are also necessary for cooperation between Th and the cytotoxic T-cell precursor (Tcp), the nature of T-cell recognition prevents native antigen being focused onto the Tcp by its receptor for subsequent processing, even if that cell were to express MHC II, which in its resting state it does not. It seems most likely that Th and Tcp bind to the same APC, for example a dendritic cell, which has processed viral antigen and displays processed viral peptides in association with both class II (for the Th cell) and class I (for the Tcp) on its surface; one cannot exclude the possibility that the APC could be the virally infected cell itself. Cytokines from the triggered Th will be released in close proximity to the Tcp which is engaging the antigen–MHC signal and will be stimulated to proliferate and differentiate into a Tc under the influence of IL-2 and -6 (figure 10.10a). However, interaction of the APC with the Th and the Tc cell can be temporally separated and, in this case, it appears that the helper T-cell 'licenses' the dendritic cell for future interaction with the cytotoxic T-cell. It does this by activating the dendritic cell through CD40, thereby upregulating costimulatory molecules and cytokine production, in particular IL-12, by the dendritic cell (figure 10.10b). An entirely Th-independent mechanism of Tc activation is also thought to occur. This has been demonstrated in, for example, the response to protein antigens given with potent adjuvants such as immunostimulatory DNA sequences (ISSs), in this case

Figure 10.10. T-helper cell activation of cytotoxic T-cells. Activation of the CD4[+] helper T-cells (Th) by the dendritic cell involves a CD40–CD40 ligand (CD154) costimulatory signal and recognition of an MHC class II peptide presented by the T-cell receptor. (a) If both the Th and the cytotoxic T-lymphocyte (Tc) are present at the same time, the release of cytokines from the activated Th cells stimulates the differentiation of the CD8[+] precursor into an activated, MHC class I-restricted Tc. However, as shown in (b), the Th and the Tc do not need to interact with the APC at the same time. In this case, the Th cell 'licenses' the dendritic cell for future interaction with a Tc cell. Thus the Th cell, by engaging CD40, drives the dendritic cell from a resting state into an activated state with upregulation of costimulatory molecules such as B7.1 and B7.2 (CD80 and CD86, respectively) and increased cytokine production, particularly of IL-12.

possibly involving adjuvant-induced production of proinflammatory cytokines and cell surface costimulatory molecules.

The lethal process

Cytotoxic T-cells (Tc) are generally of the CD8 subset, and their binding to the target cell through T-cell receptor recognition of antigen plus class I MHC is assisted by association between CD8 and class I and by other accessory molecules such as LFA-1 and CD2 (see figure 9.3).

Tc are **unusual secretory cells** which use a modified lysosome to secrete their lytic proteins. Following delivery of the TCR/CD3 signal, the **lytic granules** are driven at a rare old speed (up to 1.2 μm/sec) along the microtubule system and delivered to the point of contact between the Tc and its target (figure 10.11). This guarantees the specificity of killing dictated by TCR recognition of the target and limits any collateral damage to surrounding cells. As with NK cells, which have comparable granules (cf. p. 18), exocytosis of the granule contents, including perforins, granzymes and TNF, causes lesions in the target cell membrane and death by inducing apoptosis. Tc are endowed with a second killing mechanism involving Fas and its ligand (cf. p. 19), but the inability of perforin knockout mice to clear viruses effectively suggests that the secretory granules provide the dominant attack on virally infected cells. Videomicroscopy shows that Tc are serial killers. After the 'kiss of death', the T-cell can disengage and seek a further victim, there being rapid synthesis of new granules.

One should also not lose sight of the fact that CD8 cells synthesize other cytokines such as IFNγ which also have antiviral potential.

Inflammation must be regulated

Once the inflammatory process has cleared the inciting agent, the body needs to switch it off. IL-10 has profound anti-inflammatory and immunoregulatory effects, acting on macrophages and Th1 cells to inhibit release of factors such as IL-1 and TNF. It induces the release of soluble TNF receptors which are endogenous inhibitors of TNF, and downregulates surface TNF receptor. Soluble IL-1 receptors released during inflammation can act to 'decoy' IL-1 itself. IL-4 not only acts to constrain Th1 cells but also upregulates production of the natural inhibitor of IL-1, the IL-1 receptor antagonist (IL-1Ra). The role of TGFβ is more difficult to tease out because it has some pro- and other anti-inflammatory effects, although it undoubtedly promotes tissue repair after resolution of the inflammation.

PROLIFERATION AND MATURATION OF B-CELL RESPONSES ARE MEDIATED BY CYTOKINES

The activation of B-cells by Th, through the TCR recognition of MHC-linked antigenic peptide plus the costimulatory **CD40L–CD40 interaction**, leads to upregulation of the surface receptor for IL-4. Copious local release of this cytokine from the Th then drives powerful clonal proliferation and expansion of the activated B-cell population. IL-2 and IL-13 also contribute to this process (figure 10.12).

Under the influence of IL-4 and IL-13, the expanded clones can differentiate and mature into IgE synthesizing cells. TGFβ and IL-5 encourage cells to switch their Ig class to IgA. IgM plasma cells emerge under the tutelage of IL-4 plus -5, and IgG producers result from the combined influence of IL-4, -5, -6, -13 and IFNγ (figure 10.12).

Type 2 thymus-independent antigens can activate B-cells directly (cf. p. 171) but nonetheless still need cytokines for efficient proliferation and Ig production. These may come from accessory cells such as NK and NK-T cells which bear lectin-like receptors.

Figure 10.11. Conjugation of a cytotoxic T-cell (on left) to its target, here a mouse mastocytoma, showing polarization of the granules towards the target at the point of contact. The cytoskeletons of both cells are revealed by immunofluorescent staining with an antibody to tubulin (green) and the lytic granules with an antibody to granzyme A (red). Twenty minutes after conjugation the target cell cytoskeleton may still be intact (above), but this rapidly becomes disrupted (below). (Photographs kindly provided by Dr Gillian Griffiths.)

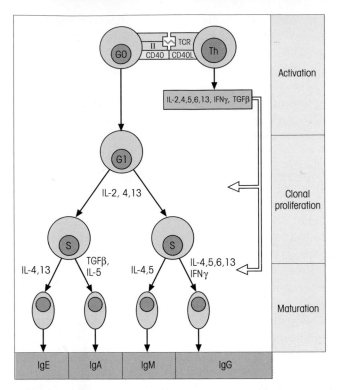

Figure 10.12. B-cell response to thymus-dependent (TD) antigen: clonal expansion and maturation of activated B-cells under the influence of T-cell-derived soluble factors. Costimulation through the CD40L–CD40 interaction is essential for primary and secondary immune responses to TD antigens and for the formation of germinal centers and memory. c-*myc* expression, which is maximal 2 hours after antigen or anti-μ stimulation, parallels sensitivity to growth factors; transfection with c-*myc* substitutes for anti-μ.

WHAT IS GOING ON IN THE GERMINAL CENTER?

The secondary follicle with its corona or mantle of small lymphocytes surrounding the pale germinal center is a striking and unique cellular structure. First, let us recall the overall events described in Chapter 8. Secondary challenge with antigen or immune complexes induces enlargement of germinal centers, formation of new ones, appearance of memory B-cells and development of Ig-producing cells of higher affinity. B-cells entering the germinal center become **centroblasts** which divide with a very short cycle time of 6 hours, and then become nondividing **centrocytes** in the basal light zone, many of which die from apoptosis (figure 10.13). As the surviving centrocytes mature, they differentiate either into **immunoblast plasma cell precursors**, which secrete Ig in the absence of antigen, or into **memory B-cells**.

What then is the underlying scenario? Following secondary antigen challenge, primed B-cells may be activated by paracortical Th cells in association with interdigitating dendritic cells or macrophages, and migrate to the germinal center. There they divide in response to powerful stimuli from complexes on follicular dendritic cells (cf. p. 160) and from cytokines released by T-cells in response to antigen-presenting B-cells. During this particularly frenetic bout of cell division, **somatic hypermutation** of B-cell Ig genes occurs. The cells also undergo **Ig class switching**. Thereafter, as they transform to centrocytes, they are vulnerable and die readily, whence they are taken up as the 'tingible bodies' by macrophages, unless rescued by association with antigen on a follicular dendritic cell. This could result from cross-linking of surface Ig receptors and is accompanied by expression of bcl-2 which protects against apoptosis. Signaling through CD40, by presentation of antigen to Th cells, would also prolong the life of the centrocyte. In either case, the interactions will only occur if the mutated surface Ig receptor still binds antigen and, as the concentration of antigen gradually falls, only if the receptor is of high affinity. In other words, the system can deliver high affinity antibody by a Darwinian process of high frequency mutation of the Ig genes and selection by antigen of the cells bearing the antibody which binds most strongly (figure 10.14). This increase of affinity as the antibody level falls late in the response is of obvious benefit, since a small amount of high affinity antibody can do the job of a large amount of low affinity (as in boxing, a small 'goodun' will generally be a match for a mediocre 'bigun').

Further differentiation now occurs. The cells either migrate to the sites of plasma cell activity (e.g. lymph node medulla) or go to expand the memory B-cell pool depending upon the cytokine and other signals received. CD40 engagement by CD40 ligand on a T-cell guides the B-cell into the memory compartment.

THE SYNTHESIS OF ANTIBODY

The sequential processes by which secreted Ig arises are illustrated in figure 10.15. In the normal antibody-forming cell there is a rapid turnover of light chains which are present in slight excess. Defective control occurs in many myeloma cells and one may see excessive production of light chains or complete suppression of heavy chain synthesis.

The variable and constant regions are spliced together in the mRNA before leaving the nucleus. Differential splicing mechanisms also provide a rational explanation for the coexpression of surface IgM and IgD with identical V regions on a single cell, and for the switch from production of membrane-bound IgM receptor to secretory IgM in the antibody-forming cell (cf. figures 4.1 and 4.2).

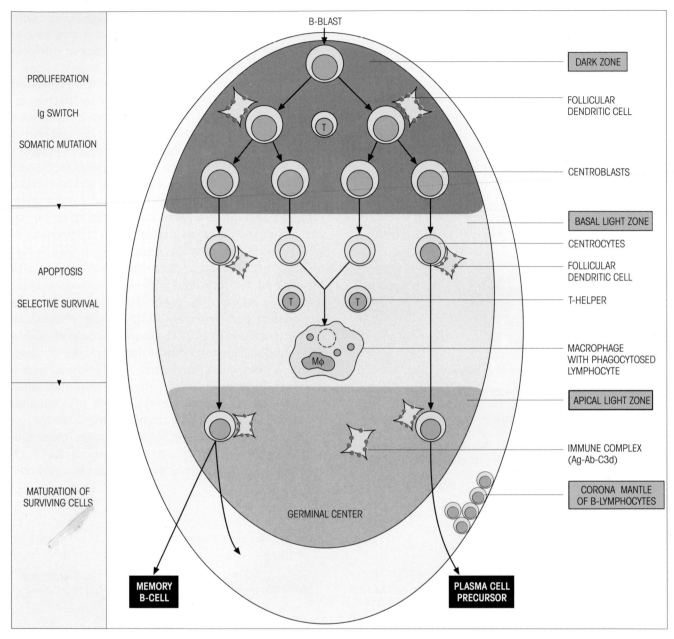

Figure 10.13. The events occurring in lymphoid germinal centers. Germinal center B-cells can be enriched through their affinity for the peanut agglutinin lectin. They show numerous mutations in the antibody genes. Expression of LFA-1 and ICAM-1 on B-cells and follicular dendritic cells (FDCs) in the germinal center makes them 'sticky'. Centroblasts at the base of the follicle are strongly CD77 positive. The Th cells bear the unusual CD57 marker. The FDCs all express CD21 and CD54; those in the apical light zone are strongly CD23 positive, those in the basal light zone express little CD23.

Through their surface receptors, FDCs bind immune complexes containing antigen and C3 which, in turn, are very effective B-cell stimulators since coligation of the surface receptors for antigen and C3 (CR2) lowers their threshold for activation. The costimulatory molecules CD40 and B7 play pivotal roles. Antibodies to CD40 prevent formation of germinal centers and anti-CD40L can disrupt established germinal centers within 12 hours. Anti-B7.2, given early in the immune response, prevents germinal center formation and, when given at the onset of hypermutation, suppresses that process.

IMMUNOGLOBULIN CLASS SWITCHING OCCURS IN INDIVIDUAL B-CELLS

The synthesis of antibodies belonging to the various immunoglobulin classes proceeds at different rates. Usually there is an early IgM response which tends to fall off rapidly. IgG antibody synthesis builds up to its maximum over a longer time period. On secondary challenge with antigen, the time-course of the IgM response resembles that seen in the primary. By contrast, the synthesis of IgG antibodies rapidly accelerates to a much higher titer and there is a relatively slow fall-off in serum antibody levels (figure 10.16). The same probably holds for IgA, and in a sense both these immunoglobulin classes provide the main immediate defense against future penetration by foreign antigens.

Individual cells can switch over from IgM to IgG production. For example, antigen challenge of irradiated recipients receiving relatively small numbers of lymphoid cells produced splenic foci of cells, each synthesizing antibodies of different heavy chain class

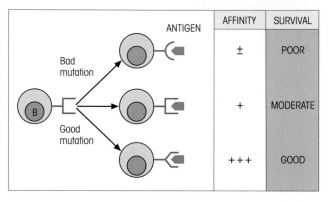

Figure 10.14. Darwinian selection by antigen of B-cells with antibody mutants of high affinity protects against cell death in the germinal center, either through cross-linking of sIg by antigen on follicular dendritic cells, or through Th cell recognition of processed antigen and signaling through CD40. In both cases, capture of antigen, particularly as the concentration falls, will be critically affected by the affinity of the surface receptor.

bearing a single idiotype; the common idiotype suggests that each focus is derived from a single precursor cell whose progeny can form antibodies of different class.

Antibody synthesis in most classes shows considerable dependence upon T cooperation in that the responses in T-deprived animals are strikingly deficient; such is true of mouse IgG1, IgG2a, IgA, IgE and part of the IgM antibody responses. T-independent antigens such as the polyclonal activator, lipopolysaccharide (LPS) endotoxin, induce synthesis of IgM with some IgG2b and IgG3. Immunopotentiation by complete Freund's adjuvant, a water-in-oil emulsion containing antigen in the aqueous phase and a suspension of killed tubercle bacilli in the oil phase (see p. 300), seems to occur, at least in part through the activation of Th cells which stimulate antibody production in T-dependent classes. The prediction from this, that the response to T-independent antigens (e.g. *Pneumococcus* polysaccharide, p. 171) should not be potentiated by Freund's adjuvant, is borne out in practice; furthermore, as mentioned previously, these antigens evoke primarily IgM antibodies and poor immunological memory, as do T-dependent antigens injected into T-cell-deficient, neonatally thymectomized hosts.

Thus, in rodents at least, the switch from IgM to IgG and other classes appears to be largely under T-cell control critically mediated by CD40 and by cytokines

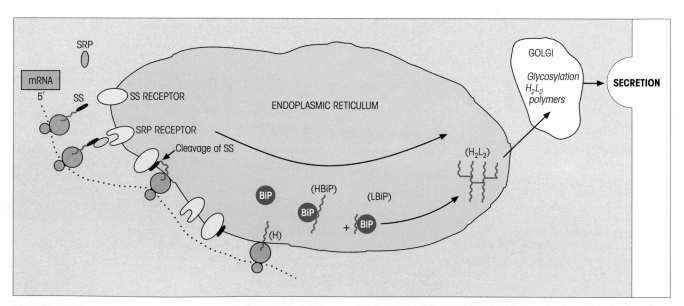

Figure 10.15. Synthesis of immunoglobulin. As mRNA is translated on the ribosome, the N-terminal signal sequence (SS) is bound by a signal recognition particle (SRP) which docks onto a receptor on the outer membrane of the endoplasmic reticulum (ER) and facilitates entry of the nascent Ig chain into the ER lumen. The SS associates with a specific membrane receptor and is cleaved; the remainder of the chain, as it elongates, complexes with the molecular chaperone BiP (heavy chain-binding protein) which binds to the heavy chain C_H1 and V_L domains to control protein folding. The unassembled chains oxidize and dissociate as the full H_2L_2 Ig molecule. The assembled H_2L_2 molecules can now leave the ER for terminal glycosylation in the Golgi and final secretion. Surface receptor Ig would be inserted by its hydrophobic sequences into the membrane of the endoplasmic reticulum as it was synthesized.

(see p. 189). Let us take another look at the stimulation of small, surface IgM-positive, B-cells by LPS. As we noted, on its own, the nonspecific mitogen evokes the synthesis of IgM, IgG3 and some IgG2b. Following addition of IL-4 to the system, there is class switching from IgM to IgE and IgG1 production, whereas IFNγ stimulates class switching from IgM to IgG2a and TGFβ induces switching from IgM to IgA or IgG2b.

Figure 10.16. Synthesis of IgM and IgG antibody classes in the primary and secondary responses to antigen.

These cytokines induce the formation of germ-line sterile transcripts which start at the I (initiation) exon 5' of the switch region for the antibody class to which switching will occur and terminate at the polyadenylation site 3' of the relevant C_H gene (figure 10.17). The transcripts are not translated but instead remain associated with the template DNA, forming RNA–DNA hybrids within the S regions of the DNA which might act as targets for enzymes involved in the recombination process. Under the influence of the recombinase, a given *VDJ* gene segment is transferred from $\mu\delta$ to the new constant region gene (figure 10.17), so yielding antibodies of the same specificity but of different class.

Class-switched B-cells are subject to high mutation rates after the initial response

The reader will no doubt recollect that this idea was raised in Chapter 4 when discussing the generation of diversity, and that the germinal center has been identified as the site of intense mutagenesis. The normal *V*-region mutation rate is of the order of 10^{-5}/base pair/cell division, but this rises to

Figure 10.17. Class switching to produce antibodies of identical specificity but different immunoglobulin isotype (in this example from IgM to IgG1) is achieved by a recombination process which utilizes the specialized switch sequences (●) and leads to a loss of the intervening DNA loop (μ, δ and γ3). Each switch sequence is 1–10 kilobases in length and comprises guanosine-rich repeats of 20–100 base pairs. Because the switch sequence associated with each C_H gene has a unique nucleotide sequence, recombination cannot occur homologously and therefore probably depends upon nonhomologous end joining. DNA repair proteins including Ku70, Ku80 and the catalytic subunit of the DNA-dependent protein kinase (DNA-PK$_{CS}$) are involved in this process.

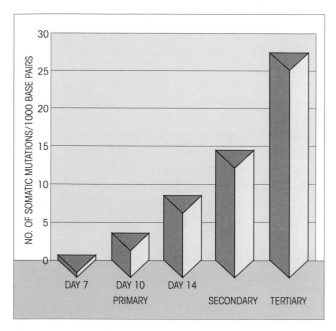

Figure 10.18. Increasing somatic mutations in the immunodominant germ-line antibody observed in hybridomas isolated following repeated immunization with phenyloxazolone. (Data from Berek C. & Apel M. (1989) In Melchers F. *et al.* (eds) *Progress in Immunology* **7**, 99. Springer-Verlag, Berlin.)

10^{-3}/base pair/generation in B-cells as a result of antigenic stimulation. This process is illustrated in figure 10.18 which charts the accumulation of somatic mutations in the immunodominant V_H/V_κ antibody structure during the immune response to phenyloxazolone. With time and successive boosting, the mutation rate is seen to rise dramatically and, in the context of the present discussion, it is clear that the strategically targeted hypermutations occurring within or adjacent to the complementarity determining hypervariable loops (figure 10.19) can give rise to cells which secrete antibodies having a different combining affinity to that of the original parent cell. Randomly, some mutated daughter cells will have higher affinity for antigen, some the same or lower and others perhaps none at all (cf. figure 10.14). Similarly, mutations in the framework regions may be 'silent' or, if they disrupt the folding of the protein, give rise to nonfunctional molecules. Pertinently, the proportion of germinal center B-cells with 'silent' mutations is high early in the immune response but falls dramatically with time, suggesting that early diversification is followed by preferential expansion of clones expressing mutations which improve their chances of reacting with and being stimulated by antigen.

Figure 10.19. An 'antigen's eye view' of sequence diversity in human antibodies. The sequence diversity has been plotted on a scale of blue (more conserved) to red (more diverse). The V_H domain is on the right and the V_κ domain on the left in both pictures. (a) Germ-line diversity prior to somatic hypermutation is focused at the center of the antigen-binding site. (b) Somatic hypermutation spreads diversity to regions at the periphery of the binding site that are highly conserved in the germ-line *V* gene repertoire.

Somatic hypermutation is therefore complementary to germ-line diversity. The V_H CDR3, which lies at the center of the antigen-binding site, was not included in this analysis and therefore is shown in gray as a loop structure. The end of the V_κ CDR3 (also excluded) lies at the center of the binding site and is not visible in this representation. (Reproduced with kind permission from Tomlinson I.M. *et al.* (1996) *Journal of Molecular Biology* **256**, 813.)

FACTORS AFFECTING ANTIBODY AFFINITY IN THE IMMUNE RESPONSE

The effect of antigen dose

Other things being equal, the binding strength of an antigen for the surface receptor of a B-cell will be determined by the affinity constant of the reaction:

$$Ag + (surface)Ab \rightleftharpoons AgAb$$

and the reactants will behave according to the law of mass action (cf. p. 86).

It may be supposed that, when a sufficient number of antigen molecules are bound to the receptors on the cell surface and processed for presentation to T-cells, the lymphocyte will be stimulated to develop into an antibody-producing clone. When only small amounts of antigen are present, only those lymphocytes with high affinity receptors will be able to bind sufficient antigen for stimulation to occur and their daughter cells will, of course, also produce high affinity antibody. Consideration of the antigen–antibody equilibrium equation will show that, as the concentration of antigen is increased, even antibodies with relatively low affinity will bind more antigen; therefore, at high doses of antigen, the lymphocytes with lower affinity receptors will also be stimulated and, as may be seen from figure 10.20, these are more abundant than those with receptors of high affinity. Furthermore, there is a strong possibility that cells with the highest affinity will bind so much antigen as to become tolerized (cf. p. 240). Thus, in summary, low amounts of antigen produce high affinity antibodies, whereas high antigen concentrations give rise to an antiserum with low to moderate affinity.

Maturation of affinity

In addition to being brisker and fatter, secondary responses tend to be of higher affinity. There are probably two main reasons for this maturation of affinity after primary stimulation. First, once the primary response gets under way and the antigen concentration declines to low levels, only successively higher affinity cells will bind sufficient antigen to maintain proliferation. Second, at this stage the cells are mutating madly in the germinal centers, and any mutants with an adventitiously higher affinity will bind well to antigen on follicular dendritic cells and be positively selected for by its persistent clonal expansion. Modification of antibody specificity by somatic point mutations allows gradual diversification on which positive selection for affinity can act during clonal expansion.

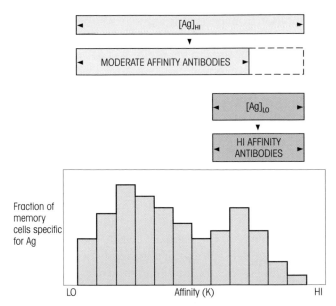

Figure 10.20. Relationship of antigen concentration to affinity of antibodies produced. Low concentrations of antigen ($[Ag]_{LO}$) bind to and permit stimulation of a range of high affinity memory cells and the resulting antibodies are of high affinity. High doses of antigen ($[Ag]_{HI}$) are able to bind sufficiently to the low affinity cells and thereby allow their stimulation, whilst the highest affinity cells may bind an excess of antigen and be tolerized (dashed line); the resulting antiserum will have a population of low to moderate affinity antibodies.

It is worth noting that responses to thymus-independent antigens, which have poorly developed memory with very rare mutations, do not show this phenomenon of affinity maturation. Overall, the ability of Th to facilitate responses to nonpolymeric, nonpolyclonally activating antigens, to induce expansive clonal proliferation, to effect class switching and, lastly, to fine-tune responses to higher affinity has provided us with bigger, better and more flexible immune responses.

MEMORY CELLS

Antibodies encoded by unmutated germ-line genes represent a form of evolutionary memory, in the sense that they tend to include specificities for commonly encountered pathogens which appear in the so-called 'natural antibody' fraction of serum. Memory acquired during the adaptive immune response requires contact with antigen and expansion of antigen-specific memory cells, as seen for example in the 20-fold increase in cytotoxic T-cell precursors after immunization of females with the male H-Y antigen.

Memory of early infections such as measles is long-lived and the question arises as to whether the memory cells are long-lived or are subject to repeated antigen stimulation from persisting antigen or subclinical reinfection. Fanum in 1847 described a measles epidemic on the Faroe Islands in the previous year in which almost the entire population suffered from infection except for a few old people who had been infected 65 years earlier. While this evidence favors the long half-life hypothesis, memory function of B-cells transferred to an irradiated syngeneic recipient is lost within a month unless antigen is given or the donor is transgenic for the *bcl-2* gene (remember that signals in the germinal center which prevent apoptosis of centrocytic B-cells also upregulate *bcl-2* expression). It is envisaged that B-cell memory is a dynamic state in which survival of the memory cells is maintained by recurrent signals from follicular dendritic cells in the germinal centers, the only long-term repository of antigen.

Recent evidence strongly suggests that memory *T-cells* can, however, persist in the absence of antigen. T-cells isolated from mice several months after they were immunized with lymphocytic choriomeningitis virus (LCMV) were transferred into two groups of genetically modified mice which lacked endogenous T-cells, one of the groups additionally lacking MHC class I expression. T-cells were parked in these mice for 10 months and then analysed *in vitro*. Functional virus-specific CD8$^+$ CTLs were still present in both groups of mice, and in similar numbers, even though those from the class I$^-$ mice could not have had antigen presented to their TCR. Indeed, these memory T-cells undergo antigen- and MHC-independent proliferation *in vivo*, their numbers controlled, at least in part, by a balance between proliferation-inducing signals from IL-15 and cell death-inducing signals from IL-2 released in the local environment, both cytokines binding to the IL-2R β chain (cf. figure 10.2). Other recent findings indicate that helper T-cell memory also does not require the continued presence of antigen or MHC and, at least in some cases, Th memory is maintained in the absence of cell division.

However, we should not lose sight of the fact that, while these experiments in transgenic and knockout animals clearly demonstrate that immunological memory *can* be maintained in the absence of antigen, usually antigen persists as complexes on follicular dendritic cells. Therefore, there is the potential for antigen-presenting cells within the germinal center to capture and process this complexed antigen and then present it to memory T-cells. Some evidence, again recent (yes, this is a very rapidly moving area of immunology!), suggests that it is a type of dendritic cell, and not the germinal center B-cells, that may subserve this function.

The memory population is not simply an expansion of corresponding naive cells

In general, memory cells are more readily stimulated by a given dose of antigen because they have a higher affinity. In the case of B-cells, we have been satisfied by the evidence linking mutation and antigen selection to the creation of high affinity memory cells within the germinal center of secondary lymph node follicles. The receptors for antigen on memory T-cells also have higher affinity but, since they do not undergo significant somatic mutation during the priming response, it would seem that cells with **pre-existing receptors of relatively higher affinity in the population of naive cells proliferate selectively through preferential binding to the antigen**.

Intuitively one would not expect to improve on affinity to the same extent that somatic hypermutation can achieve for the B-cells, but nonetheless memory T-cells augment their binding avidity for the antigen-presenting cell through increased expression of accessory adhesion molecules, CD2, LFA-1, LFA-3 and ICAM-1. Since several of these molecules also function to enhance signal transduction, the memory T-cell is more readily triggered than its naive counterpart. Indeed, memory cells enter cell division and secrete cytokines more rapidly than naive cells, and there is some evidence that they may secrete a broader range of cytokines than do naive cells.

A phenotypic change in the isoform of the leukocyte common antigen CD45R, derived by differential splicing, allows some distinction to be made between naive and memory cells. Expression of CD45RA has been used as a marker of naive T-cells and of CD45RO as a marker of memory cells capable of responding to recall antigens. However, most of the features associated with the CD45RO subset are in fact manifestations of **activated cells** and CD45RO cells can revert to the CD45RA phenotype. Memory cells, perhaps in the absence of antigenic stimulation, may therefore lose their activated status and join a resting pool. Another marker used for differentiating naive from memory cells takes one step back on the CD ladder and utilizes differences in the relative expression of the adhesion molecule CD44; naive T-cells seem to express low levels of CD44 whilst memory T-cells express high levels.

It has been proposed by Lanzavecchia and colleagues that the CCR7 chemokine receptor allows a distinction to be made between CCR7$^+$ 'central memory' T-cells, which differentiate from naive T-cells, and CCR7$^-$ 'effector memory' T-cells, which subsequently arise from the central memory T-cells (figure 10.21). Both populations are long-lived. The central

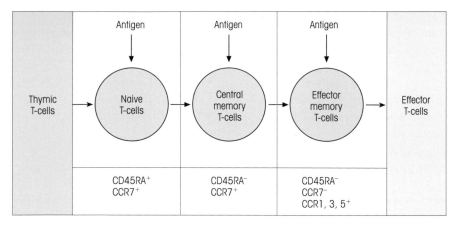

Figure 10.21. Central and effector memory T-cells. Naive T-cells bear the CD45RA splice variant of the CD45 molecule and are attracted from the thymus into secondary lymphoid tissue under the influence of CCR7-binding chemokines such as CCL19 (MIP-3β) and CCL21 (6Ckine/SLC). Upon encounter with antigen, some of these cells become effectors of the primary immune response, whilst others differentiate into central memory T-cells which retain the CCR7 chemokine receptor but lose expression of CD45RA. Subsequent re-encounter with antigen will push these cells into the effector memory compartment with replacement of CCR7 by other chemokine receptors such as CCR1, CCR3 and CCR5. This changes the homing characteristics of these cells which can now relocate as cytokine-secreting or cytotoxic T-cells to inflammatory sites under the influence of a number of chemokines including CCL3 (MIP-1α), CCL4 (MIP-1β) and CCL5 (RANTES) (see table 10.3). Note that whilst the activation and subsequent differentiation of these cells is dependent on antigen, both central memory and effector memory T-cells are thought to be long-lived in the absence of antigen.

memory cells provide a clonally expanded pool of antigen-primed cells which can travel to secondary lymphoid organs under the influence of the CCL21 (SLC) chemokine (cf. table 10.3) and, following re-encounter with antigen, can stimulate dendritic cells, help B-cells and generate effector cells. In contrast, effector memory T-cells possess CCR1, CCR3 and CCR5 receptors for proinflammatory chemokines and constitute tissue-homing cells which mediate inflammatory reactions or cytotoxicity.

Virgin B-cells lose their surface IgM and IgD and switch receptor isotype on becoming memory cells, and the differential expression of these surface markers has greatly facilitated the separation of B- and T-cells into naive and memory populations for further study. The costimulatory molecules B7.1 (CD80) and B7.2 (CD86) are rapidly upregulated on memory B-cells, and the potent ability of these cells to present antigen to T-cells could well account for the brisk and robust nature of secondary responses. A scheme similar to that outlined in figure 10.21 for T-cells may also exist for the B-lymphocyte compartment, with an initial population of memory cells possessing the B220 marker developing into B220⁻ memory B-cells which then go on to generate antibody-secreting effector cells.

SUMMARY

A succession of genes are upregulated by T-cell activation

• Within 15–30 minutes, genes for transcription factors concerned in the progression G0 to G1 and in the control of IL-2 are expressed.

• Up to 14 hours, cytokines and their receptors are expressed.

• Later, a variety of genes related to cell division and adhesion are upregulated.

Cytokines act as intercellular messengers

• Cytokines act transiently and usually at short range,

although circulating IL-1 and IL-6 can mediate release of acute phase proteins from the liver.

• They act through surface receptors belonging to six structural families.

• Cytokine-induced dimerization of individual subunits of the main (hematopoietin) receptor family activates protein tyrosine kinases, including JAKs, and leads to phosphorylation and activation of STAT transcription factors.

• Cytokines are pleiotropic, i.e. have multiple effects in the general areas of: (i) control of lymphocyte

(continued p. 198)

growth, (ii) activation of innate immune mechanisms (including inflammation), and (iii) control of bone marrow hematopoiesis (cf. figure 10.4).

• Cytokines may act sequentially, through one cytokine inducing production of another or by transmodulation of the receptor for another cytokine; they can also act synergistically or antagonistically.

• Their roles *in vivo* can be assessed by gene 'knockout', transfection or inhibition by specific antibodies.

Different T-cell subsets can make different cytokines

• As immunization proceeds, Th tend to develop into two subsets: Th1 cells concerned in inflammatory processes, macrophage activation and delayed sensitivity make IL-2 and -3, IFNγ, TNF, lymphotoxin and GM-CSF; Th2 cells help B-cells to synthesize antibody and secrete IL-3, -4, -5, -6 and -13, TNF and GM-CSF. IL-10 is secreted by Th2 cells in mice but by both Th1 and Th2 subsets in humans.

• Early interaction of antigen with macrophages or dendritic cells producing IL-12 or with a variety of cells secreting IL-4 will skew the responses to Th1 or Th2, respectively.

• Other subsets may exist, including TGFβ-secreting Th3 (Tr1) regulatory cells.

• Tc1 (IFNγ) and Tc2 (IL-4) populations can also be distinguished.

Activated T-cells proliferate in response to cytokines

• IL-2 acts as an autocrine growth factor for Th1 and paracrine for Th2 cells which have upregulated their IL-2 receptors.

• Cytokines act on cells which express the appropriate cytokine receptor.

T-cell effectors in cell-mediated immunity

• Cytokines mediate chronic inflammatory responses and induce the expression of MHC class II on endothelial cells, a variety of epithelial cells and many tumor cell lines, so facilitating interactions between T-cells and nonlymphoid cells.

• Differential expression of chemokine receptors permits selective recruitment of neutrophils, macrophages, dendritic cells and T- and B-cells.

• TNF synergizes with IFNγ in killing cells.

• Cytotoxic T-cells are generated against cells (e.g. virally infected) which have intracellularly derived peptide associated with surface MHC class I. They kill using lytic granules containing perforin, granzymes and TNF.

• T-cell-mediated inflammation is strongly downregulated by IL-4 and IL-10.

Proliferation of B-cell responses is mediated by cytokines

• Early proliferation is mediated by IL-4 which also aids IgE synthesis.

• IgA producers are driven by TGFβ and IL-5.

• IL-4 plus IL-5 promote IgM and IL-4, -5, -6 and -13 plus IFNγ stimulate IgG synthesis.

Events in the germinal center

• There is clonal expansion, isotype switch and mutation in the dark zone centroblasts.

• The B-cell centroblasts die through apoptosis unless rescued by certain signals which upregulate *bcl-2*. These include cross-linking of surface Ig by complexes on follicular dendritic cells and engagement of the CD40 receptor which drives the cell to the memory compartment.

• The selection of mutants by antigen guides the development of high affinity B-cells.

The synthesis of antibody

• RNA for variable and constant regions is spliced together before leaving the nucleus.

• Differential splicing allows coexpression of IgM and IgD with identical V regions on a single cell and the switch from membrane-bound to secreted IgM.

Ig class switching occurs in individual B-cells

• IgM produced early in the response switches to IgG, particularly with thymus-dependent antigens. The switch is largely under T-cell control.

• IgG, but not IgM, responses improve on secondary challenge.

Antibody affinity during the immune response

• Low doses of antigen tend to select high affinity B-cells and hence antibodies since only these can be rescued in the germinal center.

• For the same reasons, affinity matures as antigen concentration falls during an immune response.

Memory cells

• Memory T-cells can be maintained in the absence of antigen.

• However, immune complexes on the surface of follicular dendritic cells in the germinal centers provide a long-term source of antigen.

• Memory cells have higher affinity than naive cells, in the case of B-cells through somatic mutation, and in the case of T-cells through selective proliferation of cells with higher affinity receptors and through upregulated expression of associated molecules such as CD2 and LFA-1, which in-

(continued)

crease the avidity (functional affinity) for the antigen-presenting cell.
• Activated memory and naive T-cells are distinguished by the expression of CD45 isoforms, the former having the CD45RO phenotype, the latter CD45RA. It seems likely that a proportion of the CD45RO population reverts to a CD45RA pool of resting memory cells. CD45RA⁻ memory cells can be divided into CCR7⁺ central memory and CCR7⁻ effector memory cells.

• High levels of CD44 expression are also characteristic of memory T-cells, low level expression being associated with naive T-cells.

See the accompanying website (**www.roitt.com**) for multiple choice questions.

FURTHER READING

Camacho S.A., Kosco-Vilbois M.H. & Berek C. (1998) The dynamic structure of the germinal center. *Immunology Today* **19**, 511.

Kinoshita K. & Honjo T. (2000) Unique and unprecedented recombination mechanisms in class switching. *Current Opinion in Immunology* **12**, 195.

Moser B. & Loetscher P. (2001) Lymphocyte traffic control by chemokines. *Nature Immunology* **2**, 123.

Sallusto F., Mackay C.R. & Lanzavecchia A. (2000) The role of chemokine receptors in primary, effector, and memory immune responses. *Annual Reviews in Immunology* **18**, 593.

Sprent J. & Surh C.D. (2001) Generation and maintenance of memory T cells. *Current Opinion in Immunology* **13**, 248.

Tough D.F., Sun S., Zhang X. & Sprent J. (1999) Stimulation of naive and memory T cells by cytokines. *Immunological Reviews* **170**, 39.

Yasukawa H., Sasaki A. & Yoskimuro A. (2000) Negative regulation of cytokine signaling pathways. *Annual Reviews in Immunology* **18**, 143.

Zlotnik A. & Yoshie O. (2000) Chemokines: a new classification system and their role in immunity. *Immunity* **12**, 121.

Control mechanisms

INTRODUCTION

The acquired immune response evolved so that it would come into play when contact with an infectious agent is made. The appropriate antigen-specific cells expand, often to form a sizable proportion of the lymphocytes in the local lymphoid tissues, the effectors eliminate the antigen and then the response quietens down and leaves room for reaction to other infections. Feedback mechanisms must operate to limit the response; otherwise, after antigenic stimulation, we would become overwhelmed by the responding clones of T-cells and antibody-forming cells and their products—obviously an unwelcome state of affairs, as may be clearly seen in multiple myeloma, where control over lymphocyte proliferation is lost. It makes sense for **antigen to be a major regulatory factor** and for lymphocyte responses to be driven by the presence of antigen, falling off in intensity as the antigen concentration drops (figure 11.1). There is abundant evidence to support this view. Antigens can stimulate the proliferation of specific lymphocytes *in vitro*. Clearance of antigen *in vivo* by injection of excess antibody during the course of an immune response leads to a dramatic drop in antibody synthesis and the number of antibody-secreting cells.

ANTIGENS CAN INTERFERE WITH EACH OTHER

The presence of one antigen in a mixture of antigens can drastically diminish the immune response to the others. This is true even for epitopes within a given molecule; for example, the response to epitopes on the Fab fragment of IgG is far greater when the Fab rather than whole IgG is used for immunization due to the inhibitory nature of the Fc region. Factors which determine immunodominance include the precursor frequency of the B-cells bearing antigen receptors for different epitopes on the antigen, the relative affinity of these antigen receptors for their respective epitopes, the degree to which the surface membrane antibody protects the epitope from proteolysis following internalization of the antibody–antigen complex, and the level of competition of processed antigenic peptides for the *major histocompatibility complex* (MHC) groove. There is a clear hierarchy of epitopes with respect to this competitive binding based on differential accessibility to proteases as the molecule unfolds, and the presence or absence of particular amino acid sequences which facilitate breakdown to yield peptides in high abundance and with relatively high affinity for the MHC (figure 11.2). Thus, Sercarz envisages **dominant epitopes**, which bag the lion's share of the available MHC grooves, **subdominant epitopes**, which are less successful, and **cryptic epitopes**, which generate

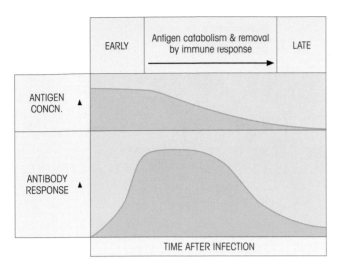

Figure 11.1. Antigen drives the immune response. As antigen concentration falls due to catabolism and elimination by antibody, the intensity of the immune response declines, but is maintained for some time at a lower level by antigen trapped on germinal center follicular dendritic cells.

Figure 11.2. Mechanisms of epitope dominance at the MHC level. The other factor which can influence dominance is the availability of reactive T-cells; if these have been eliminated, e.g. through tolerization by cross-reacting self-antigens, a peptide which may have dominated the MHC groove would be unable to provoke an immune response.

miserably low concentrations of peptide–MHC that are ignored by potentially reactive naive T-cells.

Clearly, the possibility that certain antigens in a mixture, or particular epitopes in a given antigen, may block a desired protective immune response has obvious implications for vaccine design. Contrariwise, the identification of inhibitory peptides with a predatory affinity for the MHC groove(s) should provide thera-

peutic agents to quash unwanted hypersensitivity reactions.

COMPLEMENT AND ANTIBODY ALSO PLAY A ROLE

Innate immune mechanisms are usually first on the scene and activation of the alternative pathway of complement activation will lead to C3d deposition on the microbe. When C3d-coated antigens are recognized by the B-cell, cross-linking of the BCR and the CD21 complement receptor, with its associated signal-transducing molecule CD19, enhances B-cell activation (figure 11.3a). In contrast, cross-linking of the BCR with FcγRIIB1 (cf. p. 50) delivers a negative signal by suppressing tyrosine phosphorylation of CD19 (figure 11.3b). Thus, removal of circulating antibody by plasmapheresis during an ongoing response leads to an increase in synthesis, whereas injection of preformed IgG antibody markedly hastens the fall in the number of antibody-forming cells (figure 11.4) consistent with feedback control on overall synthesis.

In complete contrast, injection of IgM antibodies enhances the response (figure 11.4), presumably by cross-linking antigen bound to the sIgM receptors without activating the Fcγ inhibitory receptor, and perhaps also via the generation of C3d by the classical pathway of complement activation. Since antibodies of this isotype are either already present amongst the broadly reactive natural antibodies, or if not will certainly appear at an early stage after antigen challenge, they would be useful in boosting the initial response.

ACTIVATION-INDUCED CELL DEATH

Although clearance of antigen from the body by the immune system will clearly lead to a downregulation of lymphocyte proliferation due to the absence of a signal through the antigen receptor, even in the presence of antigen the signals provided do not lead to the continuous proliferation of cells, but rather set off a train of events that, unless the cells are protected in some way, leads to *a*ctivation-*i*nduced *c*ell *d*eath (AICD) by apoptosis. It seems that AICD is perhaps primarily a feature of CD4 cells, allowing these cells to be cleared from the system following their proliferation. Subsequent to activation, T-cells upregulate death receptors and their ligands. If the ligands remain associated with the cell surface they can activate apoptosis in adjacent cells. However, they are often released from the cell surface by proteases, producing soluble forms which in some cases retain activity, for example the soluble version of the TNF-related apoptosis-inducing ligand (TRAIL)

Figure 11.3. Cross-linking of surface IgM antigen receptor to the CD21 complement receptor stimulates, and to the Fcγ receptor FcγRIIB1 inhibits, B-cells. (a) Following activation of complement, C3d becomes covalently bound to the microbial surface. The CD21 complement receptor binds C3d and signals through its associated CD19 molecule. The CD19, CD21 and CD81 (TAPA-1) molecules form the B-cell coreceptor and cross-linking of this complex to the surface IgM of the BCR leads to tyrosine phosphorylation of CD19 and subsequent binding of phosphatidylinositol 3-kinase (PI3-K), leading to B-cell activation. (b) The FcγRIIB1 molecule possesses a cytoplasmic immunoreceptor tyrosine-based inhibitory motif (ITIM) and, upon cross-linking to membrane Ig, becomes phosphorylated and binds the inositol polyphosphate 5′-phosphatase SHIP. This suppresses phosphorylation of CD19 and thus inhibits B-cell activation.

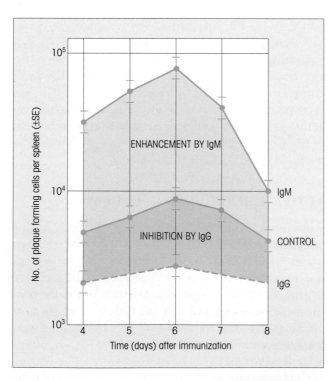

Figure 11.4. Time-course of enhancement of antibody response to sheep red blood cells (SRBC) due to injection of preformed IgM, and of suppression by preformed IgG antibodies. Mice received monoclonal IgM anti-SRBC, IgG anti-SRBC or medium alone intravenously 2 hours prior to immunization with 10^5 SRBC. (Data provided by J. Reiter, P. Hutchings, P. Lydyard and A. Cooke.)

retains the ability to signal through the receptor TRAIL-R1. Such soluble ligands can potentially mediate either paracrine or autocrine cell death. The death receptors are members of the tumor necrosis factor receptor (TNF-R) family and include TNFRI, CD95 (Fas), TRAMP (TNF receptor apoptosis-mediating protein), the aforementioned TRAIL-R1, TRAIL-R2 and death receptor (DR) 6. Apoptosis induction through these receptors initially involves cleavage of the inactive cysteine protease procaspase 8 to yield active caspase 8. Ultimately, this activation pathway converges with the apoptosis pathway induced by cellular stress, both leading to the activation of downstream effector caspases (figure 11.5). In addition to the death receptors, there are also a number of 'decoy receptors' which bind the potentially apoptosis-inducing ligands but do not signal.

When initially activated by peptide–MHC, T-cells are resistant to apoptosis but become progressively sensitive. A number of molecules are known to be protective against apoptosis; for example, bcl-2 and bcl-X_L, which appear to act as watchdogs preventing the release of pro-apoptotic proteins from the mitochondria. Of particular relevance to death receptor-mediated AICD, however, is the molecule FLIP (FLICE inhibitory protein, FLICE being an older name for caspase 8). FLIP bears structural similarity to caspase 8, and therefore by competitive inhibition prevents recruitment of this caspase into the *death-inducing signaling complex* (DISC) (figure 11.5). It appears that the

Figure 11.5. Activation-induced cell death. Receptor-based induction of apoptosis involves the trimerization of TNF-R family members (for example, Fas) by trimerized ligands (for example, Fas-ligand). This brings together cytoplasmic death domains (DD) which can recruit a number of death effector domain (DED)-containing adaptor molecules to form the death-inducing signaling complex (DISC). The different receptors use different combinations of DED-containing adaptors; Fas uses FADD (*F*as-*a*ssociated protein with *d*eath *d*omain). The DISC induces the cleavage of inactive procaspase 8 into active caspase 8, with subsequent activation of downstream effector caspases. This process eventually leads to the release of the endonuclease known as caspase-activated DNase (CAD) from a restraining protein (inhibitor of CAD; ICAD) in the cytoplasm, with subsequent translocation of the endonuclease to the nucleus. A second pathway of apoptosis induction, often triggered by cellular stress, involves a number of mitochondria-associated proteins including cytochrome *c*, Smac/DIABLO and the bcl-2 family member bax. Caspase 9 activation is the key event in this pathway and requires association of the caspase with a number of other proteins including the cofactor Apaf-1; the complex formed incorporates cytochrome *c* and is referred to as the apoptosome. The activated caspase 9 then cleaves procaspase 3. Although the death receptor and mitochondrial pathways are shown as initially separate in the figure, there is some cross-talk between them. Thus, caspase 8 can cleave the bcl-2 family member bid (not shown), a process which promotes cytochrome *c* release from mitochondria. Other members of the bcl-2 family, such as bcl-2 itself and bcl-X$_L$, inhibit apoptosis, perhaps by preventing the release of pro-apoptotic molecules from the mitochondria. M, mitochondrion.

balance between caspase 8 and FLIP levels can determine the fate of the cell when the death receptor is engaged by its ligand, but does not affect apoptosis induced by the stress-activated mitochondrial pathway (figure 11.6).

T-CELL REGULATION

T-helper cells

There is abundant evidence to suggest that different populations of Th cells are specialized for different helper functions. With respect to help for antibody production, T-cell lines derived from Peyer's patches are much better at helping IgA-producing B-cells from Peyer's patch precursors than are splenic T-cell lines. The help is for IgA-precommitted B-cells rather than for induction of the class switch to IgA, since Peyer's patch T-cells do not markedly enhance IgA production by splenic B-cells. Evidence for the production of an IgE-binding factor from Fcε receptor-bearing T-cells, which enhances B-cell secretion of IgE, has been obtained; intriguingly, a 13 kDa T-cell-derived cytokine called *g*lycosylation *i*nhibiting *f*actor (GIF) inhibits *N*-glycosylation of the IgE-binding factor so that it now becomes a suppressor of IgE synthesis. It should also be evident from the previous discussion of AICD that Th cells will not be around to expand B-cell and Tc clone sizes indefinitely.

T-cell suppression

It is perhaps inevitable that nature, having evolved a functional set of T-cells which promote immune

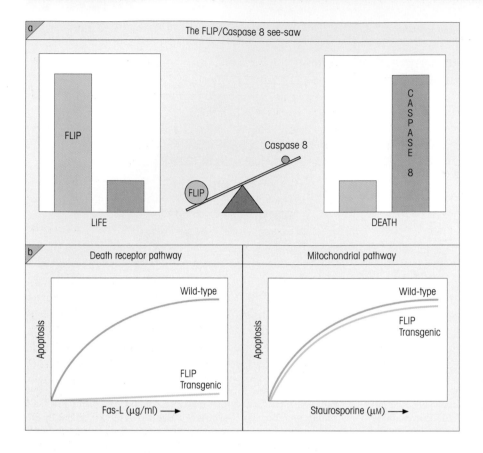

Figure 11.6. Life and death decisions. (a) The relative amounts of anti-apoptotic FLIP and pro-apoptotic caspase 8 can determine the fate of the cell. (b) Experiments involving overexpression of FLIP in a transgenic mouse model show that this protein protects T-cells from AICD stimulated through the death receptor pathway by Fas-ligand, but not from cell death triggered via the mitochondrial pathway using the drug staurosporine. (Based on data obtained by J. Tschopp and colleagues.)

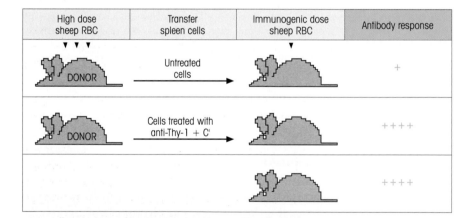

Figure 11.7. Demonstration of T-suppressor cells. A mouse of an appropriate strain immunized with an immunogenic dose of sheep erythrocytes makes a strong antibody response. However, if spleen cells from a donor of the same strain previously injected with a high dose of antigen are first transferred to the syngeneic animal, they depress the antibody response to a normally immunogenic dose of the antigen. The effect is lost if the spleen cells are first treated with a T-cell-specific antiserum (anti-Thy-1) plus complement, showing that the suppressors are T-cells. (After Gershon R.K. & Kondo K. (1971) *Immunology* **21**, 903.)

responses, should also develop a regulatory set whose job would be to modulate the helpers. T-cell suppression was first brought to the serious attention of the immunological fraternity by a phenomenon colorfully named by its discoverer, 'infectious tolerance'. Quite surprisingly it was shown that, if mice were made unresponsive by injection of a high dose of *sheep red blood cells* (SRBC), their T-cells would suppress specific antibody formation in normal recipients to which they had been transferred (figure 11.7). It may not be apparent to the reader why this result was at all surprising, but at that time antigen-induced tolerance was regarded essentially as a negative phenomenon involving the depletion or silencing of clones rather than a state of active suppression. Over the years, T-cell suppression has been shown to modulate a variety of humoral and cellular responses, the latter including delayed-type hypersensitivity, cytotoxic T-cells and antigen-specific T-cell proliferation. However, the existence of dedicated professional T-suppressor cells is a question which has generated a great deal of heat.

Suppressor and helper epitopes can be discrete

Detailed analysis of murine responses to antigens such as hen egg-white lysozyme tells us that certain determinants can evoke very strong suppressor rather than helper responses depending on the mouse strain, and also that T-suppressors directed to one determinant can switch off helper and antibody responses to other determinants on the same molecule. Thus mice of *H-2^b* haplotype respond poorly to lysozyme because they develop dominant suppression; however, if the three N-terminal amino acids are removed from the antigen, these mice now make a splendid response, showing that the T-suppression directed against the determinant associated with the N-terminal region has switched off the response to the remaining determinants on the antigen. Similar results have been obtained in several other systems. This must imply that the antigen itself acts as a form of bridge to allow communication between T-suppressor and cells reacting to the other determinants, as might occur through these cells binding to an antigen-presenting cell expressing several different processed determinants of the same antigen on its surface (figure 11.8).

Figure 11.8. Possible mechanism to explain the need for a physical linkage between suppressor and helper epitopes. The helper and putative suppressor cells can interact by binding close together on the surface of an antigen-presenting cell, which processes the antigen and displays the different epitopes on separate MHC molecules on its surface.

Characteristics of suppression

What of the effectors of suppression? In a number of experimental systems the cells which mediate suppression are far more vulnerable than helpers to adult thymectomy, X-irradiation and cyclophosphamide. For example, adult thymectomy in the mouse has little effect on the Th population, but leads to a fall in the T-suppressors, thereby increasing the response to T-independent antigens and preventing the fall-off in IgE antibody to haptens coupled with *Ascaris* extracts which occurs in intact animals.

Classically, suppressor T-cells have been described as CD8+. For example, the B10.A (2R) mouse strain has a low immune response to lactate dehydrogenase β (LDHβ) associated with the possession of the *H-2Eβ* gene of *k* rather than *b* haplotype. Lymphoid cells taken from these animals after immunization with LDHβ proliferate poorly *in vitro* in the presence of antigen, but if CD8+ cells are depleted, the remaining CD4+ cells give a much higher response. Adding back the CD8+ cells reimposes the active suppression. Human suppressor T-cells can also belong to the CD8 subset. Thus, CD8+ CD28− cells can prevent antigen-presenting B-cells from upregulating costimulatory B7 molecules in response to CD40-mediated signals from the CD40 ligand on Th cells. Following interaction with the CD8 T-cells, the APCs are then capable of inducing anergy in Th cells. This effect on B7 is mediated by inhibition of NFκB activation in the APC, an event necessary for transcription of both the B7.1 (CD80) and B7.2 (CD86) molecules.

More recently, it has become appreciated that regulatory CD4+ cells can also be major effectors of suppression. In a model of *inflammatory bowel disease* (IBD), in which transfer of CD45RB^high CD4+ T-cells from normal donor mice into mice with *severe combined immunodeficiency* (SCID) leads to the development of IBD, the disease can be prevented if CD45RB^low CD4+ regulatory T-cells (Tr) are transferred at the same time. This immunoregulatory effect could be blocked by antibodies to the IL-10 receptor or to TGFβ in mice, or to IL-4 and TGFβ in rats.

Suppressor cells of the CD4 phenotype have also been identified within the minor population which express the IL-2 receptor α chain (CD25). These suppressors are able to abrogate the responses of CD4+ CD25− T-cells by an as yet undefined cell contact-dependent, cytokine-independent mechanism.

Suppression is a regulated phenomenon

Let us look in a little more depth at some potential

TCR ▭● MHC   ● SUPPRESSOR EPITOPE   ● HELPER EPITOPE

Figure 11.9. Mutual antagonisms between T-cell subsets linked indirectly by processed antigen on an antigen-presenting cell lead to functionally distinct modes of suppression. (Leaning heavily on Bloom B.R., Salgame P. & Diamond B. (1992) *Immunology Today* **13**, 131.) Yet another mechanism may prove to be important. Unlike the mouse, many other mammalian species can express MHC class II on a proportion of their activated T-cells; presentation of processed peptide by these cells can induce CD4-positive cytotoxic cells with suppressor potential. We also need to know more about the circumstances leading to the production of TGFβ by suppressors since this cytokine inhibits T-cell proliferation.

mechanisms of suppression. We have already entertained the idea that antigen-linked T–T interactions can occur on the surface of an antigen-presenting cell (figure 11.8) and the concept of T1 and T2 CD8 subsets paralleling the Th1/Th2 dichotomy. Furthermore, the evidence for mutual antagonism (suppression) between Th1 and Th2 cells is very strong indeed. One could postulate downregulation of Th1 cells by type 2 IL-4-producing CD8 cells, and suppression of Th2 cells by type 1 IFNγ-producing CD8 cells, interacting on the surface of an antigen-presenting cell (figure 11.9). In this model, when the immune response has locked onto a particular mode, e.g. Th1-mediated cellular immunity, other types of response, such as T–B collaboration, are restricted through a cytokine inhibitory effect. Although these cells mediate T-suppression, they would not be called dedicated professional suppressors since, in a sense, their suppressive powers are a by-product of their main defensive function. Perhaps we need these cytokine-secreting Tc cells to prevent Th cells getting out of hand by excessive proliferation,

just as IgG holds back the B-cells by feedback control. There is indeed abundant evidence for such a regulatory mechanism whereby suppressors can be induced by Th1 cells.

The nature of the antigen-presenting cell, upon whose surface these interactions are thought to occur, may influence the type of cells involved and the outcome. It may be recalled that dendritic cells, macrophages, B-cells, activated T-cells and even epithelial cells with upregulated class II can all act as antigen presenters. Of interest is the finding that irradiation with UVB light inactivates dendritic cells and stimulates T-suppression; IL-2 and IFNγ are downregulated and IL-4 production is increased.

Other issues which require solutions are the mechanism by which high-dose antigen induces suppression, the role of cytotoxic CD4 and CD8 T-cells in these phenomena and the extent to which idiotype-specific T-suppressors contribute.

It is important not to lose track of the so-called 'natural suppressor cells', such as those provoked by total lymph node irradiation, and we would like to draw attention to a report that natural killer (NK) cells can inhibit the one-way mixed lymphocyte reaction (see p. 352) or the primary IgM response to sheep cells *in vitro*, by suppressing dendritic cells which have already taken up the antigen. This offers a further opportunity for feedback control since IFNγ and IL-2 produced by Th can activate NK cells.

Overall, suppression may be most commonly mediated by secretion of cytokines such as TGFβ, by secretion of yet to be defined suppressor molecules and by inactivation of APC function. Make no mistake, suppression is still a murky area, and is not for the unwary, but the light at the end of the tunnel is beckoning.

Effector T-cells are guided to the appropriate target by MHC surface molecules

Not only do MHC molecules bearing a tell-tale peptide signal the presence of an intracellular precursor (cf. p. 95, Chapter 5), they also ensure that the T-cell makes contact with the surface of the appropriate target cell.

Let us explore this point by looking at the role of Tc in viral infection. When a cell is first infected with virus, there is an eclipse phase during which the machinery of the cell is being switched for viral replication and the only marker of the complete microbe is the processed viral antigen peptide on the cell surface. At this stage, killing of the cell by a cytotoxic T-cell will prevent viral replication. The killer

T-cell knows it has reached its target when it recognizes the surface viral peptide in association with class I MHC molecules which are present on nearly every cell in the body. Thus the killer cell operates on the basis that processed viral antigen is the code for '**viral infection**' and class I molecules are the code for '**cell**' (cf. figure 5.26).

The situation is quite different with intracellular bacteria and protozoa which do not go through an eclipse phase after phagocytosis by macrophages, but are held as infectious entities; lysis by cytotoxic T-cells will merely release the organisms, not kill them. A separate strategy is required and, in this case, the effector Th1 lymphocyte recognizes the infected macrophage by the presence of microbial antigen on the surface in association with a class II molecule which is now a code for 'macrophage'. This interaction triggers the release of macrophage-stimulating cytokines, dominant among which is IFNγ. Multiple microbicidal mechanisms are triggered in the activated macrophages, including the formation of reactive oxygen intermediates and the synthesis of NO·, to the detriment of the intracellular parasites (see p. 265). Similarly, in T–B cooperation, the **B-cell** is recognized through its class II molecule associated with the foreign antigen, although in this case costimulatory signals through CD40L–CD40 interactions are required for activation. T-cells mediating **suppression** also utilize MHC molecules, but the mechanisms are unclear. In summary, each antigen-specific T-lymphocyte subset has to communicate with a particular cell type in order to make the appropriate immune response, and it does so by recognizing not only processed foreign antigen but also the particular MHC molecule used as a marker of that cell (table 11.1).

Some types of immunoregulatory cells, such as certain γδ T-cells, may recognize activation-induced, nonclassical MHC molecules, as appears to be the case with the recognition of the class Ib molecules T22 and T10 in the mouse, although the precise role of such cells is still being elucidated.

Table 11.1. Guidance of T-subpopulations to appropriate target cell by MHC molecules.

Function	Cell interaction	MHC marker on target cell
T-cell priming	T–dendritic cell	II (+*B7/CD28)
T-helper (Th1)	T–macrophage	II (+peptide)
T-helper (Th2)	T–B	II (+*CD40L/CD40)
T-suppressor	T–T	?
T-cytotoxic	T–target cell	I

*Costimulatory molecules and their ligand.

IDIOTYPE NETWORKS

Jerne's network hypothesis

The hypervariable loops on the immunoglobulin molecule which form the antigen combining site have individual characteristic shapes which can be recognized by the appropriate antibodies as idiotypic determinants (cf. p. 42). There are hundreds of thousands, if not more, different idiotypes in one individual.

Jerne reasoned brilliantly that the great diversity of idiotypes would to a considerable extent mirror the diversity of antigenic shapes in the external world. Thus, he said, if lymphocytes can recognize a whole range of foreign antigenic determinants, they should be able to recognize the idiotypes on the antigen receptors of other lymphocytes. They would therefore form a large network or series of networks depending upon **idiotype–anti-idiotype recognition** between T- and B-cells (figure 11.10), and the response to an external antigen perturbing this network would be conditioned by the state of the idiotypic interactions.

Evidence for idiotypic networks

Anti-idiotype can be induced by autologous idiotypes

There is no doubt that the elements which can form an idiotypic network are present in the body, and autoanti-idiotypes occur during the course of antigen-induced responses. For example, certain strains of mice injected with pneumococcal vaccines make an antibody response to the phosphorylcholine groups in which the germ-line-encoded idiotype T15 dominates. If the individual antibody-forming cells are examined by plaque assays at different times after immunization, waves of T15[+] and of anti-T15 (i.e. autoanti-idiotype) cells are demonstrable. Similarly, immunization with the acetylcholine agonist BISQ, followed by fusion of the spleen cells to produce hybridomas, yielded a series of anti-BISQ monoclonals (idiotypes) and a smaller number of anti-idiotypic monoclonals, of which a surprising proportion behaved as internal images of BISQ in their ability to stimulate acetylcholine receptors (figure 11.11). Anti-idiotypic reactivity has also been demonstrated in T-cell populations using various experimental systems. Indeed, anti-idiotypic T-cells recognizing peptide derived from the CDR2, CDR3 and framework regions of other TCRs appear to form a part of the normal human T-cell repertoire. Immunization of multiple sclerosis patients with myelin basic protein reactive T-cell clones induces CD8[+] cytotoxic T-cells which recognize a peptide

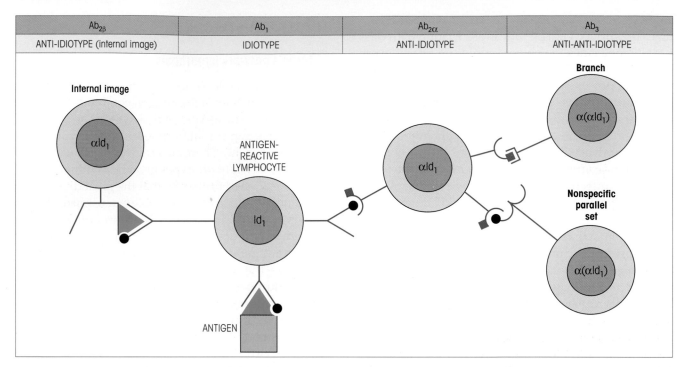

Ab$_{2\beta}$	Ab$_1$	Ab$_{2\alpha}$	Ab$_3$
ANTI-IDIOTYPE (internal image)	IDIOTYPE	ANTI-IDIOTYPE	ANTI-ANTI-IDIOTYPE

Figure 11.10. Elements in an idiotypic network in which the antigen receptors on one lymphocyte reciprocally recognize an idiotype on the receptors of another. T-helper, T-suppressor and B-lymphocytes interact through idiotype–anti-idiotype reactions producing either stimulation or suppression. T–T interactions could occur through direct recognition of one T-cell receptor (TCR) by the other, or more usually by recognition of a processed TCR peptide associated with MHC. One of the anti-idiotype sets, Ab$_{2\beta}$, may bear an idiotype of similar shape to (i.e. provides an **internal image** of) the antigen. The same idiotype (●) may be shared by receptors of different specificity, the nonspecific parallel set (since the several hypervariable regions provide a number of potential idiotypic determinants and a given idiotype does not always form part of the epitope-binding site, i.e. the paratope), so that the anti-(anti-Id$_1$) does not necessarily bind the original antigen. (The following abbreviations are often employed: α as a prefix = anti; Id = idiotype; Ab$_1$ = Id; Ab$_2\alpha$ = αId not involving the paratope; Ab$_{2\beta}$ = internal image αId involving the paratope; Ab$_3$ = $\alpha(\alpha$Id).)

derived from a TCR CDR3-associated idiotype presented by MHC class I.

A network is evident in early life

If the spleens of fetal mice which are just beginning to secrete immunoglobulin are used to produce hybridomas, an unusually high proportion are interrelated as idiotype–anti-idiotype pairs. This high level of idiotype connectivity is not seen in later life and suggests that these early cells, largely the CD5$^+$ **B-1 subset** (cf. p. 236), are programed to synthesize germ-line gene specificities which have network relationships.

Preoccupation of networks with self

Paradoxically, there is increasing evidence that preformed idiotype networks have what might seem at first sight a somewhat unhealthy interest in self-antigens. The CD5 IgM hybridomas produced from fetal mouse spleen with high idiotype connectivity have specificities similar to those of the '**natural anti-** **bodies**' which appear spontaneously in germ-free animals not exposed to exogenous antigens. Not only are many of them directed to polysaccharide antigens of common pathogens, e.g. phosphorylcholine, but a number of them have low affinity for self-components such as DNA, IgG, heat-shock proteins and cytoskeletal elements. The concept of a largely CD5 B-1 cell population forming an inward-looking world in which the component cells recognize and stimulate each other ceaselessly through their idiotypic receptor interactions to produce a range of IgM antibodies which provide an early defense against infection is most plausible. But the self-reactivity of many of these cells is enigmatic. Preset regulatory T-cell networks may also involve certain dominant autoantigens, such as heat-shock protein hsp65 and myelin basic protein from nervous tissue. Is recognition of self as important as nonself?

Irun Cohen has proposed the intriguing notion of an **immunological homunculus** (little man) in which a functional picture of the body is encoded within the immune system by regulatory network committees of

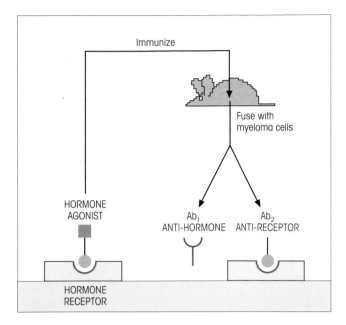

Figure 11.11. The spontaneous production of autoanti-idiotype during immunization with a hormone agonist. Hybridomas obtained from the immunized mouse secrete anti-hormone and anti-idiotype which reacts with the hormone receptor; this indicates a close relationship between hormone, receptor, anti-hormone and anti-idiotype, implying some connection between autoantibodies within the idiotype network and hormone systems.

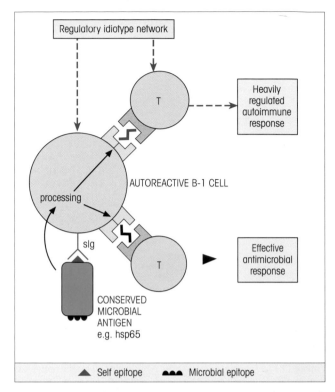

Figure 11.12. Speculation on the role of self-reacting CD5 B-1 cells in microbial infection. The surface immunoglobulin (sIg) receptor selectively captures the cross-reacting conserved bacterial antigen (in this case, heat-shock protein hsp65) and, after processing, presents self and microbe-specific epitopes associated with MHC class II. The autoreactive T-cell is heavily controlled by the idiotype regulatory network since (*ex hypothesi*) important self-antigens are dominantly encoded within the 'immunological homunculus', but the antimicrobial T-cell is free to mount a vigorous response. This accounts for the dominance of conserved antigens. (Based upon Cohen I.R. & Young D.B. (1991) *Immunology Today* **12**, 105.)

B- and T-cells which recognize certain dominant self-antigens representing the major organs in the body. (The analogy is with the neurological homunculus, a functional picture of the body in which the space occupied by a given neural network is directly related to the neurological importance of the organ it encodes, e.g. human visual and speech organs and canine olfactory organs are prominently represented.) The relevance of these ideas to the control of autoimmunity will be discussed in Chapter 19, but here we can speculate on how they might also relate to the response to infection. Consider a dominant microbial antigen such as hsp65 which is highly conserved in nature and bears several potential epitopes identical with the self-homolog. In an infection, any B-1 cells which recognize *self*-hsp65 will selectively focus the *bacterial* hsp65 onto their surface receptors (making it dominant over other bacterial antigens) and process it. The self-epitopes will be recognized by autoreactive T-cells which are highly regulated within the homunculus, whereas T-cells specific for the nonself hsp epitopes are not so constrained and will generate an effective immune response (figure 11.12).

Idiotypic regulation of immune responses

There have been a series of investigations based on the following cascade protocol. Antigen is injected into $animal_1$ and the antibody produced, Ab_1 (idiotype), is purified and injected into $animal_2$. Ab_2 (anti-idiotype) so formed is purified and used to immunize $animal_3$ and so on (figure 11.13). Consistently, it is found that Ab_2 (anti-Id_1) recognizes an idiotype (Id_1) on Ab_1 which is also strongly present in Ab_3. Ab_4 behaves like Ab_2 in seeing the common idiotype on Ab_1 and Ab_3. Nonetheless, although Ab_1 and Ab_3 share idiotypes, only a small fraction of Ab_3 reacts with the original antigen. This is the result one would expect if the idiotype was a cross-reacting Id (public Id) present on a variety of antibodies (and thus B-cell receptors) of different specificities. The anti-Id_1 (Ab_2), when injected into $animal_3$, would react with all B-cells bearing Id_1 (figure 11.13) and presumably trigger them to produce Id_1 antibodies, only a fraction of which have specificity for the original antigen.

Such frequently occurring and usually germ-line-

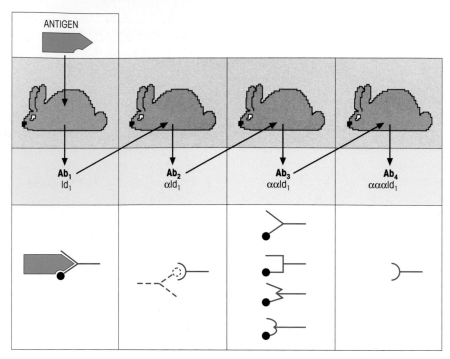

Figure 11.13. An idiotype cascade. Ab_1 produced by the antigen is injected into a second animal to produce Ab_2; this in turn is purified and injected into animal$_3$ and so on. Ab_2 and Ab_4 both react with an idiotype (●) on Ab_1 and Ab_3, but only a fraction of Ab_3 reacts with the original antigen. Bona and Paul (*Immunology Today* 1982, **3**, 230) interpret the results in terms of a common regulatory idiotype Id_1 shared by many antibodies other than those reacting with the original antigen, but recruited by the injection of anti-Id_1 (Ab_2) which stimulates the range of lymphocytes whose receptors bear this common or cross-reacting idiotype. On this basis, one can understand the paradoxical finding of Oudin and Cazenave that not all the Ig molecules bearing a given Id in response to an antigen can function as specific antibody since they belong to the nonspecific parallel set. The presence of large amounts of Id_1 in Ab_3 also suggests that the linear relationship through the cross-reacting Id_1 is dominant, with relatively insignificant branching through the variety of 'private' idiotypes on Ab_2 molecules (cf. figure 11.10) because of the low frequency of such idiotypes and their anti-idiotypes.

encoded idiotypes seem to be provoked fairly readily with anti-Id and are therefore candidates for **regulatory Id** which can be under some degree of control by a limited idiotypic network. Germane to this idea are the observations that, late in immunization, antibodies with utterly distinct specificities, directed against totally different epitopes on the same antigen, often bear a common or cross-reacting idiotype. Presumably, the first clone of B-cells to be expanded which bears a dominant cross-reacting Id can generate a population of regulatory Th cells which recognize this Id as well as antigen. Processing of internalized Ig receptor plus antigen leads to the expression of peptides derived from the idiotype and antigen in association with MHC class II; these B-cells can then access the full repertoire of antigen-specific and idiotype-specific Th cells. The latter may be of two types, one recognizing the native receptor idiotype (non-MHC-restricted) and the other, processed idiotype (MHC-restricted). From the complex mixture of B-lymphocytes activated by the other epitopes on the antigen, these Th cells will selectively recruit those with Id-positive receptors. We can now see how the antigen- and idiotype-specific Th synergize in the antibody response, the latter expanding Id-positive clones induced by the former.

The phenomenon of '**original antigenic sin**' occurs when the immune response becomes 'locked in' to particular epitopes originally encountered on a microorganism, such that it largely ignores even normally immunodominant epitopes during a subsequent encounter with an antigenically related but nonidentical microorganism. Although competition for antigen by the expanded population which forms the memory B-cells plays a major role, idiotype-specific memory Th cells could also contribute to this phenomenon.

Idiotype networks may also allow the immune response to 'tick over' for extended periods and maintain the memory cell population, while the presence of primed Th cells directed against a common Id on the various memory B-cells specific for a given antigen would increase their rate of mobilization during a secondary response.

Manipulation of the immune response through idiotypes

Quite low doses of anti-idiotype, of the order of nanograms, can greatly enhance the expression of the idiotype in the response to a given antigen, whereas doses in the microgram range lead to a suppression (figure 11.14). Thus the idiotypic network provides interesting opportunities to manipulate the immune response, particularly in hypersensitivity states such as autoimmune disease, allergy and graft rejection. However, the B-cell response is normally so diverse, suppression by anti-Id is likely to prove difficult; even when the response is dominated by a public Id and that Id is suppressed, compensatory expansion of clones bearing other idiotypes ensures that the fall in the total antibody titer is relatively undramatic (cf. figure 11.14). Conceivably, Th cells may express a narrower spectrum of idiotypes, thereby being more susceptible to suppression by Id auto-immunization. Reports that 'vaccination' with irradiated lines of Th cells specific for brain or thyroid antigens prevents the induction of experimental autoimmunity against the relevant organ are encouraging. A totally different approach would be to use monoclonal anti-Id of the 'antigen internal image'

set (figure 11.10) to stimulate antigen-specific T-suppressors capable of turning off B-cells directed to other epitopes on the antigen through bridging by the antigen itself (cf. figure 11.8).

Since we know that under suitable conditions anti-Id can also stimulate antibody production, it might be possible to use 'internal image' monoclonal anti-Ids as 'surrogate' antigens for immunization in cases where the antigen is difficult to obtain in bulk—for example, antigens from parasites such as filaria or the weak embryonic antigens associated with some cancers. Another example is where protein antigens obtained by chemical synthesis or gene cloning fail to fold into the configuration of the native molecule; this is not a problem with the anti-Id which by definition has been selected to have the shape of the antigenic epitope.

At this stage, if the reader is feeling a little groggy, try a glance at figure 11.15 which attempts to summarize the main factors currently thought to modulate the immune response.

THE INFLUENCE OF GENETIC FACTORS

Some genes affect general responsiveness

Mice can be selectively bred for high or low antibody responses through several generations to yield two lines, one of which consistently produces high-titer antibodies to a variety of antigens, and the other, antibodies of relatively low titer (figure 11.16; Biozzi and colleagues). Out of the ten or so different genetic loci involved, some give rise to a higher rate of B-cell proliferation and differentiation, while one or more affect macrophage behavior.

Antigen receptor genes are linked to the immune response

Clearly, the Ig and TCR V, D and J genes encoding the specific recognition sites of the lymphocyte antigen receptors are of fundamental importance to the acquired immune response. However, since the mechanisms for generating receptor diversity from the available genes are so powerful (cf. p. 65), immunodeficiency is unlikely to occur as a consequence of a poor Ig or TCR variable region gene repertoire. Nevertheless, just occasionally, we see holes in the repertoire due to the absence of a gene; failure to respond to the sugar polymer α1–6 dextran is a feature of animals without a particular immunoglobulin V gene, and mice lacking the $V\alpha_2$ TCR gene cannot mount a cytotoxic T-cell response to the male H-Y antigen.

Figure 11.14. Modulation of a major idiotype in the antibody response to antigen by anti-idiotype. In the example chosen, the idiotype is present in a substantial proportion of the antibodies produced in controls injected with irrelevant anti-Id plus antigen (i.e. this is a public or cross-reacting Id; see p. 44). Pretreatment with 10 ng of a monoclonal anti-Id greatly expands the Id⁺ antibody population, whereas prior injection of 10 μg of anti-Id almost completely suppresses expression of the idiotype without having any substantial effect on total antibody production due to a compensatory increase in Id⁻ antibody clones.

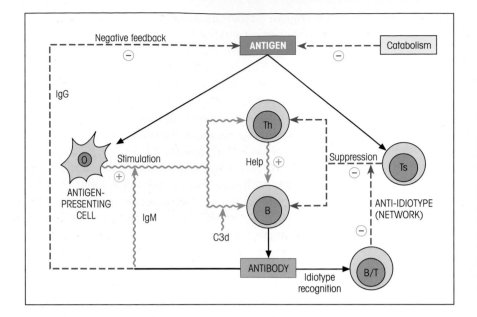

Figure 11.15. Regulation of the immune response. Th, T-helper cell; Ts, T-suppressor cell. T-help for cell-mediated immunity will be subject to similar regulation. Some of these mechanisms may be interdependent; for example, one could envisage anti-idiotypic antibody acting in concert with a suppressor T-cell by binding to its Fc receptor, or suppressor T-cells with specificity for the idiotype on Th or B-cells. To avoid too many confusing arrows, we have omitted the recruitment of B-cells by anti-idiotypic Th cells and direct activation of anti-idiotype Ts by idiotype-positive Th cells.

Figure 11.16. Selective breeding of high and low antibody responders (after Biozzi and colleagues). A foundation population of wild mice (with crazy mixed-up genes and great variability in antibody response) is immunized with sheep red blood cells (SRBC), a multi-determinant antigen. The antibody titer of each individual mouse is shown by a circle. The male and female giving the highest titer antibodies (●) were bred and their litter challenged with antigen. Again, the best responders were bred together and so on for 20 generations when all mice were high responders to SRBC and a variety of other antigens. The same was done for the poorest responders (●), yielding a strain of low responder animals. The two lines are comparable in their ability to clear carbon particles or sheep erythrocytes from the blood by phagocytosis, but macrophages from the high responders present antigen more efficiently (cf. p. 158). On the other hand, the low responders survive infection by *Salmonella typhimurium* better and their macrophages support much slower replication of *Listeria* (cf. p. 262), indicative of an inherently more aggressive microbicidal ability.

Immune response can be influenced by the MHC

There was much excitement when it was first discovered that the antibody responses to a number of thymus-dependent antigenically simple substances are determined by genes mapping to the MHC. For example, mice of the H-2^b haplotype respond well to the synthetic branched polypeptide (T,G)-A–L, whereas H-2^k mice respond poorly (table 11.2).

It was said that mice of the H-2^b haplotype (i.e. a particular set of H-2 genes) are **high responders** to (T,G)-A–L because they possess the appropriate immune response (Ir) gene. With another synthetic antigen, (H,G)-A–L, having histidine in place of tyrosine, the

Table 11.2. H-2 haplotype linked to high, low and intermediate immune responses to synthetic peptides. (T,G)-A–L, polylysine with polyalanine side-chains randomly tipped with tyrosine and glutamine; (H,G)-A–L, the same with histidine in place of tyrosine.

ANTIGEN	H-2 HAPLOTYPE				
	b	k	d	a	s
(T,G)-A–L	Hi	Lo	Int	Lo	Lo
(H,G)-A–L	Lo	Hi	Int	Hi	Lo

Table 11.3. Mapping of the *Ir* gene for (H,G)-A–L responses by analysis of different recombinant strains.

Strain	H-2 region				(H,G)-A–L Response
	K	A	E	D	
A	k	k	k	b	Hi
A.TL	s	k	k	b	Hi
B.IO.A (4R)	k	k	b	b	Hi
B.IO	b	b	b	b	Lo
A.SW	s	s	s	s	Lo

position is reversed, the 'poor (T,G)-A–L responders' now giving a good antibody response and the 'good (T,G)-A–L responders' a weak one, showing that the capacity of a particular strain to give a high or low response varies with the individual antigen (table 11.2). These relationships are only apparent when antigens of highly restricted structure are studied because the response to each single determinant is controlled by an *Ir* gene and it is less likely that the different determinants on a complex antigen will all be associated with consistently high or consistently low responder *Ir* genes; however, although one would expect an average of randomly high and low responder genes, since the various determinants on most thymus-dependent complex antigens are structurally unrelated, the outcome will be biased by the dominance of one or more epitopes (cf. p. 201). Thus H-2-linked immune responses have been observed not only with relatively simple polypeptides, but also with transplantation antigens from another strain and autoantigens where merely one or two determinants are recognized as foreign by the host. With complex antigens, in most but not all cases, H-2 linkage is usually only seen when the dose administered is so low that just one immunodominant determinant is recognized by the immune system. In this way, reactions controlled by *Ir* genes are distinct from the overall responsiveness to a variety of complex antigens which is a feature of the Biozzi mice (above).

The Ir genes map to the H-2I region and control T–B cooperation

Table 11.3 gives some idea of the type of analysis used to map the *Ir* genes. The three high responder strains have individual *H-2* genes derived from prototypic pure strains which have been interbred to produce recombinations within the H-2 region. The only genes they have in common are A^k and D^b; since the B.10 strain bearing the D^b gene is a low responder, high response must be linked in this case to possession of A^k. The I region molecules must represent the *Ir* gene

product since a point mutation in the H-2A subregion in one strain led to a change in the class II molecule at a site affecting its polymorphic specificity and changed the mice from high to low responder status with respect to their thymus-dependent antibody response to antigen *in vivo*. The mutation also greatly reduced the proliferation of T-cells from immunized animals when challenged *in vitro* with antigen plus appropriate presenting cells, and there is a good correlation between antigen-specific T-cell proliferation and the responder status of the host. The implication that **responder status may be linked to the generation of Th cells** is amply borne out by adoptive transfer studies showing that irradiated ($H-2^b \times H-2^k$) F1 mice make good antibody responses to (T,G)-A–L when reconstituted with antigen-primed B-cells from another F1 plus T-cells from a primed $H-2^b$ (high responder); T-cells from the low responder $H-2^k$ mice only gave poor help for antibody responses. This also explains why these *H-2* gene effects are seen with thymus-dependent but not T-independent antigens.

Three mechanisms have been proposed to account for class II-linked high and low responsiveness.

1 *Defective presentation.* In a high responder, processing of antigen and its recognition by a corresponding T-cell lead to lymphocyte triggering and clonal expansion (figure 11.17a). Although there is (and has to be) considerable degeneracy in the specificity of the class II groove for peptide binding, variation in certain key residues can alter the strength of binding to a particular peptide (cf. p. 98) and convert a high to a low responder because the MHC fails to present antigen to the reactive T-cell (figure 11.17b). Sometimes the natural processing of an antigen in a given individual does not produce a peptide which fits well into their MHC molecules. One study showed that a cytotoxic T-cell clone restricted to HLA-A2, which recognized residues 58–68 of influenza A virus matrix protein, could cross-react with cells from an A69 subject pulsed with the same peptide; nonetheless, the clone failed to

Figure 11.17. Different mechanisms can account for low T-cell response to antigen in association with MHC class II.

recognize A69 cells *infected* with influenza A virus. Interestingly, individuals with the HLA-A69 class I MHC develop immunity to a different epitope on the same protein.

2 *Defective T-cell repertoire.* T-cells with moderate to high affinity for self-MHC molecules and their complexes with processed self-antigens will be rendered unresponsive (cf. tolerance induction, p. 229), so creating a 'hole' in the T-cell repertoire. If there is a cross-reaction, i.e. similarity in shape at the T-cell recognition level between a foreign antigen and a self-molecule which has already induced unresponsiveness, the host will lack T-cells specific for the foreign antigen and therefore be a low responder (figure 11.17c). To take a concrete example, mice of DBA/2 strain respond well to the synthetic peptide polyglutamyl, polytyrosine (GT), whereas BALB/c mice do not, although both have identical class II genes. BALB/c B-cell blasts express a structure which mimics GT and the presumption would be that self-tolerance makes these mice unresponsive to GT. This was confirmed by showing that DBA/2 mice made tolerant by a small number of BALB/c hematopoietic cells were changed from high to low responder status. To round off the story in a very satisfying way, DBA/2 mice injected with BALB/c B-blasts, induced by the polyclonal activator lipopolysaccharide, were found to be primed for GT.

3 *T-suppression.* We would like to refer again to the MHC-restricted low responsiveness which can occur to relatively complex antigens (see p. 205), since it illustrates the notion that low responder status can arise as an expression of CD8 T-suppressor activity (figure 11.17d). Low response can be dominant in class II heterozygotes, indicating that suppression can act against Th restricted to any other class II molecule. In this it differs from models 1 and 2 above where high response is dominant in a heterozygote because the factors associated with the low responder gene cannot influence the activity of the high responder. Overall, it seems likely that each of the three models may provide the basis for class II-linked *Ir* gene phenomena in different circumstances.

Factors influencing the genetic control of the immune response are summarized in figure 11.18.

REGULATORY IMMUNONEUROENDOCRINE NETWORKS

There is a danger, as one focuses more and more on the antics of the immune system, of looking at the body as a collection of myeloid and lymphoid cells roaming around in a big sack and of having no regard to the integrated physiology of the organism. Within the wider physiological context, attention has been drawn increasingly to interactions between immunological and neuroendocrine systems.

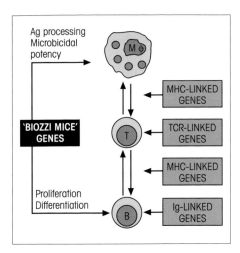

Figure 11.18. Genetic control of the immune response.

Figure 11.19. Enhancement of ACTH and corticosterone blood levels in C3H/HeJ mice 2 hours after injection of recombinant IL-1 (values are means ± SEM for groups of seven or eight mice). The significance of the mouse strain used is that it lacks receptors for bacterial lipopolysaccharide (LPS), and so the effects cannot be attributed to LPS contamination of the IL-1 preparation. (Reprinted from Besedovsky H., del Rey A., Sorkin E. & Dinarello C.A. (1986) *Science* 233, 652, with permission. Copyright © 1986 by the AAAS.)

Immunological cells have the receptors which enable them to receive signals from a whole range of hormones: corticosteroids, insulin, growth hormone, estradiol, testosterone, prolactin, β-adrenergic agents, acetylcholine, endorphins and enkephalins. By and large, glucocorticoids and androgens depress immune responses, whereas estrogens, growth hormone, thyroxine and insulin do the opposite.

A neuroendocrine feedback loop affecting immune responses

The secretion of **glucocorticoids** is a major response to stresses induced by a wide range of stimuli, such as extreme changes of temperature, fear, hunger and physical injury. They are also released as a consequence of immune responses and limit those responses in a neuroendocrine feedback loop. Thus, IL-1 (figure 11.19), IL-6 and TNF are capable of stimulating glucocorticoid synthesis and do so through the hypothalamic–pituitary–adrenal axis. This, in turn, leads to the downregulation of Th1 and macrophage activity, so completing the negative feedback circuit (figure 11.20). However, the glucocorticoid dexamethasone can prevent *a*ctivation-*i*nduced *c*ell *d*eath (AICD) in T-cells by inducing expression of GILZ (*g*lucocorticoid-*i*nduced *l*eucine zipper). The situation is therefore somewhat complex because glucocorticoids can themselves trigger apoptosis in T-cells, yet counteract apoptosis activated by peptide–MHC interaction with the TCR. In the absence of glucocorticoid, the activation of T-cells by peptide–MHC leads to a progressive loss of GILZ and eventual cell death by apoptosis. In contrast, if activation through the TCR occurs in the presence of glucocorticoids, then expression of GILZ is increased

and the cells are protected from AICD, perhaps via an effect on NFκB.

It has been shown that adrenalectomy prevents spontaneous recovery from *e*xperimental *a*llergic *e*ncephalomyelitis (EAE), a demyelinating disease with progressive paralysis produced by myelin basic protein in complete Freund's adjuvant which, however, can be blocked by implants of corticosterone. Spontaneous recovery from EAE in intact animals is associated with a dominance of Th2 autoantigen-specific clones, indicative of the view that glucocorticoids suppress Th1 and may augment Th2 cells. Individuals with a genetic predisposition to high levels of stress-induced glucocorticoids would be expected to have increased susceptibility to infections with intracellular pathogens such as *Mycobacterium leprae* which require effective Th1 cell-mediated immunity for their eradication.

Recent experiments have demonstrated that neonatal exposure to bacterial endotoxin (LPS) not only exerts a long-term influence on endocrine and central nervous system development, but substantially affects predisposition to inflammatory disease and therefore appears to program or 'reset' the functional development of both the endocrine and immune systems. Thus, in adult life, rats which had been exposed to endotoxin during the first week of life had higher basal levels of corticosterone compared with control ani-

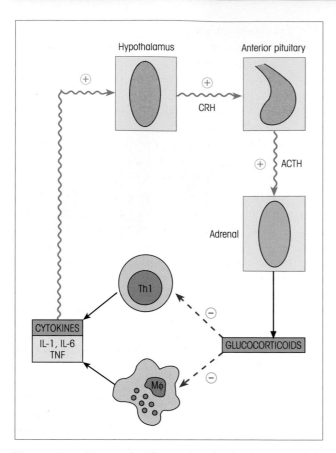

Figure 11.20. Glucocorticoid negative feedback on cytokine production. CRH, corticotropin-releasing hormone; ACTH, adrenocorticotropic hormone. Evidence for another type of circuit encompassing hormone receptor, hormone, anti-hormone and internal image anti-idiotype was presented in figure 11.11 and may be of relevance to the pathogenesis of autoimmune disorders directed against hormone receptors (see p. 422). More generally, cells of the immune system in both primary and secondary lymphoid organs can produce hormones and neuropeptides, while classical endocrine glands as well as neurons and glial cells can synthesize cytokines and appropriate receptors. Production of prolactin and its receptors by peripheral lymphoid cells and thymocytes is worthy of attention. Lymphocyte expression of the prolactin receptor is upregulated following activation and, in autoimmune disease, witness the beneficial effects of bromocriptine, an inhibitor of prolactin synthesis, in the NZB × W model of murine SLE (cf. p. 403).

mals, and showed a greater increase in corticosterone levels in response to noise stress and a more rapid rise in corticosterone levels following challenge with LPS.

Sex hormones come into the picture

Estrogen is said to be the major factor influencing the more active immune responses in females relative to males. They have higher serum Ig and secreted IgA levels, a higher antibody response to T-independent antigens, relative resistance to T-cell tolerance and greater resistance to infections. Females are also far more susceptible to autoimmune disease, an issue that will be discussed in greater depth in Chapter 19, but here let us note that oral contraceptives can induce flares of the autoimmune disorder systemic lupus erythematosus (SLE; see p. 425) and the mildly androgenic adrenal hormone, **dehydroepiandrosterone (DHEA)**, can significantly prolong the lifespan of (NZB×W) F1 females with the murine model of SLE. DHEA has positive effects on Th1 at the expense of Th2 cells and can clearly antagonize the inhibitory effects of cortisol on thymocytes and T-cell proliferation. As they say in the tabloids, watch this space.

'Psychoimmunology'

The thymus, spleen and lymph nodes are richly innervated by the sympathetic nervous system. The enzyme dopamine β-hydroxylase catalyses the conversion of dopamine to the catecholamine neurotransmitter norepinephrine which is released from sympathetic neurons in these tissues. Mice in which the gene for this enzyme has been deleted by homologous recombination exhibited enhanced susceptibility to infection with the intracellular pathogen *Mycobacterium tuberculosis* and impaired production of the Th1 cytokines IFNγ and TNF in response to the infection. Although these animals showed no obvious developmental defects in their immune system, impaired Th1 responses were also found following immunization of these mice with the hapten TNP coupled to KLH. These observations suggest that norepinephrine can play a role in determining the potency of the immune response.

Denervated skin shows greatly reduced leukocyte infiltration in response to local damage, implicating cutaneous neurons in the recruitment of leukocytes. Sympathetic nerves which innervate lymphatic vessels and lymph nodes are involved in regulating the flow of lymph and may participate in controlling the migration of β-adrenergic receptor-bearing dendritic cells from inflammatory sites to the local lymph nodes. Mast cells and nerves often have an intimate anatomical relationship and nerve growth factor causes mast cell degranulation. The gastrointestinal tract also has extensive innervation and a high number of immune effector cells. In this context, the ability of substance P to stimulate, and of somatostatin to inhibit, proliferation of Peyer's patch lymphocytes may prove to have more than a trivial significance. The pituitary hormone prolactin has also been brought to our attention by the experimental observation that inhibition of prolactin secretion by bromocriptine suppresses Th activity.

There seems to be an interaction between inflammation and nerve growth in regions of wound healing and repair. Mast cells are often abundant, IL-6 induces neurite growth and IL-1 enhances production of nerve growth factor in sciatic nerve explants. IL-1 also increases slow-wave sleep when introduced into the lateral ventricle of the brain, and both IL-1 and interferon produce pyrogenic effects through their action on the temperature-controlling center.

Although it is not clear just how these diverse neuroendocrine effects fit into the regulation of immune responses, at a more physiological level, stress and circadian rhythms modify the functioning of the immune system. Factors such as restraint, noise and exam anxiety have been observed to influence a number of immune functions including phagocytosis, lymphocyte proliferation, NK activity and IgA secretion. Amazingly, the delayed-type hypersensitivity Mantoux reaction in the skin can be modified by hypnosis. An elegant demonstration of nervous system control is provided by studies showing suppression of conventional immune responses and enhancement of NK cell activity by Pavlovian conditioning. In the classic Pavlovian paradigm, a stimulus such as food that unconditionally elicits a particular response, in this case salivation, is repeatedly paired with a neutral stimulus that does not elicit the same response. Eventually, the neutral stimulus becomes a conditional stimulus and will elicit salivation in the absence of food. Rats were given cyclophosphamide as a unconditional and saccharin as a conditional stimulus repeatedly; subsequently, there was a depressed antibody response when the animals were challenged with antigen together with just the conditional stimulus, saccharin. As more and more data accumulate, it is becoming clearer how immunoneuroendocrine networks could play a role in allergy and in autoimmune diseases such as rheumatoid arthritis, insulin-dependent diabetes mellitus and multiple sclerosis.

EFFECTS OF DIET, EXERCISE, TRAUMA AND AGE ON IMMUNITY

Malnutrition diminishes the effectiveness of the immune response

The greatly increased susceptibility of undernourished individuals to infection can be attributed to many factors: poor sanitation and personal hygiene, overcrowding and inadequate health education. But, in addition, there are gross effects of **protein-calorie malnutrition** on immunocompetence. The widespread atrophy of lymphoid tissues and the 50% reduction in circulating CD4 T-cells underlie **serious impairment of cell-mediated immunity**. Antibody responses may be intact but they are of lower affinity; phagocytosis of bacteria is relatively normal but the subsequent intracellular destruction is defective.

Deficiencies in pyridoxine, folic acid and vitamins A, C and E result in generally impaired immune responses. **Vitamin D is an important regulator**. It is produced not only by the UV-irradiated dermis, but also by activated macrophages, the hypercalcemia associated with sarcoidosis being attributable to production of the vitamin by macrophages in the active granulomas. The vitamin is a potent inhibitor of T-cell proliferation and of Th1 cytokine production. This generates a neat feedback loop at sites of inflammation where macrophages activated by IFNγ produce vitamin D which suppresses the T-cells making the interferon. It also downregulates antigen presentation by macrophages and promotes multinucleated giant cell formation in chronic granulomatous lesions. Nonetheless, as a further emphasis of the potential duality of the CD4 helper subsets, it promotes Th2 activity, especially at mucosal surfaces: quite a busy little vitamin. Zinc deficiency is rather interesting; this greatly affects the biological activity of thymus hormones and has a major effect on cell-mediated immunity, perhaps as a result. Iron deficiency impairs the oxidative burst in neutrophils since the flavocytochrome NADP oxidase is an iron-containing enzyme.

Of course there is another side to all this in that moderate restriction of total calorie intake and/or marked reduction in fat intake ameliorates age-related diseases such as autoimmunity. Oils with an *n*-3 double bond, such as fish oils, are also protective, perhaps due to increased synthesis of immunosuppressive prostaglandins.

Given the overdue sensitivity to the importance of environmental contamination, it is important to monitor the nature and levels of pollution that may influence immunity. Here is just one example: polyhalogenated organic compounds (such as polychlorinated biphenyls) steadily pervade the environment and, being stable and lipophilic, accumulate readily in the aquatic food chain where they largely resist metabolic breakdown. It was shown that Baltic herrings with relatively high levels of these pollutants, as compared with uncontaminated Atlantic herrings, were immunotoxic when fed to captive harbor seals, suggesting one reason why seals along the coasts of northwestern Europe succumbed so alarmingly to infection with the otherwise nonvirulent phocine distemper virus in 1988.

Other factors

Exercise, particularly severe exercise, induces stress and raises plasma levels of cortisol, catecholamines, IFNα, IL-1, β-endorphin and metenkephalin. It can lead to reduced IgA levels, immune deficiency and increased susceptibility to infection. Maniacal joggers and other such like masochists—you have been warned!

Multiple traumatic injury, surgery and major burns are also immunosuppressive and so contribute to the increased risk of sepsis. Corticosteroids produced by stressful conditions, the immunosuppressive prostaglandin E_2 released from damaged tissues and bacterial endotoxin derived from the disturbance of gut flora are all factors which influence the outcome after trauma.

Accepting that the problem of understanding the mechanisms of **aging** is a tough nut to crack, it is a trifle disappointing that the easier task of establishing the influence of age on immunological phenomena is still not satisfactorily accomplished. Perhaps the elderly population is skewed towards individuals with effective immune systems which give a survival advantage. Be that as it may, IL-2 production by peripheral blood lymphocytes (figure 11.21) and T-cell-mediated functions such as delayed-type hypersensitivity reactions to common skin test antigens decline with age and so, it is thought, does T-

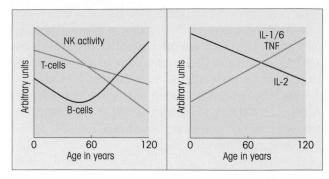

Figure 11.21. Age trends in some immunological parameters. (Based on Franceschi C., Monti D., Sansoni P. & Cossarizza A. (1995) *Immunology Today* **16**, 12.)

suppression, although this is a notoriously elusive function to measure.

Most B-cell responses to exogenous antigens are not dramatically changed with the passage of time, but one of the few well-founded observations concerns the relative increase in agalactosyl oligosaccharides on the Cγ2 domains of IgG (cf. p. 430) in parallel with a rise in IL-6 in the older age groups (figure 11.21). This is accompanied by a decrease in DHEA, and it may be significant that injection of the androgen into elderly mice leads to a fall in circulating IL-6 concentrations. Do these studies provide us with a clue to the increased prevalence of autoantibodies in our senior citizens?

SUMMARY

Control by antigen

• Immune responses are largely antigen driven. As the level of antigen falls, so does the intensity of the response.

• Antigens can compete with each other: a result of competition between processed peptides for the available MHC grooves.

Feedback control by complement and antibody

• Early IgM antibodies and C3d boost antibody responses, whereas IgG inhibits responses via the Fcγ receptor on B-cells.

T-cell regulation

• Activated T-cells express members of the TNF receptor family, including Fas, which act as death receptors and restrain unlimited clonal expansion by a process referred to as activation-induced cell death (AICD).

• At high levels of antigen, T-cells which suppress T-helpers emerge presumably as feedback control of excessive Th expansion.

• Suppressor and helper epitopes on the same molecule can be discrete.

• In some instances of suppression, the effectors are CD8 T-cells restricted either directly (which would be strange) or indirectly through a CD4 intermediary.

• Suppression may well be due to T–T interaction on the surface of antigen-presenting cells. Just as Th1 and Th2 cells mutually inhibit each other through production of their respective cytokines IFNγ and IL-4/10, so there may be two types of CD8 cells with suppressor activity: one of Tc2 type found in lepromatous leprosy patients making IL-4 and suppressing Th1 cells, and the other Tc1 cells making IFNγ capable of suppressing Th2 cells.

(continued)

Idiotype networks

• Antigen-specific receptors on lymphocytes can interact with the idiotypes on the receptors of other lymphocytes to form a network (Jerne).

• Anti-idiotypes can be induced by autologous idiotypes.

• An idiotype network involving mostly CD5 B-1 cells is evident in early life.

• T-cell idiotypic interactions can also be demonstrated.

• Preset idiotypic networks involve a number of lymphocytes with self-reactivity for dominant autoantigens. It is speculated that this preoccupation with self helps to regulate unwanted autoimmune reactions and may help to target the response to infectious agents on dominant conserved antigens like hsp65 which cross-react with self.

• Idiotypes which occur frequently and are shared by a multiplicity of antibodies (public or cross-reacting Id) are targets for regulation by anti-idiotypes in the network, thus providing a further mechanism for control of the immune response.

• The network offers the potential for therapeutic intervention to manipulate immunity.

Genetic factors influence the immune response

• Approximately 10 genes control the overall antibody response to complex antigens: some affect macrophage antigen processing and microbicidal activity and some the rate of proliferation of differentiating B-cells.

• Immunoglobulin and TCR genes are very adaptable because they rearrange to create the antigen receptors, but 'holes' in the repertoire can occur.

• Immune response genes are located in the MHC class II locus and control the interactions required for T–B collaboration.

• Class II-linked high and low responsiveness may be due to defective presentation by MHC, a defective T-cell repertoire caused by tolerance to MHC + self-peptides and T-suppression.

Immunoneuroendocrine networks

• Immunological, neurological and endocrinological systems interact, forming regulatory circuits.

• Feedback by cytokines augments the production of corticosteroids and is important because this shuts down Th1 and macrophage activity.

• Estrogens may be largely responsible for the more active immune responses in females relative to males. The male hormone, DHEA, prolongs life in females with the murine equivalent of the human autoimmune disease SLE.

Effects of diet and other factors on immunity

• Protein-calorie malnutrition grossly impairs cell-mediated immunity and phagocyte microbicidal potency.

• Exercise, trauma, age and environmental pollution can all act to impair immune mechanisms. The pattern of cytokines produced by peripheral blood cells changes with age, IL-2 decreasing and TNF, IL-1 and IL-6 increasing; the latter is associated with a lowered DHEA level.

Factors influencing the bias between Th1 and Th2 subsets

• These have figured with some prominence in this chapter and a summary of some of the major influences on the balance between Th1 and Th2 responses is presented in figure 11.22.

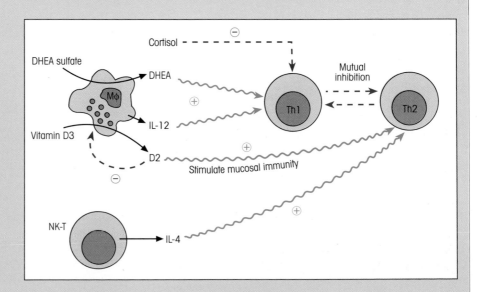

Figure 11.22. Summary of major factors affecting Th1/Th2 balance. Preferential stimulation of mucosal antibody synthesis by vitamin D involves the promotion of dendritic cell migration to the Peyer's patches. By downregulating macrophage activity, Th1 effectiveness is decreased. Cortisol and dehydroepiandrosterone (DHEA) are products of the adrenal and have opposing effects on the Th1 subset. A relative deficiency of DHEA will lead to poor Th1 performance. NK-T cells bear an αβ TCR, the natural killer cell marker NK1.1, and secrete cytokines including IL-4 which stimulate Th2 cells.

FURTHER READING

Chandra R.K. (1998) Nutrition and the immune system. In Delves P.J. & Roitt I.M. (eds) *Encyclopedia of Immunology*, 2nd edn, p. 1869. Academic Press, London. (See also other relevant articles in the *Encyclopedia*: 'Aging and the immune system', p. 59; 'Behavioral regulation of immunity', p. 336; 'Neuroendocrine regulation of immunity', p. 1824; 'Sex hormones and immunity', p. 2175; 'Stress and the immune system', p. 2220; 'Vitamin D', p. 2494.)

Cohen I.R. (2000) *Tending Adam's Garden*. Academic Press, London.

Crowley M.P. *et al.* (2000) A population of murine γδ T cells that recognize an inducible MHC class Ib molecule. *Science* **287**, 314.

Fearon D.T. & Carroll M.C. (2000) Regulation of B lymphocyte responses to foreign and self-antigens by the CD19/CD21 complex. *Annual Reviews of Immunology* **18**, 393.

Krammer P.H. (2000) CD95's deadly mission in the immune system. *Nature* **407**, 789.

Shanks N. *et al.* (2000) Early life exposure to endotoxin alters hypothalamic–pituitary–adrenal function and predisposition to inflammation. *Proceedings of the National Academy of Sciences of the United States of America* **97**, 5645.

Ontogeny and phylogeny

INTRODUCTION

Hematopoiesis originates in the early yolk sac but, as embryogenesis proceeds, this function is taken over by the fetal liver and finally by the bone marrow where it continues throughout life. The **hematopoietic stem cell which gives rise to the formed elements of the blood** (figure 12.1) can be shown to be multipotent, to seed other organs and to have a relatively unlimited capacity to renew itself through the creation of further stem cells. Thus an animal can be completely protected against the lethal effects of high doses of irradiation by injection of bone marrow cells which will repopulate its lymphoid and myeloid systems. The capacity for self-renewal is not absolute and declines with age in parallel with a shortening of the telomeres and a reduction in telomerase, the enzyme which repairs the shortening of the ends of chromosomes which would otherwise occur at every round of cell division.

HEMATOPOIETIC STEM CELLS

We have come a long way towards the goal of isolating highly purified populations of hematopoietic stem cells, although not all agree that we have yet achieved it. In the mouse, the most likely candidate, at least a *very* early progenitor, is the cell with the following surface phenotype: high expression of MHC, low positivity for Thy-1, clearly positive for Sca-1, AA4.1 and c-kit, and for the adhesion molecule PGP-1, negative or only weakly positive for Lin, and negative for B220, Mac-1, Gr-1 and CD8 (the last four being markers for B-cells, macrophages, granulocytes and cytotoxic T-cells, respectively). Impressively, less than 100 of such cells can prevent death in a lethally irradiated animal. Recently, a 'molecular phenotype' of the mouse stem cell has been obtained by analysis of subtracted cDNA libraries from highly purified fetal liver stem cells. It was revealed that there is a very high degree of precision in the control of transcription at each stage of the hematopoietic hierarchy. Certain molecules are more predominant in either fetal or adult hematopoietic

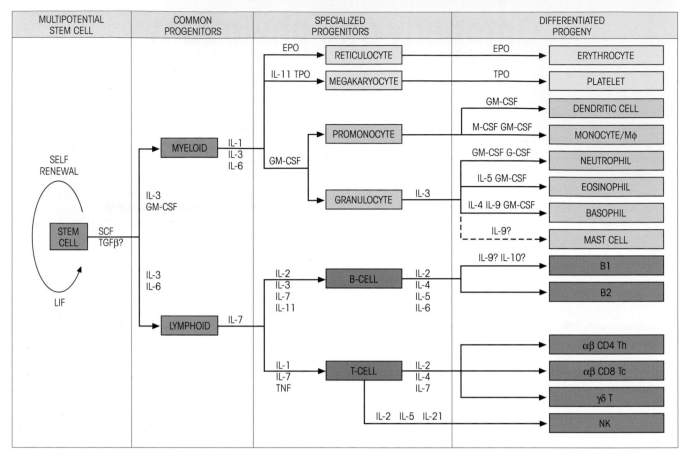

Figure 12.1. The multipotential hematopoietic stem cell and its progeny which differentiate under the influence of a series of soluble growth factors within the microenvironment of the bone marrow. The expression of various nuclear transcription factors directs the differentiation process. For example, the *Ikaros* gene encodes a zinc-fingered transcription factor critical for driving the development of a common myeloid/lymphoid precursor into a lymphoid-restricted progenitor giving rise to T-, B- and NK cells. SCF, stem cell factor; LIF, leukemia inhibitory factor; IL-3, interleukin-3, often termed the multi-CSF because it stimulates progenitors of platelets, erythrocytes, all the types of myeloid cells, and also the progenitors of B-, but not T-, cells; GM-CSF, granulocyte–macrophage colony-stimulating factor, so-called because it promotes the formation of mixed colonies of these two cell types from bone marrow progenitors either in tissue culture or on transfer to an irradiated recipient where they appear in the spleen; G-CSF, granulocyte colony-stimulating factor; M-CSF, monocyte colony-stimulating factor; EPO , erythropoietin; TPO, thrombopoietin; TNF, tumor necrosis factor; TGFβ, transforming growth factor β.

stem cells, and evidence was obtained to support an important role for TGFβ in the control of hematopoiesis. Similarly, the expression of Notch-1, our old friend NFκB and the wonderfully named Manic Fringe and Dishevelled-1 genes underscores the importance of the Notch signaling pathway in hematopoietic development. Finally, a large number of genes for cell adhesion molecules were present in the cDNA libraries, including several that implicate members of the semaphorin family in stem cell homing. In the human, CD34 is a marker of an extremely early cell but, again, there is some debate as to whether this identifies the holy pluripotent stem cell itself.

The stem cells differentiate within the microenvironment of sessile stromal cells which produce various growth factors such as IL-3, -4, -6 and -7, GM-CSF, and

so on. The importance of this interaction between undifferentiated stem cells and the microenvironment which guides their differentiation is clearly shown by studies on mice homozygous for mutations at the *w* or the *sl* loci which, amongst other defects, have severe macrocytic anemia. Bone marrow stromal cells produce stem cell factor (SCF) which remains associated with the extracellular matrix and acts on primitive stem cells through a tyrosine kinase membrane receptor, c-kit (CD117). *sl/sl* mutants have normal stem cells but defective stromal production of SCF which can be corrected by transplantation of a normal spleen fragment; *w/w* mutant myeloid progenitors lack the c-kit surface receptor for SCF, and so can be restored by injection of normal bone marrow cells (figure 12.2).

Mice with *s*evere *c*ombined *i*mmuno*d*eficiency (SCID) provide a happy environment for fragments of

	Restoration of hematopoiesis in mutant mice by normal grafts					MYELOID STEM CELLS		MICRO-ENVIRONMENT
		BONE MARROW		SPLEEN FRAGMENT				
NORMAL DONOR GRAFT	–		–		NORMAL	●	sl/sl	w/w
ANEMIC MUTANT RECIPIENT	w/w	w/w	sl/sl	sl/sl	DEFECTIVE	●	w/w	sl/sl
HEMATOPOIESIS	–	++	–	++				

Figure 12.2. Hematopoiesis requires normal bone marrow stem cells differentiating in a normal microenvironment. The *w* locus codes for c-kit, a stem cell tyrosine kinase membrane receptor for the stem cell factor (SCF) encoded by the *sl* locus. Mice which are homozygous for mutant alleles at these loci develop severe macrocytic anemia which can be corrected by transplantation of appropriate normal cells. The experiments show that the *w/w* mutant lacks normal stem cells and the *sl/sl* mutant lacks the environmental factor needed for their development.

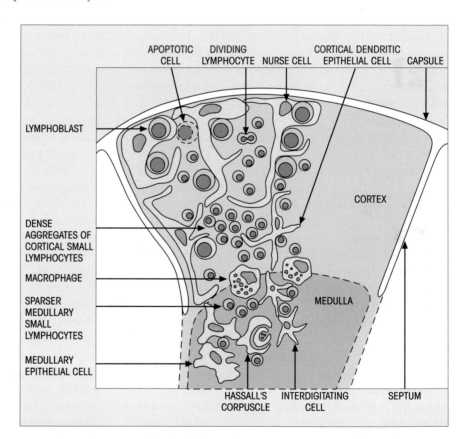

Figure 12.3. Cellular features of a thymus lobule. See text for description. (Adapted from Hood L.E., Weissman I.L., Wood W.B. & Wilson J.H. (1984) *Immunology*, 2nd edn, p. 261. Benjamin Cummings, California.)

human fetal liver and thymus which, if implanted contiguously, will produce formed elements of the blood for 6–12 months. Fetal liver provides a source of hematopoietic stem cells; but what is the role of the thymus?

THE THYMUS PROVIDES THE ENVIRONMENT FOR T-CELL DIFFERENTIATION

The thymus is organized into a series of lobules based upon meshworks of epithelial cells derived embryologically from an outpushing of the gut endoderm of the third pharyngeal pouch and which form well-defined cortical and medullary zones (figure 12.3). This framework of epithelial cells provides the microenvironment for T-cell differentiation. There are subtle interactions between the extracellular matrix proteins and a variety of integrins on different lymphocyte subpopulations produced by differential splicing and post-translational glycosylation; current musings are that the expression of these integrins, together with chemokine and chemokine receptor expression (cf. table 10.3), plays a role in the homing of progenitors to, and their subsequent migration within, the thymus. In addition, the epithelial cells produce a series of peptide hormones which mostly seem capable of promoting the appearance of T-cell differentiation markers and a variety of T-cell functions on culture with bone marrow cells *in vitro*. Several have been well characterized and sequenced, including thymulin, thymosin α_1, thymic *humoral factor* (THF) and thymopoietin (and its active pentapeptide thymopontin, TP-5). Of these, only thymulin is of exclusively thymic origin. This zinc-dependent nonapeptide tends to normalize the balance of immune responses: it restores antibody avidity and antibody production in aged mice and yet stimulates suppressor activity in animals with autoimmune hemolytic anemia induced by cross-reactive rat red cells (cf. p. 416). Thymulin may be looked upon as a true hormone, secreted by the thymus in a regulated fashion and acting at a distance from the thymus as a fine physiological immunoregulator contributing to the maintenance of T-cell subset homeostasis.

Specialized large epithelial cells in the outer cortex, known as 'nurse' cells, are associated with large numbers of lymphocytes which lie within pockets produced by the long membrane extensions of these epithelial cells. The epithelial cells of the deep cortex have branched dendritic processes, rich in class II MHC, and connect through desmosome cell junctions to form a network through which cortical lymphocytes must pass on their way to the medulla (figure 12.3). The cortical lymphocytes are densely packed compared with those in the medulla, many are in division and large numbers of them are undergoing apoptosis. On their way to the medulla, the lymphocytes pass a cordon of 'sentinel' macrophages at the corticomedullary junction. A number of bone marrow-derived interdigitating dendritic cells are present in the medulla and the epithelial cells have broader processes than their cortical counterparts and express high levels of both class I and class II MHC. Whorled keratinized epithelial cells in the medulla form the highly characteristic Hassall's corpuscles beloved of histopathology examiners. These structures may serve as a disposal system for dying thymocytes and are the only location where apoptotic cells are found in the medulla. The presence of HLA-DO and HLA-DM, molecules which mediate intracellular peptide exchange, in the epithelial cells which ring the Hassall's corpuscles suggest that they may also play a role in activation and/or tolerance of mature thymocytes, particularly given that these epithelial cells also express the peptide-presenting HLA-DR molecule.

A fairly complex relationship with the nervous system awaits discovery; the thymus is richly innervated with both adrenergic and cholinergic fibers, while the neurotransmitters oxytocin, vasopressin and neurophysin are synthesized endogenously by subcapsular, perivascular and medullary epithelial cells and nurse cells. Acute stress leads to an indecently rapid loss of cortical thymocytes and an increase in epithelial cells expressing both cortical and medullary markers—surely intrathymic epithelial stem cells? The destruction of cortical thymocytes is at least partly due to the cytolytic action of steroids, the relative invulnerability of the medullary lymphocytes being attributable to their possession of a 20α-hydroxyl steroid dehydrogenase. The distinctive nature of the two main compartments in the gland is emphasized by the selective atrophy induced by a number of agents; thus the primary target of organotin is the immature cortical thymocyte. Dioxin interacts with a receptor on cortical epithelial cells, while the immunosuppressive drug cyclosporin A causes atrophy of all the medullary elements, thereby blocking differentiation of cortical to medullary thymocytes.

In the human, thymic involution commences within the first 12 months of life, reducing by around 3% a year to middle age and by 1% thereafter. The size of the organ gives no clue to these changes because there is replacement by adipose tissue. In a sense, the thymus is progressively disposable because, as we shall see, it establishes a long-lasting peripheral T-cell pool which enables the host to withstand loss of the gland without catastrophic failure of immunological function, witness the minimal effects of thymectomy in the adult compared with the **dramatic influence in the neonate** (Milestone 12.1). Nevertheless, the adult thymus retains a residue of corticomedullary tissue containing a normal range of thymocyte subsets with a broad spectrum of TCR gene rearrangements. Adult patients receiving either T-cell-depleted bone marrow or peripheral blood hematopoietic stem cells following ablative therapy are able to generate new naive T-cells at a rate that is inversely related to the age of the individual. These observations establish that new T-cells can be generated in adult life, either in the thymus or in the still mysterious 'extrathymic' sites that have been proposed as additional locations for T-cell differentiation.

Bone marrow stem cells become immunocompetent T-cells in the thymus

The evidence for this comes from experiments on the reconstitution of irradiated hosts. An irradiated animal is restored by bone marrow grafts through the

Milestone 12.1 — The Immunological Function of the Thymus

Ludwig Gross had found that a form of mouse leukemia could be induced in low-leukemia strains by inoculating filtered leukemic tissue from high-leukemia strains provided that this was done in the immediate neonatal period. Since the thymus was known to be involved in the leukemic process, Jacques Miller decided to test the hypothesis that the Gross virus could only multiply in the neonatal thymus by infecting neonatally thymectomized mice of low-leukemia strains. The results were consistent with this hypothesis but, strangely, animals of one strain died of a wasting disease which Miller deduced could have been due to susceptibility to infection, since fewer mice died when they were moved from the converted horse stables which served as an animal house to 'cleaner' quarters.

Autopsy showed the animals to have atrophied lymphoid tissue and low blood lymphocyte levels, and Miller therefore decided to test their immunocompetence before the onset of wasting disease. To his astonishment, skin grafts, even from rats (figure M12.1.1) as well as from other mouse strains, were fully accepted. These phenomena were not induced by thymectomy later in life and, in writing up his preliminary results in 1961 (Miller J.F.A.P., *Lancet* ii, 748), Miller opined that 'during embryogenesis the thymus would produce the originators of immunologically competent cells, many of which would have migrated to other sites at about the time of birth'. All in all a superb example of the scientific method and its application by a top-flight scientist.

Figure M12.1.1. Acceptance of a rat skin graft by a mouse which had been neonatally thymectomized.

---

immediate restitution of granulocyte precursors; in the longer term, also through reconstitution of the T- and B-cells destroyed by irradiation. However, if the animal is thymectomized before irradiation, bone marrow cells will not reconstitute the T-lymphocyte population (cf. figure 7.13).

By day 11–12 in the mouse embryo, lymphoblastoid stem cells from the bone marrow begin to colonize the periphery of the epithelial thymus rudiment. If the thymus is removed at this stage and incubated in organ culture, a whole variety of mature T-lymphocytes will be generated. This is not seen if 10-day thymuses are cultured and shows that the lymphoblastoid colonizers give rise to the immunocompetent small lymphocyte progeny.

T-CELL ONTOGENY

Differentiation is accompanied by changes in surface markers

The incoming thymic lymphoid progenitors express a number of chemokine receptors and are attracted to the thymus by one or more of the numerous chemokines secreted by the thymic stromal cells—which are the critical ones is yet to be established. These progenitors express CD34 and the enzyme *ter*minal *d*eoxynucleotidyl *t*ransferase (TdT) (figure 12.4), which is involved in the insertion of nucleotide sequences at the N-terminal region of D and J variable region segments to increase diversity of the T-cell receptors (TCRs) (cf. p. 65). They also express high levels of the adhesion molecule CD44 and the stem cell factor receptor (c-kit, CD117) (p. 222), but their lack of both CD4 and CD8 designates them as **double-negative** thymocytes. They express high levels of Notch molecules. These cell surface proteins provide signals at several key points during thymocyte differentiation. Indeed, they are thought to be necessary for commitment to the T-cell lineage, T-cell development being severely impaired in $Notch^{-/-}$ knockout mice. Under the influence of IL-1 and TNF, the progenitors differentiate into prothymocytes, committed to the T-lineage, and these now undergo IL-7-mediated proliferation to form a population of $CD44^{-}$ $CD117^{-}$ pre-T-cells. At this stage, the cells begin to express various TCR chains and are then expanded, ultimately synthesizing CD3, the invariant signal transducing complex of the TCR, and becoming **double positive** for CD4+, CD8+, the markers of the helper and cytotoxic subsets respectively. Finally, again under the guiding hand of chemokines, the cells traverse the corticomedullary junction to the medulla as the CD4 and CD8 markers segregate in parallel with differentiation into separate

immunocompetent populations of **single-positive CD4+ T-helpers** and **CD8+ cytotoxic T-cell precursors** (figure 12.4). Notch-1 signaling is involved in the maturation of both of these subsets, with the Notch-1 ligands Jagged-1, Jagged-2 and δ-like-1 being expressed on thymic epithelial cells in a highly regulated way. The γδ cells remain double negative, i.e. CD4−8−, except for a small subset which express CD8.

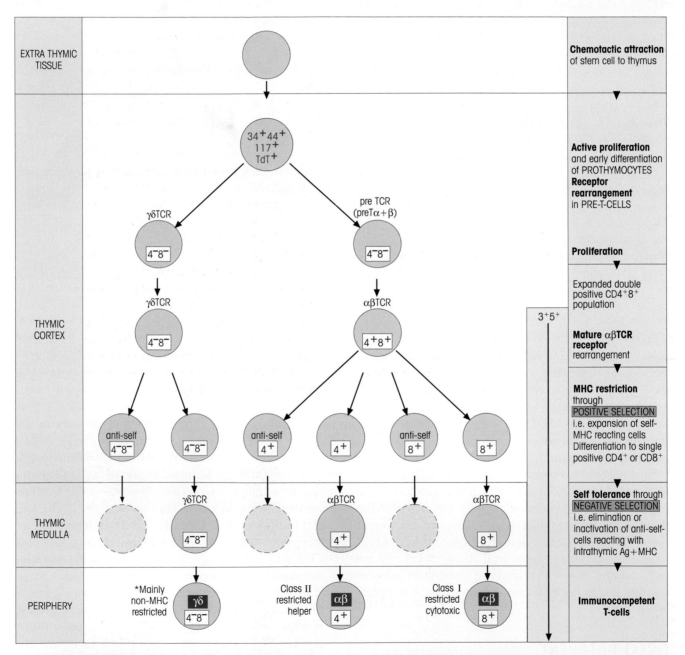

Figure 12.4. Differentiation of T-cells within the thymus. Numbers refer to CD designation. TdT, terminal deoxynucleotidyl transferase. Negatively selected cells in gray. The diagram is partly simplified for the sake of clarity. Autoreactive cells with specificity for self-antigens not expressed in the thymus may be tolerized by extrathymic peripheral contact with antigen (dashed circles). *γδ cells

mainly appear to recognize antigen directly, in a manner analogous to the antibody molecule on B-cells, although some may be restricted by nonclassical MHC class Ib or by classical MHC class II. The relatively primitive NK-T cells bearing an αβ TCR and the NK1.1 marker (cf. p. 102) are often restricted by CD1, although some are restricted by classical MHC molecules.

The factors which determine whether the double-positive cells become CD4 or CD8 cells in the thymus are still not fully established. Two major scenarios have been put forward. The **stochastic** hypothesis suggests that expression of either CD4 or CD8 is randomly switched off, whereas the **instructive** hypothesis declares that interaction of the TCR with MHC–peptide results in signals which instruct the T-cells to become either CD4$^+$ class II-restricted cells or CD8$^+$ class I-restricted cells. The weight of the evidence currently available would seem to support the instructive model, whilst not entirely excluding the possibility of a contribution from stochastic events. Thus it appears that the strength of the p56^{lck} signal (see p. 166) correlates with lineage choice and is determined by the duration of TCR engagement during the double-positive stage of thymocyte differentiation, a stronger cumulative signal favoring the generation of CD4 cells (figure 12.5).

Receptor rearrangement

The rearrangement of *V-*, *D-* and *J*-region genes required to generate the TCR (see p. 62) has not yet taken place at the prothymocyte stage. The gene for TdT and the recombinase activator genes, *RAG-1* and *RAG-2*, are transcribed at the pre-T stage and, by day 15, cells with the γδ TCR can be detected in the mouse thymus followed soon by the appearance of a '**pre-TCR**' version of the αβ TCR. Notch-1 signals (again!) appear to play a role in αβ versus γδ lineage commitment, although the details are still being worked out.

The development of αβ receptors

The *Vβ* is first rearranged in the double-negative CD4$^-$8$^-$ cells and associates with an invariant pre-α chain, pTα, to form a single 'pre-TCR' (figure 12.4). Although the pre-TCR mediates feedback inhibition on further TCR *Vβ* gene rearrangement, the extracellular domain of the pTα is not required for this inhibition, suggesting that there may not be an extracellular ligand for pTα, as had previously been assumed. A cysteine just inside the membrane on the cytoplasmic tail becomes palmitoylated and it may be this process that recruits pTα into lipid rafts containing the p56^{lck} signaling molecule. The pre-T-cells undergo a frenetic burst of proliferation controlled by thymic epithelial cells and fibroblasts, producing double-positive CD4$^+$8$^+$ cells. Further development requires rearrangement of the *Vα* gene segments so allowing formation of the mature αβ TCR. The cells are now ready for subsequent bouts of positive and negative receptor editing as will be discussed shortly.

Rearrangement of the *Vβ* genes on the sister chromatid is suppressed following the expression of the pre-TCR (remember each cell contains two chromosomes for each α and β cluster). Thus each cell only expresses a single TCR β chain and the process by which the homologous genes on the sister chromatid are suppressed is called **allelic exclusion** (cf. p. 240). The α chains appear not to always be allelically excluded, so that some T-cells may have two antigen-specific receptors, each with their own α chain but sharing a common β chain. It is not clear, however, whether both receptors can be functional.

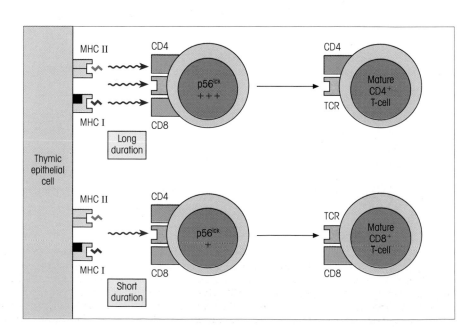

Figure 12.5. CD4 versus CD8 lineage commitment. In this model, the duration of signaling through the TCR and coreceptors on the double-positive (CD4$^+$8$^+$) thymocyte determines the intensity of the p56^{lck} signal, which in turn instructs the thymocyte to become either a CD4 T-cell if there are sustained p56^{lck} signals or a CD8 T-cell if the signals are less intense.

The development of γδ receptors

Unlike the αβ TCR, the γδ TCR in many cases seems to be able to bind directly to antigen without the necessity for antigen presentation by MHC or MHC-like molecules, i.e. it recognizes antigen directly in a manner similar to antibody. The γδ lineage does not produce a 'pre-receptor' and mice expressing rearranged γ and δ transgenes do not rearrange any further γ or δ gene segments, indicating allelic exclusion of sister chromatid genes.

γδ T-cells in the mouse, unlike the human, predominate in association with epithelial cells. A curious feature of the cells leaving the fetal thymus is the restriction in *V* gene utilization. Thus virtually all of the first wave of fetal γδ cells express the *Vγ5* gene and colonize the skin; the second wave use the same *δ* gene combination, but a different γ *V–J* pair utilizing *Vγ6*, and they seed the uterus in the female. In adult life, there is far more receptor diversity due to a high degree of junctional variation (cf. p. 65), although the intraepithelial cells in the intestine (*Vγ4*) and those in encapsulated lymphoid tissue (*Vγ4*, *Vγ1*, *Vγ2*) are again restricted with respect to *V* gene usage.

The Vγ set in the skin readily proliferates and secretes IL-2 on exposure to heat-shocked keratinocytes, implying a role in the surveillance of trauma signals. The Vγ4 cells in peripheral lymphoid tissue respond well to the tuberculosis antigen PPD ('purified protein derivative') and to conserved residues 180–196 from mycobacterial and self-heat-shock protein hsp65. However, evidence from γδ TCR knockout mice suggests that overall, in the adult, γδ T-cells may make a minor contribution to pathogen-specific protection. It has therefore been proposed that their primary role may be in the regulation of αβ T-cells, with most γδ T-cells biased towards a Th1 cytokine secretion pattern.

Two major γδ subsets predominate in the human, Vγ9,Vδ2 and Vγ1,Vδ2. The Vγ9 set rises from 25% of the total γδ cells in cord blood to around 70% in adult blood; at the same time, the proportion of Vγ1 falls from 50% to less than 30%. The majority of the Vγ9 set have the activated memory phenotype CD45RO, probably as a result of stimulation by common ligands for the Vγ9,Vδ2 TCR, such as components of mycobacteria, *Plasmodium falciparum* and the superantigen staphylococcal enterotoxin A. Vγ9 subsets of extremely limited junctional diversity were observed in the blood and bronchoalveolar lavage of two patients with sarcoidosis, a granulomatous disease with mycobacterial involvement. The conclusion that these two major γδ subpopulations are selected by powerful antigens seems inescapable.

Cells are positively selected for self-MHC restriction in the thymus

The ability of T-cells to recognize antigenic peptides in association with self-MHC is developed in the thymus. If an (H-2^k × H-2^b) F1 animal is sensitized to an antigen, the primed T-cells can recognize that antigen on presenting cells of either *H-2^k* or *H-2^b* haplotype, i.e. they can use either parental haplotype as a recognition restriction element. However, if bone marrow cells from the (H-2^k × H-2^b) F1 are used to reconstitute an irradiated F1 which had earlier been thymectomized and given an H-2^k thymus, the subsequently primed T-cells can only recognize antigens in the context of H-2^k, not of H-2^b (figure 12.6). Thus it is **the phenotype of the**

Thymectomize *b* × *k* mice	Graft with thymus of haplotype	Irradiate and reconstitute with *b* × *k* bone marrow	Prime with KLH	Proliferative response of primed T-cells to KLH on antigen-presenting cells of haplotype	
				H-2^b	H-2^k
	b × *k*	⟶		+ +	+ +
	b	⟶		+ +	−
	dGuo-treated *b*	⟶		+ +	−
	k	⟶		−	+ +
	dGuo-treated *k*	⟶		−	+ +

Figure 12.6. Imprinting of H-2 T-helper restriction by the haplotype of the thymus. Host mice were F1 crosses between strains of haplotype *H-2^b* and *H-2^k*. They were thymectomized and grafted with 14-day fetal thymuses, irradiated and reconstituted with F1 bone marrow. After priming with the antigen keyhole limpet hemocyanin (KLH), the proliferative response of lymph node T-cells to KLH on antigen-presenting cells of each parental haplotype was assessed. In some experiments, the thymus lobes were cultured in deoxyguanosine (dGuo), which destroys intrathymic cells of macrophage/dendritic cell lineage, but this had no effect on positive selection. (From Lo D. & Sprent J. (1986) *Nature* **319**, 672.)

thymus that imprints H-2 restriction on the differentiating T-cells.

It will also be seen in figure 12.6 that incubation of the thymus graft with deoxyguanosine, which destroys the cells of macrophage and dendritic cell lineage, has no effect on imprinting, suggesting that this function is carried out by epithelial cells. Confirmation of this comes from a study showing that lethally irradiated H-2^k mice, reconstituted with (b×k) F1 bone marrow and then injected intrathymically with an H-2^b thymic epithelial cell line, developed T-cells restricted by the b haplotype. The epithelial cells are rich in surface MHC molecules and the current view is that double-positive (CD4$^+$8$^+$) T-cells bearing receptors which recognize self-MHC on the epithelial cells are positively selected for differentiation to CD4$^+$8$^-$ or CD4$^-$8$^+$ single-positive cells. The evidence for this comes largely from studies in transgenic mice. Since this is a very active area, we would like to cite some experimental examples; nonprofessionals may need to hang on to their haplotypes, put on their ice-packs and concentrate.

One highly sophisticated study starts with a cytotoxic T-cell clone raised in H-2^b females against male cells of the same strain. The clone recognizes the male antigen, H-Y, and this is seen in association with the H-2D^b self-MHC molecules, i.e. it reacts with the H-2^b/Y complex. The α and β chains for the T-cell receptor of this clone are now introduced as transgenes into SCID mice which lack the ability to rearrange their own germ-line variable region receptor genes; thus the only TCR which could possibly be expressed is that encoded by the transgenes, provided of course that we are looking at females rather than males, in whom the clone would be eliminated by self-reactivity. If the transgenic SCID females bear the original H-2^b haplotype (e.g. F1 hybrids between b×d haplotypes), then the anti-H-2^b/Y receptor is amply expressed on CD8$^+$ cytotoxic precursor cells (table 12.1a), whereas H-2^d transgenics lacking H-2^b produce only double CD4$^+$8$^+$ thymocytes with no single CD4$^+$8$^-$ or CD4$^-$8$^+$ cells. Thus, as CD4$^+$8$^+$ cells express their TCR transgene, they only differentiate into CD8$^+$ immunocompetent cells if they come into contact with thymic epithelial cells of the MHC haplotype recognized by their receptor. We say that such self-recognizing thymocytes are being **positively selected**. Positive intracellular events accompany the positive selection process since the protein tyrosine kinases fyn and lck are activated in double-positive CD4$^+$8$^+$ thymocytes maturing to single-positive CD8$^+$ cells in the b haplotype background, but are low in cells which fail to differentiate into mature cells in the nonselective d haplotype.

Table 12.1. Positive and negative selection in SCID transgenic mice bearing the αβ receptors of an H-2D^b T-cell clone cytotoxic for the male antigen H-Y, i.e. the clone is of *H-2^b* haplotype and is female anti-male. (a) The only T-cells are those bearing the already rearranged transgenic TCR, since SCID mice cannot rearrange their own *V* genes. The clones are only expanded beyond the CD4$^+$8$^+$ stage when positively selected by contact with the MHC haplotype (*H-2^b*) recognized by the original clone from which the transgene was derived. Also, since the TCR recognized class I, only CD8$^+$ cells were selected. (b) When the anti-male transgenic clone is expressed on intrathymic T-cells in a male environment, the strong engagement of the TCR with male antigen-bearing cells eliminates them. (Based on data from von Boehmer H. *et al.* (1989) In Melchers F. *et al.* (eds) *Progress in Immunology* **7**, p. 297. Springer-Verlag, Berlin.)

Phenotype of thymocytes	a Positive selection		b Negative selection	
	Haplotype of transgenic females		Transgenic H-2^b mice	
	H-2$^{b/d}$	H-2$^{d/d}$	Males	Females
CD4$^-$8$^-$ TCR$^-$	+	++	+++	+
CD4$^+$8$^+$ TCR$^\pm$	++	+	−	+++
CD4$^-$8$^+$ TCR^{++}	+	−	−	+
CD4$^+$8$^-$ TCR^{++}	−	−	−	−

+, crude measure of the relative numbers of T-cells in the thymus having the phenotype indicated.

In another example, genes encoding an αβ receptor from a T-helper clone (2B4), which responds to moth cytochrome c in association with the class II molecule H-2Eα^k,β^b (remember H-2E has an α and β chain), are transfected into H-2^k and H-2^b mice. For irrelevant reasons, H-2^k mice express the H-2E molecule on the surface of their antigen-presenting cells, but H-2^b do not. In the event, the frequency of circulating CD4$^+$ T-cells bearing the 2B4 receptor was 10 times greater in the H-2^k relative to H-2^b strains, again speaking for positive selection of double-positive thymocytes which recognize their own thymic MHC. In a further twist to the story, positive selection only occurred in mice manipulated to express H-2E on their cortical rather than their medullary epithelial cells, showing that this differentiation step is effected before the developing thymocytes reach the medulla. ('Read it again Sam' as Humphrey Bogart might have said!)

T-CELL TOLERANCE

The induction of immunological tolerance is necessary to avoid self-reactivity

In essence, lymphocytes recognize foreign antigens through complementarity of shape mediated by the intermolecular forces we have described previously (see p. 85). To a large extent the building blocks used to form microbial and host molecules are the same, and so it is the assembled shapes of *self* and *nonself* mole-

Milestone 12.2—The Discovery of Immunological Tolerance

Over 40 years ago, Owen made the intriguing observation that nonidentical (dizygotic) twin cattle, which shared the same placental circulation and whose circulations were thereby linked, grew up with appreciable numbers of red cells from the other twin in their blood; if they had not shared the same circulation at birth, red cells from the twin injected in adult life would have been rapidly eliminated by an immunological response. From this finding, Burnet and Fenner conceived the notion that potential antigens which reach the lymphoid cells during their developing immunologically immature phase can in some way specifically suppress any future response to that antigen when the animal reaches immunological maturity. This, they considered, would provide a means whereby unresponsiveness to the body's own constituents could be established and thereby enable the lymphoid cells to make the important distinction between 'self' and 'nonself'. On this basis, any foreign cells introduced into the body during immunological development should trick the animal into treating them as 'self'-components in later life, and the studies of Medawar and his colleagues have shown that **immunological tolerance**, or unresponsiveness, can be artificially induced in this way. Thus neonatal injection of CBA mouse cells into newborn A strain animals suppresses their ability to reject a CBA graft immunologically in adult life (figure M12.2.1). Tolerance can also be induced with soluble antigens; for example, rabbits injected with bovine serum albumin without adjuvant at birth fail to make antibodies on later challenge with this protein.

Persistence of antigen is required to maintain tolerance. In Medawar's experiments, the tolerant state was long lived because the injected CBA cells survived and the animals continued to be chimeric (i.e. they possessed both A and CBA cells). With nonliving antigens, such as soluble bovine serum albumin, tolerance is gradually lost; the most likely explanation is that, in the absence of antigen, newly recruited immunocompetent cells which are being generated throughout life are not being rendered tolerant. Since recruitment of newly competent T-lymphocytes is drastically curtailed by removal of the thymus, it is of interest to note that the tolerant state persists for much longer in thymectomized animals.

The vital importance of the experiments by Medawar and his team was their demonstration that a state of immunological tolerance can result from exposure to an antigen. Recent studies, however, suggest that the concept of a *neonatal window* for tolerance induction is more apparent than real and stems from the relatively low number of peripheralized immunocompetent T-cells, which do not differ in behavior from resting T-cells in the adult in their tolerizability or capacity for an immune response (see papers in *Science* (1996) **271**, 1723, 1726 and 1728), albeit that resting T-cells are more readily tolerizable than memory cells. As will be discussed in the text, there is a window of susceptibility to clonal deletion of self-reacting T-lymphocytes at an immature phase in their ontogenic development within the thymus (and in the case of B-cells within the bone marrow).

Figure M12.2.1. Induction of tolerance to foreign CBA skin graft in A strain mice by neonatal injection of antigen. The effect is antigen specific since the tolerant mice can reject third-party grafts normally. (After Billingham R., Brent L. & Medawar P.B. (1953) *Nature* **172**, 603.)

cules which must be discriminated by the immune system if potentially disastrous autoreactivity is to be avoided. The restriction of each lymphocyte to a single specificity makes the job of establishing self-tolerance that much easier, simply because it just requires a

mechanism which functionally deletes self-reacting cells and leaves the remainder of the repertoire unscathed. The most radical difference between self and nonself molecules lies in the fact that, in early life, the developing lymphocytes are surrounded by self and normally only meet nonself antigens at a later stage and then within the context of the adjuventicity and cytokine release usually associated with infection. With its customary efficiency, the blind force of evolution has exploited these differences to establish the mechanisms of **immunological tolerance to host constituents** (Milestone 12.2).

Self-tolerance can be induced in the thymus

Since developing T-cells are to be found in the thymus, one might expect this to be the milieu in which exposure to self-antigens on the surrounding cells would induce tolerance. The expectation is reasonable. If stem cells in bone marrow of *H-2^k* haplotype are cultured with fetal thymus of H-2^d origin, the maturing cells become tolerant to H-2^d, as shown by their inability to give a mixed lymphocyte proliferative response when cultured with stimulators of H-2^d phenotype; third-party responsiveness is not affected. Further experiments with deoxyguanosine-treated thymuses showed that the cells responsible for tolerance induction were deoxyguanosine-sensitive, bone marrow-derived macrophages or dendritic cells which are abundant at the corticomedullary junction (table 12.2).

Intrathymic clonal deletion leads to self-tolerance

There seems little doubt that self-reactive T-cells can be physically deleted within the thymus. If we look at the experiment in table 12.1b, we can see that SCID males bearing the rearranged transgenes coding for the αβ receptor reacting with the male H-Y antigen do not possess any immunocompetent thymic cells expressing this receptor, whereas the females which lack H-Y do. Thus, when the developing T-cells react with self-

Table 12.2. Induction of tolerance in bone marrow stem cells by incubation with deoxyguanosine (dGuo)-sensitive macrophages or dendritic cells in the thymus. Clearly, the bone marrow cells induce tolerance to their own haplotype. Thus the thymic tolerance-inducing cells can be replaced by progenitors in the bone marrow inoculum (Jenkinson E.J., Jhittay P., Kingston R. & Owen J.J. (1985) *Transplantation* **39**, 331) or by adult dendritic cells from spleen, showing that it is the stage of differentiation of the immature T-cell rather than any special nature of the thymic antigen-presenting cell which leads to tolerance (Matzinger P. & Guerder S. (1989) *Nature* **338**, 74).

Bone marrow cells	Incubate with H-2^d thymus	Tolerance induction to *H-2* haplotype		
		k	d	b
k	Untreated	+	+	–
k	dGuo-treated	+	–	–
k + d	dGuo-treated	+	+	–

antigen in the thymus, they are deleted. In other words, self-reactive cells undergo a **negative selection** process in the thymus. A similar phenomenon is seen when the thymic cells bear certain self-components which act as superantigens (cf. p. 103) by reacting with a whole family of Vβ receptors through recognition of nonvariable structures on a Vβ segment. An example is the H-2E molecule which reacts with receptors belonging to the Vβ17a family; strains which cannot express H-2E because of a defect in the *Ea* gene possess mature T-cells utilizing Vβ17a, whereas strains which express H-2E normally delete their Vβ17a-positive T-cells. Likewise, mice of the *Mls^a* genotype delete Vβ6-bearing cells, the *Mls* being a locus encoding a B-cell superantigen which induces strong proliferation in Vβ6 T-cells from a strain bearing a different *Mls* allele (cf. p. 104). Even exogenous superantigens, such as staphylococcal enterotoxin B which activates the Vβ3 and Vβ8 T-cell families in the adult, will eliminate these cells when incubated with early immature thymocytes. Even more enlightening is the fact that, under these circumstances, the Vβ3 and Vβ8 thymocytes can actually be seen to undergo apoptosis (cf. p. 19).

Factors affecting positive or negative selection in the thymus

It is established that engagement of TCR by the MHC–peptide complex on some type of antigen-presenting cell underlies both positive and negative selection. But how can the same MHC–peptide signal have two totally different outcomes? Well, positive and negative selection may occur at low and high degrees of TCR ligation, respectively. For example, high concentrations of antibody to the TCR induce apoptosis in thymocytes (figure 12.7), whereas low concentrations of anti-TCR do not. Furthermore, many examples have been published showing that the same peptide will induce positive selection at low concentration and negative selection at high concentration (see legend to figure 12.8). This has led to the avidity model, which postulates that a functionally low avidity interaction between T-cell and peptide–MHC involving a relatively low number of TCRs will positively select double-positive CD4$^+$8$^+$ thymocytes, while a high avidity interaction will lead to clonal deletion (figure 12.8). Since the overall avidity of the T-cell interaction will be *inter alia* a function of ligand density × TCR density × affinity, an increase in peptide concentration will increase ligand density and hence avidity. One problem will be immediately apparent to the discerning reader in that a given peptide ligand, giving a low avidity initial stimulus for positive selection, should give a negative signal as the thymocyte differentiates and the density of TCRs increases with the change from double- to single-positive cells. This has led to the suggestion that thymic cortical cells progressively desensitize the maturing thymocyte so that it resists the more powerful stimulus of the macrophages and medullary dendritic cells, which would otherwise induce apoptosis. Evidence is also accumulating that thymic epithelium can synthesize glucocorticoids, hormones classically associated with the adrenal gland. Maybe the *gluco-corticoid-induced leucine zipper* (GILZ) (cf. p. 215)

protects the cells from a signal that would otherwise result in activation-induced cell death.

To pause for a moment, we seem to be saying that engagement of the TCR of differentiating double-positive CD4$^+$8$^+$ thymocytes with self-MHC on cortical epithelial cells leads to expansion and positive selection for clones which recognize self-MHC, perhaps with a whole range of affinities, but that engagement of the TCR with high affinity for self-MHC (+self-peptide) on bone marrow-derived medullary cells will lead to elimination and hence negative selection. Although still not fully worked out, there are also obvious differences in the biochemical pathways used for positive and negative signaling. Positive selection is cyclosporin A-sensitive and dependent on the Ras–MEK–ERK pathway (cf. p. 167), whereas negative selection is cyclosporin A-resistant and independent of this pathway. Different intensities of signaling from the TCR, and/or the types of coreceptor used, may influence which pathway is utilized. Let us finish on a cautionary note: the avidity model may be substantially correct but it could be an oversimplification. For instance, certain superantigens, which can cause clonal deletion of certain Vβ families, fail to expand them even at very low concentrations when the model would have indicated positive selection. This has spawned other models involving conformational changes, and given the complex interactions of peptides behaving as agonists, partial agonists and antagonists (cf. p. 170); the last word has not yet been spoken (not that it ever is in science!).

Figure 12.7. Electron micrograph of cells induced to undergo apoptosis in intact fetal thymus lobes after short-term exposure to anti-CD3. A and N indicate representative apoptotic and normal lymphocytes, respectively. Note the highly condensed state of the nuclei of the apoptotic lymphocytes. (Photograph kindly donated by Professor J.J.T. Owen, from Smith *et al.* (1989) *Nature* **337**, 181. Reproduced by permission from Macmillan Journals Ltd, London.)

Functional avidity T-cell/APC		THYMUS			PERIPHERY
		+ve selection	–ve selection		
		DP	SP	Death	SP
		⬤	⬤	⬤	⬤
Low	Low ligand or TCR density; low affinities*; (cryptic self)	⬤ →	⬤		→ ⬤ **Xenoreactive Autoreactive**
High	High ligand or TCR density; high affinities; (dominant self)	⬤ →	(⬤)? →	→ ⬤	**Deleted**

Figure 12.8. The avidity model of thymic positive and negative selection. It is postulated that a low avidity interaction between the T-cell and antigen-presenting cell (APC) will give positive selection and that high avidity will give deletion. DP, double-positive CD4$^+$8$^+$; SP, single-positive CD4$^+$ or CD8$^+$; *refers to affinity of peptide for the MHC or of the MHC–peptide complex for the TCR.

When Tap-1 mutant mice (cf. p. 93) are mated with mice bearing the transgenes for the TCR specific for a complex of H-2D^b with an

LCM virus peptide, the positive selection of the transgenic T-cells is impaired because of lack of MHC–peptide. However, low concentrations of the peptide added to fetal organ cultures of these mice selected the transgenic T-cells positively, while higher concentrations gave negative selection (Ljunggren H.G. & van Kaer L. (1995) *The Immunologist* **3**, 136). 'Cryptic self'-peptides (cf. p. 200) are presented at very low concentrations and will not delete potentially autoreactive clones, which may therefore escape to the periphery.

Looking again at figure 12.8, the specificities of the T-cells entering the periphery from the thymus must be moulded by the self-peptides, which drive positive selection, since normally the only peptides around must be derived from self. It is satisfying to note therefore that the T-cell repertoire tends to be biased towards peptides from extrinsic antigens which resemble self; thus, T-cell epitopes recognized on immunization with xenogeneic lysozyme corresponded with sequences having the highest homology to the syngeneic protein.

T-cell tolerance can also be due to clonal anergy

We have already entertained the idea that engagement of the TCR plus a costimulatory signal from an antigen-presenting cell are both required for T-cell stimulation, but, when the costimulatory signal is lacking, the T-cell becomes tolerized or anergic, or, if you prefer, paralysed.

Thus, anergy can be induced in **extrathymic T-cells** by peripheral antigens *in vivo* when presented by cells lacking costimulatory molecules. If a transgene construct of H-2E^b attached to an insulin promoter is introduced into a mouse which normally fails to express H-2E, the H-2E^b transgene product appears on the β-cells of the pancreas and induces tolerance to itself. Whereas the expression of H-2E on bone marrow-derived cells in the thymic medulla deletes T-cells bearing Vβ17a receptors, these cells are not lost in the tolerant transgenic mouse expressing pancreatic H-2E, i.e. there is a state of clonal anergy, not deletion. The altered immunological status of these cells is revealed by their inability to proliferate when their receptors are cross-linked by an antibody to Vβ17a.

It is unlikely that these results are due to low level expression of antigen in the thymus. Similar experiments showed that mice expressing influenza hemagglutinin on the pancreatic β-islets also became tolerant irrespective of whether the transgenic thymus was replaced by a normal gland or not. Nonetheless, anergic cells can also be generated within the thymic population as seen in mice transgenic for both an anti-K^b TCR and a K^b gene controlled by a truncated fragment of a keratin IV promoter which allowed expression on thymic medullary cells.

Peripheral T-cell anergy can occur at different levels depending upon the circumstances of antigen exposure. If the above double transgenic experiment is repeated with a full keratin IV promoter, the K^b antigen is expressed on keratinocytes and induces full tolerance, even though the same high frequency of cytotoxic T-cell precursors with the transgene TCR is seen as in single transgenic animals lacking K^b. If K^b is expressed on cells of neuroectodermal origin or hepatocytes, again the double transgenic mice are tolerant but there is dramatic downregulation of TCR and CD8 molecules; in the former but not the latter case, downregulation of TCR could be reversed by exposure to antigen *in vitro*. In some experimental models, tolerance can be abrogated by IL-2. To recapitulate, autoreactive T-cells leaving the thymus can be rendered anergic in the periphery and can display different degrees of potentially reversible unresponsiveness.

Infectious anergy

If a clone of T-helpers is subject to a limiting dilution experiment (p. 137), the minimal unit of proliferation in response to peptide on an APC is usually several cells not just one. This implies that triggering only occurs in small groups or clusters of cells and suggests that paracrine or multicellular interactions between potential responders bound to a single APC are needed to drive the cells into division (figure 12.9a). It will be appreciated that, if a newly arising extrathymic naive T-cell binds to its antigen, even on a professional APC, it will not be stimulated if its neighbors in the cluster have already been made anergic. Indeed, instead of being triggered, it will itself become anergic, so perpetuating the infectious anergic process (figure 12.9b). Recent evidence suggests that anergic T-cells can act as immunoregulatory cells by causing the downregulation of MHC class II and the costimulatory CD80 (B7.1) and CD86 (B7.2) molecules on the APC, generating an infectious anergy which does not require the simultaneous presence of the regulatory anergic cells and the cells which will themselves be made anergic (figure 12.9c). We shall see later in Chapter 17 that the induction of transplantation immunosuppression with a nondepleting anti-CD4 can be long-lasting because the production of anergic cells prevents the priming of newly immunocompetent T-lymphocytes by the transplantation antigen(s).

These anergic cells are really acting as suppressors. So far in our discussions, we have not asked the question: do dedicated T-suppressors contribute to self-tolerance? Frankly, another gray area, but experimentally we can demonstrate that, if autoimmunity is induced in a normal animal, either actively, by injection of an antigen cross-reacting with self, or passively, by injection of autoreactive T-cells (cf. p. 416 and p. 433), the self-reacting clones are usually quashed by idiotype- or antigen-specific T-suppression. In a nutshell, suppressors probably do not prevent autoimmunity but they may reverse it.

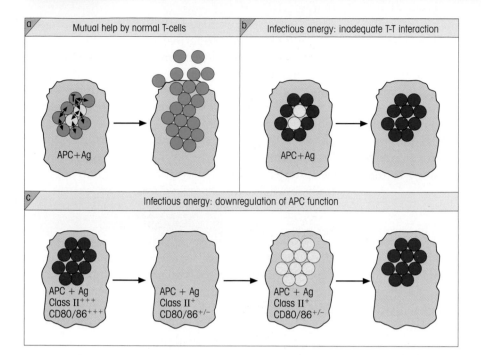

Figure 12.9. Infectious anergy. (a) Clusters of normal T-cells (green) around newly immunocompetent cells (gray) reacting with the same APC mutually support activation and proliferation. (b) Newly immunocompetent cells surrounded by anergic T-cells (red) receive no stimulatory signals from their neighbors and are themselves rendered anergic. (c) Upon being made anergic, T-cells can assume an immunoregulatory function whereby they downregulate expression of MHC class II, CD80 (B7.1) and CD86 (B7.2) molecules on the APC. This effect requires cell–cell contact between the anergic T-cells and the APC, is not blocked by neutralizing antibodies to the cytokines IL-4, IL-10 or TGFβ, and would exhibit linked suppression to other epitopes on the antigen presented by the APC. Subsequent encounter of newly immunocompetent cells with this APC will lead to anergy.

Lack of communication can cause unresponsiveness

It takes two to tango: if the self-molecule cannot engage the TCR, there can be no response. The anatomical isolation of molecules, like the lens protein of the eye and myelin basic protein in the brain, virtually precludes them from contact with lymphocytes, except perhaps for minute amounts of breakdown metabolic products which leak out and may be taken up by antigen-presenting cells, but at concentrations way below that required to trigger the corresponding naive T-cell.

Even when a tissue is exposed to circulating lymphocytes, the concentration of processed peptide on the cell surface may be insufficient to attract attention from a potentially autoreactive cell in the absence of costimulatory B7. This was demonstrated rather elegantly in animals bearing two transgenes: one for the TCR of a CD8 cytotoxic T-cell specific for LCM virus glycoprotein, and the other for the glycoprotein itself expressed on pancreatic β-cells through the insulin promoter. The result? A deafening silence: the T-cells were not deleted or tolerized, nor were the β-cells attacked. If these mice were then infected with LCM virus, the naive transgenic T-cells were presented with adequate concentrations of the processed glycoprotein within the adjuvant context of a true infection and were now stimulated. Their *primed* progeny, having an increased avidity (cf. p. 388) and thereby being able to recognize the low concentrations of processed glyco-

protein on the β-cells, attacked their targets even in the absence of B7 and caused diabetes (figure 12.10). This may sound a trifle tortuous, but the principle could have important implications for the induction of autoimmunity by cross-reacting T-cell epitopes (cf. p. 412).

Molecules that are specifically restricted to particular organs which do not normally express MHC class II represent another special case, since they would not have the opportunity clonally to delete or paralyse organ-specific CD4 T-helper cells.

Immunological silence would also result if an individual has no genes coding for lymphocyte receptors directed against particular self-determinants; analysis of the experimentally induced autoantibody response to cytochrome suggests that only those parts of the molecule which show species variation are autoantigenic, whereas the highly conserved regions where the genes have not altered for a much longer time appear to be silent, supposedly because the autoreactive specificities have had time to disappear.

B-CELLS DIFFERENTIATE IN THE FETAL LIVER AND THEN IN BONE MARROW

The B-lymphocyte precursors, pro-B-cells, are present among the islands of hematopoietic cells in fetal liver by 8–9 weeks of gestation in humans and 14 days in the mouse. Production of B-cells by the liver wanes and is mostly taken over by the bone marrow for the remain-

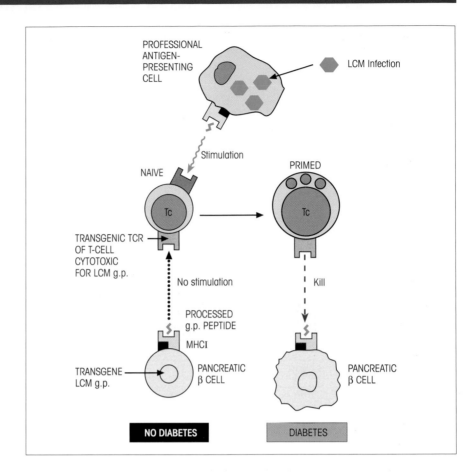

Figure 12.10. Mutual unawareness of a naive cytotoxic precursor T-cell and its B7-negative cellular target bearing epitopes present at low concentrations. Priming of the naive cell by a natural infection and subsequent attack by the higher avidity primed cells on the target tissue. LCM, lymphocytic choriomeningitis virus. (From Ohashi *et al.* (1991) *Cell* **65**, 305.)

der of life. Using the modified culture conditions introduced by Whitlock and Witte, it is now possible to grow bone marrow cells *in vitro* and achieve the differentiation of B-cells and their precursors. Stromal reticular cells, which express adhesion molecules and secrete IL-7, extend long dendritic processes making intimate contact with IL-7 receptor-positive B-cell progenitors. Although early B-cells comprise only a minor subpopulation of the cells in those cultures, it is possible to analyse the different stages in their development by rescue with the Abelson murine leukemia virus (A-MuLV), a replication-defective retrovirus capable of transforming pre-B-cells at various points in their development into clones. A series of differentiation markers associated with B-cell maturation have now been established (figure 12.11).

Pax5 is a major determining factor in B-cell differentiation

Development of hematopoietic cells along the B-cell lineage requires expression of E2A and of early B-cell factor (EBF); the absence of either of these prevents pro-B-cells progressing to the pre-B-cell stage (figure 12.12). Also required is expression of the *Pax5* gene which encodes the BSAP (*B*-cell-*s*pecific *a*ctivator *p*rotein) transcription factor. Thus, in $Pax5^{-/-}$ knockout mice, early pre-B-cells (containing partially rearranged immunoglobulin heavy chain genes) fail to differentiate into mature, surface Ig^+, B-cells (figure 12.12). However, if the pre-B-cells from $Pax5^{-/-}$ knockout mice are provided with the appropriate cytokines *in vitro*, they can be driven to produce T-cells, NK cells, macrophages, dendritic cells, granulocytes and even osteoclasts! These unexpected findings clearly show that the early pre-B-cell has the potential to be diverted from its chosen path and instead provide a source of cells for many other hematopoietic lineages. However, these pre-B-cells are not pluripotent as, unlike bone marrow stem cells, they are unable to rescue lethally irradiated mice. In the light of these findings, it has been proposed that *Pax5* acts as a master gene critical for B-cell development and functions by inhibiting, rather than activating, the expression of a set of genes. *Pax5* expression thereby suppresses alternative lineage choice in early B-cells.

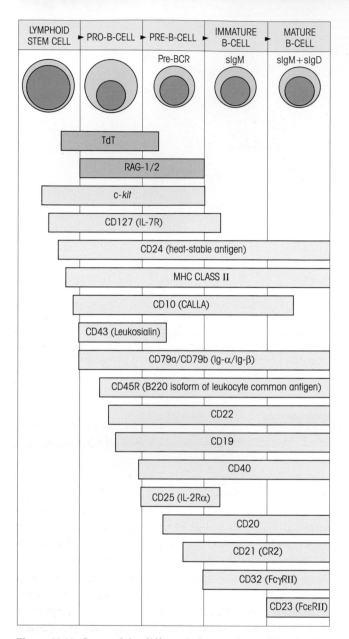

Figure 12.11. Some of the differentiation markers of developing B-cells. The time of appearance of enzymes involved in Ig gene rearrangement and diversification (blue boxes) and of surface markers defined by monoclonal antibodies (orange boxes, see table 8.1 and Appendix 1 for list of CD members) is shown.

B-1 AND B-2 CELLS REPRESENT TWO DISTINCT POPULATIONS

We have previously drawn attention to the subpopulation of B-cells which, in addition to surface IgM, express CD5 (cf. p. 208). The progenitors of this subset move from the fetal liver to the peritoneal cavity fairly early in life, at which stage they are the most abundant B-cell type and predominate in their contribution to the idiotype network and to the production of low affinity, multispecific IgM autoantibodies and the so-

Table 12.3. Comparison of two mouse B-cell subsets. (Developed from Herzenberg L.A., Stall A., Melchers F. *et al.* (eds) (1989) *Progress in Immunology* 7, p. 409. Springer-Verlag, Berlin.)

	B-1	B-2
PHENOTYPE		
IgM	+++	+
IgD	+	+++
CD5	+ or −	−
CD23	−	+
CD43	+	−
MAIN LOCATION	Peritoneal cavity	Lymphoid organs
ONTOGENY	Arise first in fetal liver	Arise later in adult bone marrow
LIFESPAN	Self-renewing Constitutive production IL-10	Replaced by IgM⁻ precursors in bone marrow
GROWTH	Propensity to expansion	Die easily
IMPAIRED DEVELOPMENT	Xid (CBA/N)[1]	me^v (motheaten)[2]
Ig GENES	Unmutated, little N-nucleotide insertion	Mutated, common N-nucleotide insertion
ANTIBODY PRODUCTION		
Serum IgM, IgG3	+++	+
IgG1	+	+++
IgG2a, IgG2b	+ to ++	++ to +++
IgM autoantibody	+++	?
IgM anti-Id	+++	?
IgM anti-bacterial Ab	+++	+ to +++
Anti-hapten/protein	?	+++
T-dependence	−	++
Affinity maturation	−	++

[1]CBA/N mice have an X-linked immunodeficiency gene (Xid) producing a defect in the Bruton tyrosine kinase (btk) associated with poor B-1 cell maturation and inadequate responses to type II T-independent antigens.
[2]Motheaten mice have the me^v mutation affecting the protein tyrosine phosphatase 1C (*PTP-1C*) gene which dramatically alters the threshold for antigen and strongly biases development toward the B-1 subpopulation. The mice have widespread autoimmunity and most of their B-cells are B-1.

called 'natural' antibodies to bacterial carbohydrates, which seemingly arise slightly later in the neonatal period without obvious exposure to conventional antigens.

The **B-1 phenotype, viz. high surface IgM, low surface IgD, CD43⁺ and CD23⁻,** is shared by a minority subpopulation which is, however, CD5⁻; these two populations are referred to as B-1a and B-1b respectively (figure 12.13). The **phenotype** of conventional **B-2 cells** (table 12.3), **low surface IgM, high surface IgD, CD5⁻, CD43⁻ and CD23⁺,** reflects the fact that they represent a separate developmental lineage (figure 12.13). Some general comments may be in order. Although B-1 cells can shift to a B-2 phenotype, and possibly vice versa, there is minimal conversion between the two lineages under normal circumstances. The B-1 cells are particularly prevalent in the peritoneal cavity, main-

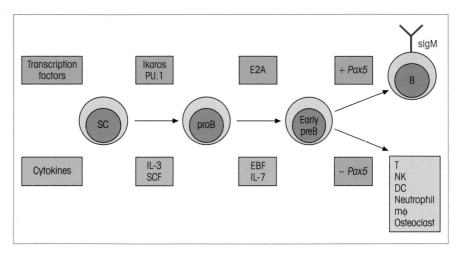

Figure 12.12. *Pax5* is required for B-cell differentiation. Hematopoietic stem cells (SC) under the influence of stem cell factor (SCF), IL-3 and the Ikaros and PU.1 transcription factors can differentiate into pro-B-cells. Further differentiation into pre-B-cells requires the E2A transcription factor together with early B-cell factor (EBF) and IL-7. Homozygous E2A mutant mice lack pre-B-cells, there being a block to $D_H J_H$ rearrangement in the Ig heavy chain locus plus severe reduction in RAG-1, Ig-α, CD19 and $λ_5$ transcripts. If at the early pre-B stage *Pax5* is not expressed, then differentiation along the B-cell lineage pathway comes to an abrupt halt. These early pre-B-cells have rearranged Ig D_H to J_H indicating their intention to become B-cells. However, even at this late stage, they can make other lineage choices as evidenced by the fact that, in the absence of *Pax5* expression, they can give rise to a number of other cell types if they are provided with appropriate cytokines. Indeed, $Pax5^{-/-}$ clones are able to develop into T-cells if transferred to immunodeficient mice, in which case they express rearranged TCR genes in addition to their initial Ig heavy chain gene rearrangement.

tain their numbers by self-replenishment and limit their *de novo* production from progenitors by feedback regulation. They can express both CD5 and its ligand CD72 on their surface, which should encourage mutual interaction, but a major factor influencing self-renewal could be the constitutive production of IL-10, since treatment of mice with anti-IL-10 from birth virtually wipes out the B-1 subset. The predisposition for self-renewal may underlie their undue susceptibility to become leukemic, with the malignant cells in chronic lymphocytic leukemia being almost invariably CD5⁺.

B-1 cells tend to use particular germ-line *V* genes, and the autoantibody response to bromelain-treated erythrocytes is restricted to this subset which utilizes the rather diminutive V_H11 and V_H12 families. Clonal expansion seems to be driven by reaction with self-antigens (see legend to figure 12.13). They tend to respond to type 2 thymus-independent antigens (cf. p. 171) and, unlike the B-2 population, they do not enter into liaisons with thymus-dependent antigens, do not enter germinal centers and hence do not undergo somatic mutation or form high affinity antibodies. This may be just as well if the harmless low affinity autoantibodies which are produced by many B-1 cells are not automatically driven to high affinity pathogenic autoantibodies. In a weak moment one sometimes hears of 'good' and 'bad' autoantibodies, with the 'good guys' possibly having the job of sweeping up broken down self-components, as envisaged by dear Pierre Grabar many years ago when he thought of them as *globulines transporteurs*.

Other functions of B-1 cells may be the generation of an idiotype network concerned in self-tolerance, the response to conserved microbial antigens, and possibly the idiotypic regulation of B-2 responses. They are certainly the source of 'natural antibodies' which provide a pre-existing first line of IgM defense against common microbes. Up to 50% of the IgA-producing cells in the lamina propria are derived from peritoneal cavity B-1 cells. These cells are therefore an important source of the mucosal IgA which coats the normal microflora of the gut.

DEVELOPMENT OF B-CELL SPECIFICITY

The sequence of immunoglobulin gene rearrangements

By analysis of A-MuLV-transformed clones of pre-B-cells, it has proved possible to unravel the orderly cascade of Ig gene rearrangements which occur during differentiation.

Stage 1. Initially, the *D–J* segments on both heavy chain coding regions (one from each parent) rearrange (figure 12.14).

Stage 2. A *V–DJ* recombinational event now occurs on one heavy chain. If this proves to be a *nonproductive* re-

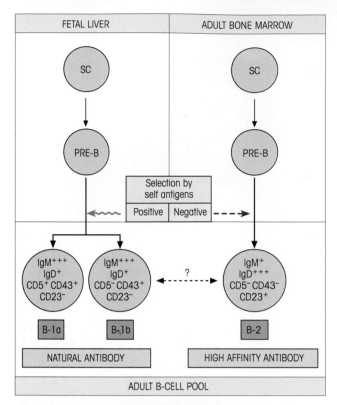

Figure 12.13. The development of separate B-cell subpopulations. It is presumed that B-1 cells of sufficiently high avidity for, say, self-surface antigens are eliminated, leaving positively selected lower affinity specificities for soluble self-antigens and the spectrum of 'natural antibody'-producing B-1 cells. In contrast, B-2 cells undergo negative, rather than positive, selection by self-antigens and the surviving B-2 cells give rise to the higher affinity IgG antibody produced by helper T-cell-dependent class-switched B-cells. It is thought that, although these subsets might be able to give rise to each other under some circumstances, generally they are maintained as separate lineages. Direct evidence that self-antigens positively select B-1 cells is provided by mice made transgenic for the $V_H 3609$ heavy chain gene. The transgene-encoded heavy chain pairs with endogenous Vκ21C light chain to produce an anti-thymocyte autoantibody associated with CD5⁺ B-cells and which recognizes a Thy-1-associated carbohydrate epitope. High levels of the transgenic B-cells and of the serum autoantibody were found only in the presence of the autoantigen, being absent in Thy-1 knockout mice. SC, stem cell; CD23, FcεRII; CD43, leukosialin.

arrangement (i.e. adjacent segments are joined in an incorrect reading frame or in such a way as to generate a termination codon downstream from the splice point), then a second $V–DJ$ rearrangement will occur on the sister heavy chain region. If a productive rearrangement is not achieved, we can wave the pre-B-cell a fond farewell.

Stage 3. Assuming that a productive rearrangement is made, the pre-B-cell can now synthesize μ chains. At around the same time, two genes, V_{preB} (*CD179a*) and $λ_5$ (*CD179b*), with homology for the V_L and C_L segments of λ light chains respectively, are temporarily tran-

scribed to form a 'pseudo-light chain' which associates with the μ chains to generate a surface surrogate 'IgM' receptor, together with the Ig-α (CD79a) and Ig-β (CD79b) chains conventionally required to form a functional B-cell receptor. Expression of this receptor is absolutely essential for further differentiation of the B-lymphocytes since disruption of the membrane exon of the μ chain or of the $λ_5$ gene by homologous recombination of embryonic stem cells (cf. p. 141) arrests development at the pre-B stage and the animal is devoid of mature B-cells. This surrogate receptor closely parallels the pre-Tα/β receptor on pre-T-cell precursors of αβ TCR-bearing cells.

Stage 4. The surface receptor is signaled, perhaps by a stromal cell, to suppress any further rearrangement of heavy chain genes on a sister chromatid. This is termed **allelic exclusion** and was first discussed in relation to the rearrangement of TCR β chains (see p. 227).

Stage 5. It is presumed that the surface receptor now initiates the next set of gene rearrangements which occur on the κ light chain gene loci. These involve $V–J$ recombinations on first one and then the other κ allele until a productive $V_κ–J$ rearrangement is accomplished. Were that to fail, an attempt would be made to achieve productive rearrangement of the λ alleles. Synthesis of conventional sIgM now proceeds.

Stage 6. The sIgM molecule now prohibits any further gene shuffling by allelic exclusion of any unrearranged light chain genes.

At the next stage of differentiation, the cell develops a commitment to producing a particular antibody class and either bears surface IgM alone or in combination with IgA or IgG. The further addition of surface IgD now marks the readiness of the virgin B-cell for priming by antigen. Some cells, therefore, bear surface Ig of three different classes: M, G and D or M, A and D; but all Ig molecules on a single cell have the same idiotype and therefore are derived from the same V_H and V_L genes, presumably by splicing of a long RNA transcript. IgD is lost on antigenic stimulation so that memory cells lack this Ig. At the terminal stages in the life of a fully mature plasma cell, virtually all surface Ig is shed. Injection of anti-μ (anti-IgM heavy chain) into chick embryos prevents the subsequent maturation of IgM and IgG antibody-producing cells, whereas anti-γ inhibits only IgG development. Although we have seen earlier that T-helpers can induce class switching, it is also the case that some isotype switching probably occurs independently of antigen as a result of microenvironmental factors. In the embryonic chicken bursa, a regular switch from IgM to IgG is observed and it seems possible that local influences in the gut will prove to be responsible for the predominant

VDJ = productive rearrangement; V~DJ = non-productive rearrangement

Figure 12.14. Sequence of B-cell gene rearrangements and postulated mechanism of allelic exclusion (see text).

development of IgA-bearing cells. These cells are generated in Peyer's patches, pass into the blood via the thoracic duct and return to populate the diffuse lymphoid tissue in the lamina propria of the gut.

The importance of allelic exclusion

Since each cell has chromosome complements derived from each parent, the differentiating B-cell has four light and two heavy chain gene clusters to choose from. We have described how, once the *VDJ* DNA rearrangement has occurred within one light and one heavy chain cluster, the *V* genes on the other four chromosomes are held in the embryonic state by an allelic exclusion mechanism so that the cell is able to express only one light and one heavy chain. This is essential for clonal selection to work since the cell is then only programed to make the one antibody it uses as a cell surface receptor to recognize antigen. Furthermore, this gene exclusion mechanism prevents the formation of molecules containing two different light or two different heavy chains which would have nonidentical combining sites and therefore be functionally monovalent with respect to the majority of antigens; such antibodies would be nonagglutinating and would tend to have low avidity as the bonus effect of multivalency could not operate.

Different specific responses can appear sequentially

The responses to given antigens in the neonatal period appear sequentially, as though each species were programed to rearrange its *V* genes in a definite order (figure 12.15). Early in ontogeny there is a bias favoring the rearrangement of the V_H genes most proximal to the *DJ* segment.

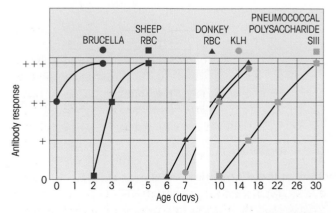

Figure 12.15. Sequential appearance of responsiveness to different antigens in the neonatal rat. RBC, red blood cell; KLH, keyhole limpet hemocyanin.

THE INDUCTION OF TOLERANCE IN B-LYMPHOCYTES

Tolerance can be caused by clonal deletion and clonal anergy

Just as for T-cells, so both mechanisms can operate on B-cells to prevent the reaction to self. Excellent evidence for deletion comes from mice bearing transgenes coding for IgM which binds to H-2K molecules of all *H-2* haplotypes except *d* and *f*. Mice of $H-2^a$ haplotype express the transgenic IgM abundantly in the serum, while 25–50% of total B-cells bear the transgenic idiotype. ($d \times k$) F1 crosses completely failed to express the transgene, either in the serum or on B-cells, i.e. B-cells programed for anti-H-2K^k were expressed in $H-2^d$ mice but deleted in mice positive for H-2K^k which in these circumstances acts as an autoantigen.

Tolerance through B-cell anergy was clearly demonstrated in another study in which double transgenic mice were made to express both lysozyme and a high affinity antibody to lysozyme. The animals were completely tolerant and could not be immunized to make anti-lysozyme; nor did the transgenic antibody appear in the serum although it was abundantly present on the surface of B-cells. These anergic cells could bind antigen to their surface receptors but could not be activated. Like the aged roué, wistfully drinking in the visual attractions of some young belle, these tolerized lymphocytes can 'see' the antigen but lack the ability to do anything about it.

Whether deletion or anergy is the outcome of the encounter with self probably depends upon the concentration and ability to cross-link Ig receptors. In the first of the two B-cell tolerance models above, the H-2K^k autoantigen would be richly expressed on cells in contact with the developing B-lymphocytes and could effectively cause cross-linking. In the second case, the lysozyme, masquerading as a 'self'-molecule, is essentially univalent with respect to the receptors on an anti-lysozyme B-cell and would not readily bring about cross-linking. The hypothesis was tested by stitching a transmembrane hydrophobic segment onto the lysozyme transgene so that the antigen would be inserted into the cell membrane. Result? B-cells expressing the high affinity anti-lysozyme transgene were eliminated.

Another self-censoring mechanism, termed receptor editing, may come into play. We have already discussed one type of receptor editing (cf. p. 66) in which secondary rearrangements substitute another *V* gene onto an already rearranged *V(D)J* segment. However, receptor editing can also occur by wholesale replacement of an entire light chain. This can best be explained by an example. If the heavy and light chain Ig genes encoding a high affinity anti-DNA autoantibody are introduced as transgenes into a mouse, a variety of light chains are produced by genetic reshuffling until a combination with the heavy chain is achieved which no longer has anti-DNA activity, i.e. the autoreactivity is edited out. This will often involve replacement of a κ light chain with a new rearrangement made on the λ light chain locus and is associated with re-expression of the *RAG-1/2* genes.

Most peripheral B-cells in mice are ligand selected as revealed by analysis of the V_H repertoire at the cDNA level of bone marrow pre-B-cells compared with mature spleen B-cells. Once peripheralized, the bulk of the B-cell pool is stable; lymph node B- (and T-) cells from unprimed mice survived comfortably for at least 20 months on transfer to H-2 identical SCID animals.

Tolerance may result from helpless B-cells

With soluble proteins at least, T-cells are more readily tolerized than B-cells (figure 12.16) and, depending upon the circulating protein concentration, a number of self-reacting B-cells may be present in the body which cannot be triggered by T-dependent self-components since the T-cells required to provide the necessary T–B help are already tolerant—you might describe the B-cells as helpless. If we think of the determinant on a self-component which combines with the receptors on a self-reacting B-cell as a hapten and another determinant which has to be recognized by a T-cell as a carrier (cf. figure 9.11), then tolerance in the T-cell to the carrier will prevent the provision of T-cell help and the B-cell will be unresponsive. Take C5 as an example; this is normally circulating at concentrations which tolerize T- but not B-cells. Some strains of mice are congenitally deficient in C5 and their T-cells can help C5-positive strains to make antibodies to C5, i.e. the C5-positive strains still have inducible B-cells but they are helpless and need nontolerized T-cells from the C5-negative strain (figure 12.17).

It is worth noting the observation that injection of high doses of a soluble antigen without adjuvant, even when given several days after primary immunization with that antigen, prevented the emergence of high affinity mutated antibodies. Transfer experiments showed the T-cells to be tolerant. This tells us that, even when an immune response is well underway, T-helpers in the germinal center are needed to permit the mutations which lead to affinity maturation of antibody and, as a further corollary, that soluble self-

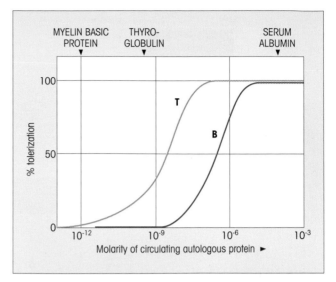

Figure 12.16. Relative susceptibility of T- and B-cells to tolerance by circulating self-antigens. Those circulating at low concentration induce no tolerance; at intermediate concentration, e.g. thyroglobulin, T-cells are moderately tolerized; molecules such as albumin which circulate at high concentrations tolerize both B- and T-cells.

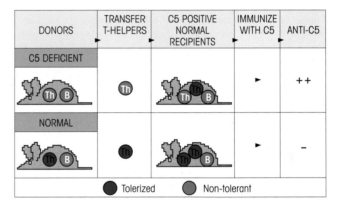

Figure 12.17. Circulating C5 tolerizes T- but not B-cells leaving them helpless. Animals with congenital C5 deficiency do not tolerize their T-helpers and can be used to break tolerance in normal mice.

antigens in the extracellular fluids can act to switch off autoreactive B-cells arising in the germinal centers by hypermutation.

Presumably, self-tolerance in both B- and T-cells involves all the mechanisms we have discussed to varying degrees and these are summarized in figure 12.18. Remember that, throughout the life of an animal, new stem cells are continually differentiating into immunocompetent lymphocytes and what is early in ontogeny for them can be late for the host; this means that self-tolerance mechanisms are still acting on early lymphocytes even in the adult, although it is always comforting to note that the threshold concentration for tolerance induction is very much lower for pre-B-cells relative to mature B-cells.

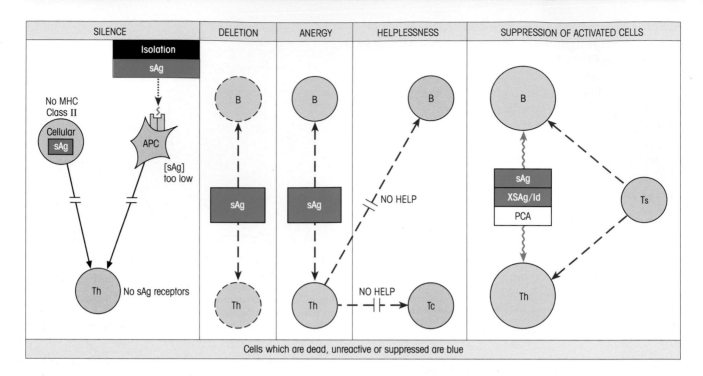

Figure 12.18. Mechanisms of self-tolerance (see text). sAg, self-antigen; XSAg/Id, cross-reacting antigen or idiotype; PCA, polyclonal activator; APC, antigen-presenting cell; Th, T-helper; Ts, T-suppressor; Tc, cytotoxic T-cell precursor.

NATURAL KILLER (NK) CELL ONTOGENY

The precise lineage of NK cells is still to be established. They share a common early progenitor with T-cells and express the CD2 molecule which is also present on T-cells. Furthermore, they have IL-2 receptors, are driven to proliferate by IL-2 and produce IFNγ. The majority of NK cells express CD56, a molecule also present on a subset of CD4+ and CD8+ T-cells. However, they do not develop in the thymus, their T-cell receptor *V* genes are not rearranged and, unlike T-cells, they express the CD16 FcγRIII. The current view is therefore that they separate from the T-cell lineage very early on in their differentiation.

THE OVERALL RESPONSE IN THE NEONATE

Lymph node and spleen remain relatively underdeveloped in the human at the time of birth, except where there has been intrauterine exposure to antigens as in congenital infections with rubella or other organisms. The ability to reject grafts and to mount an antibody response is reasonably well developed by birth, but the immunoglobulin levels, with one exception, are low, particularly in the absence of intrauterine infection. The exception is IgG which is acquired by placental transfer from the mother, a process dependent upon Fc

structures specific to this Ig class. This material is catabolized with a half-life of approximately 30 days and there is a fall in IgG concentration over the first 3 months accentuated by the increase in blood volume of the growing infant. Thereafter, the rate of synthesis overtakes the rate of breakdown of maternal IgG and the overall concentration increases steadily. The other immunoglobulins do not cross the placenta and the low but significant levels of IgM in cord blood are synthesized by the baby (figure 12.19). IgM reaches adult levels by 9 months of age. Only trace levels of IgA, IgD and IgE are present in the circulation of the newborn.

THE EVOLUTION OF THE IMMUNE RESPONSE

Invertebrates have microbial defense mechanisms

Mechanisms for the recognition and subsequent **rejection of nonself** can be identified in invertebrates as far down the evolutionary scale as marine sponges, commonly regarded as the most primitive of present-day animals (figure 12.20). Phagocytosis is of importance throughout the animal kingdom (cf. Milestone 1.1, Chapter 1). In many phyla, phagocytosis is augmented by coating with agglutinins and bactericidins capable of binding to *pathogen-associated molecular patterns* (PAMPs) on the microbial surface so providing the basis for the recognition of 'nonself'. It is notable that **infection very rapidly induces the synthesis of an impressive battery of antimicrobial peptides** in higher insects following activation of transcription factors

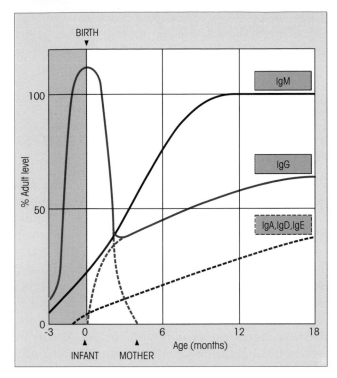

Figure 12.19. Development of serum immunoglobulin levels in the human. (After Hobbs J.R. (1969) In Adinolfi M. (ed.) *Immunology and Development*, p. 118. Heinemann, London.)

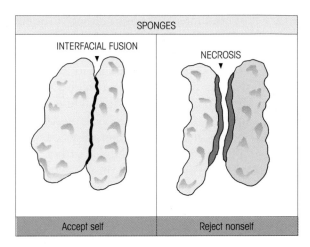

Figure 12.20. Recognition and rejection of nonself. Parabiosed fingers of a marine sponge from the same colony are permanently united but members of different colonies reject each other by 7–9 days.

which bind to promoter sequence motifs homologous to regulatory elements involved in the mammalian acute phase response. Thus, the toll molecule in drosophila is a receptor for PAMPs that activates NFκB in these flies. Drosophila with a loss-of-function mutation in *toll* are susceptible to fungal infections. Antimicrobial peptides produced by insects include disulfide-bridged cyclic peptides such as the 4 kDa anti-Gram-positive defensins and the 5 kDa antifungal peptide, drosomycin. Linear peptides inducible by infection include the cecropins and a series of anti-Gram-negative glycine- or proline-rich polypeptides. Cecropins, which have also been identified in mammals, are 4 kDa strongly cationic amphipathic α-helices causing lethal disintegration of bacterial membranes by creating ion channels.

Elements of a primordial complement system also exist among the lower orders. A protease inhibitor, an α_2-macroglobulin structurally homologous to C3 with internal thiolester, is present in the horseshoe crab. Conceivably this might represent an ancestral version of C3 which is activated by proteases released at a site of infection, deposited onto the microbe and recognized there as a ligand for the phagocytic cells. The complement receptor CR3 is an integrin, and related integrins in insects may harbor common ancestors. Mention of the horseshoe crab may have stirred a neuronal network in readers with good memories, to recall

its synthesis of limulin (cf. p. 16) which is homologous with the mammalian acute phase C-reactive protein (CRP); presumably, it acts as a lectin to opsonize bacteria and is likely to be a product of the evolutionary line leading ultimately to C1q, mannose-binding protein and lung surfactant.

The other major strategy effectively deployed by invertebrates is to wall off an invading microorganism. This is achieved, for example, through proteolytic cascades which produce a coagulum of 'gelled' hemolymph around the offender.

Please do not let us overlook plants. Higher plants develop an 'immune state' of **systemic acquired resistance** (SAR), which can be established following a localized infection with pathogens that induce lesions involving host cell death. SAR persists for several weeks and extends to a broad range of bacterial, viral and fungal pathogens beyond the initiating infective agent. A series of SAR genes encode a wide variety of microbicidal proteins which can be induced through endogenous chemical mediators such as salicylic acid and methyl-2,6-dichloroisonicotinic acid. One function of salicylic acid is to bind to a protein with catalase activity, thereby increasing H_2O_2, but, while this may contribute to an acute defensive response, other mechanisms are thought to be concerned in the induction of SAR.

Adaptive immune responses appear with the vertebrates

Lower vertebrates

Lymphocytes and genuine adaptive T- and B-responses do not emerge in the phylogenetic tree until we reach the vertebrates, although neither can be elicited in the lowliest vertebrate studied—the California hagfish. This unpleasant cyclostome (which preys upon moribund fish by entering their mouths and eating the flesh from the inside) can respond to hemocyanin provided that it is maintained at temperatures approaching 20°C (in general, poikilotherms make antibodies better at higher temperatures), but true immunoglobulins are not involved. Further up the evolutionary scale in the cartilaginous fishes, well-defined 18S and 7S immunoglobulins with heavy and light chains have now been defined, but the responses are *T-independent*.

T-cells appear

The toad, *Xenopus*, is a pliable, if unlovely, species for study since it is possible to make transgenics and cloned tadpoles fairly readily, and it has a less complex lymphoid system than mammals, characterized by a small number of lymphocytes and a restricted antibody repertoire not subject to somatic mutation. Furthermore, positive and negative thymic selection have been demonstrated in frogs.

The emergence of an honest-to-God thymus in the teleosts (bony fishes), amphibians, reptiles, birds and mammals was of course associated with MHC molecules, cell-mediated immunity, cytotoxic T-cells and allograft rejection. It could be argued that we also see phylogenetically more ancient, T-independent B-1 (CD5-positive) cells joined by a new T-dependent B-2 population. However, T-dependent, high affinity, heterogeneous, rapid secondary antibody responses are only seen with warm-blooded vertebrates such as birds and mammals, and these correlate directly with the evolution of germinal centers.

Generation of antibody diversity

Mechanisms for the generation of antibody diversity receive quite different emphasis as one goes from one species to another. We are already familiar with the mammalian system where multiple V genes are greatly amplified by a variety of recombinational events involving multiple D and J segments. The horned shark also has many V genes, but the opportunities for combinatorial joining are tightly constrained by close linkage between individual V, D, J and C segments and this may be a factor in the restricted antibody response of this species. In sharp contrast, there seems to be only one operational V gene at the light chain locus in the chicken, but this undergoes extensive somatic diversification utilizing nonfunctional adjoining V pseudo-genes in a somatic gene conversion-like process. Camel lovers should note that not only do they get by on little water but, like the llamas, they also survive on antibodies which lack light chains.

THE EVOLUTION OF DISTINCT B- AND T-CELL LINEAGES WAS ACCOMPANIED BY THE DEVELOPMENT OF SEPARATE SITES FOR DIFFERENTIATION

The differential effects of neonatal bursectomy and thymectomy in the chicken on subsequent humoral and cellular responses paved the way for our eventual recognition of the separate lymphocyte lineages which subserve these functions. Like the thymus, the bursa of Fabricius develops as an embryonic outpushing of the gut endoderm, this time from hindgut as distinct from foregut, and provides the microenvironment to cradle incoming stem cells and direct their differentiation to immunocompetent B-lymphocytes. As may be seen from table 12.4, neonatal bursectomy had a profound effect on overall immunoglobulin levels and on specific antibody production following immunization, but did not unduly influence the cell-mediated delayed-type hypersensitivity (DTH) response to tuberculin or affect graft rejection. On the other hand, thymectomy grossly impaired cell-mediated reactions and inhibited antibody production to most protein antigens.

The distinctive anatomical location of the B-cell differentiation site in a separate lymphoid organ in the chicken was immensely valuable to progress in this field because it allowed the above types of experiments to be carried out. However, many years went by in a fruitless search for an equivalent bursa in mammals before it was realized that the primary site for B-cell generation was in fact the bone marrow itself.

Table 12.4. Effect of neonatal bursectomy and thymectomy on the development of immunologic competence in the chicken. (From Cooper M.D., Peterson R.D.A., South M.A. & Good R.A. (1966) *Journal of Experimental Medicine* **123**, 75, with permission of the editors.)

All X-irradiated after birth	Peripheral blood lymphocyte count	Ig conc.	Antibody	Delayed skin reaction to tuberculin	Graft rejection
Intact	14 800	++	+++	++	+++
Thymectomized	9 000	++	+	−	+
Bursectomized	13 200	−	−	+	+

CELLULAR RECOGNITION MOLECULES EXPLOIT THE IMMUNOGLOBULIN GENE SUPERFAMILY

When nature fortuitously chances upon a protein structure ('motif' is the buzz word) which successfully mediates some useful function, the selective forces of evolution make sure that it is widely exploited. Thus, all the molecules involved in antigen recognition which we have described at such (painful!) length in Chapters 3 and 4 are members of a gene superfamily related by sequence and presumably a common ancestry. All polypeptide members of this family, which includes heavy and light Ig chains, T-cell receptor α and β chains, MHC class I and class II molecules and β_2-microglobulin, are composed of one or more immunoglobulin homology units. Each unit is roughly 110 amino acids in length and is characterized by certain conserved residues around the two cysteines found in every domain and the alternating hydrophobic and hydrophilic amino acids which give rise to the familiar antiparallel β-pleated strands with interspersed short variable lengths having a marked propensity to form reversed turns — the **'immunoglobulin fold'** in short (cf. p. 45).

Attention has been drawn to a very important feature of the Ig domain structure, namely the mutual complementarity which allows strong interdomain noncovalent interactions, such as those between V_H and V_L and the two C_H3 regions which form the IgG pFc' fragment. Gene duplication and diversification can create mutual families of interacting molecules, such as CD4 with MHC class II, CD8 with MHC class I and IgA with the poly-Ig receptor (figure 12.21). Likewise, the intercellular adhesion molecules ICAM-1 and N-CAM (figure 12.21) are richly endowed with these domains, and the long evolutionary history of N-CAM strongly suggests that these structures made an early appearance in phylogeny as mediators of intercellular recognition. In marine sponges, Ig superfamily structures are found both on the extracellular portion of the receptor tyrosine kinase (RTK) and in the more recently described cell recognition molecules (CRMs), both thought to be involved in allograft rejection. A recent trawl of the protein sequence database revealed hundreds of known members of the Ig superfamily. Some family!

The **integrins** form another structural superfamily which includes a number of hematopoietic cell surface molecules concerned with adhesion to extracellular matrix proteins and to cell surface ligands; their function is to direct leukocytes to particular tissue sites (see discussion on p. 223).

Figure 12.21. The immunoglobulin superfamily comprises a large number of surface molecules which all share a common structure, the immunoglobulin-type domain, suggesting evolution from a single primordial ancestral gene. Just a few examples are shown. (a) Multigene families involved in antigen recognition (the single copy β_2-microglobulin is included because of its association with class I). (b) Single copy genes. Thy-1 is present on T-cells and neurons. The poly-Ig receptor transports IgA across mucosal membranes. N-CAM is an adhesion molecule binding neuronal cells together. It is also found on NK cells and a subpopulation of T-cells, but its function on these lymphoid cells is unknown. (Reprinted by permission from *Nature* **323**, 15. Copyright © 1986, Macmillan Magazines Ltd with some updating.)

SUMMARY

Multipotential stem cells from the bone marrow give rise to all the formed elements of the blood

• Expansion and differentiation are driven by soluble growth (colony-stimulating) factors and contact with reticular stromal cells.

The differentiation of T-cells occurs within the microenvironment of the thymus

• Precursor T-cells arising from stem cells in the bone marrow need to travel to the thymus under the influence of chemokines in order to become immunocompetent T-cells.

T-cell ontogeny

• Differentiation to immunocompetent T-cell subsets is accompanied by changes in the surface phenotype which can be recognized with monoclonal antibodies.

• TCR genes rearrange in the thymus cortex, producing a $\gamma\delta$ TCR or a pre-$\alpha\beta$ TCR, consisting of an invariant pre-Tα associated with a conventional Vβ, before final rearrangement of the Vα to generate the mature $\alpha\beta$ TCR.

• Double-negative CD4$^-$8$^-$ pre-T-cells are driven and expanded, probably by Notch-mediated and other signals, to become double positive CD4$^+$8$^+$.

• The thymus epithelial cells **positively select** CD4$^+$8$^+$ T-cells with avidity for their MHC haplotype so that single-positive CD4$^+$ or CD8$^+$ T-cells develop that are restricted to the recognition of antigen in the context of the epithelial cell haplotype.

T-cell tolerance

• The induction of immunological tolerance is necessary to avoid self-reactivity.

• High avidity T-cells which react with self-antigens presented by corticomedullary macrophages and interdigitating dendritic cells are eliminated by **negative selection**. The paradigm that low avidity binding to MHC–peptide produces positive selection and high avidity negative, is probably broadly true but may need some amendment.

• Self-tolerance can also be achieved by anergy.

• Anergic cells attached to a dendritic cell can downregulate the antigen-presenting ability of that cell, resulting in infectious anergy.

• A state of what is effectively self-tolerance also arises when there is a failure to adequately present a self-antigen to lymphocytes, either because of compartmentalization, lack of class II on the antigen-presenting cell or low concentration of peptide–MHC (cryptic self).

• T-suppression is probably more concerned in reversing autoimmunity than preventing it.

B-cells differentiate in the fetal liver and then in the bone marrow

• They become immunocompetent B-cells after passing through pro-B-, pre-B- and immature B-cell stages.

• *Pax5* expression is essential for progression from the pre-B- to immature B-cell stage.

B-1 and B-2 represent two distinct subpopulations of B-cells

• B-1 cells represent a minor population expressing high sIgM and low sIgD. B-1a cells are CD5$^+$, B-1b are CD5$^-$. The majority of conventional B-cells, the B-2 population, are sIgM^{lo}, sIgD^{hi}, CD5$^-$. The B-1 population predominates in early life, shows a high level of idiotype–anti-idiotype connectivity, produces low affinity, IgM polyreactive antibodies, many of them autoantibodies, and is responsible for the T-independent 'natural' IgM antibacterial antibodies which appear spontaneously.

Development of B-cell specificity

• The sequence of Ig variable gene rearrangements is *DJ* and then *VDJ*.

• *VDJ* transcription produces μ chains which associate with V$_{preB}$. λ_5 chains to form a surrogate surface IgM-like receptor.

• This receptor signals allelic exclusion of unrearranged heavy chains and initiates rearrangement of V–J_κ (in the mouse) and, if unproductive, V–J_λ.

• If the rearrangement at any stage is unproductive, i.e. does not lead to an acceptable gene reading frame, the allele on the sister chromosome is rearranged.

• The mechanisms of allelic exclusion ensure that each lymphocyte is programed for only one antibody. Responses to different antigens appear sequentially with age.

The induction of tolerance in B-lymphocytes

• B-cell tolerance is induced by clonal deletion, clonal anergy, receptor editing and 'helplessness' due to preferential tolerization of T-cells needed to cooperate in B-cell stimulation.

Natural killer (NK) cell ontogeny

• NK cells share an early progenitor with T-cells but separate from the T-cell lineage early on and develop somewhere other than the thymus.

(continued)

Figure 12.22. Antigen-independent differentiation and antigen-dependent maturation of T- and B-cells. Cortical thymocytes are positively selected to recognize self-MHC haplotype. TdT, terminal deoxynucleotidyl transferase.

The overall response in the neonate

• Maternal IgG crosses the placenta and provides a high level of passive immunity at birth.

The antigen-independent differentiation within primary lymphoid organs and antigen-driven maturation in secondary lymphoid organs are summarized in figure 12.22.

The evolution of the immune response

• Recognition of self is of fundamental importance for multicellular organisms, even lowly forms like marine sponges.

• Invertebrates have defense mechanisms based on phagocytosis, killing by a multiplicity of microbicidal peptides and polyphenoloxidase metabolites, and imprisonment of the invader by coagulation of the hemolymph.

• Higher plants can establish a persisting state of systemic acquired resistance.

• B- and T-cell responses are well defined in the vertebrates and the evolution of these distinct lineages was accompanied by the development of separate sites for differentiation.

• The success of the immunoglobulin domain structure, possibly through its ability to give noncovalent mutual binding, has been exploited by evolution to produce the very large Ig superfamily of recognition molecules, including Ig, TCRs, MHC class I and II, β_2-microglobulin, CD4, CD8, the poly-Ig receptor and Thy-1. Another superfamily, the integrins, which includes LFA-1 and the VLA molecules, is concerned with leukocyte binding to endothelial cells and extracellular matrix proteins.

See the accompanying website (**www.roitt.com**) for multiple choice questions.

FURTHER READING

von Boehmer H. (2000) T-cell lineage fate: instructed by receptor signals? *Current Biology* **10**, R642.

Goldrath A.W. & Bevan M.J. (1999) Selecting and maintaining a diverse T-cell repertoire. *Nature* **402**, 255.

Hardy R.R. & Hayakawa K. (2001) B cell development pathways. *Annual Review of Immunology* **19**, 595.

Herzenberg L.A. (2000) B-1 cells, the lineage question revisited. *Immunological Reviews* **175**, 9.

Horton J. & Ratcliffe N. (1998) Evolution of immunity. In Roitt I.M., Brostoff J. & Male D.K. (eds) *Immunology*, 5th edn, p. 199. Mosby, London.

Kamradt T. & Mitchison N.A. (2001) Tolerance and autoimmunity. *New England Journal of Medicine* **344**, 655.

Nutt S.L., Heavey B., Rolink A.G. & Busslinger M. (1999) Commitment to the B lymphoid lineage depends on the transcription factor Pax5. *Nature* **401**, 556.

Phillips R.L. *et al.* (2000) The genetic program of hematopoietic stem cells. *Science* **288**, 1635.

Robey E. & Fowlkes B.J. (1998) The αβ versus γδ T-cell lineage choice. *Current Opinion in Immunology* **10**, 181.

Townsend S.E., Weintraub B.C. & Goodnow C.C. (1999) Growing up on the streets: why B-cell development differs from T-cell development. *Immunology Today* **20**, 217.

Turner R.J. (ed.) (1994) *Immunology: A Comparative Approach*. John Wiley & Sons Ltd, Chichester.

Yasutomo K., Doyle C., Miele L. & Germain R.N. (2000) The duration of antigen receptor signalling determines CD4$^+$ versus CD8$^+$ T-cell lineage fate. *Nature* **404**, 506.

Adversarial strategies during infection

INTRODUCTION

We are engaged in constant warfare with the microbes which surround us and the processes of mutation and evolution have tended to select microorganisms which have evolved means of evading our defense mechanisms. Pathogens continue to take a terrifying toll (figure 13.1), particularly in the developing world. Furthermore, the decline in mortality from infectious disease which had been seen in countries such as the USA has gone into reverse, with a rise in deaths in that country from infectious disease increasing at a rate of 4.8% per year between 1981 and 1995. There has been both the emergence of new infections and the re-emergence of some old adversaries. Among the current list of problems are Legionnaire's disease, HIV, ebola, nvCJD, *E. coli*, methicillin-resistant *Staphylococcus aureus* (MDSA), toxic shock syndrome and lyme disease. The fact that MDSA strains are becoming resistant to the drug of last resort, vancomycin, is, to put it mildly, worrying. Furthermore, it is becoming increasingly appreciated that infectious agents are related to many 'noninfectious' diseases, such as the association between *Helicobacter pylori* and peptic ulcer and of various viruses with cancer. In this chapter, we look at the varied, often ingenious, adversarial strategies which we and our enemies have developed over very long periods of time.

INFLAMMATION REVISITED

The acute inflammatory process involves a protective influx of white cells, complement, antibody and other plasma proteins into a site of infection or injury and was discussed in broad outline in the introductory chapters. Now that we are ready to look in more detail at the aggressive gambits and wily counter-attacks which characterize the conflict between microbe and host, it is appropriate to re-examine the mechanisms of inflammation in greater depth. The reader may find it helpful to have another look at the relevant sections in Chapters 1 and 2, particularly those relating to figures 1.15, 1.16, 1.17 and 2.18.

Mediators of inflammation

A complex variety of mediators are involved in acute inflammatory responses (figure 13.2). Some act directly on the smooth muscle wall surrounding the

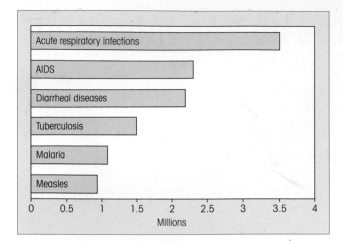

Figure 13.1. Deaths from infectious disease. These six diseases caused almost 90% of the 13 million deaths from infectious disease worldwide, as estimated by the World Health Organization for the year 1998. For more information, see http://www.who.int/infectious-disease-report.

arterioles to alter blood flow. Others act on the venules to cause contraction of the endothelial cells with transient opening of the interendothelial junctions and consequent transudation of plasma. The migration of leukocytes from the bloodstream is facilitated by mediators which upregulate the expression of adherence molecules on both endothelial and white cells and others which lead the leukocytes to the inflamed site through chemotaxis.

Leukocytes bind to endothelial cells through paired adhesion molecules

Redirecting the leukocytes charging along the blood into the site of inflammation is somewhat like having to encourage bulls stampeding down the Pamplona main street to move quietly into the side roads. We have had occasion to confront this problem when discussing lymphocyte homing (cf. p. 152, figure 8.6) and, in the present context, the adherence of leukocytes to the endothelial vessel wall through the interaction of complementary binding of cell surface molecules is an absolutely crucial step. Several classes of molecule subserve this function (cf. p. 152, table 8.3), some acting as lectins to bind a carbohydrate ligand on the complementary partner.

Initiation of the acute inflammatory response

A very early event is the upregulation of P-selectin and *p*latelet *a*ctivating *f*actor (PAF) on the endothelial cells lining the venules by histamine or thrombin released by the original inflammatory stimulus. Recruitment of

these molecules from intracellular storage vesicles ensures that they appear within minutes on the cell surface. Engagement of the lectin-like domain at the tip of the P-selectin molecule with sialyl Lewis[x] carbohydrate determinants on the mucin-like *P*-selectin *g*lyco-*p*rotein *l*igand-1 (PSGL-1) on the neutrophil surface causes the cell to slow and then **roll** along the endothelial wall and helps PAF to dock onto its corresponding receptor. This, in turn, increases surface expression of the integrins *l*ymphocyte *f*unction-*a*ssociated molecule-1 (LFA-1) and Mac-1 which now bind the neutrophil very firmly to the endothelial surface (figure 13.3).

Activation of the neutrophils also makes them more responsive to chemotactic agents and, under the influence of C5a and leukotriene-B4, they exit from the circulation by moving purposefully through the gap between endothelial cells, across the basement membrane (**diapedesis**) and up the chemotactic gradient to the inflammation site.

Damage to vascular endothelium, which exposes the basement membrane, and bacterial toxins, such as LPS, trigger other complex systems (figure 13.4). Activation of platelets by contact with basement membrane collagen or induced endothelial PAF leads to aggregation and **thrombus** formation by adherence through platelet glycoprotein Ib to von Willebrand factor on the vascular surface. Such platelet plugs are adept at stemming the loss of blood from a damaged artery, but in the venous system the damaged site is sealed by a **fibrin clot** resulting from activation of the intrinsic clotting system via contact of Hageman factor (factor XII) with the exposed surface of the basement membrane. Activated Hageman factor also triggers the kinin and plasmin systems and several of the resulting products influence the inflammatory process by increasing vascular permeability, activating endothelium, autocatalytically amplifying the production of Hageman factor XII and cleaving C3 (figure 13.4).

The ongoing inflammatory process

One must not ignore the role of the tissue macrophage which, under the stimulus of local infection or injury, secretes an imposing array of mediators. In particular, the cytokines interleukin-1 (IL-1) and tumor necrosis factor (TNF) act at a later time than histamine or thrombin to stimulate the endothelial cells and maintain the inflammatory process by upregulating E-selectin and sustaining P-selectin expression. Thus, expression of E-selectin occurs 2–4 hours after the initiation of acute inflammation, being dependent upon activation of

MEDIATOR ACTION						
	DILATATION	CONSTRICTION	INCREASE PERMEABILITY	UPREGULATE ADHESION MOL.		PMN CHEMOTAXIS
				ENDOTHELIUM	PMN	
HISTAMINE	+		+	++		
BRADYKININ	+		++			
PGE$_2$/I$_2$	+++		Potentiate other mediators			
VIP	+++					
NITRIC OXIDE	+++		+++			
LEUKOTRIENE-D4		+				
LEUKOTRIENE-C4		++	+			
C5a			++	+	++	+++
LEUKOTRIENE-B4			++		++	+++
f.Met.Leu.Phe			++		+	+
PLATELET ACTIVATING FACTOR	+		++		++	
IL-8					+++	+++
NAP-2 (CXCL7)					++	++
IL-1				++	++	
TNF				++	++	

INCREASE/DECREASE BLOOD FLOW

TRANSUDATION OF PLASMA

PMN DIAPEDESIS

ENDOTHELIAL RETRACTION

ARTERY | ARTERIOLE | CAPILLARIES | VENULE | VEIN

Figure 13.2. The principal mediators of acute inflammation. The reader should refer back to figure 1.15 to recall the range of products generated by the mast cell. The later acting cytokines such as interleukin-1 (IL-1) are largely macrophage-derived and these cells also secrete prostaglandin E$_2$ (PGE$_2$), leukotriene-B4 and the neutrophil activating chemokine NAP-2 (CXCL7). PMN, polymorphonuclear neutrophil; VIP, vasoactive intestinal peptide; TNF, tumor necrosis factor.

gene transcription. The E-selectin engages the glycoprotein E-selectin ligand-1 (ESL-1) on the neutrophil. Other later acting components are the **chemokines** (*chemo*tactic cyto*kines*) IL-8 (CXCL8) and epithelial-derived neutrophil attractant-78 (ENA-78, CXCL5) which are highly effective neutrophil chemoattractants. IL-1 and TNF also act on endothelial cells, fibroblasts and epithelial cells to stimulate secretion of another chemokine, MCP-1 (CCL2), a chemotactic protein for several different cell types which is particularly potent at attracting mononuclear phagocytes to the inflammatory site to strengthen and maintain the defensive reaction to infection.

Perhaps this is a good time to remind ourselves of the important role of chemokines (see table 10.3) in selectively attracting multiple types of leukocytes to inflammatory foci. Inflammatory chemokines are typically induced by microbial products such as lipopolysaccharide (LPS) and by proinflammatory cytokines including IL-1, TNF and IFNγ. As a very broad generalization, chemokines of the CXC subfamily, such as IL-8, are specific for neutrophils and, to varying extents, lymphocytes, whereas chemokines with the CC motif are chemotactic for T-cells, monocytes, dendritic cells, and variably for natural killer (NK) cells, basophils and eosinophils. Eotaxin (CCL11) is chemotactic for eosinophils, and the presence of significant concentrations of this mediator together

Figure 13.3. Early events in inflammation affecting neutrophil margination and diapedesis. Induced upregulation of P-selectin on the vessel walls plays the major role in the initial leukocyte–endothelial interaction (rolling) by interaction with ligands on the neutrophil such as the mucin-like P-selectin glycoprotein ligand-1 (PSGL-1, CD162). Recognition of extracellular gradients of the chemotactic mediators by receptors on the polymorphonuclear neutrophil (PMN) surface triggers intracellular signals which generate motion. The neutrophils crawl rather than swim and migration along the extracellular matrix vitronectin is dependent upon very rapid cycles of integrin-dependent adhesion and detachment regulated by calcineurin. The cytokine-induced expression of E-selectin, which is recognized by the glycoprotein E-selectin ligand-1 (ESL-1) on the neutrophil, occurs as a later event. Chemotactic factors such as IL-8, which is secreted by a number of cell types including the endothelium itself, are important mediators of the inflammatory process. (Compare events involved in homing and transmigration of lymphocytes, figure 8.6.)

with RANTES (*r*egulated upon *a*ctivation *n*ormal *T*-cell *e*xpressed and *s*ecreted, CCL5) in mucosal surfaces could account for the enhanced population of eosinophils in those tissues. The different chemokines bind to particular heparin and heparan sulfate glycosaminoglycans so that, after secretion, the chemotactic gradient can be maintained by attachment to the extracellular matrix as a form of scaffolding.

Clearly, this whole operation serves to focus the immune defenses around the invading microorganisms. These become coated with antibody, C3b and certain acute phase proteins and are ripe for phagocytosis by the granulocytes and macrophages; under the influence of the inflammatory mediators these have upregulated C3 and Ig receptors, enhanced phagocytic responses and hyped-up killing powers, adding up to bad news for the bugs.

Of course it is beneficial to recruit lymphocytes to sites of infection and we should remember that endothelial cells in these areas express VCAM-1 (cf. p. 151) which acts as a homing receptor for VLA-4-positive activated memory T-cells, while many chemokines are chemotactic for lymphocytes.

Regulation and resolution of inflammation

With its customary prudence, evolution has established regulatory mechanisms to prevent inflammation from getting out of hand. At the humoral level we have a series of complement regulatory proteins: C1

Figure 13.4. Events initiated by damaged vascular endothelium. Note that thrombin can also release platelet activating factor (PAF) which induces thrombus formation.

inhibitor, C4b-binding protein, the C3 control protein factors H and I, complement receptor CR1, *decay accelerating factor* (DAF), *membrane cofactor protein* (MCP) and immunoconglutinin, and finally the proteins which block the membrane attack complex, homologous restriction factor and CD59 (discussed further on p. 307). Some of the acute phase proteins derived from the plasma transudate would be expected to act as protease inhibitors.

At the cellular level, PGE$_2$, transforming growth factor-β (TGFβ) and glucocorticoids are powerful regulators. PGE$_2$ is a potent inhibitor of lymphocyte proliferation and cytokine production by T-cells and macrophages. TGFβ deactivates macrophages by inhibiting the production of reactive oxygen intermediates and downregulating MHC class II expression; it also quells the cytotoxic enthusiasm of both macrophages and γ-interferon (IFNγ)-activated NK cells. Endogenous glucocorticoids produced via the hypothalamic–pituitary–adrenal axis exert their anti-inflammatory effects both through the *repression* of a number of genes, including those for proinflammatory

cytokines and adhesion molecules, and the *induction* of the inflammation inhibitors lipocortin-1, secretory leukocyte proteinase inhibitor and IL-1 receptor antagonist. IL-10 inhibits antigen presentation, cytokine production and nitric oxide (NO) killing by macrophages, the latter inhibition being greatly enhanced by synergistic action with IL-4 and TGFβ.

Once the inflammatory agent has been cleared, these regulatory processes will normalize the site. When the inflammation traumatizes tissues through its intensity and extent, TGFβ plays a major role in the subsequent wound healing by stimulating fibroblast division and the laying down of new extracellular matrix elements.

Chronic inflammation

If an inflammatory agent persists, either because of its resistance to metabolic breakdown or through the inability of a deficient immune system to clear an infectious microbe, the character of the cellular response changes. The site becomes dominated by macrophages with varying morphology: many have an activated appearance, some form arrays of what are termed 'epithelioid' cells and others fuse to form giant cells. If an adaptive immune response is involved, lymphocytes in various guises will also be present. This characteristic **granuloma** walls off the persisting agent from the remainder of the body (see section on type IV hypersensitivity in Chapter 16, p. 343).

EXTRACELLULAR BACTERIA SUSCEPTIBLE TO KILLING BY PHAGOCYTOSIS AND COMPLEMENT

Bacterial survival strategies

The variety and ingenuity of these escape mechanisms are most intriguing and, as with virtually all infectious agents, if you can think of a possible avoidance strategy, some microbe will already have used it.

Evading phagocytosis

The cell walls of bacteria are multifarious (figure 13.5) and in some cases are inherently resistant to a number of microbicidal agents; but a common mechanism by which virulent forms escape phagocytosis is by synthesis of an outer **capsule**, which does not adhere readily to phagocytic cells and covers carbohydrate molecules on the bacterial surface which could otherwise be recognized by phagocyte receptors (figure 13.6a). For example, as few as 10 encapsulated pneumococci can kill a mouse but, if the capsule is removed by treatment with hyaluronidase, 10 000 bacteria are required for the job. Many pathogens evolve capsules which physically prevent access of phagocytes to C3b deposited on the bacterial cell wall.

Other organisms have actively **antiphagocytic** cell surface molecules and some go so far as to secrete **exo-**

toxins, which actually poison the leukocytes (figure 13.6b). Yet another devious ruse is to exploit binding to the surface of a nonphagocytic cell so gaining entry into a shelter from the depredations of the professional phagocyte (figure 13.6c). Presumably, some organisms try to avoid undue provocation of phagocytic cells by adhering to and *colonizing the external mucosal surfaces* of the intestine.

Challenging the complement system

Poor activation of complement. Normal mammalian cells are protected from complement destruction by regulatory proteins such as complement receptor CR1, MCP and DAF, which cause C3 convertase breakdown (see p. 307 for further discussion). Microorganisms lack these regulatory proteins so that, even in the absence of antibody, most of them would activate the alternative C pathway by stabilization of the C3bBb convertase on their surfaces. However, bacterial capsules in general tend to be poor activators of the alternative complement pathway and selective pressures have obviously favored the synthesis of capsules whose surface components do not favor stable binding of the convertase complex (figure 13.6d).

Acceleration of complement breakdown. Members of the regulators of complement activation (RCA) family which diminish C3 convertase activity include C4b-binding protein (C4BP), factor H and factor H-like protein 1 (FHL-1). Certain bacterial surface molecules, notably those rich in sialic acid, bind factor H (figure 13.6e), which then acts as a focus for the degradation of

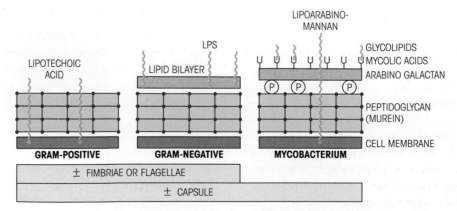

Figure 13.5. The structure of bacterial cell walls. All types have an inner cell membrane and a peptidoglycan wall which can be cleaved by lysozyme and lysosomal enzymes. The outer lipid bilayer of Gram-negative bacteria, which is susceptible to the action of complement or cationic proteins, sometimes contains lipopolysaccharide (LPS; also known as endotoxin; composed of O-specific oligosaccharide side-chains attached to a basal core polysaccharide, itself linked to the mitogenic moiety, lipid A; 148 O antigen variants of *Escherichia coli* are known). The mycobacterial cell wall is highly resistant to breakdown. When present, outer capsules may protect the bacteria from phagocytosis.

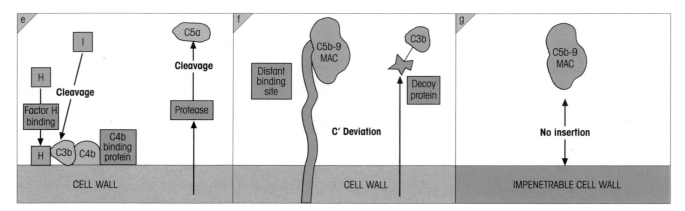

Figure 13.6. Avoidance strategies by extracellular bacteria. (a) Capsule gives poor phagocyte adherence. (b) Exotoxin poisons phagocyte. (c) Microbe attaches to surface component to enter nonphagocytic cell. (d) Capsule provides nonstabilizing surface for alternative pathway convertase. (e) Accelerating breakdown of complement by action of microbial products. (f) Complement effectors are deviated from the microbial cell wall. (g) Cell wall impervious to complement membrane attack complex (MAC).

C3b by the serine protease factor I (cf. p. 11). This is seen, for example, with *Neisseria gonorrhoeae*. Similarly, the hypervariable regions of the M-proteins of certain *Streptococcus pyogenes* (group A streptococcus) strains are able to bind FHL-1, whilst other strains downregulate complement activation by interacting with C4BP, this time acting as a cofactor for factor I-mediated degradation of the C4b component of the classical pathway C3 convertase C$\overline{4b2a}$. There is evidence that C4BP can also inhibit activation of the alternative pathway. Certain strains of group B streptococci produce a C5a-ase which may act as a virulence factor by proteolytically cleaving and thereby inactivating C5a (figure 13.6e).

Complement deviation. Some species manage to avoid lysis by deviating the complement activation site either to a secreted decoy protein or to a position on the bacterial surface distant from the cell membrane (figure 13.6f).

Resistance to insertion of terminal complement components. Gram-positive organisms (cf. figure 13.5) have evolved thick peptidoglycan layers which prevent the insertion of the lytic C5b–9 membrane attack complex into the bacterial cell membrane (figure 13.6g). Many capsules do the same.

Interfering with internal events in the macrophage

Enteric Gram-negative bacteria in the gut have developed a number of ways of influencing macrophage activity, including inducing apoptosis, enhancing the production of IL-1, preventing phagosome–lysosome fusion and affecting the actin cytoskeleton (figure 13.7).

Antigenic variation

Although the strategy of varying individual antigens in the face of a determined host antibody response is more usually associated with viruses and parasites, there are a few well-defined examples in bacteria. These include variation of surface lipoproteins in the lyme disease spirochete *Borrelia burgdorferi*, alterations in enzymes involved in synthesizing surface struc-

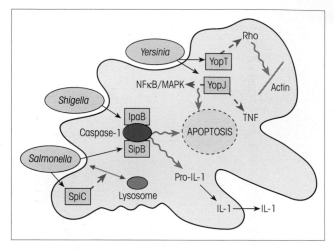

Figure 13.7. Evasion of macrophage defenses by enteric bacteria. The IpaB and SipB proteins secreted by *Shigella* and *Salmonella*, respectively, can activate caspase 1 and thereby set off a train of events that will lead to the death of the macrophage by apoptosis. Activated caspase 1 also triggers a protease which cleaves pro-IL-1, thereby causing the release of large amounts of this proinflammatory cytokine from the macrophage. Paradoxically, this may be advantageous to the bacteria because the subsequent migration of neutrophils to the intestinal lumen results in a loosening of intercellular junctions between the enterocytes, permitting cellular invasion of the basolateral surface by organisms from the lumen. The SpiC protein from *Salmonella* inhibits the trafficking of cellular vesicles, and therefore is able to prevent lysosomes fusing with phagocytic vesicles. *Yersinia* produces a number of Yop molecules (*Yersinia outer proteins*) able to interfere with the normal functioning of the phagocyte. For example, YopJ inhibits TNF production and downregulates NFκB and MAP kinases, thereby facilitating apoptosis by inhibiting anti-apoptotic pathways. YopT prevents phagocytosis by modifying the GTPase Rho involved in regulating the actin cytoskeleton. (Based on Donnenberg M.S. (2000) *Nature* **406**, 768.)

tures in *Campylobacter jejuni* and antigenic variation of the pili in *Neisseria meningitidis*. In addition, new strains can arise, as has occurred with the life-threatening *E. coli* O157:H7 which can cause hemolytic uremic syndrome and appears to have emerged about 50 years ago by incorporation of *Shigella* toxin genes into the *E. coli* 055 genome.

The host counter-attack

The defense mechanisms exploit the specificity and variability of the antibody molecule. Antibodies can defeat these devious attempts to avoid engulfment by neutralizing the antiphagocytic molecules and by binding to the surface of the organisms to focus the site for fixation of complement, so 'opsonizing' them for ingestion by neutrophils and macrophages or preparing them for the terminal membrane attack complex (Milestone 13.1). However, antibody production by B-cells usually requires T-cell help, and the T-cells need to be activated by antigen-presenting cells.

As already discussed in Chapter 1, *p*athogen-associated *m*olecular *p*atterns (PAMPs), such as the all-important lipopolysaccharide (LPS) endotoxin of Gram-negative bacteria, peptidoglycan, lipoteichoic acids, mannans, bacterial DNA, double-stranded RNA and glucans, are all molecules which are broadly expressed by microbial pathogens but are not present on the host tissues. Thus these molecules serve as an

Milestone 13.1—The Protective Effects of Antibody

The pioneering research which led to the recognition of the antibacterial protection afforded by antibody clustered in the last years of the 19th century. A good place to start the story is the discovery by Roux and Yersin in 1888, at the still famous Pasteur Institute in Paris, that the exotoxin of diphtheria bacillus could be isolated from a bacterium-free filtrate of the medium used to culture the organism. von Behring and Kitasato at Koch's Institute in Berlin in 1890 then went on to show that animals could develop an immunity to such toxins which was due to the development of specific neutralizing antidotes referred to generally as **antibodies**. They further succeeded in passively transferring immunity to another animal with serum containing the antitoxin. The dawning of an era of serotherapy came in 1894 with Roux's successful treatment of patients with diphtheria by injection of immune horse serum.

The immunological community then got its intellectual underwear in something of a twist over the next few years, first by advocates of the view that all bacterial immunity was due to antitoxins, and second by Metchnikoff's rigid espousal of phagocytosis itself as the main, if not the only, real bulwark of defense against infection. The situation was resolved by our shining knight Sir Almroth Wright in London in 1903 who proposed that the main action of the increased antibody produced after infection was to reinforce killing by the phagocytes. He called the antibodies **opsonins** (Gk. *opson*, a dressing or relish), because they prepared the bacteria as food for the phagocytic cells, and amply verified his predictions by showing that antibodies dramatically increased the phagocytosis of bacteria *in vitro*, thereby cleverly linking *innate* to *adaptive* immunity.

(continued)

Figure M13.1.1. Emil von Behring (1854–1917).

Figure M13.1.3. Sir Almroth Wright. (Slide kindly supplied by The Wellcome Centre Medical Photographic Library, London.)

Figure M13.1.2. von Behring extracting serum using a tap. Caricature by Lustigen Blättern, 1894. (Legend: 'Serum direct from the horse! Freshly drawn.') (Slide kindly supplied by The Wellcome Centre Medical Photographic Library, London.)

It was a feature of the time that major controversies were slugged out in pamphlets, books and plays, and it was impressive that Bernard Shaw should enter the fray on the side of Almroth Wright in his play *The Doctor's Dilemma*. In the preface he gave an evocative description of the function of opsonins: 'Sir Almroth Wright, following up one of Metchnikoff's most suggestive biological romances, discovered that the white corpuscles or phagocytes which attack and devour disease germs for us do their work only when we butter the disease germs appetizingly for them with a natural sauce which Sir Almroth named opsonins . . . .' (More extended and very readable accounts of immunology at the turn of the 19th century may be found in Humphrey J.H. & White R.G. (1970) *Immunology for Students of Medicine*, 3rd edn, Ch. 1. Blackwell Scientific Publications, Oxford; Craps L. (1993) *The Birth of Immunology*. Sandoz, Basel; and Silverstein A.M. (1989) *A History of Immunology*. Academic Press, San Diego.)

alerting service for the immune system, which detects their presence using a number of pattern recognition receptors (PRRs) expressed on the surface of antigen-presenting cells. Such receptors include the mannose receptor (CD206) which facilitates phagocytosis of microorganisms by macrophages and the scavenger receptor (CD204) which mediates clearance of bacteria from the circulation. Binding of LPS to the CD14 PRR on monocytes, macrophages, dendritic cells and B-cells leads to the recruitment of the toll-like receptor 4 (TLR4) molecule which is able to mediate signals activating the expression of a broad range of pro-inflammatory genes, including those for IL-1, IL-6, IL-12 and TNF and for the B7.1 (CD80) and B7.2

(CD86) costimulatory molecules. A related receptor, TLR2, recognizes Gram-positive bacterial cell wall components.

Toxin neutralization

Circulating antibodies act to neutralize the soluble antiphagocytic molecules and other exotoxins (e.g. phospholipase C of *Clostridium welchii*) released by bacteria. Combination near the biologically active site of the toxin would stereochemically block reaction with the substrate, particularly if it were macromolecular; combination distant from the active site may also cause inhibition through allosteric conformational changes. In its complex with antibody, the toxin may be unable to diffuse away rapidly and will be susceptible to phagocytosis, especially if the complex can be increased in size by the action of naturally occurring autoantibodies to complexed IgG (antiglobulin factors) and C3b (immunoconglutinin, not to be confused with bovine *conglutinin*, a nonantibody molecule which combines with the carbohydrate portion of C3b).

Opsonization of bacteria

Independently of antibody. Differences between the carbohydrate structures on bacteria and self are exploited by the **collectins**, a series of molecules with similar ultrastructure to C1q and which bear C-terminal lectin domains. These include mannose-binding protein (MBP; also referred to as mannose-binding lectin, MBL), lung surfactant proteins SP-A and SP-D and, in cattle, conglutinin, which all recognize carbohydrate ligands. Mannose-binding protein can bind to terminal mannose on the bacterial surface and then interacts with MBP-associated serine protease (MASP) which is homologous in structure to C1r and C1s. Thus the interaction is closely similar to that of C1q with C1r and s (cf. p. 22) and, in this way, leads to the antibody-independent activation of the classical pathway. SP-A, SP-D and conglutinin can all act as opsonins (see Milestone 13.1) and can mediate phagocytosis by virtue of their binding to the C1q receptor.

Augmented by antibody. Encapsulated bacteria which resist phagocytosis become extremely attractive to neutrophils and macrophages when coated with antibody and their rate of clearance from the bloodstream is strikingly enhanced (figure 13.8). The less effective removal of coated bacteria in complement-depleted animals emphasizes the synergism between antibody and complement for opsonization which is mediated

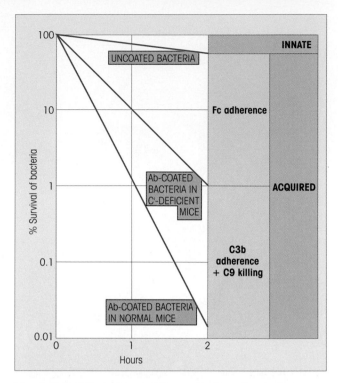

Figure 13.8. Effect of opsonizing antibody and complement on rate of clearance of virulent bacteria from the blood. The uncoated bacteria are phagocytosed rather slowly (*innate immunity*) but, on coating with antibody, adherence to phagocytes is increased manyfold (*acquired immunity*). The adherence is less effective in animals temporarily depleted of complement. This is a hypothetical but realistic situation; the natural proliferation of the bacteria has been ignored.

through specific high affinity receptors for IgG and C3b on the phagocyte surface (figure 13.9). It is clearly advantageous that the subclasses which bind strongly to these Fc receptors (e.g. IgG1 and IgG3 in the human) also fix complement well, it being appreciated that the heterodimer of C3b bound to IgG is a very efficient opsonin because it engages two receptors simultaneously. Complexes containing C3b and C4b may show immune adherence to the CR1 complement receptors on erythrocytes to provide aggregates which are transported to the liver and spleen for phagocytosis.

Some elaboration on **complement receptors** may be pertinent at this stage. The CR1 receptor (CD35) for C3b is also present on neutrophils, eosinophils, monocytes, B-cells and lymph node follicular dendritic cells. Together with the CR3 receptor (CD11b/CD18), it has the main responsibility for clearance of complexes containing C3. The *CR1* gene is linked in a cluster with C4b-binding protein and factor H, all of which subserve a regulatory function by binding to C3b or C4b to disassemble the C3/C5 convertases, and act as cofactors for the proteolytic inactivation of C3b and C4b by factor I.

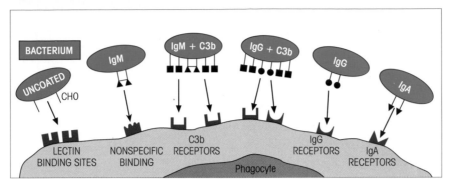

Figure 13.9. Immunoglobulin and complement coats greatly increase the adherence of bacteria (and other antigens) to macrophages and neutrophils. Uncoated bacteria adhere to lectin-like sites, including the mannose-binding receptor. There are no specific binding sites for IgM (▲▲), but there are high affinity receptors for IgG (Fc) (●) and iC3b (■) on the macrophage surface which considerably enhance the strength of binding. The aug-menting effect of complement is due to the fact that two adjacent IgG molecules can fix many C3b molecules, thereby increasing the number of links to the macrophage (cf. 'bonus effect of mul-tivalency'; p. 87). Although IgM does not bind specifically to the macrophage, it promotes adherence through complement fixation. Specific receptors for the Fcα domains of IgA have also been defined.

CR2 receptors (CD21) for iC3b, C3dg and C3d are present on B-cells and follicular dendritic cells and transduce accessory signals for B-cell activation especially in the germinal centers (cf. p. 190). Their affinity for the Epstein–Barr virus (EBV) provides the means for entry of the virus into the B-cell.

CR3 receptors (CD11b/CD18 on neutrophils, eosinophils, monocytes and NK cells) bind iC3b, C3dg and C3d. They are related to LFA-1 and CR4 (CD11c/CD18, binds iC3b and C3dg) in being members of the β_2 integrin subfamily (cf. table 8.2). CR5 is found on neutrophils and platelets and binds C3d and C3dg. A number of other complement receptors have been described including some with specificity for C1q, for C3a and C4a, and the CD88 molecule with specificity for C5a.

Some further effects of complement

Some strains of Gram-negative bacteria which have a lipoprotein outer wall resembling mammalian surface membranes in structure are susceptible to the bacteri-cidal action of fresh serum containing antibody. The antibody initiates the development of a complement-mediated lesion which is said to allow access of serum lysozyme to the inner peptidoglycan wall of the bac-terium to cause eventual cell death. Activation of com-plement through union of antibody and bacterium will also generate the C3a and C5a anaphylatoxins leading to extensive transudation of serum compo-nents, including more antibody, and to the chemotactic attraction of neutrophils to aid in phagocytosis, as de-scribed earlier under the acute inflammation umbrella (cf. figures 2.18 and 13.3).

The secretory immune system protects the external mucosal surfaces

We have earlier emphasized the critical nature of the mucosal barriers, particularly in the gut, where there is a potentially hostile interface with the microbial hordes. With an area of around $400\,\text{m}^2$, give or take a tennis court or two, the epithelium of the adult mu-cosae represents the most frequent portal of entry for common infectious agents, allergens and carcinogens. The need for well-marshaled, highly effective mucosal immunity is glaringly obvious. Awareness of such a need was evident even in bygone days. Per Brandtzaeg relates an amusing historical example.

In ancient times, kings were perpetually worried that they would be poisoned by their enemies. (One heard tell that the habit of clinking glasses together in a toast has its origin in the custom of pouring some of one's wine into the glass of the next person and so on until the operation had come full circle.) Anyway, Mithridates VI Eupator, King of Pontus (now part of Turkey) in the 1st century BC, was so frightened of being poisoned that he attempted to increase his in-testinal defenses by drinking the blood of ducks which had been fed poisonous weeds. After defeat by the Ro-mans and mutiny in his army he tried unsuccessfully to poison himself, testimony to the effectiveness of oral immunization. As a grisly negative control, his two daughters had no difficulty in committing suicide using the same poison, whereupon the desperate king was forced to order his bodyguard to kill him with a more conventional weapon.

The gut mucosal surfaces are defended by both antigen-specific and nonantigen-specific mechanisms.

Figure 13.10. Defense of the mucosal surfaces. (a) IgA opsonizes organisms and prevents adherence to the mucosa. (b) IgE recruits agents of the immune response by firing the release of mediators from mast cells.

Among the nonspecific mechanisms, those provided by antimicrobial peptides are worth highlighting. These are produced not only by neutrophils and macrophages but also by mucosal epithelium, where they serve as a primary bacterial defense barrier. As described in Chapter 1, the group of antimicrobial peptides called defensins cause lysis of bacteria via disruption of their surface membranes. Specific immunity is provided by secretory IgA and IgM, with IgA1 predominating in the upper areas and IgA2 in the large bowel. Most other mucosal surfaces are also protected predominantly by IgA with the surprising exception of the reproductive tract tissues of both male and female, where the dominant antibody isotype is IgG. The size of the task is highlighted by the fact that 80% of the Ig-producing B-cells in the body are present in the secretory mucosae and exocrine glands. IgA antibodies afford protection in the external body fluids, tears, saliva, nasal secretions and those bathing the surfaces of the intestine and lung by coating bacteria and viruses and preventing their adherence to the epithelial cells of the mucous membranes, which is essential for viral infection and bacterial colonization. Secretory IgA molecules themselves have very little innate adhesiveness for epithelial cells, but high affinity Fc receptors for this Ig class are present on macrophages and neutrophils and can mediate phagocytosis (figure 13.10a).

If an infectious agent succeeds in penetrating the IgA barrier, it comes up against the next line of defense of the secretory system (see p. 154) which is manned by

IgE. There are obvious parallels between the ways in which complement-derived anaphylatoxins and IgE utilize the mast cell to cause local amplification of the immune defenses. It is worth noting that most serum IgE arises from plasma cells in mucosal tissues and in the lymph nodes that drain them. Although present in low concentration, IgE is bound very firmly to the Fc receptors of the mast cell (see p. 55) and contact with antigen leads to the release of mediators which effectively recruit agents of the immune response and generate a local acute inflammatory reaction. Thus histamine, by increasing vascular permeability, causes the transudation of IgG and complement into the area, while chemotactic factors for neutrophils and eosinophils attract the effector cells needed to dispose of the infectious organism coated with specific IgG and C3b (figure 13.10b). Engagement of the Fcγ and C3b receptors on local macrophages by such complexes will lead to secretion of factors which further reinforce these vascular permeability and chemotactic events. Broadly, one would say that immune exclusion in the gut is noninflammatory, but immune elimination of organisms which penetrate the mucosa is proinflammatory.

Where the opsonized organism is too large to be engulfed, phagocytes can kill by an extracellular mechanism after attachment by their Fcγ receptors. This phenomenon, termed *antibody-dependent cellular cytotoxicity* (ADCC), has been discussed earlier (see p. 32) and there is evidence for its involvement in parasitic infections (see p. 271).

The mucosal tissues contain a variety of T-lymphocyte species, but their role and that of the mucosal epithelial cells, other than in a helper function for local antibody production, is of less relevance for the defense against extracellular bacteria.

Some specific bacterial infections

First let us see how these considerations apply to defense against infection by common organisms such as streptococci and staphylococci. β-Hemolytic **streptococci** were classified by Lancefield according to their carbohydrate antigen, and the most important for human disease are those belonging to group A. *Streptococcus pyogenes* posed a major worldwide health threat; in 1981, more than six million children suffered from associated rheumatic disease in India alone, and resurgence of a highly virulent strain causing rheumatic fever and toxic shock syndrome has occurred in the USA.

The most important virulence factor is the surface M-protein (variants of which form the basis of the Griffith typing). This protein is an acceptor for factor H which facilitates C3b breakdown, and binds fibrinogen and its fragments which cover sites that may act as complement activators (figure 13.11). It thereby inhibits opsonization and the protection afforded by antibodies to the M-component is attributable to the striking increase in phagocytosis which they induce. The ability of group A streptococci to elicit cross-reactive autoantibodies which bind to cardiac myosin is thought to be involved in poststreptococcal autoimmune disease. High titer antibodies to the streptolysin O exotoxin (ASO), which damages membranes, are indicators of recent streptococcal infection. The streptococcal *pyrogenic exotoxins* SPE A, B and C are superantigens associated with scarlet fever and toxic shock syndrome. The toxins are neutralized by antibody and the erythematous intradermal reaction to injected toxin (the Dick reaction) is only seen in individuals lacking antibody. Antibody can also neutralize bacterial enzymes like hyaluronidase which act to spread the infection.

Streptococcus mutans is an important cause of both endocarditis and dental caries. The organism has a constitutive enzyme, glucosyltransferase, able to convert sucrose to dextran which is utilized for adhesion to the tooth surface. Passive transfer of IgG, but not IgA or IgM, antibodies to *S. mutans* in monkeys conferred protection against caries. It is thought that IgG antibody and complement in the gingival crevicular fluid bathing the tooth opsonize the bacteria to facilitate phagocytosis and killing by neutrophils. Curiously, a single treatment with a monoclonal anti-*S. mutans* kept teeth free of the microorganism for 1 year, perhaps due to a shift in bacterial ecology, with the place vacated by *S. mutans* being filled with another organism from the oral flora.

Virulent forms of **staphylococci**, of which *Staphylo-*

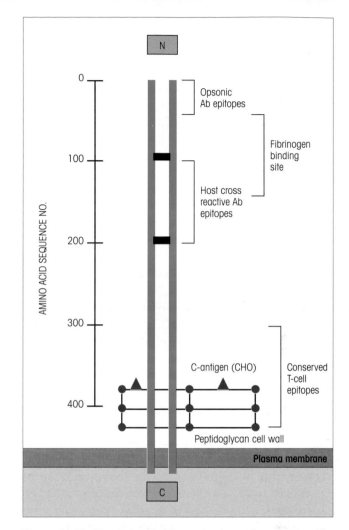

Figure 13.11. Streptococcal M-protein from *S. pyogenes*. The coiled-coil dimers are approximately 50 nm long. (Based on Robinson J.H. & Kehoe M.A. (1992) *Immunology Today* **13**, 362.)

coccus aureus is perhaps the most common, resist phagocytosis. This may be due partly to capsule formation *in vivo* and partly to the elaboration of factors such as a coagulase enzyme which could protect the bacterium by a barrier of fibrin. It has been suggested that the ability of a cell wall component, protein A, to combine with the Fc portion of IgG (other than subclass IgG3) is responsible for inhibition of phagocytosis by virulent strains, but IgG–protein A complexes fix complement and one study reports that protein A actually increases complement-mediated phagocytosis. We must return an open verdict on that issue. It seems to be accepted that *S. aureus* is readily phagocytosed in the presence of *adequate* amounts of antibody, but a small proportion of the ingested bacteria survives and they are difficult organisms to eliminate completely. Where the infection is inadequately controlled, severe lesions may occur in the immunized host as a consequence of type IV delayed hypersensitivity reactions. Thus, staphylococci were found to be avirulent when injected into mice passively immunized with antibody, but caused extensive tissue damage in animals previously given sensitized T-cells.

Other examples where antibodies are required to overcome the inherently antiphagocytic properties of **bacterial capsules** are seen in immunity to infection by pneumococci, meningococci and *Haemophilus influenzae*. *Bacillus anthrax* possesses an antiphagocytic capsule composed of a γ-polypeptide of D-glutamic acid but, although anticapsular antibodies effectively promote uptake by neutrophils, the exotoxin is so potent that vaccines are inadequate unless they also stimulate antitoxin immunity. In addition to releasing such lethal exotoxins, *Pseudomonas aeruginosa* also produces an elastase that inactivates C3a and C5a; as a result, only minimal inflammatory responses are made in the absence of neutralizing antibodies.

The ploy of **diverting complement activation** to insensitive sites is seen rather well with different strains of Gram-negative *Salmonella* and *Escherichia coli* organisms which vary in the number of O-specific oligosaccharide side-chains attached to the lipid-A-linked core polysaccharide of the endotoxin (cf. figure 13.5). Variants with long side-chains are relatively insensitive to killing by serum through the alternative complement pathway (see p. 11); as the side-chains become shorter and shorter, the serum sensitivity increases. Although all variants activate the alternative pathway, only those with short or no side-chains allow the cytotoxic membrane attack complex to be inserted near to the outer lipid bilayer (figure 13.6f). On the other hand, antibodies focus the complex to a more vulnerable site.

The destruction of gonococci by serum containing antibody is dependent upon the formation of the membrane attack complex, and rare individuals lacking C8 or C9 are susceptible to *Neisseria* infection. *N. gonorrhoeae* (gonococci) specifically binds complement proteins and prevents their insertion in the outer membranes, but antibody, like a ubiquitous 'Mr Fixit', corrects this situation, at least so far as the host is concerned. With respect to the infective process itself, IgA produced in the genital tract in response to these organisms inhibits the attachment of the bacteria, through their pili, to mucosal cells, but seems unable to afford adequate protection against reinfection. This seems to be due to a very effective antigenic shift mechanism which alters the sequence of the expressed pilin by gene conversion. The outer membrane protein P or B inhibits phagocyte microbicidal activity and induces apoptosis in the target cells. Failure to achieve good protection might also be a reflection of the ability of the gonococci to produce a protease which cleaves a proline-rich sequence present in the hinge region of IgA1 (but not of IgA2), although the presence in most individuals of neutralizing antibodies against this protease may interfere with its proteolytic activity. Meningococci, which frequently infect the nasopharynx, *H. influenzae* and *S. pneumoniae* have similar unfair proteases.

Cholera is caused by the colonization of the small intestine by *Vibrio cholerae* and the subsequent action of its enterotoxin. The B subunits of the toxin bind to specific GM1 monosialoganglioside receptors and translocate the A subunit across the membrane where it activates adenyl cyclase. The increased cAMP then causes fluid loss by inhibiting uptake of sodium chloride and stimulating active Cl⁻ secretion by intestinal epithelial cells. Locally synthesized IgA antibodies against *V. cholerae* lipopolysaccharide and the toxin provide independent protection against cholera, the first by inhibiting bacterial adherence to the intestinal wall, the second by blocking attachment of the toxin to its receptor. In accord with this analysis are the epidemiological data showing that children who drink milk with high titers of IgA antibodies specific for either of these antigens are less likely to develop clinical cholera.

Yersinia and *Salmonella* are among the select number of bacterial pathogens which have evolved special mechanisms to enter, survive and replicate within normally **nonphagocytic host cells**. The former gains entry through binding of its outer membrane protein, invasin, to multiple β₁ integrin receptors on the host cell. *Salmonella*, on the other hand, induces membrane ruffling on the target cell, linked in some way to signaling events which lead to bacterial uptake.

The ways in which antibody can parry the different facets of bacterial invasion are summarized in figure 13.12.

BACTERIA WHICH GROW IN AN INTRACELLULAR HABITAT

Bacterial gambits

Some strains of bacteria, such as the tubercle and leprosy bacilli and *Listeria* and *Brucella* organisms, escape the wrath of the immune system by cheekily fashioning an intracellular life within one of its strongholds, the macrophage no less. Mononuclear phagocytes are a good target for such organisms in the sense that they are very mobile and allow wide dissemination throughout the body. Entry of opsonized bacteria is facilitated by phagocytic uptake after attachment to

Figure 13.12. Antibody defenses against bacterial invasion.

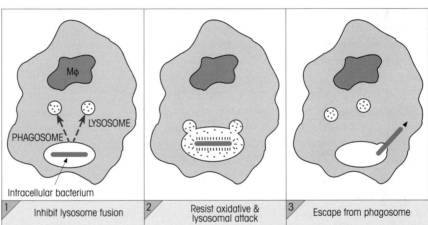

Figure 13.13. Evasion of phagocytic death by intracellular bacteria.

Fcγ and C3b receptors but, once inside, many of them defy the mighty macrophage by subverting the innate killing mechanisms in a variety of ways. Organisms such as *Mycobacterium tuberculosis* inhibit fusion of the lysosomes with the phagocytic vacuole containing the ingested bacterium (figure 13.13). Mycobacterial lipids, such as lipoarabinomannan, obstruct priming and activation of the macrophage and also protect the bacteria from attack by scavenging reactive oxygen intermediates such as superoxide anion, hydroxyl radicals and hydrogen peroxide (cf. p. 6). Organisms such as *Listeria monocytogenes* use a special lysin to escape from their phagosomal prison to lie happily free within the cytoplasm; some rickettsiae and the protozoan *Trypanosoma cruzi* can do the same. If there is a mechanism available to inhibit, some microorganisms will eventually find a way to do it.

Defense is by T-cell-mediated immunity (CMI)

In an elegant series of experiments, Mackaness demonstrated the importance of CMI reactions for the killing of intracellular parasites and the establishment of an immune state. Animals infected with moderate doses of *M. tuberculosis* overcome the infection and are immune to subsequent challenge with the bacillus. The immunity can be transferred to a normal recipient with T-lymphocytes but not macrophages or serum from an immune animal. Supporting this view, that specific immunity is mediated by T-cells, is the greater susceptibility to infection with tubercle and leprosy bacilli of mice in which the T-lymphocytes have been depressed by thymectomy plus anti-T-cell monoclonals, or in which the TCR genes have been disrupted by homologous gene recombination (knockout mice).

Activated macrophages kill intracellular parasites

When monocytes first settle down in the tissue to become 'resident' macrophages they are essentially downregulated with respect to the expression of surface receptors and function. They can be activated in several stages (figure 13.14), but the ability to kill obligate intracellular microbes only comes after stimulation by macrophage activating factor(s), such as IFNγ released from stimulated cytokine-producing T-cells. Foremost amongst the killing mechanisms which are upregulated are those mediated by reactive oxygen intermediates and NO·. The activated macrophage is undeniably a remarkable and formidable cell, capable of secreting the 60 or so substances which are concerned in chronic inflammatory reactions (figure 13.15)—not the sort to meet in an alley on a dark night!

The mechanism of T-cell-mediated immunity in the Mackaness experiments now becomes clear. Specifically primed T-cells react with processed antigen derived from the intracellular bacteria present on the surface of the infected macrophage in association with MHC II; the subsequent release of cytokines activates the macrophage and endows it with the ability to kill the organisms it has phagocytosed (figure 13.16).

Examples of intracellular bacterial infections

Listeria

Undoubtedly, T-helper-1 (Th1)-activated macrophages are crucially important for the ultimate elimination

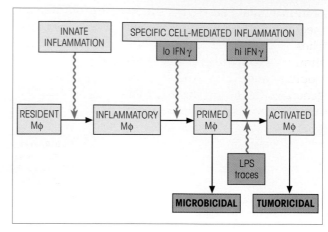

Figure 13.14. Stages in the activation of macrophages (Mφ) for microbicidal and tumoricidal function. Macrophages taken from sites of inflammation induced by complement or nonimmunological stimuli, such as thioglycollate, are considerably increased in size, acid hydrolase content, secretion of neutral proteinases and phagocytic function. If we may give one example, the C3b receptors on resident Mφ are not freely mobile in the membrane and so cannot permit the 'zippering' process required for phagocytosis (see p. 6); consequently, they bind but do not ingest C3b-coated red cells. Inflammatory Mφ, on the other hand, have C3 receptors which display considerable lateral mobility and the C3-opsonized erythrocytes are readily phagocytosed. In addition to the dramatic upregulation of intracellular killing mechanisms, striking changes in surface components accompany activation. In mouse macrophages there is an increase in class II MHC (dramatic), Fc receptors for IgG2b and binding sites for tumor cells; in contrast, the mannose receptor (CD206), the F4/80 marker and IgG2a receptors all decline, while the Mac-I (CD11b) component of the CR3 iC3b receptor remains unchanged.

Figure 13.15. The role of the activated macrophage in the initiation and mediation of chronic inflammation with concomitant tissue repair, and in the killing of microbes and tumor cells. It is possible that macrophages differentiate along distinct pathways to subserve these different functions. The electron micrograph shows a highly activated macrophage with many lysozomal structures which have been highlighted by the uptake of thorotrast; one (arrowed) is seen fusing with a phagosome containing the protozoan *Toxoplasma gondii*. (Courtesy of Professor C. Jones.)

of intracellular *Listeria*, but the complex role of innate mechanisms early in infection must be considered. These are outlined in figure 13.17, where attention should be drawn to the bactericidal action of neutrophils and the central action of IL-12, which generates the macrophage activator IFNγ through its stimulation of NK cells and recruitment of Th1 helpers. Mutant mice lacking αβ and/or γδ T-cells reveal that

Figure 13.16. The 'cytokine connection': nonspecific murine macrophage killing of intracellular bacteria triggered by a specific T-cell-mediated immunity reaction. (a) Specific CD4 Th1 cell recognizes mycobacterial peptide associated with MHC class II and releases Mφ activating IFNγ. (b) The activated Mφ kills the intracellular TB, mainly through generation of toxic NO·. (c) A 'senile' Mφ, unable to destroy the intracellular bacteria, is killed by CD8 and CD4 cytotoxic cells and possibly by IL-2-activated NK cells. The Mφ then releases live tubercle bacilli which are taken up and killed by newly recruited Mφ susceptible to IFNγ activation (d). Human monocytes require activation by both IFNγ and IL-4 plus a CD23-mediated signal for induction of iNO synthase and production of NO·.

these two cell types make comparable contributions to resistance against primary *Listeria* infection, but that the αβ TCR set bears the major responsibility for conferring protective immunity. γδ T-cells control the local tissue response at the site of microbial replication and γδ knockout mutants develop huge abscesses when infected with *Listeria*.

Tuberculosis

Tuberculosis (TB) is on the rampage, aided by the emergence of multidrug-resistant strains of *Mycobacterium tuberculosis*. It is predicted that a total of 225 million new cases and 79 million deaths will occur between 1998 and 2030. This is not helped by the fact that human immunodeficiency virus (HIV)-infected individuals with low CD4 counts have increased susceptibility to *M. tuberculosis* infection.

With respect to host defense mechanisms, as seen with *Listeria* infection, murine macrophages activated by IFNγ can destroy intracellular mycobacteria with magisterial ease, largely through the generation of toxic NO·. Some parasitized macrophages reach a stage at which they are too incapacitated to be stirred into action by T-cell messages, and here a somewhat ruthless strategy has evolved in which the host deploys cytotoxic CD8, and possibly CD4 and NK cells, to execute the helpless macrophage and release the live mycobacteria; these should now be taken up by newly immigrant phagocytic cells susceptible to activation by IFNγ and summarily disposed of (figure 13.16).

The position is more complicated in the human. IFNγ-stimulated human monocytes cannot eliminate intracellular TB, although there is some stasis and IFNγ does upregulate expression of the 1-hydroxylase which converts vitamin D_3 into the 1,25-dihydroxy form, a potent activator of antimycobacterial mechanisms. However, there is no induction of NO· synthase (iNOS type II) unless IL-4 is also added to the system, whereupon there is copious production of NO· in a CD23-dependent reaction.

A further plethora of potential defensive mechanisms is emerging. The TB products Ag85B (a mycolyl transferase) and ESAT-6 are potent inducers of IFNγ from CD4 cells. CD4$^-$8$^-$ αβ T-cells proliferate in response to mycolic acid and lyse cells presenting the acid in the context of CD1b, while human $V\gamma_2V\delta_2$ T-cells recognize protein antigens, isopentenyl pyrophosphates and prenyl pyrophosphates from *M. tuberculosis*. The γδ T-cells have an eerie, almost compelling, relationship to mycobacterial antigens. A substantial proportion of them can lyse target cells presenting mycobacterial antigens and, in the mouse, a

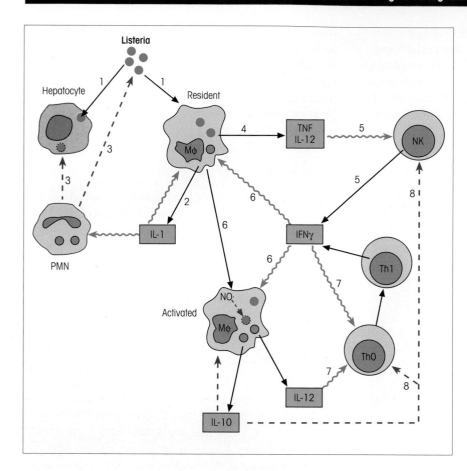

Figure 13.17. Immune response to *Listeria* infection. (1) *Listeria* infects resident macrophages and hepatocytes; (2) the Mφ release IL-1 which activates polymorphs; (3) the activated PMN destroy *Listeria* bacilli by direct contact and are cytotoxic for infected hepatocytes; (4) the infected Mφ release TNF and IL-12 which stimulate NK cells; (5) NK cells secrete IFNγ, which (6) activates the macrophage to produce NO· and kill intracellular *Listeria*; (7) IFNγ plus Mφ-derived IL-12 recruit Th1 cells which reinforce Mφ activation through the production of IFNγ. (8) Eventual synthesis of IL-10, encouraged by the action of immune complexes, downregulates Mφ, NK and Th1 activity. (Based on an article by Rogers H.W., Tripps C.S. & Unanue E.R. (1995) *The Immunologist* **3**, 152.)

high percentage react to the 65 kDa heat-shock protein. A vital role for these cells in murine TB is indicated by the death of γδ TCR deletion mutants after an infection with *M. tuberculosis* which was still tolerated by immunocompetent animals.

Given these potential CMI defenses, why do some individuals fail to eradicate their infections with mycobacteria and other intracellular facultative bacteria and so suffer from diseases such as TB and leprosy even though they have established Th1 responses? One important clue is provided by the demonstration that inbred strains of mice differ dramatically in their susceptibility to infection by various mycobacteria, *Salmonella typhimurium* and *Leishmania donovani*. Resistance is associated with a T-cell-independent enhanced state of macrophage priming for bactericidal activity involving oxygen and nitrogen radicals. Moreover, macrophages from resistant strains have increased MHC class II expression and a higher respiratory burst, are more readily activated by IFNγ, and induce better stimulation of T-cells, whereas macrophages from susceptible strains tend to have suppressor effects on T-cell proliferation to mycobacterial antigens. Susceptibility and resistance to *Mycobacterium tuberculosis* in murine models depend upon a number of genes, including *sst1* (susceptibility

to *tuberculosis 1*) and *Nramp1* (*natural resistance-associated macrophage protein 1*). At least 11 polymorphisms have been identified in the human *Nramp1* homolog and studies are underway to link individual polymorphisms to susceptibility.

Where the host has difficulty in effectively eliminating these organisms, the chronic CMI response to local antigen leads to the accumulation of densely packed macrophages which release angiogenic and fibrogenic factors and stimulate the formation of granulation tissue and ultimately fibrosis. The activated macrophages, perhaps under the stimulus of IL-4, transform to epithelioid cells and fuse to become giant cells. As suggested earlier, the resulting granuloma represents an attempt by the body to isolate a site of persistent infection.

Leprosy

In human leprosy, the disease presents as a spectrum ranging from the **tuberculoid** form, with lesions containing small numbers of viable organisms, to the **lepromatous** form, characterized by an abundance of *M. leprae* within the macrophages. The tuberculoid state is associated with good cell-mediated dermal hypersensitivity reactions and a bias towards Th1-

type responses, although these are still not good enough to eradicate the bacilli completely. In the lepromatous form, there is poor T-cell reactivity to whole bacilli and poor lepromin dermal responses, although there are numerous plasma cells which contribute to a high level of circulating antibody and indicate a more prominent Th2 activity. Clearly, CMI rather than humoral immunity is important for the control of the leprosy bacillus, but reasons for the inadequate responses of the lepromatous patients are still uncertain.

IMMUNITY TO VIRAL INFECTION

Genetically controlled constitutional factors which render a host or certain of their cells nonpermissive (i.e. resistant to takeover of their replicative machinery by virus) play a dominant role in influencing the vulnerability of a given individual to infection. Macrophages may readily take up viruses nonspecifically and kill them. However, in some instances, the macrophages allow replication and, if the virus is capable of producing cytopathic effects in various organs, the infection may be lethal; with noncytopathic agents, such as lymphocytic choriomeningitis, Aleutian mink disease and equine infectious anemia viruses, a persistent infection may result. Viruses can avoid recognition by the host's immune system by latency or by sheltering in privileged sites, but they have also evolved a maliciously cunning series of evasive strategies.

Immunity can be evaded by antigen changes

Changing antigens by drift and shift

In the course of their constant duel with the immune system, viruses are continually changing the structure of their surface antigens. They do so by processes termed 'antigenic drift' and 'antigenic shift', the nature of which may be made more apparent by consideration of different influenza strains. The surface of the influenza virus contains a hemagglutinin, by which it adheres to cells prior to infection, and a neuraminidase, which releases newly formed virus from the surface sialic acid of the infected cell; of these, the hemagglutinin is the more important for the establishment of protective immunity. Minor changes in antigenicity of the hemagglutinin occur through point mutations in the viral genome (**drift**), but major changes arise through wholesale swapping of genetic material with reservoirs of different viruses in other animal hosts (**shift**) (figure 13.18). When alterations in the hemagglutinin are sufficient to render previous

Figure 13.18. Antigenic drift and shift in influenza virus. The changes in hemagglutinin structure caused by drift may be small enough to allow protection by immunity to earlier strains. This may not happen with radical changes in the antigen associated with antigenic shift and so new virus epidemics break out. There have been 31 documented influenza pandemics (widespread epidemics occurring throughout the population) since the first well-described pandemic of 1580. In the last century there were three, associated with the emergence by antigenic shift of the Spanish flu in 1918 with the structure H_1N_1 (the official nomenclature assigns numbers to each hemagglutinin and neuraminidase major variant), Asian flu in 1957 (H_2N_2) and Hong Kong flu in 1968 (H_3N_2); note that each new epidemic was associated with a fundamental change in the hemagglutinin. The pandemic in 1918 killed an estimated 40 million people.

immunity ineffective, new influenza epidemics break out.

Mutant forms can be favored by selection pressure from antibody. In fact, one current strategy for generating mutants in a given epitope is to grow the virus in tissue culture in the presence of a monoclonal antibody which reacts with that epitope; only mutants which do not bind the monoclonal will escape and grow out. This principle underlies the antigenic variation characteristic of the common cold rhinoviruses. The site for attachment and penetration of mucosal cells bearing ICAM-1 is a hydrophobic pocket lying on the floor of a canyon which antibodies were thought to be too large to penetrate. Many antibodies react with the rim of the viral canyon and mutations in the rim would thus enable the virus to escape from the host immune response without affecting the conserved site for binding to the target cell. However, one recent structural study identified three neutralizing antibodies which bear Fabs that contact a significant proportion of the canyon directly overlapping with the ICAM-1-binding site. Hydrophobic drugs have been synthesized which fit the rhinovirus canyon and cause a change in conformation which prevents binding to cells and, since host proteins have very different folds to those of the viral capsid molecule, the drugs have limited cytotoxicity. A more recent drug has been designed to slot into the substrate-binding site of the neuraminidase, so inhibiting its biological activity.

Mutation can produce antagonistic T-cell epitopes

Hepatitis B virus isolates from chronically infected patients can present variant epitopes which act as TCR antagonists capable of inhibiting naturally occurring antiviral cytotoxic T-cells. Mutations which modify residues critical for recognition by MHC or TCR may generate partial agonists that can induce a profound and long-lasting state of T-cell anergy (cf. p. 233 and figure 9.8). Either strategy can lead to persistent infection.

Some viruses can affect antigen processing

Virtually every step in processing and presentation can be sabotaged by one virus or another. Thus, EBNA-1, the Epstein–Barr virus (EBV) nuclear antigen-1, contains glycine–alanine repeats which inhibit proteasome-mediated processing of the virus. Peptide binding to TAP is prevented by the infected cell protein 47 (ICP47) of herpes simplex virus, whilst the US6 protein of cytomegalovirus (CMV) prevents peptide transport through the TAP pore. Other CMV proteins can bind to and thereby retain MHC class I molecules in the endoplasmic reticulum; yet others redirect the molecules to degradation pathways. The K3 and K5 proteins of herpes virus downregulate expression of class I molecules. The net effect is a lack of surface target for cytotoxic T-cells. With respect to NK cells, which kill cells lacking MHC class I, CMV-encoded homologs of class I proteins can prevent NK-mediated lysis.

The MHC class II pathway is not exempt from such interference. HIV Nef affects vesicle traffic and endocytic processing involved in the generation of peptides, whilst the EIA protein of adenovirus interferes with IFNγ-mediated upregulation of MHC class II expression.

Viruses can interfere with immune effector mechanisms

Playing games with the host's humoral responses

Just as bacteria possess proteins capable of binding the Fc region of antibody (cf. p. 261), so certain viruses also possess Fcγ receptors. Herpes simplex virus (HSV) types 1 and 2, coronavirus and murine cytomegalovirus all bear such molecules which, by binding antibody 'the wrong way round', may inhibit Fc-mediated effector functions.

As we saw for bacteria (cf. p. 255), viruses can block complement-mediated induction of the inflammatory response and thereby prevent viral killing. Pox viruses encode a complement control protein VCP (IMP) which binds C3b and C4b, making both the classical (C$\overline{4b2a}$) and alternative (C$\overline{3bBb}$) C3 convertases susceptible to factor I-mediated destruction. For its part, herpes simplex type 1 subverts the complement cascade by virtue of its surface glycoprotein C which binds C3b, interfering with its interaction with C5 and properdin.

Several viruses utilize complement receptors to gain entry into cells, especially since engagement of the complement receptor alone on a macrophage is a feeble activator of the respiratory burst. Flavivirus coated with iC3b enters through the CR3 receptors. Members of the *regulators of the complement activation* (RCA) family are used as cellular receptors for various viruses, such as CD46 (membrane cofactor protein) by measles virus and human herpes virus-6 (HHV-6), and CD55 (decay accelerating factor) used by echoviruses and coxsackie viruses. As noted previously, EBV infects B-cells by binding to the CR2 surface receptors. Ominously, HIV coated with antibody and complement is more virulent than unopsonized virus.

Cell-mediated immunity can also be manipulated

Parainfluenza virus type 2 strongly inhibits Tc cells by downregulating granzyme B expression (cf. p. 19). Numerous viral open reading frames encode proteins homologous to host cytokines and their receptors. Anti-IFN strategies are particularly abundant, with many viruses producing proteins able to block IFN-induced JAK/STAT pathway activation. A prime viral target is also the activation of the double-stranded RNA-dependent protein kinase (PKR) and other components of the cell thought to be involved in setting up an antiviral state in cells following their exposure to IFN. The macrophage tropic African swine fever virus encodes a homolog of IκB and thereby blocks the NFκB-mediated transcription of cytokine genes. Some viruses, including ectromelia (mousepox) virus, produce homologs of semaphorin molecules which bind to semaphorin receptors on macrophages, thereby inducing these signaling pathways in the host cells, a process which may facilitate viral replication. Human poxvirus-encoded proteins can bind IL-18 and thereby inhibit IL-18-induced IFNγ production and NK responses. The list just goes on and on. Apoptosis of a cell could be considered bad news for a virus living very comfortably inside that cell. Therefore it is yet again not surprising that viruses have come up with ways of preventing apoptosis. Just a couple of examples. The adenovirus *14.7K* gene encodes a protein which binds to and thereby inhibits caspase 8. Various herpesviruses encode homologs of the anti-apoptotic protein bcl-2. In contrast, some viral proteins may be pro-apoptotic, in this case perhaps aiding dissemination of virus particles.

An EBV product with 84% identity to human IL-10 helps the virus to escape the antiviral effects of IFNγ by downregulating Th1 cells. Poxviruses encode soluble homologs of the IFNα/β receptor and the IFNγR, thereby competitively inhibiting the action of all three interferons. Others, particularly herpesviruses and poxviruses, possess several genes encoding chemokine-like and chemokine receptor-like proteins which can subvert the action of numerous chemokines.

Protection by serum antibody

The antibody molecule can neutralize viruses by a variety of means. It may stereochemically inhibit combination with the receptor site on cells, thereby preventing penetration and subsequent intracellular multiplication, the protective effect of antibodies to influenza viral hemagglutinin providing a good example. Similarly, antibodies to the measles hemagglutinin prevent entry into the cell, but the spread of virus from cell to cell is stopped by antibodies to the fusion antigen. Antibody may destroy a free virus particle directly through activation of the classical complement pathway or produce aggregation, enhanced phagocytosis and intracellular death by the mechanisms already discussed.

Relatively low concentrations of circulating antibody can be effective and one is familiar with the protection afforded by poliomyelitis antibodies, and by human γ-globulin given prophylactically to individuals exposed to measles. The most clear-cut protection is seen in diseases with long incubation times where the virus has to travel through the bloodstream before it reaches the tissue which it finally infects. For example, in poliomyelitis, the virus gains access to the body via the gastrointestinal tract and eventually passes through the circulation to reach the brain cells which become infected. Within the blood, the virus is neutralized by quite low levels of specific antibody, while the prolonged period before the virus infects the brain

allows time for a secondary immune response in a primed host.

Local factors

With other viral diseases, such as influenza and the common cold, there is a short incubation time, related to the fact that the final target organ for the virus is the same as the portal of entry and no intermediate stage involving passage through the body occurs. There is little time for a primary antibody response to be mounted and in all likelihood the **rapid production of interferon** is the most significant mechanism used to counter the viral infection. Experimental studies certainly indicate that, after an early peak of interferon production, there is a rapid fall in the titer of live virus in the lungs of mice infected with influenza (figure 13.19). Antibody, as assessed by the serum titer, seems to arrive on the scene much too late to be of value in aiding recovery. However, antibody levels may be elevated in the local fluids bathing the infected surfaces, e.g. nasal mucosa and lung, despite low serum titers, and it is the production of **antiviral antibody** (most prominently IgA) by locally deployed immunologically primed cells which is of major importance for the **prevention of subsequent infection**. Unfortunately, in so far as the common cold is concerned, a subsequent infection is likely to involve an antigenically unrelated virus so that general immunity to colds is difficult to achieve.

Cell-mediated immunity gets to the intracellular virus

In Chapter 2, we emphasized the general point that, to a first approximation, antibody deals with extracellu-

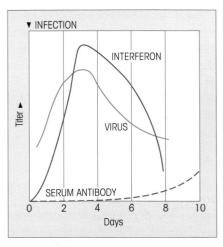

Figure 13.19. Appearance of interferon and serum antibody in relation to recovery from influenza virus infection of the lungs of mice. (From Isaacs A. (1961) *New Scientist* **11**, 81.)

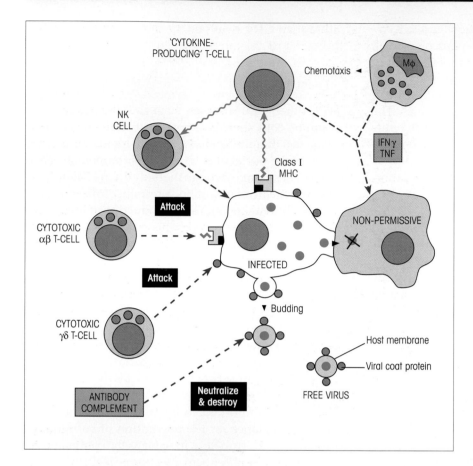

Figure 13.20. Control of infection by 'budding' viruses. Free virus released by budding from the cell surface is neutralized by antibody. Specific cytotoxic T-cells kill virally infected targets directly. Interaction with a (separate?) subpopulation of T-cells releases cytokines which attract macrophages, prime contiguous cells with IFNγ and TNF to make them resistant to viral infection and activate cytotoxic NK cells. NK cells are powerful producers of IFNγ and GM-CSF. They can recognize a lack of MHC class I on the infected cell membrane or partake in antibody-dependent cellular cytotoxicity (ADCC) if antibody to viral coat proteins is bound to the infected cell. Included in this group of budding viruses are: oncorna (=oncogenic RNA virus, e.g. murine leukemogenic), orthomyxo (influenza), paramyxo (mumps, measles), toga (dengue), rhabdo (rabies), arena (lymphocytic choriomeningitis), adeno, herpes (simplex, varicella zoster, cytomegalo, Epstein–Barr, Marek's disease), pox (vaccinia), papova (SV40, polyoma) and rubella viruses.

lar infective agents and CMI with intracellular ones. The same holds true for viruses which try to shelter from antibody in an intracellular habitat. Local or systemic antibodies can block the spread of cytolytic viruses which are released from the host cell they have just killed, but alone they are usually inadequate to control those viruses which bud off from the surface as infectious particles because they are also capable of spreading to adjacent cells without becoming exposed to antibody (figure 13.20). The importance of CMI for recovery from infection with these agents is underlined by the inability of children with primary T-cell immunodeficiency to cope with such viruses, whereas patients with Ig deficiency but intact CMI are not troubled in this way.

NK cells can kill virally infected targets

In earlier chapters, we have explained how early recognition and killing of a virally infected cell before replication occurs is of obvious benefit to the host. The importance of the NK cell in this role as an agent of preformed innate immunity can be gauged from observations on the exceedingly rare patients with complete absence of these cells who suffer recurrent life-threatening viral infections, including EBV, varicella and cytomegaloviruses (CMVs). The surface of a virally infected cell undergoes modification, probably in its surface carbohydrate structures, making it an attractive target for NK cells, which can be shown to be cytotoxic *in vitro* to cells infected with a number of different viruses. The NK cell possesses two families of surface receptors. One, killer activating receptors, binds to carbohydrate and other structures expressed collectively by all cells; the other, killer inhibitory receptors, recognizes MHC class I molecules and overrules the signal from the activating receptor. Thus, the sensitivity of the target cell is closely related to self-MHC class I expression; sensitive targets have low class I, but transfection with the self-MHC molecule will generally protect them. Karrer has suggested that, whereas T-cells search for the presence of foreign shapes, NK cells survey tissues for the absence of self as indicated by aberrant or absent expression of MHC class I, which might occur in tumorigenesis or in certain viral infections. The ability of EBV to downregulate class I would explain the drastic nature of this infection in NK-deficient patients mentioned above. The production of IFNα during viral infection not only protects surrounding cells, but also activates NK cells and upregulates MHC expression on the adjacent cells, making them more resistant to cytotoxicity.

Cytotoxic T-cells (Tc) are crucial elements in immunity to infection by budding viruses

T-lymphocytes from a sensitized host are directly cytotoxic to cells infected with viruses, the new MHC-associated peptide antigens on the target cell surface being recognized by specific αβ receptors on the aggressor lymphocytes. There is a quite surprising frequency of dual specificities in target cell recognition by virus-specific Tc clones, which can lyse uninfected allogeneic cells or targets expressing peptides with little homology from different regions of the same viral protein, from different proteins of the same virus, or even from different unrelated viruses. Thus activation by a second virus may help to maintain memory, and there may be a spontaneous immunity to an unrelated virus after initial infection with a cross-reacting strain. Downregulation of MHC class I poses no problems for **TCR1 γδ Tc** which recognize native viral coat protein (e.g. herpes simplex virus glycoprotein) on the cell surface (figure 13.20).

Tc cells can usually be detected in the peripheral blood lymphocytes of individuals who have recovered from infection with influenza, CMV or EBV by re-exposure *in vitro* to appropriately infected cells. In the case of CMV, for example, the targets are cells with the 'early antigen' on their surface expressed within 6 hours of infection. As discussed above, it is clearly advantageous for the cytotoxic cell to strike so soon after infection. Studies on volunteers, showing that high levels of cytotoxic activity before challenge with live influenza correlated with low or absent shedding of virus, speak in favor of the importance of Tc in human viral infection.

After a natural infection, both antibody and Tc cells are generated; subsequent protection is long-lived without reinfection, possibly being reinforced by bystander activation through cytokines released from other stimulated T-cells, or perhaps by random triggering with unrelated viruses based on the dual specificity described earlier. By contrast, injection of killed influenza produces antibodies but no Tc and protection is only short term.

Cytokines recruit effectors and provide a 'cordon sanitaire'

A number of studies on the transfer of protection to influenza, lymphocytic choriomeningitis, vaccinia, ectromelia and CMV infections have focused on CD8 rather than CD4 T-cells as the major defensive force. The knee-jerk response would be to implicate cytotoxicity, but remember that CD8 cells also produce cytokines. This may well be crucial when viruses escape the cytotoxic mechanism and manage to sidle laterally into an adjacent cell. CMI can now play some new cards: if T-cells stimulated by viral antigen release cytokines such as IFNγ and macrophage or monocyte chemokines, the mononuclear phagocytes attracted to the site will be activated to secrete TNF, which will synergize with the IFNγ to render the contiguous cells nonpermissive for the replication of any virus acquired by intercellular transfer (figure 13.20). In this way, the site of infection can be surrounded by a cordon of resistant cells. Like IFNα, IFNγ increases the nonspecific cytotoxicity of NK cells (see p. 18) for infected cells. This generation of 'immune interferon' (IFNγ) and TNF in response to non-nucleic acid viral components provides a valuable back-up mechanism when dealing with viruses which are intrinsically poor stimulators of interferon synthesis.

Antibody has a part too

The neutralization of free virus particles by antibody is relatively straightforward but the interaction with infected cells is rather more complex. Access to the surface antigens by αβ T-cells cannot be blocked by antibody since these cells recognize processed antigen, whereas antibody binds native antigen. Antibodies can, however, block γδ Tc by reacting with surface antigen on incipiently budding virions, but should be able to initiate ADCC (p. 32) as has been reported with herpes-, vaccinia- and mumps-infected target cells.

Do not forget the importance of antibody in **preventing reinfection** with most viruses.

IMMUNITY TO FUNGI

Not too much is known about this subject. Many fungal infections become established in immunocompromised hosts or when the normal commensal flora are upset by prolonged administration of broad-spectrum antibiotics. T-cells are important in defense and can recognize antigens from organisms such as *Cryptococcus neoformans* and *Candida albicans*, killing them by the granzyme system. NK cells can also lyse *C. neoformans*.

IMMUNITY TO PARASITIC INFECTIONS

The diverse organisms responsible for the major parasitic diseases are listed in figure 13.21. The numbers af-

Figure 13.21. **The major parasites in humans** and the sheer enormity of the numbers of people infected. (Data from World Health Organization, 1990.)

fected are truly horrifying and the sum of misery these organisms engender is too large to comprehend. The consequences of parasitism could be, at one extreme, a lack of immune response leading to overwhelming superinfection, and, at the other, an exaggerated life-threatening immunopathologic response. To be successful, a parasite must steer a course *between* these extremes, avoiding wholesale killing of the human host and yet at the same time escaping destruction by the immune system. In practice, each type of parasite is virtually a world unto itself in the complexity of the mechanisms by which this is achieved.

The host responses

A wide variety of defensive mechanisms are deployed by the host, but the rough generalization may be made that a humoral response develops when the organisms invade the bloodstream (malaria, trypanosomiasis), whereas parasites which grow within the tissues (e.g. cutaneous leishmaniasis) usually elicit CMI (table 13.1). Often, a chronically infected host will be resistant to reinfection with fresh organisms, a situation termed **concomitant immunity**. This is seen particularly in schistosomiasis but also in malaria, where historically the phenomenon was called 'premunition'. The resident and the infective forms must differ in some way yet to be pinpointed.

Humoral immunity

Antibodies of the right specificity present in adequate concentrations and affinity are reasonably effective in providing protection against blood-borne parasites, such as *Trypanosoma brucei*, and the sporozoite and

Table 13.1. The relative importance of antibody and cell-mediated responses in protozoal infections.

PARASITE	TRYPANOSOMA BRUCEI	PLASMODIUM	TRYPANOSOMA CRUZI	LEISHMANIA
HABITAT	Free in blood	Inside red cell	Inside macrophage	Inside macrophage
ANTIBODY				
Importance	++++	+++	++	+
Mechanism	Lysis with complement Opsonizes for phagocytosis	Blocks invasion Opsonizes for phagocytosis	Limits spread in acute infection	Limits spread
Means of evasion	Antigenic variation	Intracellular habitat Antigenic variation	Intracellular habitat	Intracellular habitat
CELL-MEDIATED				
Importance	–	+	+++ (Chronic phase)	++++
Mechanism	–	Cytokine-mediated activation of macrophages and NK cells	Macrophage activation by cytokines and killing by TNF, metabolites of O_2 and NO· Role for cytotoxic T-cells	

merozoite stages of malaria. Thus, individuals receiving IgG from solidly immune adults in malaria endemic areas are themselves temporarily protected against infection, the effector mechanisms being opsonization and phagocytosis, and complement-dependent lysis.

A marked feature of the immune reaction to helminthic infections, such as *Trichinella spiralis* in humans and *Nippostrongylus brasiliensis* in the rat, is the eosinophilia and the high level of IgE antibody produced. In humans, serum levels of IgE can rise from normal values of around 100 ng/ml to as high as 10 000 ng/ml. These changes have all the hallmarks of response to Th2-type cytokines (cf. p. 181) and it is notable that, in animals infected with helminths, injection of anti-IL-4 greatly reduces IgE production and anti-IL-5 suppresses the eosinophilia. This exceptional increase in IgE has encouraged the view that it represents an important line of defense. One can see that antigen-specific triggering of IgE-coated mast cells would lead to exudation of serum proteins containing high concentrations of protective antibodies in all the major Ig classes and the release of eosinophil chemotactic factor. It is relevant to note that schistosomula, the early immature form of the schistosome, have been killed in cultures containing both specific IgG and eosinophils, which induce a form of ADCC by binding through their FcγRII receptors to the IgG-coated organism (figure 13.22); after 12 hours or so, the major basic protein forming the electron-dense core of the eosinophilic granules is released onto the parasite and brings about its destruction. A contribution to this process from CMI is emerging, since eosinophils can express class II MHC and their IgG-mediated ADCC is strongly enhanced by granulocyte–macrophage colony-stimulating factor (GM-CSF) and TNF. Further evidence for an involvement of this cell comes from the experiment in which the protection afforded by passive transfer of antiserum *in vivo* was blocked by pretreatment of the recipient with an anti-eosinophil serum. It has also been found that eosinophils can kill IgE-coated schistosomula, but the mechanism is different because activation of the IgE (FcεRI) receptors now triggers release of platelet activating factors and the eosinophil peroxidase. This dichotomy in Fcγ and Fcε receptor pathways is also evident from reports that IgE but not IgG can mediate schistosome killing by macrophages or platelets.

Two further points are in order. The IgE-mediated reactions may be vital for recovery from infection, whereas the resistance in vaccinated hosts may be more dependent upon preformed IgG and IgA antibodies.

Cell-mediated immunity

Just like mycobacteria, many parasites have adapted to life within the macrophage despite the possession by that cell of potent microbicidal mechanisms includ-

Figure 13.22. Electron micrograph showing an eosinophil (E) attached to the surface of a schistosomulum (S) in the presence of specific antibody. The cell develops large vacuoles (V) which appear to release their contents on to the parasite (×16 500). (Courtesy of Drs D.J. McLaren and C.D. Mackenzie.)

Figure 13.23. Role of NO· in macrophage leishmanicidal activity. The NO· synthase inhibitor L-NMMA (50 mM) inhibits the ability of macrophages to kill intracellular *Leishmania* where growth is monitored by [^{3}H]thymidine incorporation (a) and also blocks NO production measured by accumulation of NO$_2^-$ in the culture supernatant at 72 hours (b). The D-isomer, D-NMMA, used as a control does not inhibit the enzyme. (Data taken from Liew F.Y. & Cox F.E.G. (1991) *Immunology Today* **12**, A17.)

ing NO· (figure 13.23). Intracellular organisms, such as *Toxoplasma gondii*, *Trypanosoma cruzi* and *Leishmania* spp., use a variety of ploys to subvert the macrophage killing systems (see below) but again, as with mycobacterial infections, cytokine-producing T-cells are crucially important for the stimulation of macrophages to release their killing power and dispose of the unwanted intruders.

In vivo, the balance of cytokines produced is of the utmost importance. Infection of mice with *Leishmania major* is instructive in this respect; the organism produces fatal disease in susceptible mice but other strains are resistant. This is partly controlled by alleles of the *Nramp-1* gene (cf. p. 266) but, as discussed earlier in Chapter 10, in susceptible mice there is excessive stimulation of Th2 cells producing IL-4 which do not help to eliminate the infection, whereas resistant strains are characterized by the expansion of Th1 cells which secrete IFNγ in response to antigen presented by macrophages harboring *living* protozoa. Combined therapy of susceptible strains with the leishmanicidal drug, Pentostam, plus IL-12, which recruits Th1 cells, provides promise that Th2 activities which exacerbate disease can be switched to protective Th1 responses. CD4 clones which recognize only *lysates* of the organism do not confer protection even though they produce IFNγ, a point to be borne in mind in designing vaccines. Experiments in knockout mice suggest that perforins, granzyme B and FasL are not necessary for the protection afforded to mice by vaccination with irradiated sporozoites. Of particular importance for protection, however, is the induction of IFNγ and CD8$^+$ T-cells. Interleukin-12 and nitric oxide are also required, and NK cells may play a subsidiary role.

Organisms such as malarial plasmodia, and incidentally rickettsiae and chlamydiae, that live in cells which are not professional phagocytes, may be eliminated through activation of intracellular defense mechanisms by IFNγ released from CD8$^+$ T-cells or even by direct cytotoxicity. This is very much the case in hepatic cells harboring malarial sporozoites, and it is pertinent to note that, following the recognition of an association between HLA-B53 and protection against severe malaria, B53-restricted Tc reacting with a conserved nonamer from a liver stage-specific antigen were demonstrated in the peripheral blood of resistant individuals. A large case control study of malaria in Gambian children showed that the protective B53 class I antigen is common in West African children but rare in other racial groups, lending further credence to the hypothesis that MHC polymorphism has evolved primarily through natural selection by infectious pathogens.

Eliminating worm infestations of the gut is a more tricky operation and the combined forces of cellular and humoral immunity are required to expel the unwanted guest. One of the models studied is the response to *Nippostrongylus brasiliensis*; transfer studies in rats showed that, although antibody produces some damage to the worms, T-cells from *immune* donors are also required for vigorous expulsion, which is proba-

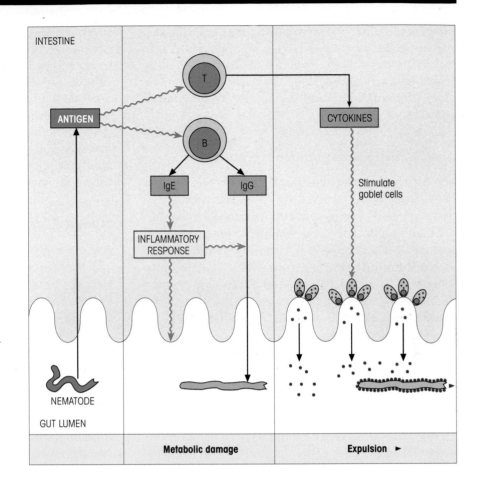

Figure 13.24. The expulsion of nematode worms from the gut. The parasite is first damaged by IgG antibody passing into the gut lumen, perhaps as a consequence of IgE-mediated inflammation and possibly aided by accessory ADCC cells. Cytokines released by antigen-specific triggering of T-cells stimulate proliferation of goblet cells and secretion of mucous materials, which coat the damaged worm and facilitate its expulsion from the body by increased gut motility induced by mast cell mediators, such as leukotriene-D4, and diarrhea resulting from inhibition of glucose-dependent sodium absorption by mast cell-derived histamine and PGE_2.

bly achieved through a combination of mast cell-mediated stimulation of intestinal motility and cytokine activation of the innumerable intestinal goblet cells. These secrete a complex mixture of densely glycosylated high molecular weight molecules which form a viscoelastic gel around the worm, so protecting the colonic and intestinal surfaces from invasion (figure 13.24). Another model, this time of *Trichinella spiralis* infection in mice, again hints at a duality of T-subset cytokine responses. One strain, which expels adult worms rapidly, makes large amounts of IFNγ and IgG2a antibody, while, in contrast, more susceptible mice make miserly amounts of IFNγ and favor IgG1, IgA and IgE antibody classes. Clearly, the protective strategy varies with the infection.

Evasive strategies by the parasite

Resistance to effector mechanisms

Some tricks to pre-empt the complement defenses are of interest. *T. cruzi* has elegantly created a DAF-like molecule (cf. p. 307) which accelerates the decay of C3b. The cercariae of *Schistosoma mansoni* activate com-

plement directly, but eject the bound C3 by shedding their glycocalyx. The *Plasmodium falciparum* protein PfEMP1 is expressed on the surface of infected erythrocytes and can bind to CR1 (CD35) on other infected erythrocytes leading to rosette formation, which may facilitate spread of the parasite with minimal exposure to the host immune system. In a similar fashion, malarial sporozoites shed their circumsporozoite antigen when it binds antibody, and *Trypanosoma brucei* releases its surface antigens into solution to act as decoy proteins (p. 255). In each case, these shedding and decoy systems are well suited to parasites or stages in the parasite life cycle which are only briefly in contact with the immune system.

We have already mentioned the way in which different protozoal parasites hide away from the effects of antibody by using the interior of a macrophage as a sanctuary. To do this they must block the normal microbicidal mechanisms and they use similar methods to those deployed by intracellular obligate and facultative bacteria (cf. p. 263). *Toxoplasma gondii* inhibits phagosome–lysosome fusion by lining up host cell mitochondria along the phagosome membrane. *Trypanosoma cruzi* escapes from the confines of the phagosome into the cytoplasm, while *Leishmania* parasites are surrounded by a lipophosphoglycan which protects them from the oxidative burst by scavenging oxygen radicals. They also downregulate expression of MHC and B7 so diminishing T-cell stimulation.

Avoiding antigen recognition by the host

Some parasites **disguise** themselves to look like the host. This can be achieved by molecular mimicry as demonstrated by cross-reactivity between *Ascaris* antigens and human collagen. Another way is to cover the surface with host protein. Schistosomes are very good at that; the adult worm takes up host red-cell glycoproteins, MHC molecules and IgG and lives happily in the mesenteric vessels of the host, despite the fact that the blood which bathes it contains antibodies which can prevent reinfection.

Another very crafty ruse, rather akin to moving the goalposts in football, is **antigenic variation**, in which the parasites escape from the cytocidal action of humoral antibody on their cycling blood forms by the ingenious trick of altering their antigenic constitution. Figure 13.25 illustrates how the trypanosome continues to infect the host, even after fully protective antibodies appear, by switching to the expression of a new antigenic variant which these antibodies cannot inactivate; as antibodies to the new antigens are synthesized, the parasite escapes again by changing to yet a further variant and so on. In this way, the parasite can remain in the bloodstream long enough to allow an opportunity for transmission by blood-sucking insects or blood-to-blood contact. The same phenomenon has been observed with *Plasmodium* spp. and this may explain why, in hyperendemic areas, children are subjected to repeated attacks of malaria for their first few years and are then solidly immune to further infection. Immunity must presumably be developed against all the antigenic variants before full protection can be attained, and indeed it is known that IgG from individuals with solid immunity can effectively terminate malaria infections in young children.

Deviation of the host immune response

Immunosuppression has been found in most of the parasite infections studied. During infection by trypanosomes, for example, antibody and CMI are only 5–10% of the normal values while T-suppressor activity mediated by IL-10 and IFNγ is prominent, presumably related to an excessive load of antigen. *Schistosoma mansoni* possesses a gene with homology for proopiomelanocortin which, in the human, is a prohormone that is cleaved to generate adrenocorticotropic hormone (ACTH), melanocyte-stimulating hormone (MSH) and the opioid β-endorphin. All have immunomodulatory properties and both ACTH and β-endorphin have been demonstrated in culture when adult worms were incubated at 37°C in minimum essential medium; if neutrophils are added to the system, α-MSH, derived from ACTH by the cell's neutral endopeptidase (CD10; CALLA, p. 387), is also formed.

Parasites may also manipulate T-cell subsets to their own advantage. Filariasis provides a case in point: it

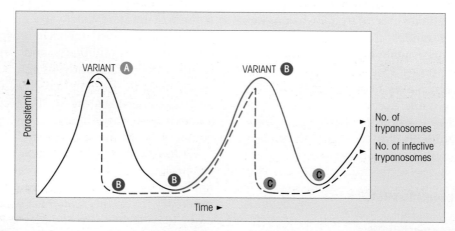

Figure 13.25. Antigenic variation during chronic trypanosome infection. As antibody to the initial variant A is formed, the blood trypanosomes become complexed prior to phagocytosis and are no longer infective, leaving a small number of viable parasites which have acquired a new antigenic constitution. This new variant (B) now multiplies until it, too, is neutralized by the primary antibody response and is succeeded by variant C. At any time, only one of the variant surface glycoproteins (VSGs) is expressed and covers the surface of the protozoan to the exclusion of all other antigens. Nearly 9% of the genome (approximately 1000 genes) is devoted to generation of VSGs. Switching occurs by insertion of a duplicate gene into a new genomic location in proximity to the promoter.

has been suggested that individuals with persistent microfilariae fail to mount presumably protective immediate hypersensitivity responses, including IgE and eosinophilia, as a result of active suppression of Th2 cells.

Epidemiological surveys accord with a protective role for IgE antibodies in schistosomiasis, but they also reveal a susceptible population producing IgM and IgG4 antibodies which can block ADCC dependent upon IgE. The ability of certain helminths to activate IgE-producing B-cells polyclonally is good for the parasite and correspondingly not so good for the host, since a high concentration of irrelevant IgE binding to a mast cell will crowd out the parasite-specific IgE molecules and diminish the possibility of triggering the mast cell by specific antigen to initiate a protective defensive reaction.

Transmissible spongiform encephalopathies

New *v*ariant Creutzfeldt–*J*akob *d*isease (nvCJD) was first described in 1996 and, in common with sheep scrapie and *b*ovine *s*pongiform *e*ncephalopathy (BSE), is classed as a *t*ransmissible *s*pongiform *e*ncephalopathy (TSE) caused by prions. The role of the immune system in prion diseases seems to be one of helping the disease rather than combating it. These infectious diseases lead to abnormally folded, relatively protease-resistant forms of host prion protein (PrP). Infectivity usually replicates to high levels in lymphoid tissues before spreading to the central nervous system, and there is evidence to suggest that *f*ollicular *d*endritic *c*ells (FDCs) in spleen, lymph node and Peyer's patches may be involved in this replication. This may be because FDCs naturally express high levels of the normal PrP which then becomes abnormal following exposure

to the TSE agent. B-lymphocytes may play a subsidiary role via their production of lymphotoxin, a cytokine necessary for the maintenance of a differentiated state in the FDCs. Furthermore, in addition to FDCs, macrophages have been proposed as providing a reservoir of infectivity.

Immunopathology

Where parasites persist chronically in the face of an immune response, the interaction with foreign antigen frequently produces tissue-damaging reactions. One example is the immune complex-induced nephrotic syndrome of Nigerian children associated with quartan malaria. Increased levels of TNF are responsible for pulmonary changes in acute malaria, cerebral malaria in mice and severe wasting of cattle with trypanosomiasis. Another example is the liver damage resulting from IL-4-mediated granuloma formation around schistosome eggs (cf. figure 16.28); one of the egg antigens directly induces IL-10 production in B-cells, thereby contributing to Th2 dominance. Remarkably, the hypersensitivity reaction helps the eggs to escape from the intestinal blood capillaries into the gut lumen to continue the cycle outside the body, an effect mediated by TNFα.

Cross-reaction between parasite and self may give rise to autoimmunity, and this has been proposed as the basis for the cardiomyopathy in Chagas' disease. It is also pertinent that the nonspecific immunosuppression which is so widespread in parasitic diseases tends to increase susceptibility to bacterial and viral infections and, in this context, the association between Burkitt's lymphoma and malaria has been ascribed to an inadequate host response to the Epstein–Barr virus.

SUMMARY

Immunity to infection involves a constant battle between the host defenses and the mutant microbes trying to evolve evasive strategies.

Inflammation revisited

• Inflammation is a major defensive reaction initiated by infection or tissue injury.
• The mediators released upregulate adhesion molecules on endothelial cells and leukocytes, which pair together causing, first, rolling of leukocytes along the vessel wall

and then passage across the blood vessel up the chemotactic gradient to the site of inflammation.
• IL-1, TNF and chemokines such as IL-8 are involved in maintaining the inflammatory process.
• Inflammation is controlled by complement regulatory proteins, PGE$_2$, TGFβ, glucocorticoids and IL-10.
• LPS is bound by LBP which transfers the LPS to the CD14–TLR4 complex, thereby activating genes in the APC which encode proinflammatory molecules.
• Inability to eliminate the initiating agent leads to a

(*continued p. 278*)

chronic inflammatory response dominated by macrophages often forming granulomas.

Extracellular bacteria susceptible to killing by phagocytosis and complement

• Bacteria try to avoid phagocytosis by surrounding themselves with capsules, secreting exotoxins which kill phagocytes or impede inflammatory reactions, deviating complement to inoffensive sites or by colonizing relatively inaccessible locations.

• Antibody combats these tricks by neutralizing the toxins, making complement deposition more even on the bacterial surface, and overcoming the antiphagocytic nature of the capsules by opsonizing them with Ig and C3b.

• The secretory immune system protects the external mucosal surfaces. IgA inhibits adherence of bacteria and can opsonize them. IgE bound to mast cells can initiate the influx of protective IgG, complement and polymorphs to the site by a miniature acute inflammatory response.

Bacteria which grow in an intracellular habitat

• Intracellular bacteria such as tubercle and leprosy bacilli grow within macrophages. They defy killing mechanisms by blocking macrophage activation, scavenging oxygen radicals, inhibiting lysosome fusion, having strong outer coats and by escaping from the phagosome into the cytoplasm.

• They are killed by CMI: specifically sensitized T-helpers release cytokines on contact with infected macrophages which powerfully activate the formation of nitric oxide (NO·), reactive oxygen intermediates (ROIs) and other microbicidal mechanisms.

Immunity to viral infection

• Viruses try to avoid the immune system by changes in the antigenicity of their surface antigens. Point mutations bring about minor changes (antigenic drift), but radical changes leading to endemics can result from wholesale swapping of genetic material with different viruses in other animal hosts (antigenic shift).

• Some viruses subvert the function of the complement system to their own advantage.

• Antibody neutralizes free virus and is particularly effective when the virus has to travel through the bloodstream before reaching its final target.

• Where the target is the same as the portal of entry, e.g. the lungs, IFN is dominant in recovery from infection.

• Antibody is important in preventing reinfection.

• 'Budding' viruses which can invade lateral cells without becoming exposed to antibody are combated by CMI.

Infected cells express a processed viral antigen peptide on their surface in association with MHC class I a short time after entry of the virus, and rapid killing of the cell by cytotoxic αβ T-cells prevents viral multiplication which depends upon the replicative machinery of the intact host cell. γδ Tc recognize native viral coat protein on the target cell surface. NK cells are also cytotoxic.

• T-cells and macrophages producing IFNγ and TNF bathe the contiguous cells and prevent them from becoming infected by lateral spread of virus.

Immunity to parasitic infections

• Diseases involving *protozoal parasites* and *helminths* affect hundreds of millions of people. Antibodies are usually effective against the blood-borne forms. IgE production is notoriously increased in worm infestations and can lead to mast cell-mediated influx of Ig and eosinophils; schistosomes coated with IgG or IgE are killed by adherent eosinophils through extracellular mechanisms involving the release of cationic proteins and peroxidase.

• Organisms such as *Leishmania* spp., *Trypanosoma cruzi* and *Toxoplasma gondii* hide from antibodies inside macrophages, use the same strategies as intracellular parasitic bacteria to survive, and like them are killed when the macrophages are activated by Th1 cytokines produced during cell-mediated immune responses. NO· is an important killing agent.

• CD8 cells also have a protective role.

• Expulsion of intestinal worms usually depends heavily on Th2 responses and requires the coordinated action of antibody, the release of mucin by cytokine-stimulated goblet cells and the production of intestinal contraction and diarrhea by mast cell mediators.

• Some parasites avoid recognition by disguising themselves as the host, either through molecular mimicry or by absorbing host proteins to their surface.

• Other organisms such as *Trypanosoma brucei* and various malarial species have the extraordinary ability to cover their surface with a dominant antigen which is changed by genetic switch mechanisms to a different molecule as antibody is formed to the first variant.

• Most parasites also tend to produce nonspecific suppression of host responses.

• Chronic persistence of parasite antigen in the face of an immune response often produces tissue-damaging immunopathological reactions such as immune complex nephrotic syndrome, liver granulomas and autoimmune lesions of the heart. Generalized immunosuppression increases susceptibility to bacterial and viral infections.

(continued)

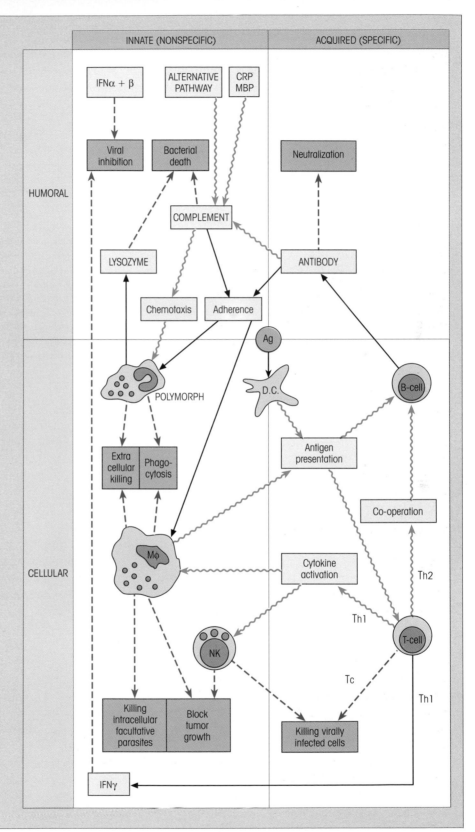

Figure 13.26. Simplified scheme to emphasize the interactions between innate and acquired immunity mechanisms. The dendritic cell which presents antigen to B-cells in the form of immune complexes is the follicular dendritic cell in germinal centers, whereas the MHC class II-positive interdigitating dendritic cell presents antigen to T-cells. (Developed from Playfair J.H.L. (1974) *British Medical Bulletin* **30**, 24.)

(*continued p. 280*)

- As the features of the response to infection are analysed, we see more clearly how the specific acquired response operates to amplify and enhance innate immune mechanisms; the interactions are summarized in figure 13.26.

Prion diseases
- Scrapie, BSE and nvCJD are transmissible spongiform encephalopathies caused by prions.

- Abnormally folded, protease-resistant forms of host prion protein (PrP) develop.
- FDCs in lymphoid tissues become infected prior to spread of the infectious agent to the CNS.

See the accompanying website (**www.roitt.com**) for multiple choice questions.

FURTHER READING

Alcami A. & Koszinowski U.H. (2000) Viral mechanisms of immune evasion. *Immunology Today* **21**, 447.

Donnenberg M.S. (2000) Pathogenic strategies of enteric bacteria. *Nature* **406**, 768.

Gudmundsson G.H. & Agerberth B. (1999) Neutrophil antibacterial peptides, multifunctional effector molecules in the mammalian immune system. *Journal of Immunological Methods* **232**, 45.

Kramnik I., Dietrich W.F., Demant P. & Bloom B.R. (2000) Genetic control of resistance to experimental infection with virulent *Mycobacterium tuberculosis*. *Proceedings of the National Academy of Sciences of the United States of America* **97**, 8560.

Lindahl G., Sjöbring U. & Johnsson E. (2000) Human complement regulators: a major target for pathogenic microorganisms. *Current Opinion in Immunology* **12**, 44.

Medzhitov R. & Janeway C. (2000) Innate immunity. *New England Journal of Medicine* **343**, 338.

Mims C.A., Playfair J.H.L., Roitt I.M., Wakelin D. & Williams R. (1998) *Medical Microbiology*, 2nd edn. Mosby, London.

Prophylaxis

INTRODUCTION

The control of infection is approached from several directions. One method of breaking the chain of infection has been achieved in the UK with rabies and psittacosis by controlling the importation of dogs and parrots, respectively. Improvements in public health—water supply, sewage systems, education in personal hygiene—prevent the spread of cholera and many other diseases; and of course when other measures fail we can fall back on the induction of immunity (Milestone 14.1).

PASSIVELY ACQUIRED IMMUNITY

Temporary protection against infection can be established by giving preformed antibody from another individual of the same or a different species (table 14.1; figure 14.1). As the acquired antibodies are utilized by combination with antigen or catabolized in the normal way, this protection is gradually lost.

Horse globulins containing antitetanus and antidiphtheria toxins have been extensively employed prophylactically, but at the present time the practice is more restricted because of the complication of serum sickness developing in response to the foreign protein. This is more likely to occur in subjects already sensitized by previous contact with horse globulin; thus individuals who have been given horse antitetanus (e.g. for immediate protection after receiving a wound out in the open) are later advised to undergo a course of active immunization to obviate the need for further injections of horse protein in any subsequent emergency.

Maternally acquired antibody

In the first few months of life, while the baby's own lymphoid system is slowly getting under way, protection is afforded to the fetus by maternally derived IgG antibodies acquired by placental transfer and to the neonate by intestinal absorption of colostral immunoglobulins (figure 14.1). The major immunoglobulin in milk is secretory IgA and this is not absorbed by the baby but remains in the intestine to protect the mucosal surfaces. In this respect it is quite striking that the sIgA antibodies are directed against bacterial and viral antigens often present in the intestine, and it is presumed that IgA-producing cells, responding to gut

Milestone 14.1—Vaccination

The notion that survivors of serious infectious disease seldom contract that infection again has been embedded in folklore for centuries. In an account of the terrible plague which afflicted Athens, Thucydides noted that, in the main, those nursing the sick were individuals who had already been infected and yet recovered from the plague. Deliberate attempts to ward off infections by inducing a minor form of the disease in otherwise healthy subjects were common in China in the Middle Ages. There, they developed the practice of inhaling a powder made from **smallpox** scabs as protection against any future infection. The Indians inoculated the scab material into small skin wounds, and this practice of **variolation** (Latin *varus*, a pustular facial disease) was introduced into Turkey where the inhabitants of Circassia were determined to prevent the ravages of smallpox epidemics interfering with the lucrative sale of their gorgeous daughters to the harems of the wealthy.

Voltaire, in 1773, tells us that the credit for spreading the practice of variolation to Western Europe should be attributed to Lady Wortley Montague, a remarkably enterprising woman who was the wife of the English Ambassador to Constantinople in the time of George I. With little scruple, she inoculated her daughter with smallpox in the face of the protestations of her Chaplain who felt that it could only succeed with infidels, not Christians. All went well however and the practice was taken up in England despite the hazardous nature of the procedure which had a case fatality of 0.5–2%. These dreadful risks were taken because, at that time, as Voltaire recorded '… three score persons in every hundred have the smallpox. Of these three score, twenty die of it in the most favorable season of life, and as many more wear the disagreeable remains of it on their faces so long as they live.'

Edward Jenner (1749–1823), a country physician in Gloucestershire, suggested to one of his patients that she might have smallpox, but she assured him that his diagnosis was impossible since she had already contracted cowpox through her chores as a milkmaid (folklore again!). This led Jenner to the series of experiments in which he showed that prior inoculation with cowpox, which was nonvirulent (i.e. nonpathogenic) in the human, protected against subsequent challenge with smallpox (cf. p. 30). His ideas initially met with violent opposition but were even-

Figure M14.1.1. Edward Jenner among patients in the Smallpox and Inoculation Hospital at St Pancras. Etching after J. Gillray, 1802. (Kindly supplied by The Wellcome Centre Medical Photographic Library, London.)

tually accepted and he achieved world fame; learned societies everywhere elected him to membership, although it is intriguing to note that the College of Physicians in London required him to pass an examination in classics and the Royal Society honored him with a Fellowship on the basis of his work on the nesting behavior of the cuckoo. In the end he inoculated thousands in the shed in the garden of his house in Berkeley, Gloucestershire, which now functions as a museum and venue for small symposia organized by the British Society for Immunology (rather fun to visit if you get the chance).

The next seminal development in vaccines came through the research of Louis Pasteur who had developed the germ theory of disease. A culture of chicken cholera bacillus, which had accidently been left on a bench during the warm summer months, lost much of its ability to cause disease; nonetheless, birds which had been inoculated with this old culture were resistant to fresh virulent cultures of the bacillus. This **attenuation** of **virulent** organisms was reproduced by Pasteur for anthrax and rabies using abnormal culture and passage conditions. Recognizing the relevance of Jenner's research for his own experiments, Pasteur called his treatment **vaccination**, a term which has stood the test of time.

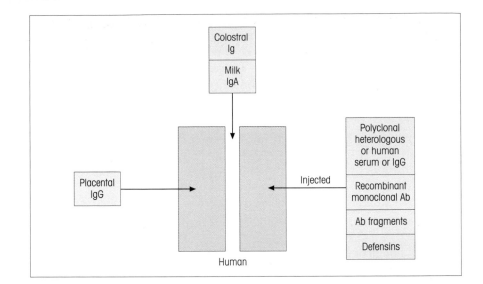

Figure 14.1. Passive immunization produced by: transplacental passage of IgG from mother to fetus, acquisition of IgA from mother's colostrum and milk by the infant, and injection of polyclonal antibodies, recombinant monoclonal antibodies expressed in prokaryotes or plants, antibody fragments (Fab or scFv) derived from phage libraries and, in the future, synthetic polymorph defensins.

Table 14.1. Passive immunotherapy with antibody.

INFECTION	SOURCE OF ANTIBODY		USE
	HORSE	HUMAN	
Tetanus Diphtheria	√	√	Prophylaxis Treatment
Botulism Gas gangrene Snake or scorpion bite	√	–	Treatment
Varicella zoster	–	√	Treatment immunodeficiency
Rabies	–	√	Post-exposure to vaccine
Hepatitis B	–	√	Treatment
Hepatitis A	–	√	Prophylaxis (Travel)
Measles	–	√	Treatment
Cytomegalovirus	–	√	Prophylaxis in patients receiving immunosuppression

antigens, migrate and colonize breast tissue (as part of the MALT immune system; see p. 154), where the antibodies they produce appear in the milk. The case for mucosal vaccination of future mothers against selected infections is inescapable.

Pooled human γ-globulin

Regular injection of pooled human adult γ-globulin is an essential treatment for patients with long-standing immunodeficiency. The preparations are also of value to modify the effects of chickenpox or measles in other individuals with defective immune responses, such as premature infants, children with protein malnutrition or patients on steroid treatment. Contacts with

cases of infectious hepatitis may also be afforded protection by γ-globulin. Human antitetanus immunoglobulin is preferable to horse antitoxin serum, which may cause hypersensitivity reactions. Curiously, pooled γ-globulin is being increasingly used as a treatment for autoimmune diseases such as idiopathic thrombocytopenic purpura, possibly acting through anti-idiotypic mechanisms.

Isolated γ-globulin preparations tend to form small aggregates spontaneously and these can lead to severe anaphylactic reactions when administered intravenously, on account of their ability to aggregate platelets and to activate complement and generate C3a and C5a anaphylatoxins. For this reason, the material is always injected intramuscularly. Preparations free of aggregates are available, and separate pools with raised antibody titers to selected organisms such as vaccinia, herpes zoster, tetanus and perhaps rubella would be welcome. This need may ultimately be satisfied as it becomes possible to produce human monoclonal antibodies on demand.

Cultured antibodies made to order

The techniques for producing *human* monoclonal antibodies to predetermined specificities from hybridoma cells (cf. p. 122) still leave something to be desired and restlessly we look to recombinant DNA technology to satisfy the need (figure 14.1). There are several approaches to the production of antibodies which do not depend upon the human immune system, such as the Fab and single chain Fv (V_H–V_L) constructs (cf. p. 124) selected from phage libraries. Single V_H domain antibodies, being so small, may well be capable of reaching cell receptors on viruses which are tucked away at the bottom of protein canyons where they might be inaccessible to the Fv of an intact antibody, but the sticky nature of these V_H domains has to be addressed. Some antibodies possess peptidase activity, particularly where the light chains have homology to serum proteases, and this could lead to enhanced degradation of the antigen. Expression of **antibody genes in plants** is going to be big business; the technology is now in place to produce recombinant IgA antibodies coupled to secretory pieces in plants, and these should provide an invaluable supplement to dried cows' milk baby food in cases where the mother's milk is of poor quality.

Never neglect innate immune mechanisms. Defensins, the broad-range antimicrobial peptides present in polymorphonuclear neutrophil (PMN) granules (cf. p. 9), are now being engineered in tobacco plants and it is planned to use them for fungal and bacterial infections which become refractory to conventional antibiotics. A good example of lateral thinking by the project leaders.

Adoptive transfer of cytotoxic T-cells

This is a labor-intensive operation and will be restricted to instances where the donor shares an MHC class I allele. To give one example, up to 30% of recipients of bone marrow allografts from mismatched family members or matched unrelated donors develop Epstein–Barr virus (EBV) lymphoma. Pilot studies aimed at potential prophylaxis showed that EBV-induced cytotoxic T-cell (Tc) lines transferred to the bone marrow recipients reconstituted the patients' immune responses to EBV for at least 18 months.

VACCINATION

Herd immunity

In the case of tetanus, active immunization is of benefit to the individual but not to the community since it will not eliminate the organism which is found in the feces of domestic animals and persists in the soil as highly resistant spores. Where a disease depends on human transmission, immunity in just a proportion of the population can help the whole community if it leads to a fall in the reproduction rate (i.e. the number of further cases produced by each infected individual) to less than one; under these circumstances the disease will die out: witness, for example, the disappearance of diphtheria from communities in which around 75% of the children have been immunized (figure 14.2). But

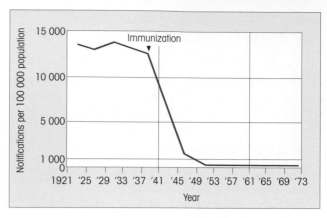

Figure 14.2. Notification of diphtheria in England and Wales per 100 000 population showing dramatic fall after immunization. (Reproduced from Dick G. (1978) *Immunisation*. Update Books; with kind permission of the author and publishers.)

this figure must be maintained; there is no room for complacency. In contrast, focal outbreaks of measles have occurred in communities which object to immunization on religious grounds, raising an important point for parents in general. Each individual must compare any perceived disadvantage associated with vaccination in relation to the increased risk of disease in their unprotected child.

Strategic considerations

The objective of vaccination is to provide effective immunity by establishing adequate levels of antibody and a primed population of memory cells which can rapidly expand on renewed contact with antigen and so provide protection against infection. Sometimes, as with polio infection, a high blood titer of antibody is required; in mycobacterial diseases, such as tuberculosis (TB), a macrophage-activating cell-mediated immunity (CMI) is most effective, whereas with influenza virus infection, cytotoxic T-cells probably play a significant role. The site of the immune response evoked by vaccination may also be most important. For example, in cholera, antibodies need to be in the gut lumen to inhibit adherence to and colonization of the intestinal wall.

Eradication of the infectious agent is not always the most practical goal. To take the example of malaria, the blood-borne form releases molecules which trigger tumor necrosis factor (TNF) and other cytokines from monocytes, and the secretion of these mediators is responsible for the unpleasant effects of the disease. Accordingly, an antibody response targeted to these

Table 14.2. Factors required for a successful vaccine.

FACTOR	REQUIREMENTS
Effectiveness	Must evoke protective levels of immunity: at the appropriate site of relevant nature (Ab, Tc, Th1,Th2) of adequate duration
Availability	Readily cultured in bulk or accessible source of subunit
Stability	Stable under extreme climatic conditions, preferably not requiring refrigeration
Cheapness	What is cheap in the West may be expensive in developing countries but WHO and others try to help
Safety	Eliminate any pathogenicity

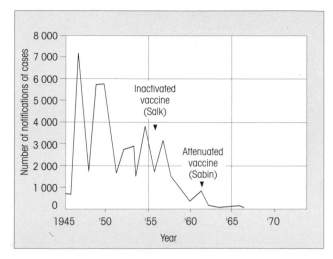

Figure 14.3. Notifications of paralytic poliomyelitis in England and Wales showing the beneficial effects of community immunization with killed and live vaccines. (Reproduced from Dick G. (1978) *Immunisation.* Update Books; with kind permission of the author and publishers.)

released antigens with structurally conserved epitopes may be a realistic holding strategy, while the search for a global vaccine aimed at the more elusive antigen-swapping parasite itself is grinding forward. Under these circumstances life with the parasite might be acceptable.

In addition to an ability to engender effective immunity, a number of mundane but nonetheless crucial conditions must be satisfied for a vaccine to be considered successful (table 14.2). The antigens must be readily available, and the preparation should be stable, cheap and certainly, safe, bearing in mind that the recipients are most often healthy children. Clearly, the first contact with antigen during vaccination should not be injurious and the maneuver is to avoid the pathogenic effects of infection, while maintaining protective immunogens.

KILLED ORGANISMS AS VACCINES

The simplest way to destroy the ability of microbes to cause disease, yet maintain their antigenic constitution, is to prevent their replication by killing in an appropriate manner. Parasitic worms and, to a lesser extent, protozoa are extremely difficult to grow up in bulk to manufacture killed vaccines. This problem does not arise for many bacteria and viruses and, in these cases, the inactivated microorganisms have generally provided safe antigens for immunization. Examples are typhoid (in combination with the relatively ineffective paratyphoid A and B), cholera and killed poliomyelitis (Salk) vaccines. The success of the Salk vaccine was slightly marred by a small rise in the incidence of deaths from poliomyelitis in 1960–61 (figure 14.3), but this has now been attributed to poor antigenicity of one of the three different strains of virus used, and present-day vaccines are far more potent. Care has to be taken to ensure that important protec-

tive antigens are not destroyed in the inactivation process. During the production of an early killed measles vaccine, the fusion antigen, which permits cellular spread of virus, was inactivated; as a result, incomplete immunity was produced and this left the individual susceptible to the development of immunopathological complications on subsequent natural infection. The dangers of incomplete immunity are especially worrying in areas where measles is endemic and the immune response is relatively enfeebled due to protein malnutrition. Since the widespread correction of this dietary deficiency is unlikely in the near future, it is worth considering whether nonspecific stimulation by immunopotentiating drugs or thymus hormones at the time of vaccination might provide a feasible solution.

LIVE ATTENUATED ORGANISMS HAVE MANY ADVANTAGES AS VACCINES

The objective of attenuation is to produce a modified organism which mimics the natural behavior of the original microbe without causing significant disease. In many instances the immunity conferred by killed vaccines, even when given with adjuvant (see below), is often inferior to that resulting from infection with live organisms. This must be partly because the replication of the living microbes confronts the host with a **larger and more sustained dose of antigen** and that, with budding viruses, infected cells are required for the establishment of good **cytotoxic T-cell memory**.

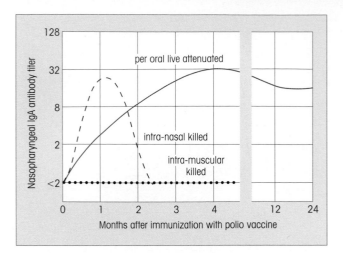

Figure 14.4. Local IgA response to polio vaccine. Local secretory antibody synthesis is confined to the specific anatomical sites which have been directly stimulated by contact with antigen. (Data from Ogra P.L. *et al.* (1975) In Notkins A.L. (ed.) *Viral Immunology and Immunopathology*, p. 67. Academic Press, New York.)

Another significant advantage of using live organisms is that the immune **response takes place largely at the site of the natural infection.** This is well illustrated by the nasopharyngeal IgA response to immunization with polio vaccine. In contrast with the ineffectiveness of parenteral injection of killed vaccine, intranasal administration evoked a good local antibody response; however, whereas this declined over a period of 2 months or so, per oral immunization with *live attenuated* virus established a persistently high IgA antibody level (figure 14.4).

There is in fact a strong upsurge of interest in strategies for mucosal immunization. Remember, the MALT system involves mucous membranes covering the aerodigestive and urogenital tracts as well as the conjunctiva, the ear and the ducts of all exocrine glands which are essentially protected by sIgA antibodies. Resident T-cells in these tissues produce large amounts of transforming growth factor-β (TGFβ), and the interleukins IL-10 and IL-4, which promote the B-cell switch to IgA, and note also that human intestinal epithelial cells themselves are major sources of TGFβ and IL-10.

Classical methods of attenuation

The objective of attenuation, that of producing an organism which causes only a very mild form of the natural disease, can be equally well attained if one can identify heterologous strains which are virulent for another species, but avirulent in humans. The best example of this was Jenner's seminal demonstration that cowpox would protect against smallpox. Since then, a truly remarkable global effort by the World Health Organization (WHO), combining extensive vaccination and selective epidemiological control methods, **has completely eradicated the human disease**—a wonderful achievement. Emboldened by this success, the WHO embarked upon a program to eradicate polio and, despite setbacks caused by armed conflict limiting access to local populations, it is hoped to declare the world free of polio by 2005. One can even follow the progress of this campaign on http://www.polioeradication.org.

Attenuation itself was originally achieved by empirical modification of the conditions under which an organism grows. Pasteur first achieved the production of live but nonvirulent forms of chicken cholera bacillus and anthrax (cf. Milestone 14.1) by such artifices as culture at higher temperatures and under anerobic conditions, and was able to confer immunity by infection with the attenuated organisms. A virulent strain of *Mycobacterium tuberculosis* became attenuated by chance in 1908 when Calmette and Guérin at the Institut Pasteur, Lille, added bile to the culture medium in an attempt to achieve dispersed growth. After 13 years of culture in bile-containing medium, the strain remained attenuated and was used successfully to vaccinate children against tuberculosis. The same organism, BCG (bacille Calmette–Guérin), is widely used today for the immunization of tuberculin-negative individuals. Attenuation by cold adaptation of influenza and other respiratory viruses seems hopeful; the organism can grow at the lower temperatures (32–34°C) of the upper respiratory tract, but fails to produce clinical disease because of its inability to replicate in the lower respiratory tract (37°C).

Attenuation by recombinant DNA technology

It must be said that many of the classical methods of attenuation are somewhat empirical and the outcome is difficult to control or predict. With knowledge of the genetic makeup of these microorganisms, we can apply the molecular biologist's delicate scalpel to deliberately target the alterations in life-style which are needed for successful attenuation. Thus genetic recombination is being used to develop various attenuated strains of viruses, such as influenza, with lower virulence for humans and some with an increased multiplication rate in eggs (enabling newly endemic strains of influenza to be adapted for rapid vaccine production). Not surprisingly, strains of HIV-1, with vicious deletions of the regulatory genes, are being investigated as protective vaccines. The potential is clearly quite enormous.

The **tropism** of attenuated organisms for **the site** at which **natural infection** occurs is likely to be exploited dramatically in the near future to establish gut immunity to typhoid and cholera using attenuated forms of *Salmonella* strains and *Vibrio cholerae* in which the virulence genes have been identified and modified by genetic engineering.

Microbial vectors for other genes

An ingenious trick is to use a virus as a 'piggy-back' for genes encoding a vaccine immunogen. Incorporation of such 'foreign' genes into attenuated recombinant viral vectors, such as fowlpox virus and modified vaccinia virus Ankara strain, which infect mammalian hosts but are unable to replicate effectively, provides a powerful vaccination strategy with many benefits. The genes may be derived from organisms which are difficult to grow or inherently dangerous, and the constructs themselves are replication deficient, nonintegrating, stable and relatively easy to prepare. The proteins encoded by these genes are appropriately expressed *in vivo* with respect to glycosylation and secretion, and are processed for *m*ajor *h*istocompatibility *c*omplex (MHC) presentation by the infected cells, thus effectively endowing the host with both humoral immunity and CMI.

A wide variety of genes have been expressed by vaccinia virus vectors, and it has been demonstrated that the products of genes coding for viral envelope proteins, such as influenza virus hemagglutinin, vesicular stomatitis virus glycoprotein, human immunodeficiency virus (HIV)-1 gp120 and herpes simplex virus glycoprotein D, could be correctly processed and inserted into the plasma membrane of infected cells. Hepatitis B surface antigen (HBsAg) was secreted from recombinant vaccinia virus-infected cells as the characteristic 22 nm particles (figure 14.5). It is an impressive approach and chimpanzees have been protected against the clinical effects of hepatitis B virus, while mice inoculated with recombinant influenza hemagglutinin generated cytotoxic T-cells and were protected against influenza infection.

Attention has turned to BCG as a vehicle for antigens required to evoke CD4-mediated T-cell immunity. The organism is avirulent, has a low frequency of serious complications, can be administered any time after birth, has strong adjuvant properties, gives long-lasting CMI after a single injection and is a bargain at around US $0.05 a shot. The development of shuttle vectors which can replicate in *E. coli* as plasmids and in

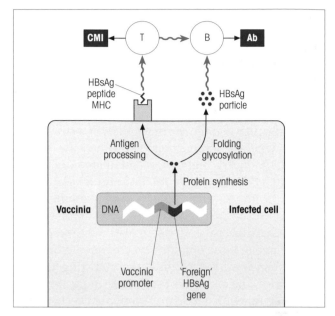

Figure 14.5. Hepatitis B surface antigen (HBsAg) vaccine using an attenuated vaccinia virus carrier. The HBsAg protein is synthesized by the machinery of the host cell: some is secreted to form the HBsAg 22 nm particle which stimulates antibody (Ab) production, and some follows the antigen processing pathway to stimulate cell-mediated immunity (CMI) and T-helper activity.

mycobacteria as phages has allowed foreign DNA to be introduced into *M. smegmatis* and BCG vaccine strains. We can expect many advances on this front: thus incorporation of a gene for kanamycin resistance into the plasmid provides a selectable marker for transformed bacteria, while inclusion of a signal sequence permits secretion of the recombinant protein. Recombinant BCG, engineered to express the outer surface protein A (OspA) of *Borrelia* in its cell membrane, induced excellent antibody titers. For those interested, *Borrelia burgdorferi* is the cause of lyme disease associated with an arthritic condition.

The ability of *Salmonella* to elicit **mucosal responses by oral immunization** has been exploited by the design of vectors which allow the expression of any protein antigen linked to *E. coli* enterotoxin, a powerful mucosal immunostimulant. There is an attractive possibility that the oral route of vaccination may be applicable not only for the establishment of gut mucosal immunity but also for providing systemic protection. For example, *Salmonella typhimurium* not only invades the mucosal lining of the gut, but also infects cells of the mononuclear phagocyte system throughout the body, thereby stimulating the production of humoral and secretory antibodies as well as CD4 and CD8 cell-mediated immunity. Since attenuated *Salmonella* can be made to express proteins from *Shigella*, cholera, malaria sporozoites and so on, it is entirely feasible to consider these as potential oral vaccines. *Salmonella* may also carry 'foreign genes' within separate DNA plasmids and, after phagocytosis by antigen-presenting cells, the plasmids can be released from the phagosome into the cytosol if the plasmid bears a recombinant lysteriolysin gene or the bacterium is an auxotrophic mutant whose cell walls disintegrate within the phagosome; the plasmid then moves to the nucleus where it is transcribed to produce the desired antigen. Quite strikingly, these attenuated organisms are very effective when inhaled; for example, intranasal immunization with recombinant BCG expressing the OspA lipoprotein (*vide supra*) elicited substantive mucosal and systemic immune responses comparable to those obtained by the parenteral route. Vaccinologists are still confidently predicting **'the age of the nose'** and we should soon hear more of human trials with this wide variety of attenuated vectors.

Constraints on the use of attenuated vaccines

Attenuated vaccines for poliomyelitis (Sabin), measles and rubella have gained general acceptance. However, with live viral vaccines there is a possibility that the nucleic acid might be incorporated into the host's genome or that there may be reversion to a virulent form, as seen recently with the reactivation of the live attenuated form of varicella zoster virus (chickenpox) in individuals with a relatively low titer response. Reversion is less likely if the attenuated strains contain several mutations. Another disadvantage of attenuated strains is the difficulty and expense of maintaining appropriate cold-storage facilities, especially in out-of-the-way places. In diseases such as viral hepatitis, AIDS and cancer, the dangers associated with live vaccines are daunting, as witnessed by the experience with attenuated simian immunodeficiency virus in monkeys (see p. 319). As discussed above, with certain vaccines there is a very small, but still real, risk of developing complications and it cannot be emphasized too often that this **risk must be balanced against the expected chance of contracting the disease with its own complications**. Where this is minimal, some may prefer to avoid general vaccination and to rely upon a crash course backed up if necessary by passive immunization in the localities around isolated outbreaks of infectious disease.

It is important to recognize those children with immunodeficiency before injection of live organisms; a child with impaired T-cell reactivity can become overwhelmed by BCG and die. Perhaps this is only a sick story, but it is said that in one particular country at a certain time there were no adults with T-cell deficiency.

The reason? All children had been immunized with live BCG as part of a community health program(!). The extent to which children with partial deficiencies are at risk has yet to be assessed. It is also inadvisable to give live vaccines to patients being treated with steroids, immunosuppressive drugs or radiotherapy or who have malignant conditions such as lymphoma and leukemia; pregnant mothers must also be included here because of the vulnerability of the fetus.

Use in a veterinary context

For veterinary use, of course, there is a little less concern about minor side-effects and excellent results have been obtained using existing vaccinia strains with rinderpest in cattle and rabies in foxes, for example. In the latter case, a recombinant vaccinia virus vaccine expressing the rabies surface glycoprotein was distributed with bait from the air and immunized approximately 80% of the foxes in that area. No cases of rabies have since been seen, but epidemiological considerations indicate that, with the higher fox density that this leads to, the higher the percentage which have to be made immune; thus, either one has to increase the efficacy of the vaccine, or culling of the animals must continue—an interesting consequence of interference with ecosystems. Less complicated is the use of such immunization to control local outbreaks of rabies in rare mammalian species, such as the African wild dog in certain game reserves which are threatened with extinction by the virus.

SUBUNIT VACCINES CONTAINING INDIVIDUAL PROTECTIVE ANTIGENS

A whole parasite or bacterium usually contains many antigens which are not concerned in the protective response of the host but may give rise to problems by suppressing the response to protective antigens or by provoking hypersensitivity, as we saw in the last chapter. Vaccination with the isolated protective antigens may avoid these complications, and identification of these antigens then opens up the possibility of producing them synthetically in circumstances where bulk growth of the organism is impractical or isolation of the individual components too expensive.

Identification of protective antigens is greatly facilitated if one has an experimental model. If protection is antibody-mediated, one can try out different monoclonal antibodies and use the successful ones to pull out the antigen. Where antigenic variation is a major factor, desperate attempts are being made to identify some element of constancy which could provide a basis for vaccination, again using monoclonal antibodies with their ability to recognize a single specificity in a highly complex mixture. If protection is based primarily on T-cell activity, the approach would then be through the identification of individual T-cell clones capable of passively transferring protection. Switching back to humans, one seeks encouragement that the experimental models have kept the focus on the right target by confirming that the immune response to the antigen identified in the models correlates with protection in naturally infected individuals.

The use of purified components

Bacterial exotoxins such as those produced by diphtheria and tetanus bacilli have long been used as immunogens. First, they must of course be detoxified and this is achieved by formaldehyde treatment, which fortunately does not destroy the major immunogenic determinants (figure 14.6). Immunization with the **toxoid** will therefore provoke the formation of protective antibodies, which neutralize the toxin by stereochemically blocking the active site, and encourage removal by phagocytic cells. The toxoid is generally given after adsorption to aluminum hydroxide which acts as an adjuvant and produces higher antibody titers.

The emphasis now is to move towards gene cloning of individual proteins once they have been identified immunologically and biochemically. In general, a protein subunit used in a vaccine should contain a sufficient number of T-cell epitopes to avoid human leukocyte antigen (HLA)-related unresponsiveness within the immunized population. In order to maintain a pool of memory B-cells over a reasonable period of time, persistence of antigen on the follicular dendritic cells in a form resistant to proteolytic degradation with retention of the native three-dimensional configuration is needed. Glycosylation of the protein contributes to this stability, but by the same token might not give a good T-cell response, so that the vaccine may need to be supplemented with a separate

denatured source of T-cell epitopes. Purified polysaccharide vaccines are in a different category in that they normally require coupling to some immunogenic carrier protein, such as tetanus toxoid or mycobacterial heat-shock protein (figure 14.7), since they fail to stimulate T-helpers or induce adequate memory. This maneuver can give respectable antibody titers, but these will only be boosted by a natural infection if the carrier is derived from or related to the infecting agent itself.

Antigens can be synthesized through gene cloning

Recombinant DNA technology enables us to make genes encoding part or the whole of a protein peptide chain almost at will, and express them in an appropriate vector. We have already ruminated upon vaccinia virus and other recombinant vectors. Another strategy is to fuse the gene with the Ty element of yeast which self-assembles into a highly immunogenic virus-like particle. In a similar fashion, peptides can be fused with the core antigen of hepatitis B virus, which spontaneously polymerizes into 27 nm particles capable of eliciting strong T-cell help. However, we often wish to develop vaccines which utilize the gene product on its own, incorporated in an adjuvant. Baculovirus vectors in moth cell lines produce large amounts of glycosylated recombinant protein, while the product secreted by yeast cells expressing the *HBsAg* gene is available as a commercial vaccine. Stably transformed transgenic bananas are now being developed to express

Figure 14.7. The carrier effect of mycobacterial heat-shock protein (hsp70) without adjuvant. Antibody responses to group C meningococcal polysaccharide (MenC) conjugated to hsp70 injected into mice with and without priming to the attenuated *Mycobacterium* BCG. (From Lambert P.-H., Louis J.A. & del Giudice G. (1992) In Gergely *et al.* (eds) *Progress in Immunology* **VIII**, pp. 683–689. Springer-Verlag, Budapest.)

Figure 14.6. Modification of toxin to harmless toxoid without losing many of the antigenic determinants. Thus antibodies to the toxoid will react well with the original toxin.

protein vaccines. Bananas are cheap and easy to grow in the developing world and children like to eat them raw so avoiding inactivation by cooking. It is a sobering thought that a few hectares of the fruit could satisfy the annual global requirement for a single dose of oral immunogen.

The potential of gene cloning is clearly vast and, in principle, economical, but there are sometimes difficulties in identifying a good expression vector, in obtaining correct folding of the peptide chain to produce an active protein, and in separating the required product from the culture *mélange* in an undenatured state. One restriction is that carbohydrate antigens cannot be synthesized directly by recombinant DNA technology, although many of the cohort of genes which encode the cascade of enzymes needed to produce complex carbohydrates have themselves now been cloned.

The naked gene itself acts as a vaccine

Teams working with J. Wolff and P. Felgner experimented with a new strategy for gene therapy which involved binding the negatively charged DNA to cationic lipids which would themselves attach to the negatively charged surface of living cells and then presumably gain entry. The surprise was that controls injected with DNA without the lipids actually showed an *even higher uptake of DNA* and expression of the protein it encoded, so giving rise to the whole new technology of **naked DNA therapy**. As Wolff put it: 'We tried it again and it worked. By the fourth or fifth time we knew we were onto something big. Even now I get a chill down my spine when I see it working.' Well, there is the real excitement of a blockbuster finding, even if, as usually happens to be the case, it arises from serendipity. It was quickly appreciated that the injected DNA functions as a source of immunogen *in situ* and can induce strong immune responses. So, now, vaccinologists everywhere are scurrying around trying to adapt the new technology.

The transcription unit composed of the cDNA gene with a poly A terminator is stitched in place in a DNA plasmid with a cytomegalovirus promoter and a CpG bacterial sequence as a very potent adjuvant. It is usually injected into muscle where it can give prolonged expression of protein. Undoubtedly, the pivotal cell is the dendritic antigen-presenting cell which may be transfected directly, could endocytose soluble antigen secreted into the interstitial spaces of the muscle, and could take up cells that have been killed or injured by the vaccine. The CpG immunostimulatory sequences provoke the synthesis of IFNα and β, IL-12 and IL-18 which promote the formation of Th1 cells; this in turn

generates good cell-mediated immunity, helps the B-cell synthesis of certain antibody classes (e.g. IgG2a in the mouse) and induces good cytotoxic T-cell responses, presumably reflecting the cytosolic expression of the protein and its processing with MHC class I. Let's look at an example. It will be recalled that frequent point mutations (drift; p. 267) in antigenically important regions of influenza surface hemagglutinin give rise to substantial antigenic variation, whereas the major internal proteins which elicit T-cell-mediated immunity responses have been relatively conserved over the last 60 years. On this line of reasoning, nucleoprotein DNA should give broad protection against other influenza strains and indeed it does (figure 14.8). A combination of DNAs encoding the hemagglutinin (included only for statutory reasons) and nucleoprotein genes gave nonhuman primates and ferrets good protection against infection, and protected ferrets against challenge with an antigenically distinct epidemic human virus strain more effectively than the contemporary clinically licensed vaccine. Excellent antibody responses to the viral hemagglutinin were also readily obtained in monkeys. Vaccination can also be achieved by coating the plasmids onto minute gold particles and shooting them into skin cells by the high-pressure 'biolistic' helium gun (cf. p. 141). This technique uses 100-fold less plasmid DNA than the muscle injection and the response is skewed more towards Th2-dependent antibody production, possibly because the antigen dose is too low to foster Th1 cells.

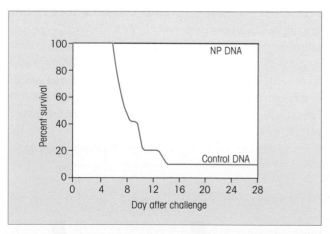

Figure 14.8. Protection from cross-strain influenza challenge after vaccination with nucleoprotein DNA. Mice were immunized three times at 3-week intervals with 200 μg of nucleoprotein (NP) or vector (control) DNA and lethally challenged with a heterologous influenza strain 3 weeks after the last immunization. Survival of mice given NP DNA was significantly higher than in mice receiving vector ($p = 0.0005$). (Data kindly provided by Dr Margaret A. Liu and colleagues from *DNA and Cell Biology* (1993) **12**(9), and reproduced by permission of Mary Ann Liebert Inc.)

Figure 14.9. Induction of memory cells by DNA vaccine and boost of antibody production with the protein immunogen, human chorionic gonadotropin-β (β-hCG). Groups of five (C57BL/6×BALB/c)F1 mice each received 50 μg of the β-hCG DNA plasmid at weeks 0 and 2; one group received a further injection of the plasmid, while the other was boosted with 5 μg of the β-hCG protein antigen in RIBI (cf. p. 300) adjuvant. Dilutions of serum were tested for antibodies to β-hCG by indirect ELISA. Mean titers + SE are shown. (Data from Laylor R., Lund T. *et al.* (1999) *Clinical and Experimental Immunology* **117**, 106.)

The persistent but low level of expression of the protein antigen by naked DNA vaccines establishes a pool of relatively high affinity memory B-cells which can readily be revealed by boosting with protein antigen (figure 14.9). This has given rise to a rather impressive **'prime and boost'** strategy where these memory cells are expanded by boosting with a nonreplicating viral vector, such as fowlpox virus or Ankara strain-modified vaccinia virus, bearing a gene encoding the antigen. Mice immunized in this fashion with influenza virus hemagglutinin produced satisfyingly high levels of IgG2a antibody and were protected against challenge with live virus. Remarkably, up to 30% of circulating CD8 T-cells were specific for the immunizing epitope as shown by MHC class I tetramer binding (cf. p. 138). A similar strategy with *Plasmodium berghei* produced high levels of peptide-specific CD8 cells secreting IFNγ which protected against challenge by sporozoites.

A new generation of genetic vaccines overcomes the poor efficacy of some DNA- and RNA-based vaccines by incorporating the replicating machinery used by members of the alphavirus genus, which includes the Sindbis and Semliki Forest viruses, into the DNA plasmid. The **alphaviral genome** consists of a single positive-stranded RNA encoding structural genes, one of which can be substituted by the antigen gene, and an RNA replicase. Cells transfected with the plasmid replicon become loaded with alphavirus and antigen and meet a sticky apoptotic end whereupon they are taken up by antigen-presenting cells to initiate a powerful immune response.

There is a lot going for DNA vaccines. Considering influenza virus, for example, the DNA needed to prepare a vaccine can be obtained directly from current clinical material without having to select specific mutant strains. Altogether, the speed and simplicity mean that the 2 years previously needed to make a recombinant vaccine can be reduced to months. DNA vaccines do not need the cumbersome and costly protein synthesis and purification procedures that subunit formulations require; almost identical production facilities can be used for totally different vaccine candidates; and they can be prepared in a highly stable powder form which does not depend on the cold complex chain logistically needed for heat-sensitive vaccines, such as the oral polio vaccine in tropical countries. But, above all, they are incredibly cheap. The $3 required for an injection of recombinant hepatitis B represents the whole health budget for a single individual in some countries, whereas the single shot of DNA vaccine would be a tiny fraction of that. Current trials are addressing a number of safety considerations, such as the possibility of permanent incorporation of a plasmid into the host genome. The widespread use of DNA vaccines in humans will depend upon the results of such trials, although observations to date have generally been very encouraging.

EPITOPE-SPECIFIC VACCINES MAY BE NEEDED

Most immunogens, especially proteins, present a variety of B- and T-cell epitopes to the immune system.

Most, if not all, will elicit protective responses, but some may have undesirable characteristics. For example, if there is cross-reaction with a self-epitope, as between *Trypanosoma cruzi* and heart muscle, potentially pathogenic autoimmune reactions may result. Sometimes an immunodominant region, such as the V3 loop in HIV gp120, hogs the antibody response at the expense of the more weakly immunogenic conserved regions, but continually escapes from capture by a high mutation rate. Similar escape mutants crop up in the Tc response to highly mutating dominant T-cell epitopes in malaria and various viral protein antigens. Unwanted epitope effects are seen in the phenomenon of '**original antigenic sin**', in which a second infection with influenza virus involving an antigenically related but not identical strain generates antibodies with a higher titer for the strain which produced the first infection. It is conceivable also that certain epitopes may bias T-helpers towards an inappropriate subset or may engender a predominantly suppressive, antagonistic or anergic response which could downregulate T-cell reactivity to linked epitopes on the same immunogen (figure 14.10).

Frequently, a natural infection gives rise to a poorly functional protective antibody response and discourages the search for vaccine candidates which could generate effective humoral immunity. Nonetheless, in many of these infections, a deliberately selected monoclonal antibody specific for more weakly immunogenic conserved regions of the microbe can be protective, as has been demonstrated in models of HIV, Ebola virus and *Candida* infections. In other words, the epitope giving rise to the protective monoclonal antibody is subdued as an immunogen when present as a component of the infectious microbe, but potentially might be exploited to stimulate high levels of protective antibodies if it could be extracted from the molecular 'woodwork' so to speak.

Bearing in mind the many different circumstances we have discussed, the requirement may arise for a vaccine in which the good protective epitopes can be brought into the front line and dissociated from the molecular environment of the 'bad guys' which compromise the protective responses. In other words, we need to construct **epitope-specific vaccines**, preferably based on conserved regions, which provide broad defense. Several approaches are possible.

Epitopes can be mimicked by synthetic peptides

B-cell epitopes

Small peptide sequences corresponding to important epitopes on a microbial antigen can be synthesized readily and economically; long ones are rather expensive to manufacture. One might predict that, although the synthetic peptide has the correct linear *sequence* of amino acids, its random structure would make it a poor model for the *conformation* of the parent antigen and hence a poor vaccine for evoking humoral immunity. Curiously, this does not always seem to be a serious drawback. The 20-amino acid peptide derived from the foot and mouth virus-specific protein (VP1) evokes a good neutralizing response. The explanation has been forthcoming from X-ray structural analysis which shows the peptide sequence to be in a 'loop' region with blurred electron density indicative of dramatic disorder. In this case, the epitope is linear and evidently the flexibility of the loop structure may approach that of the free peptide which can thus mimic the epitope on the native VP1 molecule and stimulate a protective antibody response when used as a vaccine (figure 14.11a and b). Where the epitope is linear but is restricted in conformation by adjacent structures in the intact protein, immunization with free peptide tends to produce antibodies of disappointing affinity for the protein itself for the reasons outlined in figure 14.11c.

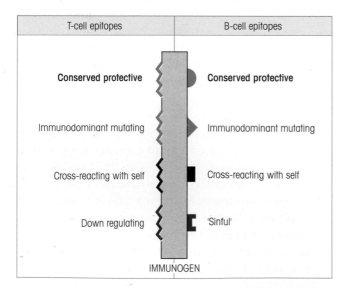

Figure 14.10. Desirable (green) and unwanted (red) epitopes on a protein immunogen. Conserved epitopes give broader protection against mutant variant strains although they may sometimes be weakly immunogenic when present in the whole microbe. Epitopes may be unwanted because: (i) they are immunodominant and attract the main immune response but continually escape by mutation; (ii) they cross-react with self-epitopes and can trigger autoimmunity; (iii) they are responsible for 'original antigenic sin' (see text); or (iv) they downregulate or antagonize T-cell-mediated immunity.

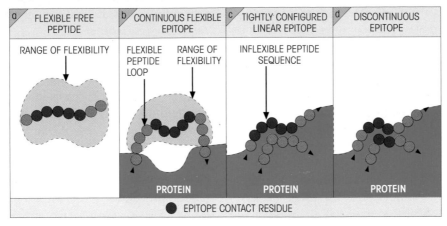

Figure 14.11. Structural basis for peptide mimicry of protein epitopes. (a) The free peptide is very flexible and can adopt a large number of structures in solution. (b) If the peptide sequence is present as a linear epitope on a part of a protein which is a flexible loop or chain, this will also exist in a variety of structures resembling the free peptide to a fair extent, and will behave comparably as an antigen and as an immunogen (vaccine) so that the peptide will raise antibodies which react well with the native protein. (c) If the linear epitope on the protein is structurally constrained (i.e. inflexible), it represents only one of the many structures adopted by the free peptide; thus if this peptide is used for immunization, only a minority of the B-cells stimulated will be complementary in shape to the native protein, so the peptide would be a poor vaccine for humoral immunity to microbes containing the protein antigen. (Note, however, that the antibodies produced would be good for Western immunoblots where the protein has been denatured after sodium dodecyl sulfate (SDS) treatment and the peptide structure is relatively free.) Preformed antibodies to the protein would react with the peptide, albeit with lower affinity, because energy must be used to constrain the peptide to the one structure which fits the antibody—just like the force used to restrain a madman in a strait-jacket. Where the sequence has a comparable degree of constraint in both peptide and protein, as in the disulfide-bonded loops in diphtheria toxin and hepatitis B surface antigen, antipeptide sera react reasonably well with the native protein. (d) Most commonly, the epitopes are discontinuous and, even if with difficulty we can predict the contact residues, the techniques for designing a peptide with appropriate structure are not robust, although some progress is being made using antibody to select from a random bacteriophage library in which the peptides are constrained on a structural scaffold, such as that supporting the Ig CDR3 loop.

T-cell epitopes

Although short peptides may not have the conformation to stimulate adequate B-cell responses, they can prime antigen-specific T-cells which recognize the primary sequence rather than the tertiary configuration of the protein. If the primed T-cells mediate CMI and possibly act to help B-cells make antibody, they could enable the host to have a head start in mounting an effective response on subsequent exposure to natural infection, and this would prove to be a useful prophylactic strategy.

We have already alluded to T-cell epitopes, often dominant and subject to high mutation rates, which can downregulate or subvert protective CMI responses. Under these circumstances, conserved peptide sequences which form **subdominant or cryptic epitopes** (cf. p. 201) **can function as effective vaccines**. The ineffectiveness of these sequences in providing adequate MHC–peptide levels to *prime* resting T-cells when the whole protein is processed by antigen-presenting cells can be side-stepped by immunizing with adequate doses of the preformed synthetic peptide. Because **primed**, as compared with **resting**, T-cells can be stimulated by much lower concentrations of MHC–peptide and do not necessarily require major costimulatory signals, they will react with infected cells which have processed and presented the cryptic epitopes; furthermore, because the primed T-cells will be directed against conserved sequences, they will therefore provide broad CMI protection against mutated strains.

A major worry about peptides as T-cell vaccines is the variation in ability to associate with the different polymorphic forms of MHC molecules present in an outbred population, which contributes to the immune response (*Ir*) gene effect described earlier (see p. 213). This is not quite as serious as it might be owing to groupings of HLA types with consensus structures of the main B and F pockets in the peptide-binding groove, enabling them to recognize very similar peptide motifs. So far, three of these so-called **HLA supertypes**, linked to HLA-A2, -A3 and -B7 respectively, have been identified, covering in total around 90% of the population. Residues 378–398 of the malaria circumsporozoite protein provide an exception in being virtually a universal T-cell epitope recognizable by all individuals so far tested. Other examples are residues 307–319 in influenza hemagglutinin and both 830–843 and 947–967 in tetanus toxin. These sequences, and possibly the highly conserved heat-shock proteins, can provide promiscuous (i.e. HLA-independent) T-cell helper epitopes to conjugate with peptide vaccines.

Making the peptides immunogenic

The immunogenicity of peptides for B-cells is invariably bound up with a dependence on T-cell help, and failure to provide linked T-cell epitopes is thought to be responsible for poor antibody responses to the foot and mouth disease VP1 loop peptide in cattle and pigs, and to polymers of the tetrapeptide asparagylalanyl-asparagylproline (NANP) of malarial circumsporozoite antigens in humans (cf. p. 297). When the general T-cell carrier, peptide 378–398 (see above), was coupled to $(NANP)_3$ tetramer repeat, good antibody responses were obtained in all strains of mice tested. Furthermore, after priming with this synthetic peptide, whole sporozoites would boost antibody titers. This brings up two points: first, as we have already noted, in order for the natural infection to boost, the T- and B-cell epitopes must both be present and, second, they must be linked so that the T-cell epitope is taken up for processing by the lymphocyte which recognizes the B-cell epitope (figure 9.12). This does not always imply that the link in the infectious agent must be covalent, since mice primed with the core antigen of hepatitis B virus gave excellent responses to the surface antigen when challenged with whole virions, i.e. an interstructural relationship may function in this regard as well as an intramolecular one. In contrast, animals immunized with an HBs B-cell peptide coupled with a streptococcal peptide T-cell carrier require boosting with the original vaccine but do not receive a boost from natural infection. Mycobacterial heat-shock proteins are excellent carriers for peptides even in the absence of adjuvants and irrespective of BCG priming (figure 14.7), possibly due to the preprogramming of responses to cross-reacting self-heat-shock proteins in the 'immunological homunculus' (cf. p. 208). In some cases, responses induced by protein carriers might suppress the ability of a second injection of the vaccine to boost peptide antibody levels through antigenic competition and, in this respect, peptides providing the carrier T-cell epitope have a distinct advantage. It is worth noting that the presentation of a peptide, such as the foot and mouth disease virus VP1 loop, in the form of an octamer coupled to a poly-L-lysine backbone produces responses of far greater magnitude than the monomer, a strategy which has proved successful when multiple clusters of peptides are linked to a small central oligolysine core in what has been labeled 'the multiple antigen peptide (MAP)

system'. Are not the multiple peptide units acting as carriers for each other?

Notwithstanding these considerations, **the majority of protein determinants are discontinuous**, i.e. involve amino acid residues far apart in the primary sequence but brought close to each other by peptide folding (figure 14.11d; cf. p. 293). In such cases, peptides which represent linear sequences of the primary structure will, at best, only mimic part of a determinant and will generate low affinity responses. Defining a discontinuous determinant by X-ray crystallography and site-related mutagenesis takes a long time and, by computer analysis, perhaps even longer. Even when armed with this information, synthesis of a configured peptide which will topographically mimic the contact residues that constitute such an epitope still remains a serious challenge. Progress is being made in using monoclonal antibodies to select peptide epitopes binding with higher affinity from bacteriophage libraries of random hexa- or heptapeptides, which are constrained on a structural scaffold such as that holding the CDR3 loop in the immunoglobulin variable region. Well, we have already encountered this type of epitope. Since it would be selected by an antibody we would class it as an **anti-idiotype** and, likewise, if we used it as an immunogen it would be acting as an **idiotype**.

Anti-idiotypes can be exploited as epitope-specific vaccines

In principle, **internal image anti-idiotypes** provide surrogates for discontinuous B-cell epitopes through possession of an innate structure capable of binding with the antigen combining site of the idiotype antibody. Knowledge of the contact residues within the epitope is not necessary. Since antigen–antibody binding is wholly dependent upon noncovalent intermolecular forces, which only become significant when the interacting molecular surfaces are very close together (cf. p. 85), all that is required is that, from the spectrum of millions of different antibody shapes available, one selects those that have a closely complementary three-dimensional topographical configuration which facilitates the intimate contact needed for these forces to permit effective binding. If the reader trundles back to figure 11.10, it will be seen that there are two main categories of anti-idiotype: $Ab_{2\alpha}$, which recognize cross-reacting, presumably regulatory, idiotypes, and $Ab_{2\beta}$, which are thought to behave as internal images of the antigenic determinant. In those instances in which the major Id is mostly associated with a given specificity (e.g. murine T15 Id is largely present on antibodies to phosphorylcholine), then $Ab_{2\alpha}$ anti-Ids could provide useful potential vaccines, particularly for carbohydrates which are notoriously poor immunogens in the very young. They might also be applicable to the expansion of specific antitumor clones with their own private idiotypes in cancer patients. In general, however, the internal image $Ab_{2\beta}$ anti-idiotypes are capable of stimulating a wider range of lymphocytes and must be the strategy of choice. Figure 14.12 maps out how to go about generating $Ab_{2\alpha}$ anti-idiotypic vaccines which mimic epitopes defined by high affinity monoclonal antibodies (i.e. idiotypes). We would call this **reverse immunization**, in the sense that we are reversing the normal progression from antigen to antibody by using antibody to generate antigen. The approach is eminently feasible, and a number of examples of mimicry of epitopes on molecules such as hepatitis B surface antigen and yeast killer toxins have been reported.

B-cell lymphomas each produce a single characteristic immunoglobulin whose hypervariable regions represent unique targets for immunotherapy. How encouraging to read that, after many years of toil, protective immunity against a surface Ig-negative myeloma has been achieved by injection of a DNA vaccine with the myeloma Ig scFv linked to fragment C of tetanus toxoid, which acts as a danger signal to stimulate the anti-Id response. Curiously, the effectors appeared to be CD4 rather than CD8 T-cells.

Mutants which have lost unwanted epitopes can correctly fold desired discontinuous B-cell epitopes

The most natural way to achieve a correctly configured discontinuous B-cell epitope is to allow the protein to fold spontaneously. If the gene encoding the protein antigen is mutated so that the unwanted epitope is eliminated by replacement of its amino acid side-chains, without affecting the folding of the protein chain which generates the epitopes we wish to preserve, our object is achieved. Preservation of the desired epitopes and destruction of the 'bad' epitopes by 'genetic sandpapering' can obviously be monitored by following the reactivity of the mutants with the appropriate monoclonal antibody (figure 14.13). It will be apparent that 'bad' T-cell epitopes can also be eliminated by targeted mutations.

Sometimes, it should be possible to mask an undesirable epitope by introducing a glycosylation site into the sequence. In other cases, one can eliminate large unwanted segments of the antigen if the remaining peptide sequence can still fold correctly. Thus, immunization with the highly conserved extracellular domain of the influenza virus M2 protein fused to the N-terminus of the hepatitis B core protein gave 90–100% protection against lethal viral challenge and, bearing in mind the conserved nature of the antigen, this ought to cover a variety of influenza strains.

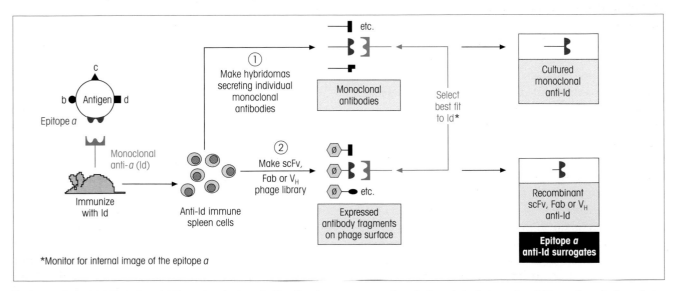

Figure 14.12. Derivation of anti-idiotypic mimics of a B-cell epitope. A high affinity monoclonal antibody (idiotype; Id) specific for the *a* epitope on the antigen is injected to generate an anti-Id response. Spleen cells from the immunized mice are used (1) to make a range of hybridomas, each secreting an individual monoclonal antibody, a small proportion of which will be internal image anti-Id, or (2) a phage library expressing surface antibody fragments. These are screened with the original monoclonal Id to select the best fitting anti-Id monoclonals or antibody fragments. These, in turn, are monitored for behavior as internal image of *a* through ability to block binding of the original Id to *a*, to bind to other anti-*a* monoclonals and to be recognized by a polyclonal antiserum raised against the antigen in other species. A successful candidate can then be produced in bulk to provide a surrogate vaccine for epitope *a*.

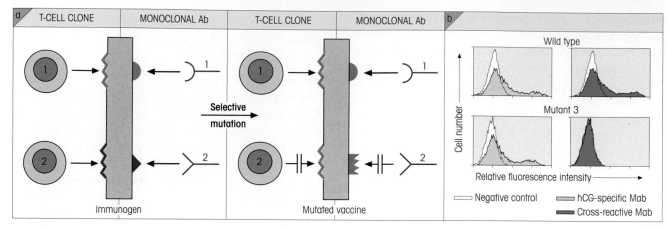

Figure 14.13. (a) Selective mutation of unwanted (dark blue) with retention of desirable (green) epitopes in a protein vaccine. Success of the mutation strategy can be monitored by reactivity with monoclonal antibodies (B-epitopes) and T-cell clones (T-epitopes). Our immunoprotein engineering group at University College London has used this strategy to mutate human chorionic gonadotropin-β (β-hCG) so that it still retains β-hCG-specific epitopes but has lost those shared with human luteinizing hormone (hLH). β-hCG has been investigated as a contraceptive vaccine to aid population control, since antibodies to β-hCG neutralize the hormone and prevent successful pregnancy. However, the production of antibodies to hLH is undesirable since this hormone is present all the time, not just during pregnancy as is essentially the case for hCG (cf. figure 17.21). The mutant epitopes (orange) avoid this unwanted LH cross-reactivity. The C-terminal end of the construct can be extended to encode suitable T-helper carrier epitopes. For simplicity, the T-cell recognition of MHC–peptide has been ignored. (b) FACS analysis of cells transfected to express β-hCG on their surface, showing a mutant which retains the β-hCG-specific epitope but has lost the cross-reactive epitopes characteristic of the wild-type protein.

Likewise, the isolated 19 kDa C-terminal fragment of the merozoite-specific protein MSP-1 confers antibody-mediated protection on monkeys to challenge with the blood stage of the malaria parasite.

CURRENT VACCINES

The established vaccines in current use and the schedules for their administration are set out in tables 14.3 and 14.4.

Because of the pyrogenic reactions and worries about possible hypersensitivity responses to the whole-cell component of the conventional pertussis vaccine, a new generation of vaccines containing one or more purified components of *Bordetella pertussis*, and therefore termed 'acellular' vaccines, has been licensed in the USA. The combination of diphtheria and tetanus toxoids with acellular pertussis (DTP) is recommended for the later fourth and fifth 'shots' and for children at increased risk for seizures. Children under 2 years of age make inadequate responses to the T-independent *H. influenzae* capsular polysaccharide, so they are now routinely immunized with the antigen conjugated with tetanus or diphtheria toxoids.

A resurgence of **measles** outbreaks in recent years has prompted recommendations for the reimmunization of children, at the age of school entry or at the change to middle school, with measles. The considerable morbidity and mortality associated with hepatitis B infection, its complex epidemiology and the diffi-

culty in identifying high-risk individuals have led to recommendations for vaccination in the 6–18-month age group.

Maternally derived IgG antibody can inhibit *de novo* immune responses through feedback control (cf. p. 201). Preliminary results suggest that infants of 4–6 months can be seroconverted by inhaled aerosol measles vaccine which presumably evades the maternal antibody; this will have singular relevance in endemic measles areas, where almost split-second timing is required with conventional immunization as passively acquired antibody wanes. Naked DNA vaccines may also have a role to play here.

Tuberculosis is the largest cause of death in the world from a single infectious disease and, while it remains a truly major problem in developing countries, cases have also increased by around one-third in Western countries. There is an alarmingly heightened susceptibility to TB of individuals with HIV, and worldwide multidrug-resistant strains are appearing. Thus, although BCG has been in use for 70 years and is reasonably efficacious and safe in healthy non-T-cell-deficient subjects, there is certainly a vital need for the development of new drugs and vaccines. It remains to be seen whether the disappointing degree of protection against TB and *Mycobacterium leprae* found with BCG in field trials in certain parts of the globe is due to the use of high doses, deficient strains or subversion of the response to group i cross-reacting antigens by suppressive mycobacterial species in the local environment.

Table 14.3. Current and experimental vaccines.

Type	Established	Experimental
BACTERIAL VACCINES		
Live attenuated	*Mycobacterium tuberculosis (BCG)*	● *Vibrio cholerae* ● *Salmonella typhi* (Ty21a: Vi⁻ mutant) ● *S. typhi* (aroA: aromatic pathway mutant)
Inactivated	*V. cholerae* *B. pertussis* *S. typhi*	● *V. cholerae* + toxin B subunit *M. leprae*
Subunit	*Haemophilus influenzae* *Neisseria meningitidis* *Streptococcus pneumoniae*	*S. typhi* (capsular Vi⁻carrier) *H. Influenzae* (dip/tet toxoid) *M. tuberculosis* (naked DNA)
Toxoid	Tetanus, diphtheria	
VIRAL VACCINES		
Live attenuated	Vaccinia Measles Mumps Rubella ● Polio (Sabin) Varicella zoster ● Adeno Yellow fever	Cytomegalovirus Hepatitis A Influenza Dengue ● Rota Parainfluenza Japanese encephalitis
Inactivated	Polio (Salk) Influenza Rabies Japanese encephalitis Hepatitis A	
Subunit	Hepatitis B, influenza	HIV, influenza, hepatitis B/C, herpes, cytomegalovirus, rabies (all naked DNA in experimental animals)

● Given orally

Table 14.4. Current vaccination practice.

VACCINE		ADMINISTRATION		
		UK	USA	OTHER COUNTRIES
CHILDREN				
Triple (DTP) vaccine: diphtheria, tetanus, pertussis	Primary	2–6 mo (3x/4 weekly)		Japan: 2 yr
	Boost DT	3–5yr	15 mo/4 yr DT every 10 yr	
Polio: live	Primary	Concomitant with DTP		
	Boost	4/6 yr	15 mo, 4 yr high-risk adult	
killed		Immunocompromised		
MMR vaccine: measles, mumps rubella	Primary	12–15 mo		Africa: 6 mo
	Boost	4–5yr 10–14 yr seronegative girls selectively with rubella		
BCG (TB, leprosy)		10–14 yr	high risk only	Tropics: at birth
Haemophilus		Concomitant with DTP		
Varicella		Neonates at risk, immunocompromised		
ELDERLY				
Pneumococcal polysaccharide serotypes		Aged & high risk		
Influenza		Aged & high risk		
SPECIAL GROUPS				
Hepatitis B		Travellers, high risk groups		
Hepatitis A Meningitis (A+C)		Travellers to endemic areas		
Yellow fever Typhoid		Travellers to endemic areas		Tropics: infants Yellow fever: boost residents and frequent visitors every 10 yr
Rabies		Prophylactically in high risk groups Post-exposure to contacts in endemic areas		

EXPERIMENTAL VACCINES IN DEVELOPMENT

Malaria

Don't sneer at low technology. The major advance in malaria control has been the finding that the impregnation of bed nets with the insecticide pyrethroid reduces *Plasmodium falciparum* deaths by 40%. However, with the emergence of drug-resistant strains of mosquito, vaccines must be developed. The goal is achievable since, although children are very susceptible, adults resident in highly endemic areas acquire a protective but nonsterilizing immunity probably mediated by antibodies specific for the blood stages.

Antigen variation poses a big problem for vaccine development and a number of investigators in the malaria field have turned their attention to the invariant antigens of the **sporozoite**, which is the form with which the host is first infected; this rapidly reaches the liver to emerge later as merozoites which infect the red cells (figure 14.14). Because the sporozoite only takes 30 minutes to reach the liver, the antibody has to act fast, so that inactivation is limited by diffusion events and hence dependent on the concentration of antibody molecules. The sporozoite has a characteristic antigen with multiple tetrapeptide repeats. *Plasmodium falciparum*, for example, has 37 repeats of NANP. Field trials of vaccines with polymers of NANP and similar tetrapeptides from other species have not so far been spectacularly successful, but building in powerful T-cell help in the form of the promiscuous 378–398

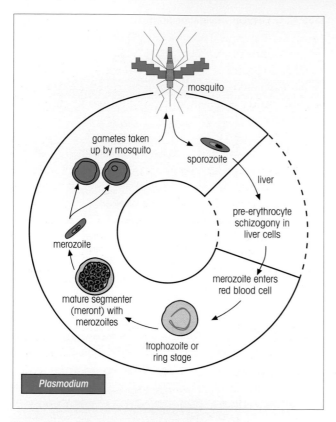

Figure 14.14.   The life cycle of the malaria parasite.

STAGE	VACCINE	STRATEGY
SPOROZOITES	CIRCUMSPOROZOITE (CS) PROTEIN OR PEPTIDES	Ab blocks infection of liver
LIVER STAGE	CS PROTEIN OR PEPTIDES	T-cell mediated immunity destroys liver stage
MEROZOITES	MEROZOITE ANTIGENS	Block infection of red cells
ASEXUAL ERYTHROCYTE STAGE / TOXIC ANTIGEN	ASEXUAL STAGE RBC	Destroy infected red cells
	TOXIC PRODUCT	Ab neutralizes toxin
GAMETOCYTES	SEXUAL STAGES	Ab blocks transmission
GAMETES		
MOSQUITO	MOSQUITO TRYPSIN	

Figure 14.15. Strategies for a malaria vaccine. A vaccine incorporating a yeast-derived polypeptide representing the zygote-specific antigen Pfs25, which can induce transmission-blocking antibodies, looks like the next candidate for big field trials of efficacy. If antibodies to the mosquito midgut trypsin are taken into the blood meal with the gametocytes, they block the trypsin-mediated activation of the parasite prochitinase enzyme required for penetration of the chitin layer lining the midgut by the ookinates (differentiated from the gametocyte stage).

epitope (see p. 294) or a mycobacterial heat-shock protein hsp70 carrier (which obviates the need for adjuvant) should improve efficacy. Mice immunized with radiation-attenuated sporozoites or circumsporozoite protein linked to attenuated *Salmonella* were resistant to live challenge with sporozoites, which should be useful for nonimmune travelers visiting areas where malaria is endemic. Immunity is mediated by noncytotoxic CD8 cells which target infected hepatocytes through the production of IFNγ, NO· and IL-12; the latter cosily initiates a positive feedback loop by stimulating IFNγ secretion by NK cells.

Many laboratories have been targeting the various antigens associated with the **blood stages**, and much publicity has been given to trials using the vaccine SPf66, which consists of three peptide epitopes from three blood stage proteins intercalated with NANP sequences. Some clear protection was originally obtained in large-scale trials in South America, but two further trials in other areas were unfortunately ineffective. The C-terminal fragment of the merozoite-specific protein, MSP-1$_{19}$, mentioned earlier, has considerable promise. One of the products of the infected erythrocytes is a glycophospholipid with features of the insulin second messenger. This may be responsible

for many of the secondary features of malaria by acting as an excessive stimulator of TNF production. A strategy based on using the molecule as a vaccine would resemble the well-established approach to tetanus and diphtheria, where the toxin rather than the organism is attacked. Other groups are focusing on antigens which elicit antibodies able to **block transmission** (see legend to figure 14.15); these would be altruistic vaccines in that they only help the next guy down the line and finally the community as a whole.

A brief summary of the many different vaccine strategies being deployed to counter this complex parasite is presented in figure 14.15, and there may be a consensus that, ultimately, vaccines will contain antigens from all stages probably presented as a mixture of the naked DNA genes which encode them. Perhaps the time has come to introduce a radically new attack on the problem, side-stepping the relatively small-scale studies currently in progress. A gigantic shotgun approach to the identification of protective sporozoite vaccine candidates requiring a hefty input of governmental investment has been proposed. The strategy envisages the following stages: (i) identify putative open reading frames (ORFs) from the genomic sequence of the parasite, (ii) immunize mice with DNA vaccine plasmids derived from each ORF, (iii) use the antisera to screen hepatocytes infected with irradiated sporozoites, (iv) select those plasmids shown by the selection process to encode antigens expressed in the hepatocytes, (v) predict degenerate HLA superfamily binding T-cell epitopes, (vi) validate them as targets of CD8 responses in volunteers immunized with irradiated sporozoites, (vii) string the resulting T-cell epitopes together in a single vaccine plasmid. Phew! This 'big picture' post human-genome style may well be the blueprint for the future.

Schistosomiasis

The morbidity in this chronic and debilitating disease is related to the remarkable fecundity of the female worm which lays hundreds of eggs every day. These are deposited in numerous mucous membranes and tissues, and the granulomas which form around them (cf. figure 16.28) lead to the development of severe fibrotic and often irreversible lesions. Specific IgE can produce worm damage through antibody-dependent cellular cytotoxicity (ADCC) mechanisms (cf. p. 32 and figure 13.22) involving eosinophils and possibly mononuclear phagocytes as effector cells, and may be regarded as a factor in recovery from infection together with Th1 CMI, schistosomes being susceptible to the lethal effects of NO· produced by activated macrophages. IgE, G and A antibodies correlate with resistance to reinfection in drug-cured patients, while IgA appears to control fecundity as shown by passive transfer experiments. Our abilities to stimulate IgE and, to a lesser extent, IgA antibodies at will are, to put it mildly, still somewhat underdeveloped, but it is encouraging to note that a monoclonal antibody to the glutathione-S-transferase of S. mansoni inhibits the enzyme, protects against challenge and dramatically reduces the laying and viability of eggs.

Another protective monoclonal to a different epitope has no effect on enzymic activity or on the production and viability of eggs, but does reduce the worm burden. The recombinant enzyme, possibly in a cocktail with other schistosome antigens and cercarial proteases, could provide a promising future vaccine.

Cholera

In the case of **cholera**, an oral vaccine which combines the B subunit of cholera toxin with killed vibrios has been reported in a big field trial in Bangladesh to stimulate excellent gut mucosal antibody formation, the response being said to equal that seen after clinical cholera. The vaccine also afforded cross-protection against the enterotoxin of E. coli, responsible for travelers' diarrhea.

Tuberculosis

Extensive field trials of the nonvirulent *Mycobacterium vaccae* are underway using the killed organisms which generate strong Th1 responses. To obviate the potential adverse effects of live BCG vaccine in immunodeficient subjects (e.g. HIV-positive), auxotrophic strains which fail to grow in the absence of essential amino acids, such as methionine and leucine, were created by insertional mutagenesis. The strains died out within 16–32 weeks in mice and severe combined immunodeficient (SCID) mice survived for at least 230 days compared with 8 weeks for a conventional BCG vaccine. These auxotrophic strains gave excellent protection against challenge with virulent bacilli and so offer a potentially safe vaccine against TB for populations at risk for HIV.

At the subunit level, as might now be anticipated, naked DNA vaccines for heat-shock and other common mycobacterial antigens are being developed and seem to be highly effective, in mice at least.

ADJUVANTS

For practical and economic reasons, prophylactic immunization should involve the minimum number of injections and the least amount of antigen. We have referred to the undoubted advantages of replicating attenuated organisms in this respect, but nonliving organisms, and especially purified products, frequently require an adjuvant which, by definition, is a substance incorporated into or injected simultaneously with antigen which potentiates the immune response (Latin *adjuvare*—to help). It is interesting that bacterial structures provide the major source of immunoadjuvants, presumably because they provide danger signals of infection, and it is no accident that the 'piggy-back' incorporation of the gene encoding an immunogen into attenuated *Salmonella* and BCG can be so effective. In a sense, the basis of adjuvanticity is often the recognition of these signals by phylogenetically ancient receptors on accessory cells. The mode of action of adjuvants may be considered under several headings.

Depot effects

Free antigen usually disperses rapidly from the local tissues draining the injection site, and an important function of the so-called repository adjuvants is to counteract this by providing a long-lived reservoir of antigen, either at an extracellular location or within macrophages. The most common adjuvants of this type used in humans are **aluminum compounds** (phosphate and hydroxide). Empirically, it has long been realized that hydrophobic substances tend to augment immune responses, and Freund's incomplete adjuvant, in which the antigen is incorporated in the aqueous phase of a stabilized water-in-paraffin oil emulsion, usually produces higher and far more sustained antibody levels with a broadening of the response to include more of the epitopes in the antigen preparation. However, because of the lifelong persistence of oil in the tissues and the occasional production of sterile abscesses, and the unpalatable fact that paraffin oil produces tumors in mice, the replacement of incomplete Freund's with different types of oil, such as squalene or biodegradable peanut oil, has been considered. It is reassuring that the recent analysis of large-scale trials of vaccines containing emulsified mineral oils, performed 30–40 years ago, has shown that such procedures do not increase the incidence of neoplasms or autoimmune disease.

Activation of antigen-presenting cells

Under the influence of the repository adjuvants, macrophages form granulomas which provide sites for interaction with antibody-forming cells. The maintenance by the depot of consistent antigen concentrations ensures that, as antigen-sensitive cells divide within the granuloma, their progeny are highly likely to be further stimulated by antigen. Virtually all adjuvants deliver antigens to antigen-presenting cells and stimulate them by improving immunogenicity through an increase in the concentration of processed antigen on their surface and the efficiency of its presentation to lymphocytes, by the provision of accessory costimulatory signals to direct lymphocytes towards

an immune response rather than tolerance, and by the secretion of soluble stimulatory cytokines which influence the proliferation of lymphocytes. For example, quite apart from the ability of mycobacterial hsp70 to act as a powerful carrier, its innate adjuvanticity (figure 14.7) is mediated by upregulating expression of the proinflammatory cytokines, TNF, IL-1β and IL-6, through a CD14/NFκB pathway. One of the most potent stimulators of antigen-presenting cells is lipid A from Gram-negative bacterial lipopolysaccharide (LPS), but it has many side-effects and interest has shifted to its derivative, monophosphoryl lipid A (MLA), which is less toxic. The **Ribi adjuvant**, perhaps one of the most commonly used formulations in experimental work (and hopefully in humans), is a water-in-oil emulsion incorporating MLA and an MDP derivative (see below).

Effects on lymphocytes

In mice, alum tends to stimulate helper cells of the Th2 family, whereas complete Freund's adjuvant favors the Th1 subset. It will be recalled that complete Freund's is made from the incomplete adjuvant by addition of killed mycobacteria (cf. p. 192), but the immunopathological effects of the mycobacterial component in complete Freund's are so striking that its use in humans is not normally countenanced; fortunately, the active component has been identified as the water-soluble **muramyl dipeptide** (MDP; *N*-acetyl-muramyl-L-alanyl-D-isoglutamine) and a number of acceptable derivatives are now available. Hydrophilic MDP analogs with aqueous antigen preferentially stimulate antibody responses, but if administered in a hydrophobic microenvironment, such as mineral oil, or incorporated into liposomes, CMI is the major outcome.

The role of modulatory cytokines in these early immunologic interactions is important, and several experimental approaches are exploring the effect of cytokines administered simultaneously with antigen. In one study, a construct of the macrophage stimulator *g*ranulocyte–*m*acrophage *c*olony-*s*timulating *f*actor (GM-CSF), linked to a monoclonal immunoglobulin, successfully induced anti-idiotypic responses relevant to the treatment of chronic lymphocytic leukemia. IL-2 has an adjuvant activity in unresponsive leprosy patients and a single injection in dialysis patients effectively induced their seroconversion to hepatitis B surface antigen. The potential of IL-12 to encourage Th1 responses is also being actively pursued.

The need for adjuvants which stimulate mucosal immunity is being met by exploiting the ability of *E. coli*

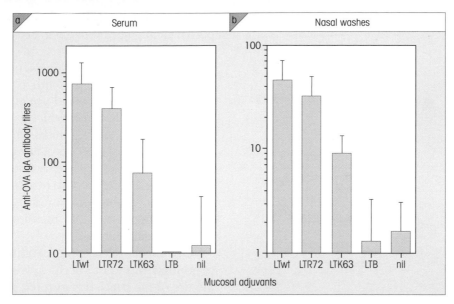

Figure 14.16. Mucosal adjuvanticity of mutants of *E. coli* heat-labile enterotoxin (LT) with reduced toxicity. Ovalbumin-specific IgA antibody titers (mean + SD) in mice immunized intranasally three times with ovalbumin alone or in combination with wild-type LT (LTwt), an A → R mutant of the A chain at position 72 (LTR72) retaining only 0.6% of the toxic ADP-ribosyltransferase activity, a non-toxic S → K mutant of the A chain at position 63 (LTK63), and the recombinant B chain (LTB) which targets the monosialoganglioside (GMI) receptor-binding site. LTR72 has comparable adjuvanticity to LTwt but only very low toxicity (LTwt is responsible for travelers' diarrhea). Even higher titers of antibody are recovered from lung washes and lesser amounts from vaginal washes. (Data from Giuliani M.M. *et al.* (1998) *Journal of Experimental Medicine* **187**, 1123, reproduced with permission.)

heat-labile enterotoxin (LT) and cholera toxin to target intestinal cells. LT is very immunogenic when given by the oral route and a nontoxic mutant of comparable potency as an adjuvant (figure 14.16) has been developed for ultimate use in humans. Coupling a protein antigen to cholera toxin B subunit targets the vaccine to the epithelial cells of the intestinal tract and usually produces good IgG and IgA antibodies which appear also in the saliva, tears and milk, indicating that the antigen-specific IgA precursor cells become disseminated throughout the MALT system. Whether the immune response to the cholera precludes its use as a carrier for immunization with further antigens remains an open question. Speaking of cholera toxin, it was reported that a soluble antigen, such as diphtheria toxoid, applied to the skin of mice together with cholera toxin produced persistent high levels of IgG antibodies, a not entirely predictable outcome.

Newer approaches to the presentation of antigen

Recent interest has centered on the use of small lipid membrane vesicles (**liposomes**) as agents for the presentation of antigen to the immune system. It may be that the liposome acts as a storage vacuole within the macrophage or perhaps fuses with the macrophage membrane to provide a suitably immunogenic complex. The differing pathways for processing peptides within antigen-presenting cells can be turned to advantage by encapsulating antigen in acid-resistant liposomes so that they can only enter the MHC class I route and stimulate CD8 T-cells. Antigens within acid-sensitive liposomes become associated with both class I and class II molecules. Proteins anchored in the lipid membrane by hydrophobic means give augmented CMI. Short synthetic peptides coupled covalently to monophosphoryl lipid A or tripalmitoyl-*S*-glyceryl-cysteinyl-seryl-serine (P3CSS) have high priming efficiency. One can readily envisage the possibility of a single-shot liposome vaccine with multiple potentialities which incorporate several antigens, different adjuvants and specialized targeting molecules (figure 14.17).

Another innovation is the **Iscom** (immunostimulating complex), a hydrophobic matrix of the surfactant saponin, with antigen, cholesterol and phosphatidylcholine. Antigens with a transmembrane hydrophobic region, such as surface molecules of lipid-containing viruses, are powerfully immunogenic in this vehicle and may engender cytotoxic T-cell responses. Iscoms are extremely resistant to acid and bile salts and are immunogenic by the oral route, producing systemic immunity and good local secretory IgA. Intranasal exposure established protective immunity to influenza

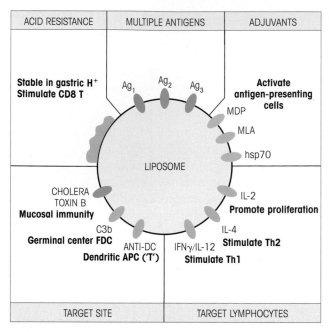

Figure 14.17. The 'do-it-all-in-one' omnipotent liposome particle illustrating some possible ways to build immunogenic flexibility into a single-shot liposome vaccine. The interior of the liposome may also contain depots of certain components. MDP, muramyl dipeptide; MLA, monophosphoryl lipid A; hsp70, mycobacterial heat-shock protein 70.

in mice. Saponin itself, initially purified from the bark of the tree *Quillaja saponaria*, is too toxic for human use. A less toxic derivative, Quil A, is widely used for veterinary vaccines, but an even less toxic derivative, QS21, is being evaluated for safety and efficacy in clinical trials. Another group of surfactants, the non-ionic block copolymers having a hydrophobic poly-oxypropylene core linked to hydrophilic polymers of polyoxyethylene, are likely to be acceptable for use in humans.

It may be useful to focus on the notion floated earlier that polymeric antigens tend to be more immuno-genic, and to note a novel form of solid matrix of the Cowan strain of *S. aureus* which can bind several molecules of monoclonal antibody, which can, in turn, immobilize several molecules of antigen. Using a variety of monoclonals, one can purify onto their binding sites appropriate antigens from a mixture to give a multivalent subunit vaccine. One could also incorporate the *E. coli* enterotoxin mutants mentioned above to give good mucosal immunity.

With respect to the practicability and convenience of administration of vaccines, we should not ignore the use of the **biolistics gun** (cf. p. 141) to introduce gold microspheres coated with plasmids of the gene encoding the vaccine antigen or antigens (cf. p. 290).

There have been some very important advances in the design of controlled-release systems for antigen delivery *in vivo*. Polymers of polylactic–polyglycolic esters are nontoxic biodegradable vehicles which can be prepared in a mixture of different formulations to provide **slow release** of an antigen (or any active drug or hormone) for periods up to several months.

There are exciting times ahead for vaccine development, but it should always be borne in mind that no matter how successful these clever strategies prove to be in experimental animals, the acid test which destroys so many promising approaches is the long-term effect in the human.

SUMMARY

Passively acquired immunity

- Passive immunity can be acquired by maternal antibodies or from homologous pooled γ-globulin.
- Horse antisera are more restricted because of the danger of serum sickness.
- Antibodies are being constructed to order using recombinant DNA technology and can be produced in bulk in plants.

Vaccination

- Active immunization provides a protective state through contact with a harmless form of the disease organism.
- A good vaccine should be based on antigens which are easily available, cheap, stable under extreme climatic conditions and nonpathogenic.

Killed organisms as vaccines

- Killed bacteria and viruses have been widely used.

Live attenuated organisms

- The advantages are: replication gives a bigger dose, the immune response is produced at the site of the natural infection.
- Attenuated vaccinia or polio can provide a 'piggy-back' carrier for genes from other organisms which are difficult to attenuate.
- BCG is a good vehicle for antigens requiring CD4 T-cell

(continued)

immunity and salmonella constructs may give oral and systemic immunity. Intranasal immunization is fast gaining popularity.

• The risk with live attenuated organisms is reversion to the virulent form and danger to immunocompromised individuals.

Subunit vaccines

• Whole organisms have a multiplicity of antigens, some of which are not protective, may induce hypersensitivity or might even be frankly immunosuppressive.

• It makes sense in these cases to use purified components.

• There is greatly increased use of recombinant DNA technology to produce these antigens. Expression in bananas provides a very cheap way of achieving oral immunization in the developing world.

• Naked DNA encoding the vaccine subunit can be injected directly into muscle, where it expresses the protein and produces immune responses. The advantages are stability, ease of production and cheapness.

• Epitope-specific vaccines based on conserved structures have the advantage that they can provide broad protection and may avoid the possible deleterious effects of other epitopes (autoimmunity, T-downregulation, original antigenic sin, escape by mutation of immunodominant epitopes) when certain whole antigens are used for immunization.

• Epitope-specific vaccines can be based on peptides, internal image anti-idiotypes or epitope-loss mutants.

• Peptides may only usefully mimic the native protein for vaccination to produce antibody if the epitope is linear and relatively unconstrained in structure. Carriers such as tetanus toxoid or mycobacterial heat-shock proteins are needed to make the peptide immunogenic. Linear peptides can mimic T-cell epitopes in the whole protein.

• Epitope-loss mutants have undesirable epitopes replaced but still fold correctly to produce the wanted discontinuous B-cell epitope(s).

Current vaccines

• Children in the USA and UK are routinely immunized with diphtheria and tetanus toxoids and pertussis (DTP triple vaccine) and attenuated strains of measles, mumps and rubella (MMR) and polio. BCG is given at 10–14 years.

• Subunit forms of pertussis lacking side-effects are being introduced.

• The capsular polysaccharide of *H. influenzae* has to be linked to a carrier.

• The elderly receive vaccines of influenza and *Pneumococcus* polysaccharides.

• Vaccines for hepatitis A and B, meningitis, yellow fever, typhoid, cholera and rabies are available for travelers and high-risk groups.

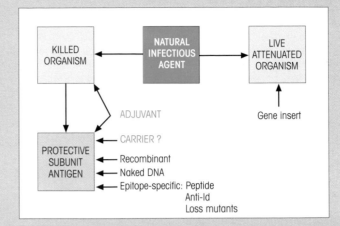

Figure 14.18. Strategies for vaccination.

Vaccines in development

• In malaria, the experimental vaccines are targeted at the *sporozoite and blood stages*, the *toxin* producing serious side-effects, the *gametes* and the insect gut trypsin.

• Recombinant glutathione-*S*-transferase is a promising candidate for a vaccine against schistosomiasis.

• An oral vaccine composed of cholera toxin B subunit and killed vibrios induced good mucosal immunity to cholera.

Adjuvants

• Adjuvants work by producing depots of antigen, and by activating macrophages; they sometimes have direct effects on lymphocytes.

• Adjuvants such as the muramyl dipeptide analogs derived from mycobacterial cell walls and the monophosphoryl lipid A derivative from Gram-negative LPS may soon be in general use.

• New methods of delivery include linking the antigen to small lipid membrane vesicles (liposomes) or a special glycoside matrix (Iscom). These delivery particles can be furnished with many factors which improve their immunogenicity and flexibility. One can build in several antigens into the same particle, adjuvants such as MDP and MLA, cytokines to influence lymphocyte subset responses and molecules such as cholera toxin B and *E. coli* enterotoxin to target particular sites in the body.

• Antigens built into biodegradable polymers of varying half-life can provide single-shot vaccines which mimic a conventional course of immunization requiring several injections.

The overall strategies for vaccination are summarized in figure 14.18.

See the accompanying website (**www.roitt.com**) for multiple choice questions.

FURTHER READING

Del Giudice G., Covacci A., Telford J.L., Montecucco C. & Rappuoli R. (2001) The design of vaccines against *Heliobacter pylori* and their development. *Annual Review of Immunology* **19**, 523.

Featherstone C. (1996) Vaccines by agriculture. *Molecular Medicine Today* **2**, 278.

Harding C.V., Collins D.S., Kanagawa O. & Unanue E.R. (1991) Liposome-encapsulated antigens engender liposomal processing for class II MHC presentation and cytosolic processing for class I presentation. *Journal of Immunology* **147**, 2860.

Kumar V. & Sercarz E. (1996) Genetic vaccination: the advantages of going naked. *Nature Medicine* **2**, 857.

Lambert P.H. (1993) New vaccines for the world—needs and prospects. *The Immunologist* **1**, 50.

Mims C.A., Playfair J.H.L., Roitt I.M., Wakelin D. & Williams R. (1998) *Medical Microbiology*, 2nd edn. Mosby, London.

Nicholson B.H. (ed.) (1994) *Synthetic Vaccines*. Blackwell Science, Oxford.

Nossal G.J.V. (2000) The global alliance for vaccines and immunization—a millennial challenge. *Nature Immunology* **1**, 5.

Peter G. (1992) Current concepts: childhood immunizations. *New England Journal of Medicine* **327**, 1794.

Powell M.F. & Newman M.J. (eds) (1995) *Vaccine Design*. Plenum Publishing, New York.

Sherwood J.K. *et al.* (1996) Controlled release of antibodies for long-term topical passive immunoprotection of female mice against genital herpes. *Nature Biotechnology* **14**, 468.

Whittum-Hudson J.A. *et al.* (1996) Oral immunisation with anti-idiotype to exoglycolipid antigen protects against *Chlamydia trachomatis* infection. *Nature Medicine* **2**, 1116.

Yap P.L. (ed.) (1992) *Clinical Applications of Intravenous Immunoglobulin Therapy*. Churchill Livingstone, Edinburgh.

Zinkernagel R. & Lambert P.H. (1992) Immunity to infection. *Current Opinion in Immunology* **4**, 385 (also 1993, **5**, issue 4).

Immunodeficiency

INTRODUCTION

In accord with the dictum that 'most things that can go wrong, do so', a multiplicity of immunodeficiency states in humans, which are **not secondary** to environmental factors, have been recognized. These 'experiments of nature' provide valuable clues regarding the function of the defective factors concerned. We have earlier stressed the manner in which the interplay of complement, antibody and phagocytic cells constitutes the basis of a tripartite defense mechanism against pyogenic (pus-forming) infections with bacteria which require prior opsonization before phagocytosis. It is not surprising, then, that deficiency in any one of these factors may predispose the individual to repeated infections of this type. Patients with T-cell deficiency of course present a markedly different pattern of infection, being susceptible to those viruses and moulds which are normally eradicated by cell-mediated immunity (CMI).

A relatively high incidence of malignancies, and of autoantibodies with or without autoimmune disease, has been documented in patients with immunodeficiency possibly due to failure of T-cell regulation or inability to control key viral infections.

The following sections examine various forms of these **primary immunodeficiencies** which have a genetic basis.

DEFICIENCIES OF INNATE IMMUNE MECHANISMS

Phagocytic cell defects

In **chronic granulomatous disease** the monocytes and polymorphs fail to produce reactive oxygen intermediates (figure 15.1) due to a defect in the cytochrome b_{558} oxidase system (cf. p. 4) normally activated by phagocytosis. The cytochrome has 92 and 22 kDa subunits and, in the X-linked form of the disease, there are mutations in the gene encoding the larger of these subunits. In the majority of cases, no cytochrome is produced, but one variant gp92 mutation permits the synthesis of low levels of the protein (figure 15.1) and the condition can be improved by treatment with γ-interferon. The 30% of chronic granulomatous disease patients who inherit their disorder in an autosomal recessive pattern express a defective form of the oxidase resulting from mutations in the smaller p22^{phox} cy-

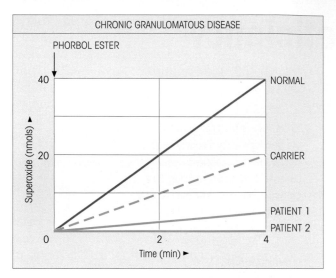

Figure 15.1. Defective respiratory burst in neutrophils of patients with chronic granulomatous disease. The activation of the NADP/cytochrome oxidase is measured by superoxide anion ($\cdot O_2^-$; cf. figure 1.10) production following stimulation with phorbol myristate acetate. Patient 2 has a p92^{phox} mutation which prevents expression of the protein, whilst patient 1 has the variant p92^{phox} mutation producing very low but measurable levels. Many carriers of the X-linked disease express intermediate levels, as in the individual shown who is the mother of patient 2. (Data from Smith R.M. & Curnutte J.T. (1991) *Blood* **77**, 673.)

tochrome subunit and in the cytosolic p47^{phox} and p67^{phox} (*phox* = phagocyte oxidase) components of the total reduced nicotinamide adenine dinucleotide phosphate (NADPH) oxidase system. Not unexpectedly, the knockout of gp92^{phox} provides a handy mouse model (cf. figure 1.10).

Curiously, the range of infectious pathogens which trouble these patients is relatively restricted. The most common pathogen is *Staphylococcus aureus*, but certain Gram-negative bacilli and fungi such as *Aspergillus fumigatus* and *Candida albicans* are frequently involved. The factors underlying this restriction are two-fold. First, many bacteria help to bring about their own destruction by generating H_2O_2 through their own metabolic processes, but if they are catalase positive, the peroxide is destroyed and the bacteria will survive. Thus polymorphs from these patients readily take up catalase-positive staphylococci in the presence of antibody and complement but fail to kill them intracellularly. Second, the organisms which are most virulent tend to be those that are highly resistant to the oxygen-independent microbicidal mechanisms of the phagocyte.

Lack of the CD18 β subunit of the $β_2$ integrins produces a **leukocyte adhesion deficiency** causing impaired neutrophil chemotaxis and recurrent bacterial infection. Emigration of monocytes, eosinophils and lymphocytes is unaffected since these can fall back on the alternative VCAM-1/VLA-4 $β_1$ integrin system. Two cases (remember these primary immunodeficiencies tend to be pretty rare) of leukocyte adhesion deficiency associated with mental retardation and Bombay hh blood group phenotype had defective neutrophil motility due to a failure to produce sialyl Lewis^x, the ligand used to bind to the selectins on endothelial cells. The defect in the synthesis of blood group H antigen, which is also a fucosylated carbohydrate, suggests a defect in fucose metabolism. In the not too distant future, these deficiencies will be treated by gene replacement but, in the meantime, allogeneic bone marrow grafts used to correct the CD18-linked disease are surprisingly well tolerated, possibly because of the LFA-1 defect.

In **Chediak–Higashi** disease and the 'beige' murine counterpart, dysfunction of NK cells and neutrophils is associated with the accumulation of giant intracytoplasmic granules which result from defective trafficking of the late endosomal/lysosomal compartment. The patients suffer from sometimes fatal pyogenic infections, particularly with *Staphylococcus aureus*. Infection often triggers a mysterious 'accelerated phase' of unremitting T-cell proliferation, but this can be brought under control by bone marrow transplantation.

Mendelian susceptibility to mycobacterial infection in humans involving BCG or nontuberculous mycobacteria can be traced to recessive mutations in four genes, two affecting the chains of the IFNγ receptor (IFNγR1 and IFNγR2) and, the others, the IL-12 p40 and IL-12R β1 subunits. Apart from some increased susceptibility to *Salmonella*, no other opportunistic infections were observed, highlighting the selectivity of the IFNγ protective role. To put things in perspective, mycobacteria induce IL-12 secretion by macrophages and dendritic cells which then activates both NK and T-cells; these then produce IFNγ which turns on the macrophage mechanisms providing protection against less pathogenic mycobacteria.

There is a group of so-called **'autoinflammatory' disorders** characterized by apparently unprovoked inflammation unrelated to high titer autoantibodies or antigen-specific T-cells. One such, **TNF receptor-associated periodic syndrome** (TRAPS), presents with prolonged fever bouts and severe localized inflammation caused by dominantly inherited mutations in the *TNFRSFIA* gene encoding the 55 kDa TNF receptor. Impaired cleavage of the receptor ectodomain with diminished shedding of the potentially antagonistic soluble receptor may account for the persistent inflammatory signal, and it is salutary to note the beneficial effects of treatment with a recombinant p75 TNFR-Fcγ fusion protein or anti-TNF. Yet another hereditary periodic fever syndrome is **familial Mediterranean fever** due to mutations in the *MEFV* gene that encodes a 95 kDa inflammatory regulator denoted as pyrin or marenostrin, expressed predominantly in neutrophils and Th1 cytokine-activated monocytes.

Complement system deficiencies

Defects in control proteins

The importance of complement in defense against infections is emphasized by the occurrence of repeated life-threatening infection with pyogenic bacteria in patients lacking factor I, the C3b inactivator. Because of this inability to destroy C3b, there is continual activation of the alternative pathway through the feedback loop, leading to very low C3 and factor B levels with normal C1, C4 and C2.

Each red blood cell is bombarded daily with 1000 molecules of C3b generated through the formation of fluid phase alternative pathway C3 convertase from the spontaneous hydrolysis of the internal thiolester of C3. There are several regulatory components on the red cell surface to deal with this. The C3 convertase complex is dissociated by decay accelerating factor (DAF; CD55) and by CR1 complement receptors (not forgetting factor H from the fluid phase; cf. p. 11), after which the C3b is dismembered by factor I in concert with CR1, membrane cofactor protein (MCP) or factor H (figure 15.2). There are also two inhibitors of the membrane attack complex, homologous restriction factor (HRF) and the abundant protectin molecule (CD59) which, by binding to C8, prevent the unfolding of the first C9 molecule needed for membrane insertion. DAF, HRF and CD59 bind to the membrane through glycosyl phosphatidylinositol anchors. In a condition known as **paroxysmal nocturnal hemoglobinuria (PNH)**, there is a defect in the ability to synthesize these anchors, caused by a mutation in the X-linked *PIG-A* gene encoding the enzyme required for adding *N*-acetyl glucosamine to phosphatidylinositol. In the absence of these complement regulators, serious lysis of the red cells occurs. In the less severe type II PNH, there is a defect in DAF, but in the type III form, associated also with deficiency of CD59, susceptibility to spontaneous complement-mediated lysis is greatly increased (figure 15.2). The erythrocytes can be normalized by adding back the deficient factors.

In **acute myocardial infarction**, the expression of

Figure 15.2. Paroxysmal nocturnal hemoglobinuria (PNH). A mutation in the *PIG-A* gene, which encodes α-1,6-*N*-acetyl glucosaminyl-transferase, results in an inability to synthesize the glycosyl phosphatidylinositol anchors, deprives the red cell membrane of complement control proteins and renders the cell susceptible to complement-mediated lysis. Type II is associated with a DAF defect and the more severe type III with additional CD59 deficiency. DAF, decay accelerating factor; CR1, complement receptor type 1; MCP, membrane cofactor protein; HRF, homologous restriction factor; MAC, membrane attack complex.

the CD59 protectin decreases, perhaps due to the shedding of small membrane vesicles, and this sensitizes the injured myocardial cells to attack by the membrane attack complex (MAC) leading to a clear demarcation between nonviable and viable tissue areas.

An inhibitor of active C1 is grossly lacking in **hereditary angioedema** and this can lead to recurring episodes of acute circumscribed noninflammatory

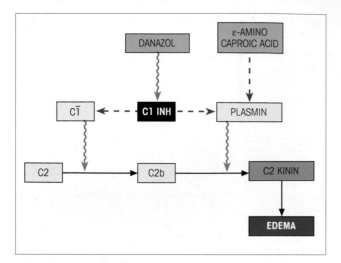

Figure 15.3. C1 inhibitor deficiency and angioedema. C1 inhibitor stoichiometrically inhibits C1, plasmin, kallikrein and activated Hageman factor and deficiency leads to formation of the vasoactive C2 kinin by the mechanism shown. The synthesis of C1 inhibitor can be boosted by methyltestosterone or preferably the less masculinizing synthetic steroid, danazol; alternatively, attacks can be controlled by giving ε-aminocaproic acid to inhibit the plasmin.

edema mediated by a vasoactive C2 fragment (figure 15.3). The patients are heterozygotes and synthesize small amounts of the inhibitor which can be raised to useful levels by administration of the synthetic anabolic steroid danazol or, in critical cases, of the purified inhibitor itself. ε-Aminocaproic acid, which blocks the plasmin-induced liberation of the C2 kinin, provides an alternative treatment.

Deficiency of components of the complement pathway

Deficiencies in C1q, C1r, C1s, C4 and C2 predispose to the development of immune complex diseases such as SLE (cf. p. 425), perhaps due to a decreased ability to mount an adequate host response to infection with a putative etiologic agent or, more probably, to eliminate antigen–antibody complexes effectively (cf. p. 337). Bearing in mind the focus of the autoimmune response in SLE on the molecular constituents of the blebs appearing on the surface of apoptotic cells (cf. p. 427), the importance of C1q in binding to and clearing these apoptotic bodies becomes paramount. So it is that C1q-deficient mice develop high titer antinuclear antibodies and die with severe glomerulonephritis. In another twist to the story, apoptotic bodies coated with C1q and C4 migrate to the bone marrow where they bind the C4b receptor and negatively select self-

reactive B-cells, as evidenced by the activation of antinuclear B-cells in C4-deficient animals.

Permanent deficiencies in C5, C6, C7, C8 and C9 have all been described in humans, yet in virtually every case the individuals are healthy and not particularly prone to infection, apart from an increased susceptibility to disseminated *Neisseria gonorrhoeae* and *N. meningitidis*. Thus full operation of the terminal complement system does not appear to be essential for survival, and adequate protection must be largely afforded by opsonizing antibodies and the immune adherence mechanism.

PRIMARY B-CELL DEFICIENCY

X-Linked (Bruton-type) a-γ-globulinemia is due to early B-cell maturation failure

Bruton's congenital a-γ-globulinemia is one of several immunodeficient syndromes which have been mapped to the X chromosome (figure 15.4). The defect occurs at the pre-B-cell stage and the production of immunoglobulin in affected males is grossly depressed, there being few lymphoid follicles or plasma cells in lymph node biopsies. Mutations occur in Bruton's tyrosine kinase (*Btk*) gene, which is also responsible for the *xid* defect in mice. The children are subject to repeated infection by pyogenic bacteria—*Staphylococcus aureus*, *Streptococcus pyogenes* and *S. pneumoniae*, *Neisseria meningitidis*, *Haemophilus influenzae*—and by a rare protozoan, *Pneumocystis carinii*, which produces a strange form of pneumonia. Cell-mediated immune responses are normal and viral infections such as measles and smallpox are readily brought under control. Therapy involves the repeated administration of human γ-globulin to maintain adequate concentrations of circulating immunoglobulin.

Mutations in either the μ heavy chain or the λ_5 chain, which contribute to the surrogate IgM receptor on pre-B-cells (cf. p. 238), result in a phenotype similar to that seen in Bruton's a-γ-globulinemia with arrest at the pro-B stage. The implication would be that *Btk* provides the signal for pro- to pre-B differentiation through this pre-B-cell receptor complex.

IgA deficiency and common variable immunodeficiency (CVID) have a similar genetic basis

These diseases, which are the first and second most common primary immunodeficiencies, represent the extreme ends of a spectrum of immunoglobulin defi-

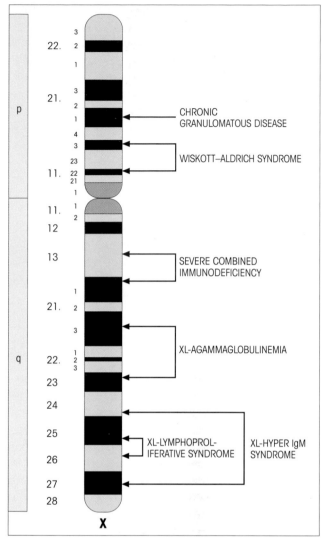

Figure 15.4. Loci of the X-linked (XL) immunodeficiency syndromes. Males are more likely to be affected by X-linked recessive genes because, unlike the situation with females where there are two X chromosomes, homozygosity is not needed.

and Fas by CD4 cells and an increased rate of apoptosis. CVID patients have to be protected against recurrent pyogenic infections with intravenous γ-globulin but, strangely, HIV infection restores the production of IgG and IgM, but not IgA, antibodies. This could mean that CVID is potentially reversible by immunoregulatory factors and lends support to the notion that selective IgA deficiency predisposes to CVID.

Transient hypo-γ-globulinemia is seen in early life

A degree of immunoglobulin deficiency occurs naturally in human infants as the maternal IgG level wanes, and may become a serious problem in very premature babies. A more protracted **transient hypo-γ-globulinemia of infancy**, characterized by recurrent respiratory infections, is associated with low IgG levels which often return somewhat abruptly to normal by 4 years of age. There is a deficiency in the number of circulating lymphocytes and in their ability to generate help for Ig production by B-cells activated by pokeweed mitogen, but this becomes normal as the disease resolves spontaneously.

PRIMARY T-CELL DEFICIENCY

Patients with no T-cells or poor T-cell function are vulnerable to opportunistic infections and, since B-cell function is to a large extent T-dependent, T-cell deficiency also impacts negatively on humoral immunity. Dysfunctional T-cells often permit the emergence of allergies, lymphoid malignancies and autoimmune syndromes, the latter presumably arising from inefficient negative selection in the thymus or the failure to generate appropriate regulatory cells.

Some deficiencies affect early T-cell differentiation

The **DiGeorge** and **Nezelof syndromes** are characterized by a failure of the thymus to develop properly from the third and fourth pharyngeal pouches during embryogenesis (DiGeorge children also lack parathyroids and have severe cardiovascular abnormalities). Consequently, stem cells cannot differentiate to become T-lymphocytes and the 'thymus-dependent' areas in lymphoid tissue are sparsely populated; in contrast, lymphoid follicles are seen but even these are poorly developed (figure 15.5). Cell-mediated immune responses are undetectable and, although the infants can deal with common bacterial infections, they

ciencies. IgA deficiency, which may include IgG2, and CVID often occur within the same family with frequent sharing of HLA haplotype, and individual family members may gradually convert from one disease to the other. This suggests a common genetic basis, but the heterogeneity of the disease complicates the search for candidate genes which has not so far progressed beyond the identification of one or more susceptibility loci within the TNF/lymphotoxin region of the MHC class III genes. Likewise, the cellular defects have not been satisfactorily pinpointed: the majority of patients have a defect in T-cell priming by antigen which *might* be attributable to an antigen-presenting cell dysfunction, and most patients reveal a pattern of raised CD8 IFNγ production, increased expression of HLA-DR

Figure 15.5. Lymph node cortex. (a) From patient with DiGeorge syndrome showing depleted thymus-dependent area (TDA) and small primary follicles (PF); (b) from normal subject: the populated T-cell area and the well-developed secondary follicle with its mantle of small lymphocytes (M) and pale-staining germinal center (GC) provide a marked contrast. (DiGeorge material kindly supplied by Dr D. Webster; photograph by Mr C.J. Sym.) In the murine model, the athymic nude mouse, there is an abnormality in the winged helix protein.

may be overwhelmed by vaccinia (figure 15.6) or measles, or by bacille Calmette–Guérin (BCG) if given by mistake. Humoral antibodies can be elicited, but the response is subnormal, presumably reflecting the need for the cooperative involvement of T-cells. (The similarity of this condition to neonatal thymectomy and of B-cell deficiency to neonatal bursectomy in the chicken should not go unmentioned.) Treatment by grafting neonatal thymus leads to restoration of immunocompetence, but some matching between the major histocompatibility antigens on the nonlymphocytic thymus cells and peripheral cells is essential for the proper functioning of the T-lymphocytes (p. 228). Complete absence of the thymus is pretty rare and more often one is dealing with a 'partial DiGeorge' in which the T-cells may rise from 6% at birth to around 30% of the total circulating lymphocytes by the end of the first year; antibody responses are adequate.

Mutation of the purine degradation enzyme, **purine nucleoside phosphorylase**, results in the accumulation of the metabolite deoxy-GTP which is toxic to T-cell precursors through its ability to inhibit ribonucleotide reductase, an enzyme required for DNA synthesis and hence cell replication. Targeting of the T-cell lineage by this deficiency could well be linked to a relatively low level of 5'-nucleotidase. Some T-cells 'leak through' but they give inadequate protection against infection and the disease is usually fatal unless a bone marrow transplant life-line is offered.

Mutations in the recombinase enzymes, RAG-1 and RAG-2 (cf. figure 3.8), which initiate *VDJ* recombination events, usually result in complete failure to generate mature antigen-specific lymphocyte receptors and give rise to the severe combined immunodeficiency (SCID) phenotype (see below). In **Omenn's syndrome**, the particular RAG mutants allow some T-cells, apparently of Th2 phenotype, to sneak through, although they are not capable of preventing a failure to thrive and relatively early death.

MHC class II deficiency, previously known by its more sleazy appellation, 'bare lymphocyte syndrome', is associated with recurrent bronchopulmonary infections and chronic diarrhea occurring within the first year of life, with death from overwhelming viral infections at a mean age of 4 years. The condition arises from mutations affecting the RFX-B, CIITA, RFX-5 and RFXAP promoter proteins that bind to the 5'-untranslated region of the class II genes. Feeble expression of class II molecules on thymic epithelial cells grossly impedes the positive selection of CD4 T-helpers, and those that do leak through will not be encouraged by the lack of class II on antigen-presenting cells and B-lymphocytes. Note also that rare patients with mutations in *TAP-1* or *TAP-2* have an MHC class I bare lymphocyte syndrome.

Figure 15.6. A child with severe combined immunodeficiency showing skin lesions due to infection with vaccinia gangrenosum resulting from smallpox immunization. Lesions were widespread over the whole body. (Reproduced by kind permission of Professor R.J. Levinsky and the Medical Illustration Department of the Hospital for Sick Children, Great Ormond Street, London.)

Deficiencies leading to dysfunctional T-cells

Cell-mediated immunity (CMI) is depressed in immunodeficient patients with **ataxia telangiectasia** or with thrombocytopenia and eczema (**Wiskott–Aldrich syndrome**). The *Wiskott–Aldrich syndrome protein* (**WASP**) plays a critical role in signal transduction by interacting with Src-homology 3 (SH3) domains and in the regulation of cytoskeletal reorganization. WASP clusters physically with actin through the GTPase Cdc42 and possibly other molecules which regulate actin polymerization. Mutations in the *WASP* gene thus adversely affect cell motility, phagocyte chemotaxis, dendritic cell trafficking and the polarization of the T-cell cytoskeleton towards the B-cells dur-

ing T–B collaboration. Poor cell-mediated immunity and impaired antibody production in affected boys are hardly surprising consequences.

Ataxia telangiectasia is a human autosomal recessive disorder of childhood which has been recognized as a **chromosomal breakage syndrome** characterized by progressive cerebellar ataxia with degeneration of Purkinje cells, a hypersensitivity to X-rays and an unduly high incidence of cancer. The mutated gene, *ATM*, encodes a protein kinase (Atm) which is a member of the phosphatidylinositol 3-kinase family. Following ultraviolet or ionizing radiation, the normal gene acts through the tumor suppressor protein p53 and thence p21 to arrest the cell cycle at the G1–S border, and through the Chk2 kinase and Cdc25 to block the G2–M transition. Presumably, the cellular DNA repair mechanisms now have a chance to operate. Regrettably, the relationship of the Atm defect to immunodeficiency is not clear. Another disease characterized by immune dysfunction, radiation sensitivity and increased incidence of cancer is the **Nijmegen breakage syndrome** where a mutation in the *NBS1* gene leads to a defective protein, nibrin, which normally functions as a component of a double-stranded DNA repair complex.

It is exciting to see the molecular basis of diseases being unraveled and an excellent example of nature yielding its secrets has been provided by studies on the **XL hyper-IgM syndrome**, a rare disorder characterized by recurrent bacterial infections, very low levels or absence of IgG, IgA and IgE and normal to raised concentrations of serum IgM and IgD. It transpires that point mutations and deletions in the T-cell CD40L (CD154) map to the part of the molecule thought to be concerned in the interaction with B-cell CD40 (cf. p. 174), thereby rendering the T-cells incapable of transmitting the signals needed for Ig class switching in B-cells. Maybe a note of caution regarding gene therapy would not be amiss at this point. CD40L knockout mice mimicking human X-linked hyper-IgM syndrome were injected with transduced BM or thymic cells using a retroviral vector containing the *CD40L* gene. Low level constitutive expression stimulated humoral and cellular immune functions, but 12 of 19 mice developed T-lymphoproliferative disorders, suggesting that current methods of gene therapy may be inappropriate for disorders involving highly regulated genes in essential positions in proliferative cascades.

Also for the collector are the rare cases of severe T-cell deficiency arising from mutation in the ε and γ chains of the CD3 complex and the ZAP-70 kinase (p. 166) which generate dysfunctional T-cells and preferentially impair the differentiation of CD8 T-cells.

COMBINED IMMUNODEFICIENCY

Severe combined immunodeficiency disease (SCID) involving B-, T- and NK cells represents the most severe form of primary immunodeficiency, affecting one child in approximately every 80 000 live births. These infants exhibit profound defects in cellular and humoral immunity, with death occurring within the first year of life due to severe and recurrent opportunistic infections. Prolonged diarrhea resulting from gastrointestinal infections and pneumonia due to *Pneumocystis carinii* are common; *Candida albicans* grows vigorously in the mouth or on the skin. If vaccinated with attenuated organisms (figure 15.6), these infants usually die of progressive infection. SCID infants must be rescued by a bone marrow transplant if they are to survive.

Reticular dysgenesis is a rapidly fatal variant of severe combined immunodeficiency associated with a lack of both myeloid and lymphoid cell precursors, but SCID can arise from a variety of circumstances which selectively target lymphoid cell differentiation.

Mutations in the IL-7 signaling pathway cause SCID

Over half of the cases of severe combined immunodeficiency (SCID), which affects both B- and T-cell development, derive from mutations in the γ_c chain of the receptors for interleukins IL-2, -4, -7, -9 and -15. Of these, IL-7R is the most crucial for lymphocyte differentiation, and mutations in the interleukin-specific IL-7R α chain, or in JAK3 which transduces the γ_c signal, produce similar phenotypes. Mutations in the γ_c cytokine receptor gene were completely rescued with autologous bone marrow stem cells cultured with growth factors on fibronectin fragments (the magic ingredient needed for success) and transfected with a retroviral vector carrying the normal gene. While the T-cell defects can be corrected by transplantation of haplotype-matched allogeneic marrow within the first 3 months of life without the need for myeloablative pretreatment, and with survival rates of as high as 96%, donors may not always be readily accessible and, in a proportion of cases, the B- and NK cell defects are not corrected; these would benefit from the transfected autologous cell strategy.

SCID can arise from grossly deficient *VDJ* recombination

Unlike the sneak through of immunocompetent cells which accompanies the partial *RAG* deficiency in Omenn's syndrome, grossly dysfunctional mutations in the recombinase enzymes, which catalyse the introduction of the double-stranded breaks permitting subsequent recombination of the *V*, *D* and *J* segments, prevent the emergence of any mature lymphocytes. Failure of the *VDJ* recombination mechanism is also a feature of the radiosensitive cells from SCID patients with defective DNA-dependent protein kinase, a component of the complex which realigns and repairs the free coding ends created by the RAG enzymes. Just a snippet—naturally occurring SCID with a similar phenotype has been identified in Arabian foals.

SCID can be due to mutations in the purine salvage pathway enzyme, adenosine deaminase

Many SCID patients have a genetic deficiency of the purine degradation enzyme, adenosine deaminase (ADA), which results in the accumulation of the metabolite, dGTP, which is toxic to early lymphoid stem cells. The comparable immunodeficiency seen in acute lymphocytic leukemia patients treated with the ADA inhibitor deoxycoformacin attests to the validity of this analysis. Half the ADA-deficient SCID patients do reasonably well on transfusions of normal red cells containing the enzyme, whereas others with a longer standing more severe deficiency, which might have affected the thymus epithelium, also require treatment with the enzyme modified by polyethylene glycol which extends its half-life. These patients are excellent candidates for gene therapy. Children have been treated with periodic infusion of their own T-cells corrected by transfection with the *ADA* gene linked to a retroviral vector. Significant reconstitution of antibody responses and delayed-type skin tests to environmental antigens has been achieved without apparent complications. Hematopoietic stem cells from umbilical cord blood transfected with the *ADA* gene could be detected up to 18 months of age, but the level of expression was very low and, until the technology is improved, such patients must be maintained on enzyme replacement therapy.

Combined immunodeficiency resulting from inherited defective control of lymphocyte function

X-linked lymphoproliferative disease (XLP), previously known as Duncan's syndrome, is a progressive immunodeficiency disorder characterized by fever, pharyngitis, lymphadenopathy and dysgammaglobulinemia, with a particular vulnerability to Epstein–Barr viral infection. Mutations have been uncovered in the *SH2DIA/SAP* gene encoding SAP (signaling lymphocytic activation molecule (SLAM)-associated protein) which binds to SLAM through its SH2 domain. Since triggering of SLAM leads to strong induction of IFNγ in both Th1 and Th2 cells and acts on B-cells to enhance proliferation and increase susceptibility to apoptosis, mutations in SAP which adversely affect the activation of SLAM will weaken the immune response, especially with regard to EBV infection where viral replication with B-cells is heavily controlled by host T-cells. Mutation in another signal regulatory protein, the CD45 protein tyrosine phosphatase, gave rise to the SCID seen in a child with feeble lymphocyte responses at 2 months of age.

Mice with the *lpr* gene exhibit a **progressive lymphoproliferative syndrome** reflecting an accumulation of abnormal CD4$^-$8$^-$ T-cells with variable autoimmune features (cf. table 19.4). The mutation encodes an incompetent Fas (CD95) molecule and thereby defective Fas-triggered lymphocyte apoptosis. The homozygous deficiency is extremely rare in humans. Impaired T- and B-cell development and excessive production of autoantibodies by B-1 cells are the consequences of mutations in **motheaten** mice (cf. p. 417), affecting the *h*ematopoietic *c*ell *p*hosphatase (HCP) which regulates phosphorylation events triggered by engagement of antigen receptors.

RECOGNITION OF IMMUNODEFICIENCIES

Defects in immunoglobulins can be assessed by quantitative estimations; levels of 2 g/l arbitrarily define the practical lower limit of normal. The humoral immune response can be examined by first screening the serum for natural antibodies (A and B isohemagglutinins, heteroantibody to sheep red cells, bactericidins against *E. coli*) and then attempting to induce active immunization with diphtheria, tetanus, pertussis and killed poliomyelitis—but no live vaccines. CD19, 20 and 22 are the main markers used to enumerate B-cells by immunofluorescence.

Patients with T-cell deficiency will be hypo- or unreactive in skin tests to such antigens as tuberculin, *Candida*, trichophytin, streptokinase/streptodornase and mumps. Active skin sensitization with dinitrochlorobenzene may be undertaken. The reactivity of peripheral blood mononuclear cells to phytohemagglutinin is a good indicator of T-lymphocyte reactivity as is also the one-way mixed lymphocyte reaction (see Chapter 17). Enumeration of T-cells is most readily achieved by cytofluorimetry using CD3 monoclonal antibody.

In vitro tests for complement and for the bactericidal and other functions of polymorphs are available, while the reduction of nitroblue tetrazolium (NBT) or the stimulation of superoxide production provides a measure of the oxidative enzymes associated with active phagocytosis.

SECONDARY IMMUNODEFICIENCY

Immune responsiveness can be depressed nonspecifically by many factors. CMI in particular may be impaired in a state of malnutrition, even of the degree which may be encountered in urban areas of the more affluent regions of the world. Iron deficiency is particularly important in this respect, as are zinc and selenium deficiencies.

Viral infections are not infrequently immunosuppressive, and the profound fall in cell-mediated immunity which accompanies **measles infection** has been attributed to specific suppression of IL-12 production by viral cross-linking of monocyte surface CD46 (the complement regulator also known as membrane cofactor protein; cf. p. 307). The most notorious immunosuppressive virus, human immunodeficiency virus (HIV), will be elaborated upon in the next major section. In lepromatous leprosy and malarial infection there is evidence for a constraint on immune responsiveness imposed by distortion of the normal lymphoid traffic pathways and, additionally, in the latter instance, macrophage function appears to be aberrant. Skewing of the balance between Th1 and Th2 cells as a result of infection may also depress the subset most appropriate for immune protection.

Many therapeutic agents, such as X-rays, cytotoxic drugs and corticosteroids, although often used in a nonimmunological context, can nonetheless have dire effects on the immune system (see p. 382). **B-lymphoproliferative disorders**, such as chronic lymphatic leukemia, myeloma and Waldenström's macroglobulinemia, are associated with varying degrees of hypo-γ-globulinemia and impaired antibody responses. Their common infections with pyogenic bacteria contrast with the situation in Hodgkin's disease where the patients display all the hallmarks of defective CMI—susceptibility to tubercle bacillus, *Brucella*, *Cryptococcus* and herpes zoster virus.

ACQUIRED IMMUNODEFICIENCY SYNDROME (AIDS)

Clinical features

AIDS is a particularly unpleasant fatal disease caused by infection with the human immunodeficiency virus

Figure 15.7. Viral pneumonia due to cytomegalovirus; radiograph showing extensive diffuse pneumonitis in both lung fields, characteristic of viral infection. (Reproduced from Lambert H.P. & Farrar W.E. (eds) (1982) *Infectious Diseases Illustrated*, p. 2.2. W.B. Saunders and Gower Medical Publishing, with permission.)

(HIV). It has reached endemic proportions and has thereby caused widespread alarm (and knowledge of immunology) amongst the public. Transmission is usually through infection with blood or semen containing HIV-1 or the related virus, HIV-2. In parts of Africa, where the incidence is frightful, transmission is largely by heterosexual contact. Prostitutes constitute a pivotal major initial reservoir of the infection, unlike their counterparts in developed countries, such as Japan, Australia, New Zealand, and the West, in whom the prevalence of AIDS has remained surprisingly low, and the majority of cases have occurred in male homosexuals, with other groups at risk including intravenous drug abusers, hemophiliacs receiving factor VIII derived from pooled plasma and infants of sexually promiscuous or drug-addicted mothers. Nevertheless, the number of infected heterosexuals is increasing. Death is usually due to pulmonary infection, but serious complications involving the nervous system are appearing in about 30% of cases. In essence, usually after a protracted latent period, there is a sudden onset of immunodeficiency associated with opportunistic infections involving, most commonly, *Pneumocystis carinii*, but also cytomegalovirus (figure 15.7), Epstein–Barr (EB) and herpes simplex viruses, fungi such as *Candida*, *Aspergillus* and *Cryptococcus*, and the protozoan *Toxoplasma*; additionally, there is exceptional susceptibility for Kaposi's sarcoma. There is also an AIDS-related complex (ARC), characterized by fever, weight loss and lymphadenopathy.

Characteristics of HIV

HIV-1/2 are members of the lentivirus group, which produce disease with a long latency and are adept at evading the immune system. They are RNA retroviruses with a relatively complex and tightly compressed genome (figure 15.8a) and the many virion proteins are generated by RNA splicing and cleavage by the viral protease (figure 15.8c).

The infection of cells by HIV

The envelope glycoprotein gp120 of HIV **binds avidly to cell surface CD4** molecules, but only initiates gp41-dependent fusion with the cell leading to infection when chemokine coreceptors are engaged (figure 15.8b). Helper T-cells with their abundant CD4 are a major target for infection, but the presence of even relatively low densities of CD4 on macrophages and microglia makes them susceptible to infection, and in the latter case is suspected to be a major factor in the cerebral complications of the disease. Different virus isolates vary in their relative tropism for T-cells and macrophages. Early in infection, the viruses utilize the CCR5 coreceptor for entry into memory T-cells and macrophages; these 'M-tropic' strains are usually unable to induce syncytia when cultured with CD4 T-cells (NSI, nonsyncytium inducing). These frequently evolve into 'T-tropic' strains which can infect resting T-cells using the CXCR4 coreceptor and are syncytium inducing (SI). Immature dendritic cells expressing CCR5 are attracted by the CC chemokines RANTES, MIP-1α and MIP-1β (see Table 10.3) which are released from cytotoxic T-lymphocytes (CTLs) when they encounter viral antigen. The dendritic cells capture HIV through a surface protein DC-SIGM and migrate to lymphoid tissue, where they form unique syncytia with T-cells which explosively drive replication of the virions by providing the two transcription factors needed: **Sp1** derived from unstimulated T-cells and **NFκB** proteins constitutively expressed by the dendritic cells. Undoubtedly, '*une liaison dangereuse*'! Possibly of crucial importance has been the discovery that suspensions of single *follicular* dendritic cells (FDCs) from human tonsil can be directly infected with HIV by a process which does not involve CD4. The infected cells permit viral replication and can reinfect T-cells *in vitro*. As we shall see, FDCs are a major reservoir of HIV in AIDS.

On gaining entry into a cell, HIV, as an RNA retrovirus, utilizes a **reverse transcriptase** to convert its genetic RNA into the corresponding DNA which is integrated into the host genome where it can remain

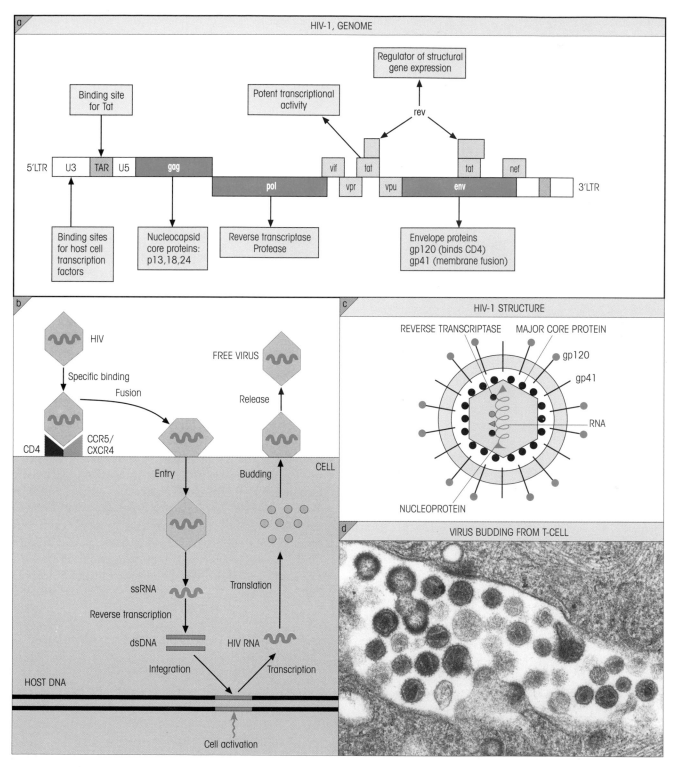

Figure 15.8. Characteristics of the HIV-1 AIDS virus. (a) HIV-1 genome and gene products. Tat, master switch, turns on all viral gene expression; *rev*, gene responsible for expression of structural proteins; *vif*, gene controlling infectivity by free, not cell-bound, virus; Vpr, weak transcriptional activator; Vpu, required for efficient virion budding and env processing; Nef, uncertain function linked to pathogenesis *in vivo*; LTR, long terminal repeats concerned in regulation of viral expression; contain regions reacting with products of *tat* and *nef* genes and in addition the *TATAAA* (the TATA box) promoter sequence, NFκB core enhancer elements and Sp-1-binding sites. Mice bearing the *tat* transgene develop Kaposi sarcoma-like skin lesions. (b) Intracellular life cycle of HIV. (c) HIV-1 structure. (d) Electron micrograph of mature and budding HIV-1 particles at the surface of human PHA blasts. (Courtesy of Dr Carol Upton and Professor S. Martin.)

latent for long periods (figure 15.8b). Stimulation of latently infected T-cells or macrophages activates HIV replication through an increase in the intracellular concentration of NFκB dimers, which bind to consensus sequences in the HIV enhancer region (figure 15.9). It is significant that tumor necrosis factor (TNF), which upregulates HIV replication through this NFκB pathway,

is present in elevated concentrations in the plasma of HIV-infected individuals, particularly in the advanced stage. Perhaps, also, the greater susceptibility of Africans to AIDS may be linked to activation of the immune system through continual microbial insult. Infectious virus is finally released from the cell by budding (figure 15.8d).

Natural history of the disease

The sequence of events following HIV-1 infection is charted in figure 15.10. An acute early retroviral syndrome with fever, myalgia, arthralgia and so forth is accompanied by viremia and positive tests for blood p24, a dominant nucleocapsid antigen. An immune response to the virus identifiable by circulating antibodies to p24 and the envelope proteins gp120 and gp41, and by the production of gp120-specific cytotoxic T-cells, curtails the viremia and leads to **sequestration of HIV in lymphoid tissue**. Trapping of viral particles complexed with antibody and complement stimulates follicular hyperplasia and infection of the FDC. In effect, the follicles become the principal site for viral replication and infection of other cells of the immune system (figure 15.11). Eventually, follicular involution leads to a gradual degeneration of the FDC network with an increase in viral burden and replication in peripheral blood mononuclear cells. Crucially, in patients with progressive disease, **circulating CD4 T-cell numbers fall steadily** but, only when there is profound depletion with levels below, say, $50\,\text{mm}^{-3}$, do the consequences for CMI responses, as exemplified by the depressed delayed-type skin reactivity to common antigens (figure 15.12) and the failure to produce

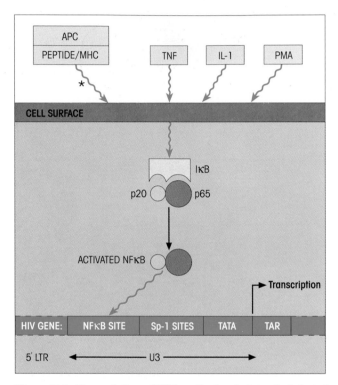

Figure 15.9. Upregulation of HIV replication in latently infected cell through external stimulation. *, T-cells only; IκB, inhibitor of NFκB.

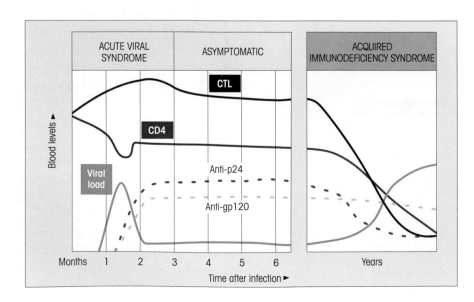

Figure 15.10. The natural history of HIV-1 infection.

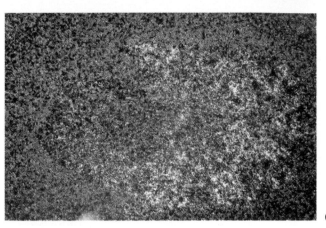

(a)

(b)

Figure 15.11. Abundance of HIV in lymphoid tissue demonstrated by *in situ* hybridization of lymph node sections from a representative HIV-infected patient in early stage disease. (a) Dark field image of a lymph node section after protease digestion. Location of HIV RNA is indicated by the silver grains which appear as white dots. An intense hybridization signal is predominantly restricted to the area of the germinal centers. (b) Higher magnification of a protease-digested section showing the intense distribution of silver grains in the light zone of a germinal center. (Reproduced from photos kindly provided by Dr A.S. Fauci with permission; cf. Pantaleo G., Graziosi C. & Fauci A.S. (1993) The role of the lymphoid organs in the pathogenesis of HIV infection. *Seminars in Immunology* **5**, 157.)

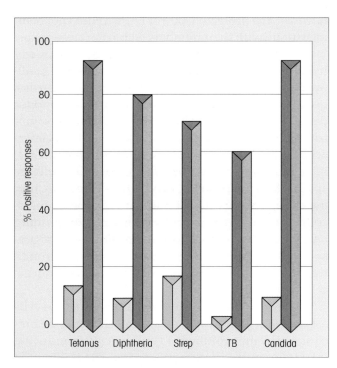

Figure 15.12. Skin test reactivity to common microbial antigens among AIDS patients (▢; *n* = 20) **and controls** (▮; *n* = 10). Other studies with more advanced patients have reported completely negative skin tests. (Reproduced from Lane H.C. & Fauci A.S. (1985) *Annual Reviews of Immunology* **3**, 477, with permission.)

cytomegalovirus-specific cytotoxic T-cells (Tc), become quite devastating. The patient is now wide open to life-threatening infections caused by normally nonpathogenic (i.e. opportunistic) agents such as *Pneumo-* *cystis carinii* and cytomegalovirus, characteristic of AIDS.

The diagnostic features of AIDS are pretty unmistakable

An individual with opportunistic infections, lymphopenia, low CD4 but relatively normal CD8 in the peripheral blood, raised IgG and IgA levels and poor skin tests to common recall antigens (figure 15.12) may well have AIDS, particularly if he or she comes from a group at risk. γ-Interferon (IFNγ) and neopterin, a degradation product of guanosine triphosphate (GTP) induced in macrophages by IFNγ, are good indicators of CMI and are significantly increased in AIDS infection preceding a subsequent loss of CD4 cells. Confirmation of the diagnosis comes from lymph node biopsy, showing profound abnormalities and drastic changes in germinal centers, and the demonstration of viral antibodies by enzyme-linked immunosorbent assay (ELISA) and by 'immunoblotting' (cf. pp. 113 and 117). Serum p24 antigen is often positive in active disease but isolation of virus or demonstration of the HIV genome provides the final confirmation of infection.

Factors affecting the progression of AIDS
(figure 15.13)

By looking for correlations between the speed with which infected individuals develop disease and the various parameters of the immune response, one hopes to gain insight into those elements which afford

Figure 15.13. Factors affecting HIV progression. *Neutralizing antibody more effective against HIV-2. HAART, highly active antiretroviral drug therapy.

some degree of protection and could guide the attempts to produce effective vaccines. Bearing in mind the discovery of the importance of CCR5 as a chemokine coreceptor for the infection of cells with NSI HIV clades, it is gratifying to note the 10-fold reduced risk of HIV infection in individuals **homozygous for the *CCR5Δ32* allele**, where the 32 base deletion encodes a nonfunctional product. Homozygotes represent 1–3% of northern Europeans, declining as one goes south, and absent in African, Asiatic and Oceanic populations. It has been speculated that the mutation may have been fixed in northwest Europe in the 14th century to provide a selective advantage against bubonic plague. The progression of HIV infection is delayed even in the heterozygotes.

As mentioned above, a powerful early **CD8 CTL response** can drastically reduce the viral load with beneficial effects long term. An important role for CTLs is implied by the extended survival of 28–40% of HIV-1-infected Caucasians who were fully heterozygous at HLA class I loci *lacking* B35 or CW4 alleles or both. Furthermore, viral load increased dramatically following CD8 depletion in macaque monkeys infected with simian immunodeficiency virus (SIV) which causes an AIDS-like syndrome. Being an RNA retrovirus, HIV is subject to a ferociously high mutation rate, and longitudinal studies in this model showed that CTL evasion by epitope mutation is an important escape strategy for compromising the antiviral immune response.

In addition to their capacity as CTL effectors, CD8 cells from infected patients produce a number of factors which suppress HIV replication in cultured CD4 cells. One of these factors is IL-16 which cross-links the membrane-proximal D4 domain of CD4 and blocks infection by the virus. It is relevant that high serum levels of IL-16 correlate well with slow progression of the disease.

Enumeration with HLA class I/peptide tetramers has revealed that up to 5% of total CD8 cells in the acute phase are specific for a single epitope and the numbers inversely correlate with viral load. As time goes on, however, the protective power of the cells is not commensurate with their numbers; in boxing jargon, they 'punch below their weight'. Whether they are purely dysfunctional or represent anergic or regulatory IL-10-producing cells is not clear, but on one point there is a general consensus: a sustained healthy **CD8 response depends heavily on robust CD4 Th1 effectors** contributing IFNγ, chemokines and useful cell to cell interactions. And here is the root of the problem since, initially, although more than 0.5% of total CD4 cells are specific for viral proteins, these are deleted soon after infection. There is no shortage of hypotheses to account for this depletion, but money tends to be riding on the induction of apoptosis in proliferating antigen-specific CD4 cells infected either directly or through the intimacy of syncytium formation with dendritic cells harboring the virus.

The horrendous fall in overall numbers of CD4 cells associated with the onset of clinical AIDS may be precipitated by the evolution of T-cell syncytium inducing (SI) strains as the disease progresses. The ability of SI virus to infect thymocytes might exacerbate an already precarious situation by cutting off the admittedly low volume supply of new T-cells still generated by an aged thymus. (Enthusiastic readers can ferret out even more hypothetical mechanisms for HIV-mediated T-depletion, e.g. in *Essential Immunology*, 9th edn, pp. 323–324, and Hazenberg M.O. *et al.* (2000) *Nature Immunology* **1**, 285.)

Antibodies to variable loop 3 (V3) of the envelope gp120 protein arise during disease and are frequently capable of preventing viral infection of CD4 T-cells *in vitro*. Nonetheless, they are rarely protective *in vivo*, partly because monkey experiments showed that very high titers are required and masking of epitopes by overhanging carbohydrate groups may blunt the immunogenicity, perhaps because virus may be directly transmitted from follicular dendritic cells to CD4 T-cells without exposure to antibody, and certainly because the V3 sequences undergo extensive mutation.

Neutralizing antibodies are more effective in **HIV-2** infection where progression to death is much slower than with HIV-1, and asymptomatic individuals commonly reveal deletions in the *Nef* gene, a slow or negligible decline in CD4 cells and strong CTL responses.

Therapeutic strategies for controlling AIDS

Highly active antiretroviral drug therapy (HAART) is very effective when given early in the disease and can reduce plasma viral load to undetectable levels. But the virus persists in a latent form in resting CD4 T-cells with a decay half-life of 40 months. Supposing that the reservoir of latent cells is as small as 1×10^5 cells, effective eradication could take as long as 60 years and, in any case, the treatment is very costly and not without side-effects. The sensible strategy is to keep this residual virus under control by the immune system. One approach is to use an intermittent drug regimen. This allows a re-emergence of virus capable of boosting reasonably robust immune responses which, in turn, would synergize with the reinstallation of combination drug therapy. The goal, though, is to develop a vaccine which could contain the infection following the initial HAART without the need for further antiviral drugs.

Given the relative efficacy of CD8 T-cells early in infection and their dependence on robust CD4 helpers, together with the evidence for the protective role of cell-mediated immunity in the SIV rhesus monkey model, effort is being directed towards Th1-biased vaccines. Logically, this should go hand-in-hand with the eradication of any concurrent worm infestation which would favor Th2 responses. Trials are in progress with vaccines incorporating a large number of T-cell epitope peptide sequences to minimize the chance of the infecting strains evading immune recognition by mutation and, where prophylactic immunization is contemplated, to take advantage of the fair degree of cross-clade recognition of defined CTL epitopes. In a series of studies in rhesus macaques, it tran-

spired that the most promising containment of challenge by a highly virulent virus with an envelope heterologous to the immunizing strain was achieved by intradermal priming with envelope *gag*, *pol* and *Nef* DNA, followed by boosting with recombinant fowlpox virus. Oral immunization with an **attenuated** recombined SIV/HIV vaccine in which the *Vpu* and *Nef* genes were deleted led to protection against vaginally transmitted infection, but there was a disturbing tendency for even the attenuated strains to be pathogenic. This underscores the importance of mucosal defense against initial infection and must give some credence to the idea that the presence of antiviral antibodies in mucosal secretions could be a significant factor in primary defense. In fact, despite the discouraging comments raised earlier, the identification of a strongly neutralizing monoclonal antibody directed to a conserved region of the gp160 envelope precursor suggests that, in a normal infection, antibodies to this potentially protective epitope might be overwhelmed by non-neutralizing responses to other adjacent B-cell epitopes; if this were so, an epitope which mimicked this conserved epitope could be an additional valuable vaccine candidate.

Some other approaches, still in their formative stages, are in the wings. Now that techniques of transfecting bone marrow cells are more successful, one looks for advances in 'intracellular immunization' through the introduction of genes encoding potentially anti-HIV molecules which will protect the future differentiated CD4 T-cell from infection. In one approach, bone marrow cells are transfected with a sequence of the CD4 gene coding for an HIV-blocking peptide; on regrafting, some of the stem cells will become CD4$^+$ T-cells, secreting a surrounding barrier of the blocking peptide which protects the lymphocyte from infection by the virus. Another group have transfected the stem cells with an scFv (cf. p. 125) gene encoding a single HIV-specific antibody combining site which disrupts the viral replication cycle. Using a similar system, one could also envisage the transfection of antisense genes to block the expression of HIV regulatory genes. Despite this frantic activity, a change in social behavior patterns would have a major impact on the relentless spread of AIDS. One cannot help recalling the aggrieved request by God to the supplicant, frustrated by the failure of his prayers to win him a lottery prize, to help Him by buying a lottery ticket.

SUMMARY

Primary immunodeficiency states (table 15.1)

• These occur in the human, albeit somewhat rarely, as a result of a defect in almost any stage of differentiation in the whole immune system.

• Rare X-linked mutations produce disease in males.

• Defects in phagocytic cells, the complement pathways or the B-cell system lead in particular to infection with bacteria which are disposed of by opsonization and phagocytosis.

• Patients with T-cell deficiencies are susceptible to viruses and moulds which are normally eradicated by CMI.

Table 15.1. Summary of primary immunodeficiency states.

DEFECTIVE GENE PRODUCT(S)	DISORDER
COMPLEMENT DEFICIENCES	
C1, C2, C4	Immune complex disease (SLE)
C1 inhibitor	Angioedema
DAF, HRF, CD59 (GPI anchor regulatory proteins)	Paroxysmal nocturnal hemoglobinuria
C3, Fact H, Fact I	Recurrent pyogenic infections
C5, C6, C7, C8 Properdin	Recurrent *Neisseria* infections
PHAGOCYTIC DEFECTS	
NADPH oxidase	Chronic granulomatous disease
CD18 (β_2-integrin β chain)	Leukocyte adhesion deficiency
?	Chediak–Higashi disease
IFNγR1/2, IL-12 p40, IL-12Rβ1	Mendelian susceptibility to mycobacterial infection
TNFR	TNF-receptor associated periodic syndrome
Pyrin	Familial Mediterranean fever
PRIMARY B-CELL DEFICIENCY	
Bruton's tyrosine kinase	Bruton congenital a-γ-globulinemia
μ heavy chain, λ_5 chain	Pro-B arrest; Bruton phenotype
?	IgA deficiency and common variable immunodeficiency
?	Transient infant hypo-γ-globulinemia
PRIMARY T-CELL DEFICIENCY	
?	DiGeorge and Nezelof syndromes; failure of thymic development
PNP	Purine nucleoside phosphorylase deficiency toxic to T-cells
RAG-1/2	Omenn's syndrome; partial *VDJ* recombination
MHC class II promoters	'Bare lymphocyte syndrome'
WASP	Wiskott–Aldridge syndrome; defective cytoskeletal regulation
Atm	Ataxia telangiectasia; defective DNA repair
CD154 (CD40L)	X-linked hyper-IgM syndrome
CD3 ε and γ chains, ZAP-70	Severe T-cell deficiency
COMBINED IMMUNODEFICIENCY	
?	Reticular dysgenesis; defective production of myeloid and lymphoid precursors
IL-7Rα, γ_c, Jak3	SCID due to defective IL-7 signaling
RAG-1/2	Complete failure of *VDJ* recombination
ADA	Adenosine deaminase deficiency; toxic to early lymphoid stem cells
SAP	X-linked lymphoproliferative disease; defective cell signaling

(continued)

Secondary immunodeficiency

• Immunodeficiency may arise as a secondary consequence of malnutrition, lymphoproliferative disorders, agents such as X-rays and cytotoxic drugs, and viral infections.

Acquired immunodeficiency syndrome (AIDS)

• AIDS results from infection by the RNA retroviruses HIV-1 and HIV-2.

• HIV infects T-helper cells through binding of its envelope gp120 to CD4 and either CCR5 or CXCR4 chemokine receptor cofactors. It also infects macrophages, microglia, T-cell-stimulating dendritic cells and FDCs, the latter through a CD4-independent pathway.

• Within the cell, the RNA is converted by the reverse transcriptase to DNA, which can be incorporated into the host's genome, where it lies dormant until the cell is activated by stimulators such as TNF which increase NFκB levels.

• There is usually a long asymptomatic phase after the early acute viral infection has been curtailed by a CD8 CTL immune response and the virus is sequestered to the FDC in the lymphoid follicles where it progressively destroys the dendritic cell meshwork.

• A disastrous fall in CD4 T-helpers destroys cell-mediated defenses and leaves the patient open to life-threatening infections through opportunist organisms such as *Pneumocystis carinii* and cytomegalovirus.

• There is a tremendous battle between the immune system and the virus, with extremely high rates of viral destruction and CD4 T-cell replacement.

• CD4 T-cell depletion may eventually occur as a result of direct pathogenicity, syncytium formation, susceptibility to apoptosis and possibly other mechanisms.

• AIDS is diagnosed in an individual with opportunistic infections, by low CD4 but normal CD8 T-cells in blood, poor delayed-type skin tests, positive tests for viral antibodies and p24 antigen, lymph node biopsy and isolation of live virus or demonstration of HIV genome by the polymerase chain reaction (PCR).

• Highly active antiretroviral drug therapy (HAART), combining inhibitors of reverse transcriptase and protease, can eliminate detectable virus early in disease, although latent virus remains.

• Vaccines are being targeted to Th1 responses but it is a very difficult virus to control.

See the accompanying website (**www.roitt.com**) for multiple choice questions.

FURTHER READING

Austen K.F., Burakoff S.J., Rosen F.S. & Strom T.B. (eds) (1996) *Therapeutic Immunology*. Blackwell Science, Oxford.

Brostoff J., Scadding G.K., Male D. & Roitt I.M. (eds) (1991) *Clinical Immunology*, Chapters 23–25. Gower Medical Publishing, London.

Buckley R.H. (2000) Advances in immunology: primary immunodeficiency diseases due to defects in lymphocytes. *New England Journal of Medicine* **343**, 1313.

Burton D.R. & Parren P.W. (2000) Vaccines and the induction of functional antibodies: time to look beyond the molecules of natural infection? *Nature Medicine* **6**, 123.

Chapel H., Haeney M., Misbah S. & Snowden N. (1999) *Essentials of Clinical Immunology*, 4th edn. Blackwell Science, Oxford.

Fauci A.S. (1996) Host factors and the pathogenesis of HIV-induced disease. *Nature* **384**, 529.

Fischer A. *et al.* (1997) Naturally occurring primary deficiencies of the immune system. *Annual Reviews of Immunology* **15**, 93.

Hammarstrom L., Vorechovsky I. & Webster D. (2000) Selective IgA deficiency (SigAD) and common variable immunodeficiency (CVID). *Clinical and Experimental Immunology* **120**, 225.

Ho D.D., Neumann A.U., Perelson A.S., Chen W., Leonard J.M. & Markowitz M. (1995) *Nature* **373**, 123; and Wei X., Ghosh S.K., Taylor M.E. *et al.* (1995) *Nature* **373**, 117. (Both study the effect of initial treatment with antiviral drugs and show the very high rate of viral replication and CD4 repletion.)

Huss R. (1996) Inhibition of cyclophilin function in HIV-1 infection by cyclosporin A. *Immunology Today* **17**, 259.

Leonard W.J. (ed.) (2000) Genetic effects on immunity. *Current Opinion in Immunology* **12**, 465. (Critical reviews appearing annually.)

Lokki M.-L. & Colten H.R. (1995) Genetic deficiencies of complement. *Annals of Medicine* **27**, 451.

McMichael A. (ed.) (2000) HIV. *Current Opinion in Immunology* **12**, 367. (Critical reviews appearing annually.)

Ochs H.D., Smith C.I.E. & Puck J.M. (eds) (2000) *Primary Immunodeficiency Diseases—A Molecular and Genetic Approach*. Oxford University Press, New York and Oxford.

Poignard P., Klasse P.J. & Sattentau Q.J. (1996) Antibody neutralization of HIV-1. *Immunology Today* **17**, 239.

Rosen F.S. *et al.* (1997) Primary immunodeficiency diseases: report of WHO Scientific Group. *Clinical and Experimental Immunology* **109**, S1.

Stiehm E.R. (ed.) (1989) *Immunological Disorders in Infants and Children*, 3rd edn. W.B. Saunders, Philadelphia.

Hypersensitivity

INTRODUCTION

When an individual has been immunologically primed, further contact with antigen leads to secondary boosting of the immune response. However, the reaction may be excessive and lead to gross tissue changes (hypersensitivity) if the antigen is present in relatively large amounts or if the humoral and cellular immune state is at a heightened level. It should be emphasized that the mechanisms underlying **these inappropriate immune responses leading to tissue damage**, which we speak of as **hypersensitivity reactions**, are those normally employed by the body in combating infection as discussed in Chapter 13. Hypersensitivity can also arise from direct interaction of the inciting agent with elements of the innate immune system without intervention by acquired responses.

ANAPHYLACTIC HYPERSENSITIVITY (TYPE I)

The phenomenon of anaphylaxis

The earliest accounts of inappropriate responses to foreign antigens relate to **anaphylaxis** (Milestone 16.1). The phenomenon can be readily reproduced in guinea-pigs which, like humans, are a highly susceptible species. A single injection of 1 mg of an antigen such as egg albumin into a guinea-pig has no obvious effect. Repeat the injection 2–3 weeks later and the sensitized animal reacts very dramatically with the symptoms of generalized anaphylaxis; almost immediately, the guinea-pig begins to wheeze and within a few minutes dies from asphyxia. Examination shows intense constriction of the bronchioles and bronchi and generally there is: (i) contraction of smooth muscle, and (ii) dilatation of capillaries. Similar reactions do occur in human subjects and have been observed following wasp and bee stings or injections of penicillin in appropriately sensitive individuals. In many instances only a timely injection of epinephrine to counter the smooth muscle contraction and capillary dilatation can prevent death.

Sir Henry Dale recognized that histamine mimics the systemic changes of anaphylaxis and, furthermore, that exposure of the uterus from a sensitized guinea-pig to antigen induces an immediate contraction associated with an explosive degranulation of mast cells (figure 1.14) responsible for the release of histamine and a number of other mediators (figure 1.15).

Anaphylaxis is triggered by clustering of IgE receptors on mast cells through cross-linking

Two main types of mast cell have been recognized, exemplified in the rat by those in the intestinal mucosa and those in the peritoneum and other connective tissue sites. They differ in a number of respects, for example in the type of protease and proteoglycan in their granules, and in the proliferative response of the mucosal mast cell to the T-cell cytokine IL-3 (table 16.1). This last point is made rather tellingly by the striking proliferation of mast cells in the intestinal mucosa dur-

Milestone 16.1 — The Discovery of Anaphylaxis

People are not equal. Idiosyncratic responses to given stimuli have been recognized from time immemorial and hypersensitive reactions in some individuals to normally innocuous environmental agents have been frequently observed. As Lucretius remarked two thousand years ago, 'Differences are so great that one man's meat is another man's poison'. Sir Thomas More records that the future King Richard III was aware that strawberries gave him urticaria and arranged to be served a bowl of the fruit at a banquet attended by an arch-enemy. When he broke out in a spectacular rash, he accused his guest of attempted poisoning and had him summarily executed.

Scientific interest in hypersensitivity was aroused by the observations of Richet and Portier. During a South Sea cruise on Prince Albert of Monaco's yacht, the Prince, presumably smarting from an encounter with *Physalia* (the jelly-fish known as the Portugese-Man-of-War with very nasty tentacles), suggested that toxin production by the fish might be of interest. Let Richet and Portier take up the story in their own words (1902).

'On board the Prince's yacht, experiments were carried out proving that an aqueous glycerin extract of the filaments of *Physalia* is extremely toxic to ducks and rabbits.

On returning to France, I could not obtain *Physalia* and decided to study comparatively the tentacles of *Actinaria* (sea anemone). While endeavouring to determine the toxic dose (of extracts), we soon discovered that some days must elapse before fixing it; for several dogs did not die until the fourth or fifth day after administration or even later. We kept those that had been given insufficient to kill, in order to carry out a second investigation upon these when they had recovered. At this point an unforeseen event occurred. The dogs which had recovered were intensely sensitive and died a few minutes after the administration of small doses. The most typical experiment, that in which the result was indisputable, was carried out on a particularly healthy dog. It was given at first 0.1 ml of the glycerin extract without becoming ill: 22 days later, as it was in perfect health, I gave it a second injection of the same amount. In a few seconds it was extremely ill; breathing became distressful; it could scarcely drag itself along, lay on its side, was seized with diarrhea, vomited blood and died in 25 minutes.'

The development of sensitivity to relatively harmless substances was termed by these authors **anaphylaxis**, in contrast to **prophylaxis**.

Table 16.1. Comparison of two types of mast cell.

CHARACTERISTICS	MUCOSAL MAST CELL	CONNECTIVE TISSUE MAST CELL
GENERAL		
Abbreviation*	MC$_t$	MC$_{tc}$
Distribution	Gut & lung	Most tissues**
Differentiation favored by	IL-3	Fibroblast factor
T-cell dependence	+	−
High affinity Fcε receptor	2×10^5/cell	3×10^4/cell
GRANULES		
Alcian blue and Safranin staining	Blue & brown	Blue
Ultrastructure	Scrolls	Gratings/lattices
Protease	Tryptase	Tryptase & chymase
Proteoglycan	Chondroitin sulfate	Heparin
DEGRANULATION		
Histamine release	+	++
LTC$_4$: PGD$_2$ release	25 : 1	1 : 40
Blocked by disodium cromoglycate/theophylline	−	+

*Based on protease in granules.
**Predominate in normal skin and intestinal submucosa.

ing infection with certain parasites in intact, but not in T-depleted, rodents, the effect being mediated by a combination of IL-3 and IL-4. The two types have common precursors and are interconvertible depending upon the environmental conditions, with mucosal MC$_t$ (*t*ryptase) phenotype favored by IL-3 and connective tissue MC$_{tc}$ (*t*ryptase *c*hymotryptase) being promoted by a fibroblast factor. However, both types display a high affinity receptor for IgE (FcεRI: cf. figure 3.18), a property shared with their circulating counterpart, the basophil. The strength of binding to the mast cell is evident from the retention of IgE antibodies at a site of intradermal injection for several weeks; IgG4 in the human also binds to the mast cell receptor, but more weakly, and disperses from the injection site within a day or so. It has long been established that the anaphylactic antibodies in the human are mainly of the IgE class.

Anaphylaxis is mediated by the reaction of allergen with IgE antibodies bound strongly through their Cε3 domains to the α chain of the high affinity receptor (FcεRI; $K_d = 10^{-9}$ to 10^{-10} M) on the surface of the mast cell (figure 16.1). Cross-linking of these IgE antibodies by a multivalent hapten will trigger media-

Fcε

Cε4

Cε4

Cε3

N

N

Binding site 2

Binding site 1

d2

d1

*

Membrane
anchor

FCεR

Figure 16.1. The structural basis of the binding of IgE to the high affinity mast cell receptor FcεRI. Side view of the complex with the two Fc chains in yellow and red and the FcεRIα chain in blue; carbohydrate residues are shown as sticks. The two Cε3 domains of the heavy chain dimer of IgE bind asymmetrically to two distinct interaction sites on the α chain of the receptor. The β-turn loop on one Cε3 binds along one side of the d2 domain, while surface loops plus the Cε2–Cε3 linker region on the other Cε3 interact with the top of the d1–d2 interface. The 1 : 1 stoichiometry of this asymmetric binding precludes the linkage of one IgE to two receptor molecules and ensures that triggering due to α–α aggregation only occurs through multivalent binding to surface IgE (see figure 16.2). The cleft between the d2 and d1 domains facing the plasma membrane is probably connected in some way to the receptor β chain to provide information on the aggregation status of the α chain. (Photograph kindly provided by Dr Ted Jardetzky and reproduced by permission of the Nature Publishing Group.)

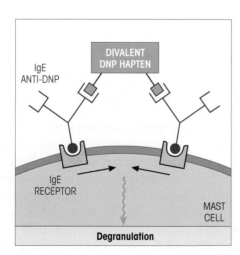

IgE
ANTI-DNP

DIVALENT
DNP HAPTEN

IgE
RECEPTOR

MAST
CELL

Degranulation

Figure 16.2. Clustering of IgE receptors either by multivalent hapten or antibody to the receptors themselves leads to mast cell degranulation. Studies using preformed aggregates of IgE of known size which stimulate mast cells showed that the reaction could be terminated by addition of selective kinase inhibitors. Small stable clusters of receptors continue to initiate signals for at least 1 hour. Lyn, which is the first tyrosine kinase to be activated, is normally present in caveolae membrane domains and only cosediments with the FcεRI when the latter are aggregated.

tor release (figure 16.2); trimers are more effective than dimers and tetramers even more so. The critical event is aggregation of the receptors by cross-linking as clearly shown by the ability of divalent antibodies reacting directly with the receptor to trigger the mast cell.

The FcεRIγ subunit resembles the ζ chain of the T-cell receptor (TCR) and part of the low affinity FcγRIII on macrophages. The cytoplasmic domain on the β and γ subunits shares a common *i*mmunoreceptor *t*yrosine-based *a*ctivation *m*otif (ITAM) with CD3γ, δ, ε, TCR ζ, η and B-cell receptor-associated Ig-α and Ig-β, and truncation of this domain abolishes receptor-mediated activation in a reconstituted system. Aggregation of the FcεRIα chains through cross-linking of the bound IgE antibodies activates the Lyn protein tyrosine kinase associated with the β chains and, if the aggregates persist, this leads to transphosphorylation of the β and γ chains of other receptors within the cluster and recruitment of the Syk kinase (figure 16.3). The subsequent series of phosphorylation-induced activations leads to the recruitment of the phospholipase C and the GTPase-linked Ras and Rac pathways as set out in figure 16.3. The net result of the biochemical cascade is degranulation with release of preformed mediators and the synthesis of arachidonic acid metabolites

Figure 16.3. Mast cell triggering. (a) Early events in signaling through the high affinity IgE receptor, FcεRI. Aggregation of the FcεRIα chains through cross-linking of bound IgE by multivalent antigen (allergen) alerts the β and γ chains of the receptor, leading to activation of the linked Lyn and Syk protein tyrosine kinases. They in turn phosphorylate and activate the PI(3) kinase, Bruton's tyrosine kinase (Btk) and the membrane adaptor protein LAT which recruits phospholipase Cγ1 and adaptor molecules concerned in the activation of GTPase/kinase cascades. (b) The activated phospholipase Cγ1 generates diacylglycerol (DAG) which targets protein kinase C, while inositol $(1,4,5)P_3$ (IP_3) elevates cytoplasmic Ca^{2+} by depleting the ER stores. The raised calcium concentration activates transcriptional factors and causes granule exocytosis. The Grb-2/Sos and Slp-76/Vav complexes also associated with the LAT adaptor trigger the Ras and Rac/Rho GTPase-induced serial kinase cascades, respectively, leading to the activation of transcription factors and rearrangements of the actin cytoskeleton. (Figure essentially designed by Dr Helen Turner, based on the article by Turner H. & Kinet J.-P. (1999) *Nature* (Supplement on Allergy and Asthma) **402**, B24.)

formed by the cyclo-oxygenase and lipoxygenase pathways (cf. figure 1.15). To recapitulate, the preformed mediators released from the granules include histamine, heparin, neutral protease, eosinophil and neutrophil chemotactic factors and platelet activating factor, while leukotrienes LTB4, LTC4 and LTD4, the prostaglandin PGD2 and thromboxanes are all newly synthesized. We now know that IL-3, IL-4, IL-5 and IL-6 and *granulocyte–macrophage colony-stimulating factor* (GM-CSF), a typical Th2 pattern of cytokines cells, are also released.

Under normal circumstances, these mediators help to orchestrate the development of a defensive acute inflammatory reaction (and in this context let us not for-

get that complement fragments C3a and C5a can also trigger mast cells, although not through IgE receptors). When there is a massive release of these mediators under abnormal conditions, as in atopic disease, their bronchoconstrictive and vasodilatory effects predominate and become distinctly threatening.

Atopic allergy

Clinical responses to extrinsic allergens

At least 10% of the population suffer to a greater or lesser degree with allergies involving localized IgE-mediated anaphylactic reactions to allergens such

Figure 16.4. House dust mite—a major cause of allergic disease. The electron micrograph shows the rather nasty looking mite graced by the name *Dermatophagoides pteryonyssinus* and fecal pellets on the bottom left which are the major source of allergen. The biconcave pollen grains (top left) shown for comparison indicate the size of particle which can become airborne and reach the lungs. The mite itself is much too large for that. (Reproduced by courtesy of Dr E. Tovey.)

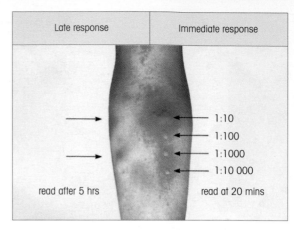

Figure 16.5. Atopic allergy. Skin prick tests with grass pollen allergen in a patient with typical summer hay fever. Skin tests were performed 5 hours (left) and 20 minutes (right) before the photograph was taken. The tests on the right show a typical end-point titration of a type I immediate wheal and flare reaction. The late phase skin reaction (left) can be clearly seen at 5 hours, especially where a large immediate response has preceded it. Figures for allergen dilution are given.

as grass pollens, animal danders, the feces from mites in house dust (figure 16.4) and so on. An increasing number of allergens have now been cloned and expressed including **Der p1** from mites and **Lol pI–V** from rye grass pollen. Der p1 proves to be a protease which increases the permeability of the bronchial mucosa, thereby facilitating its own passage along with other allergens across the epithelium and allowing access to and sensitization of cells of the immune system. It splits the low affinity IgE receptor, CD23, on B-cells so reducing its negative impact on IgE synthesis when occupied by IgE; it also cleaves the IL-2 receptor α chain which biases the immune response to Th2-dependent IgE production. Short cuts to allergen purification can be achieved by screening cDNA libraries for IgE-binding proteins using immunoblotting techniques. This was a godsend for the purification of the allergen from the venom of the Australian jumper ant, *Myrmecia pilosula*; just think of trying to accumulate ants by the kilogram to isolate the allergen using conventional protein fractionation.

The local anaphylactic reaction to injection of antigen into the skin of atopic patients is manifest as a wheal and flare (figure 16.5) which is short lived and resolves within an hour or so; it may be succeeded by a late phase response involving eosinophil infiltrates which peak at around 5 hours. Contact of the allergen with cell-bound IgE in the bronchial tree, the nasal mucosa and the conjunctival tissues releases mediators of anaphylaxis and produces the symptoms of **asthma** or **allergic rhinitis and conjunctivitis** (hay fever) as the case may be. A proportion of the patients who experi-

ence late phase responses after bronchial challenge with allergen eventually develop chronic **asthma**. This disease affects 155 million individuals worldwide and costs $6 billion a year to treat in the USA alone. Patients fall into three main categories.

1 The majority who are **extrinsic asthmatics** associated with **atopy**, i.e. the genetic predisposition to synthesize inappropriate levels of IgE specific for external allergens.

2 Nonatopic intrinsic asthmatics.

3 **Occupational asthmatics** exposed to specific proteins or small molecular weight chemicals.

Bronchial biopsy and lavage of asthmatic patients reveal an unequivocal involvement of **mast cells and eosinophils** as the major mediators secreting effector cells, while T-cells provide the microenvironment required to sustain the chronic inflammatory response which is an essential feature of the histopathology in each category (figure 16.6). The resulting variable airflow obstruction and bronchial hyper-responsiveness are the cardinal clinical and physiological features of the disease.

The atopic trait can also manifest itself as an **atopic dermatitis** (figure 16.7), with house dust mite, domestic cats and German cockroaches often proving to be the environmental offenders. Recalling the inflammation in asthma, skin patch tests with Der p1 in these eczema patients produce an infiltrate of eosinophils, T-cells, mast cells and basophils. The number of individuals affected is comparable to the number affected by asthma which may be a surprise to some.

Awareness of the importance of IgE sensitization to

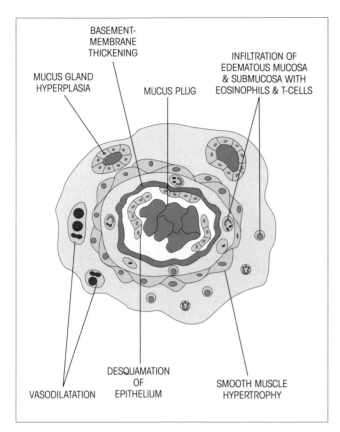

Figure 16.6. Pathological changes in asthma. Diagram of cross-section of an airway in severe asthma.

Figure 16.7. An atopic eczema reaction on the back of a knee of a child allergic to rice and eggs. (Kindly provided by Professor J. Brostoff.)

Figure 16.8. The role of gut sensitivity in the development of asthma to food allergens. A patient challenged by feeding with egg developed asthma within hours, as shown here by the depressed lung function test of measuring peak air flow; the symptoms at the end-organ stage were counteracted by the β-adrenoreceptor agonist, isoprenaline. However, oral sodium cromoglycate (SCG), which prevents antigen-specific mast cell triggering, also prevented the onset of asthma after oral challenge with egg. Note that SCG taken orally has no effect on the response of an asthmatic to inhaled allergen. (From Brostoff J. (1986) In Brostoff J. & Challacombe S.J. (eds) *Food Allergy*, p. 441. Baillière Tindall, London, reproduced with permission.)

food allergens in the gut has increased dramatically. Sensitization to egg white and cows' milk may even occur in early infancy through breast-feeding, with antigen passing into the mother's milk. Food additives such as sulfiting agents can also cause adverse reactions. Contact of the food with specific IgE on mast cells in the gastrointestinal tract may produce local reactions such as diarrhea and vomiting, or may allow the allergen to enter the body by causing a change in gut permeability through mediator release; the allergen may complex with antibodies and cause distal lesions by depositing in the joints, for example, or it may diffuse freely to other sensitized sites, such as the skin (figure 16.7) or lungs, where it will cause a further local anaphylactic reaction. Thus eating strawberries may produce urticarial reactions and egg may precipitate an asthmatic attack in appropriately sensitized individuals. The role of the sensitized gut in acting as a 'gate' to allow entry of allergens is strongly suggested by experiments in which oral sodium cromoglycate, a mast cell stabilizer, prevented subsequent asthma after ingestion of the provoking food (figure 16.8).

Anaphylactic drug allergy is manifest in the dramatic responses to drugs such as penicillin which haptenate body proteins by covalent coupling to induce

IgE synthesis. In the case of penicillin, the β-lactam ring links to the ε-amino of lysine to form the penicilloyl determinant. The fine specificity of the IgE antibodies permits discrimination between closely similar drugs, such that some patients may be allergic to amoxicillin but tolerate benzylpenicillin which differs by only very minor modifications of the side-chains.

Pathologic mechanisms in asthma

We should now look in more depth at those events

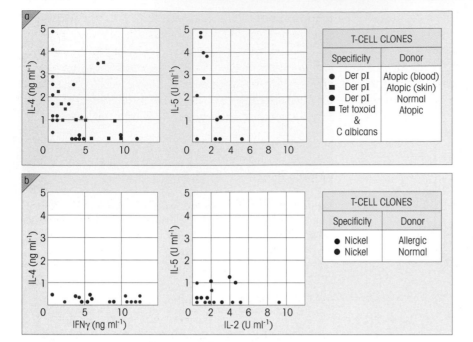

Figure 16.9. Th2 dominance in atopic allergy shown by cytokine profiles of antigen-specific CD4[+] T-cell clones from (a) patients with type I atopic allergy and (b) subjects with type IV contact sensitivity, compared with normal controls. Each point represents the value for an individual clone. Archetypal Th1 clones have high IFNγ and IL-2 and low IL-4 and IL-5; Th2 clones show the converse. The high level of IL-4 drives the switch to IgE production by B-cells and further promotes the Th2 bias, which is reinforced by suppression of Th1 cells by NO· derived from cytokine-stimulated airway epithelial cells. (Data from Kapsenberg M.L., Wierenga E.A., Bos J.D. & Jansen H.M. (1991) *Immunology Today* **12**, 392.)

which generate the chronicity of asthma. Remember that there is an *early phase* bronchial response to inhaled antigen essentially involving mast cell mediators, and an inflammatory *late phase* dominated by eosinophils. **Both phases are IgE-dependent** as shown by their marked attenuation in the great majority of asthmatics treated for around 9 weeks with a humanized monoclonal antibody (RhuMAb-E25) specific for the binding site of human IgE to its high affinity receptor, which reduces IgE to almost undetectable levels and downregulates FcεRI expression. Activated mast cells make some contribution to eosinophil recruitment by secretion of an eosinophil chemoattractant and tryptase, which can switch on a protease-activated receptor (PAR-2) on the surface of endothelial and epithelial cells, leading to cytokine production and the expression of adhesion molecules which selectively recruit eosinophils and basophils. The most important trigger of the late phase reaction is now thought to be **activation of alveolar macrophages** through the interaction of allergen with IgE bound to the low affinity receptors (FcεRII; CD23), leading to a significant increase in the production of TNF and IL-1β. These cytokines then stimulate the release of the powerful **eosinophil chemoattractants**: eotaxin (CCL11), RANTES (CCL5) and MCP5 (CCL12) (cf. p. 187) from bronchial epithelial cells and fibroblasts. Note also that eotaxin and RANTES can contribute directly to local inflammation by IgE-independent degranulation of basophils.

A new player now enters the field: primed T-cells traffic into the inflamed site and are strongly attracted by eotaxin. Since the T-cell response is heavily skewed towards the **Th2 subset in asthma** (figure 16.9), encounter with the allergen on antigen-presenting cells will promote the synthesis of IL-4, -5 and -13. IL-4 stimulates further eotaxin release, while IL-5 upregulates chemokine receptors on eosinophils, maintains their survival through an inhibitory effect on natural apoptosis and is involved in their longer term recruitment from bone marrow.

Things now look bad for the bronchial tissues and a multitude of factors contribute to allergen-induced airway dysfunction: (i) a virtual soup of bronchoconstrictors, the leukotrienes being especially important, bathe the smooth muscle cells, (ii) edema of the airway wall, (iii) altered neural regulation of airway tone through binding of eosinophil major basic protein (MBP) to M2 autoreceptors on the nerve endings with increased release of acetylcholine, (iv) airway epithelial cell desquamation due to the toxic action of MBP, there being a strong correlation between the number of desquamated cells in bronchoalveolar lavage fluid and the concentration of MBP, (v) mucus hypersecretion due to IL-13 and, to a lesser extent, IL-4, leukotrienes and platelet activating factor acting on submucosal glands and their controlling neural elements, and finally (vi) a repair-type response involving the production of fibroblast growth factor, TGFβ and platelet-derived growth factor, the laying down of collagen, scar and fibrous tissue and hypertrophy of smooth muscle, leading to an exaggerated narrowing of the airways in response to a variety of environmental stimuli (figure 16.6). The wide range of cytokines and mediators produced by lung epithelial and endothelial cells, fibroblasts and smooth muscle cells may account for the persistence of airway inflammation and the permanent structural changes in chronic disease sufferers, even in the absence or apparent absence of ongoing exposure to inhalant allergens to which subjects are sensitized, a state where conventional immunotherapy might not be expected to be beneficial.

Unlike atopic asthmatics, **intrinsic asthmatics** have negative skin tests to common aeroallergens, no clinical or family history of allergy, normal levels of serum IgE and no detectable specific IgE antibodies to common allergens. Nonetheless, they resemble the atopics in important respects: bronchial biopsies show enhanced expression of IL-4, IL-13, RANTES and eotaxin, and of the mRNA for the ε germ line transcript and the ε heavy chain, suggestive of local IgE synthesis. Is there a role for virus-specific IgE or for IgE autoantibodies to the FcεRI?

The inflammatory infiltrate in **atopic dermatitis** closely resembles that in asthma. The epidermal dendritic cells have markedly upregulated FcεRI expression, and an incoming allergen will activate them either directly or as allergen–IgE complexes; the TNF, IL-1β and GM-CSF which they produce will, in turn, promote the release of the eosinophil chemoattractants, RANTES and eotaxin, from keratinocytes and fibroblasts. A newly identified keratinocyte CC chemokine, CTACK (CCL27; cf. p. 187), preferentially attracts skin-homing CLA⁺ memory T-cells; these make up 80–90% of the T-cells in the infiltrate and account for the specific response to the offending allergen.

Etiological factors in the development of atopic allergy

There is a strong familial predisposition to the development of atopic allergy (figure 16.10). One factor is undoubtedly the overall ability to synthesize the IgE isotype—the higher the level of IgE in the blood, the greater the likelihood of becoming atopic (figure 16.10). Genetic studies show this to be linked to chromosome 13q. Linkages have also been established for other factors contributing to atopy: to chromosome 11q involving the FcεRIβ chain, to 2q containing the IL-1 cluster, and to 5q within the IL-4, -9, -13, GM-CSF and CD14 gene cluster. A C → T base change 159 bases upstream of the transcription start site for CD14, the high affinity receptor for bacterial LPS endotoxin, is significantly associated with high levels of soluble CD14 and low levels of IgE. What relevance might this have for atopic disease? Well, excessive exposure of babies to

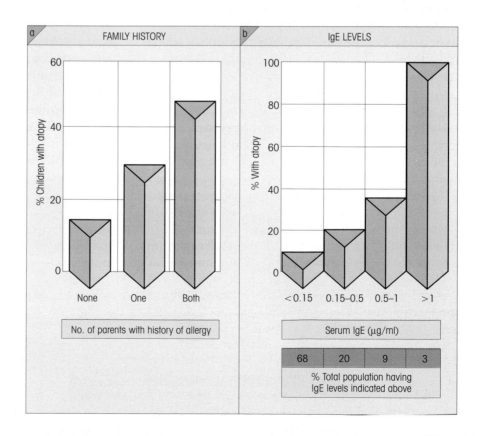

Figure 16.10. Risk factors in allergy: (a) family history; (b) IgE levels —the higher the serum IgE concentration, the greater the chance of developing atopy.

bacterial LPS in dirty homes, farms and households with dogs will tend to stimulate Th1 responses at the expense of Th2 and could account for the much lower incidence of atopy in these children. Indeed, a study of BCG vaccination in Japanese children revealed a strong inverse correlation between the development of delayed-type tuberculin reactions and the susceptibility to asthma. The current notion is that good hygiene in the early years is bad for you and is responsible for the steady increase in prevalence of atopy, the exposure to IL-12/Th1-inducing infections skewing the infant 'immunostat' more firmly towards the Th1 end of the spectrum and away from a Th2-related propensity to synthesize IgE. This may be oversimplified but it does make a good story—sorry, hypothesis. Other environmental influences, such as smoking and the use of beta-blockers during pregnancy, increase the incidence of atopy in the offspring, as does contact with highly allergenic proteins such as cows' milk, eggs, fish, nuts and Der p1 before mucosal protective mechanisms, especially IgA, are reasonably established. The old wives' tale that 'breast is best' would seem to have merit, although in some cases small amounts of dietary allergens may find their way into the mother's milk.

Clinical tests for allergy

Sensitivity is normally assessed by the response to intradermal challenge with antigen. The release of histamine and other mediators rapidly produces a **wheal and erythema** (figure 16.5), maximal within 30 minutes and then subsiding. These immediate wheal and flare reactions may be followed by a late phase reaction (cf. figure 16.5) which sometimes lasts for 24 hours, redolent of those seen following challenge of the bronchi and nasal mucosa of allergic subjects and similarly characterized by dense infiltration with eosinophils and T-cells.

The correlation between skin prick test responses and the **radioallergosorbent test** (RAST, see p. 113) for allergen-specific serum IgE is fairly good. In some instances, intranasal challenge with allergen may provoke a response even when both of these tests are negative, probably as a result of local synthesis of IgE antibodies.

The presence of proteins secreted from mast cells or eosinophils in the serum or urine could provide important surrogate markers of disease and might predict exacerbations.

Therapy

If one considers the sequence of reactions from initial exposure to allergen right through to the production of atopic disease, it can be seen that several points in the chain provide legitimate targets for therapy (figure 16.11).

Allergen avoidance. Avoidance of contact with *potential* allergens is often impractical, although, to give one example, feeding infants cows' milk at too early an age is discouraged. After sensitization, avoidance where possible is obviously worthwhile, but the reluctance of some parents to dispose of the family cat to stop little Algernon's wheezing is sometimes quite surprising.

Figure 16.11. Atopic allergies and their treatment: sites of local responses and possible therapies. Events and treatments relating to local anaphylaxis in green and to chronic inflammation in red.

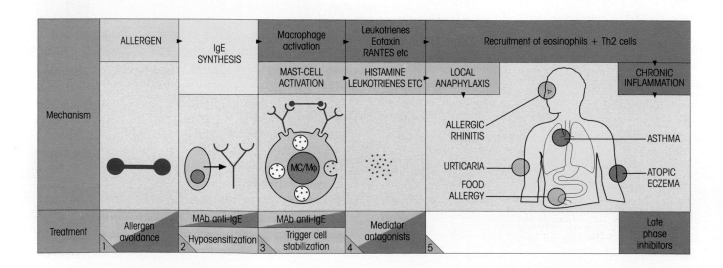

Modulation of the immunological response. Attempts to desensitize patients immunologically by repeated subcutaneous injection of small amounts of allergen have at least the merit of a long history and can lead to worthwhile improvement in individuals subject to insect venom anaphylaxis or hay fever, but are less effective in asthma. Injection of naked DNA coding for house dust mite allergen directly into the muscle, or oral administration of chitosan-coated plasmid DNA containing a dominant peanut allergen gene, reduced IgE synthesis and gave good protection against anaphylactic challenge in mice, but the long-term endogenous expression of allergen in sensitized humans might lead to precarious situations. The purpose of allergen hyposensitization therapy was originally to boost the synthesis of 'blocking' antibodies, whose function was to divert the allergen from contact with tissue-bound IgE. While this may well prove to be a contributory factor, downregulation of IgE synthesis by engagement of the FcγRIIB receptor (cf. p. 50) on B-cells by allergen-specific IgG linked to allergen molecules bound to surface IgE receptors also seems likely (cf. p. 202; see Chapter 11 on IgG regulation of Ab production). Additionally, if T-lymphocyte cooperation is important for IgE synthesis and eosinophil-mediated pathogenesis, the beneficial effects of antigen injection may also be mediated through induction of tolerant, anergic or suppressor T-cells. A switch from Th2 to Th1 by injection of heat-killed *Mycobacterium vaccae* or the administration of tolerizing or antagonist peptide epitopes represent other possible therapeutic modalities. Fortunately, most patients respond to a remarkably limited number of T-cell epitopes on any given allergen, and so it may not be necessary to tailor the therapeutic peptide to each individual. Clinical trials with high doses of Fel d 1-derived peptides from cat allergen have resulted in decreased sensitivity, although isolated late responses to allergen by direct T-cell activation may be induced. A case can be made for future prophylactic hyposensitization of children with two asthmatic parents who have at least a 50% probability of developing the disease.

The humanized anti-IgE monoclonal, RhuMAb-E25, directed against the FcεRI-binding domain of IgE (cf. p. 324) may provide an exciting new therapy for severe forms of asthma and atopic dermatitis, because it impacts the disease process at several points. It reduces the circulating IgE levels almost to vanishing point by direct neutralization, and decreases IgE synthesis through binding to the inhibitory FcγRIIB as it cross-links the surface immunoglobulin on IgE-producing B-cells (cf. the effect of allergen-specific IgG mentioned above).

Stabilization of the triggering cells. This precipitous fall in circulating IgE caused by RhuMAb-E25 decreases the occupancy of mast cell FcεRI receptors, and reduces receptor synthesis, perhaps through the lack of positive feedback mediated by the β chains; an additional nudge to the downregulation of receptor biosynthesis may be provided by cross-linking of the free Fcε-binding domain on the mast cell surface (cf. figure 16.1) and subsequent engagement of the FcγRIIB. Signaling through allergen will obviously be far less effective because only a small number of receptors per cell will be activated. Last and by no means least, similar mechanisms will operate to limit the allergen-induced activation of macrophages and hence eosinophil recruitment. At the drug level, much relief has been obtained with agents such as inhalant isoprenaline and **sodium cromoglycate**, a member of the chromone family, which render mast cells resistant to triggering. Sodium cromoglycate blocks chloride channel activity and maintains cells in a normal resting physiological state, which probably accounts for its inhibitory effects on a wide range of cellular functions, such as mast cell degranulation, eosinophil and neutrophil chemotaxis and mediator release, and reflex bronchoconstriction. Some or all of these effects are responsible for its anti-asthmatic actions. Strangely, it also inhibits the release of IgE from tonsils of nonatopic subjects stimulated with IL-4.

The triggering of macrophages through allergen interaction with surface-bound IgE is clearly a major initiating factor for late reactions, as discussed above, and resistance to this stimulus can be very effectively achieved with corticosteroids. Unquestionably, **inhaled corticosteroids** have revolutionized the treatment of asthma. Their principal action is to suppress the transcription of multiple inflammatory genes, including in the present context those encoding cytokine production.

Mediator antagonism. **Histamine H_1-receptor antagonists** have for long proved helpful in the symptomatic treatment of atopic disease. Newer drugs such as loratadine and fexofenadine are effective in rhinitis and in reducing the itch in atopic dermatitis, although they have little benefit in asthma. Cetirizine additionally has useful effects on eosinophil recruitment in the late phase reaction. An important recent advance has been the introduction of long-acting inhaled **β_2-agonists** such as salmeterol and formoterol which are bronchodilators and protect against bronchoconstriction for over 12 hours. Potent **leukotriene antagonists** such as Pranlukast also block constrictor challenges and show striking efficacy in certain patients, particularly aspirin-sensitive asthmatics (logical if you think about it). At the experimental level, an antibody to IL-5 had an effect on an allergy model in primates lasting several months.

Theophylline was introduced for the treatment of asthma more than 50 years ago and remains the single most prescribed drug for asthma worldwide. As a **phosphodiesterase (PDE) inhibitor** it increases intracellular cAMP, thereby causing bronchodilatation, inhibition of IL-5-induced prolongation of eosinophil survival and probably suppression of eosinophil migration into the bronchial mucosa. Good news for the patient. There are many isoenzyme forms of PDE, and bronchodilators such as benafentrine are currently being developed.

Attacking chronic inflammation. Certain drugs impede atopic disease at more than one stage. **Cetirizine** is a case in point with its dual effects on the histamine receptor and on eosinophil recruitment. **Corticosteroids** seem to do almost everything; apart from their role in stabilizing macrophages, they solidly inhibit the activation and proliferation of the Th2 cells, which are the dominant underlying driving force in chronic asthma, and may call a halt to the development of irreversible narrowing of the airways. So it is that new generation inhaled steroids (e.g. budesonide, mometasone furoate, fluticasone propionate) with high anti-inflammatory potency but minimal side-effects due to hepatic metabolism, provide first-line therapy for most chronic asthmatics, with supplementation by long-acting β_2-agonists and theophylline.

ANTIBODY-DEPENDENT CYTOTOXIC HYPERSENSITIVITY (TYPE II)

Where an antigen is present on the surface of a cell, combination with antibody will encourage the demise of that cell by promoting contact with phagocytes, either by reduction in surface charge, or by **opsonic adherence** to Fcγ or C3b receptors. Cell death may also occur through activation of the full **complement** system up to C8 and C9 producing **direct membrane damage** (figure 16.12). Although, in the case of hemolytic antibodies, the generation of a single active complement site is enough to cause erythrocyte lysis, other cells appear to have repair mechanisms and it is likely that several complement sites need to be recruited in order to overwhelm the cell's defenses.

The operation of a quite distinct cytotoxic mechanism derives from the finding that target cells coated with low concentrations of IgG antibody can be killed 'nonspecifically' through an extracellular nonphagocytic mechanism involving nonsensitized leukocytes which bind to the target by their specific receptors for the Cγ2 and Cγ3 domains of IgG Fc (figures 16.12 and 16.13). It should be noted that this so-called **antibody-dependent cellular cytotoxicity (ADCC)** may be exhibited by both phagocytic and nonphagocytic myeloid cells (polymorphs and monocytes) and by large granular lymphocytes with Fc receptors dubbed 'K-cells', which are almost certainly identical with the natural killer (NK) cells (see p. 32). Contact between the effector and target cells is essential and activity is inhibited by cytochalasin B which interferes with cell

Figure 16.12. Antibody-dependent cytotoxic hypersensitivity (type II). Antibodies directed against cell surface antigens cause cell death not only by C-dependent lysis but also by Fcγ and C3b adherence reactions leading to phagocytosis, or through nonphagocytic extracellular killing by certain lymphoid and myeloid cells (antibody-dependent cellular cytotoxicity). IgG cytotoxic antibodies directed to tumors or to glomerular basement membrane are 10–100 times more pathogenic in animals deficient in FcγRIIB relative to their wild-type controls, pointing to a balance of activating and inhibitory signals controlling the dominant effector pathway in these responses, and implicating the macrophage as the critical cell type involved.

Figure 16.13. Killing of Ab-coated target by antibody-dependent cellular cytotoxicity (ADCC). Fcγ receptors bind the effector to the target which is killed by an extracellular mechanism. Human monocytes and IFNγ-activated neutrophils kill Ab-coated tumor cells using their FcγRI receptors; lymphocytes (NK cells) kill hybridoma targets through FcγRIII receptors. (a) Diagram of effector and target cells. (b) Electron micrograph of attack on Ab-coated chick red cell by a mouse large granular lymphocyte showing close apposition of effector and target and vacuolation in the cytoplasm of the latter. ((b) Courtesy of P. Penfold.)

Figure 16.14. The ABO system. The allelic genes A and B code for transferases which add either *N*-acetylgalactosamine (NAcGal) or galactose (Gal), respectively, to H substance (Fuc, fucose). The oligosaccharide is anchored to the cell membrane by coupling to a sphingomyelin called ceramide. Eighty-five per cent of the population secrete blood group substances in the saliva, where the oligosaccharides are present as soluble polypeptide conjugates formed under the action of a secretor (*se*) gene.

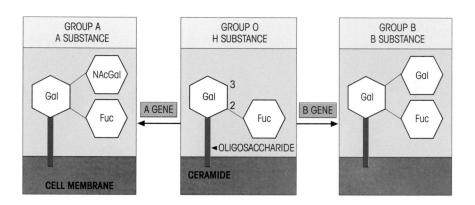

movement, and by aggregated IgG which binds firmly to the Fc receptors and blocks their ability to interact with antibody on the surface of the target.

ADCC can be readily observed as a phenomenon *in vitro*; to give examples, human K-cells have been shown to be strikingly unpleasant to chicken red cells coated with rabbit antibody, while schistosomules coated with either IgG or IgE can be killed by eosinophils (cf. figure 13.22). Whether ADCC plays a positive role *in vivo* remains a tricky question, but functionally this extracellular cytotoxic mechanism would be expected to be of significance where the target is too large for ingestion by phagocytosis, e.g. large parasites and solid tumors. It could also act as a back-up system for T-cell killing.

Type II reactions between members of the same species (alloimmune)

Transfusion reactions

Of the many different polymorphic constituents of the human red cell membrane, **ABO blood groups** form the dominant system. The antigenic groups A and B are derived from H substance (figure 16.14) by the action

of glycosyltransferases encoded by *A* or *B* genes, respectively. Individuals with both genes (group AB) have the two antigens on their red cells, while those lacking these genes (group O) synthesize H substance only. Antibodies to A or B occur spontaneously when the antigen is absent from the red cell surface; thus a person of blood group A will possess anti-B and so on. These **isohemagglutinins** are usually IgM and probably belong to the class of 'natural antibodies'; they would be boosted through contact with antigens of the gut flora which are structurally similar to the blood group carbohydrates, so that the antibodies formed cross-react with the appropriate red cell type. If an individual is blood group A, he/she would be tolerant to antigens closely similar to A and would only form cross-reacting antibodies capable of agglutinating B red cells; similarly an O individual would make anti-A and anti-B (table 16.2). On transfusion, mismatched red cells will be coated by the isohemagglutinins and will cause severe complement-mediated intravascular hemolysis.

Clinical refractoriness to platelet transfusions is frequently due to HLA alloimmunization, but one can usually circumvent this problem by depleting the platelets of leukocytes.

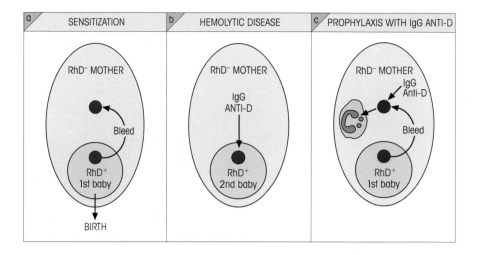

Figure 16.15. Hemolytic disease of the newborn due to rhesus incompatibility. (a) RhD+ve red cells from the first baby sensitize the RhD−ve mother. (b) The mother's IgG anti-D crosses the placenta and coats the erythrocytes of the second RhD+ve baby causing type II hypersensitivity hemolytic disease. (c) IgG anti-D given prophylactically at the first birth removes the baby's red cells through phagocytosis and prevents sensitization of the mother.

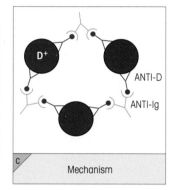

Figure 16.16. The Coombs' test for antibody-coated red cells used for detecting rhesus antibodies and in the diagnosis of autoimmune hemolytic anemia (cf. table 19.2, Note 5, p. 402). (Photographs courtesy of Professor A. Cooke.)

Table 16.2. ABO blood groups and serum antibodies.

BLOOD GROUP (PHENOTYPE)	GENOTYPE	ANTIGEN	SERUM ANTIBODY
A	AA, AO	A	ANTI-B
B	BB, BO	B	ANTI-A
AB	AB	A and B	NONE
O	OO	H	ANTI-A ANTI-B

Rhesus incompatibility

The **rhesus (Rh) blood groups** form the other major antigenic system, the RhD antigen being of the most consequence for isoimmune reactions. A mother with an RhD−ve blood group (i.e. *dd* genotype) can readily be sensitized by red cells from a baby carrying RhD antigens (*DD* or *Dd* genotype). This occurs most often at the birth of the first child when a placental bleed can release a large number of the baby's erythrocytes into the mother. The antibodies formed are predominantly of the IgG class and are able to cross the placenta in any subsequent pregnancy. Reaction with the D-antigen on the fetal red cells leads to their destruction through

opsonic adherence, giving hemolytic disease of the newborn (figure 16.15).

These anti-D antibodies fail to agglutinate RhD+ve red cells *in vitro* ('incomplete antibodies') because the low density of antigenic sites does not allow sufficient antibody bridges to be formed between the negatively charged erythrocytes to overcome the electrostatic repulsive forces. Erythrocytes coated with anti-D can be made to agglutinate by addition of albumin or of an anti-immunoglobulin serum (Coombs' reagent; figure 16.16).

If a mother has natural isohemagglutinins which can react with any fetal erythrocytes reaching her circulation, sensitization to the D-antigens is less likely due to 'deviation' of the red cells away from the antigen-sensitive cells. For example, a group O RhD−ve mother with a group A RhD+ve baby would destroy any fetal erythrocytes with her anti-A before they could immunize to produce anti-D. In an extension of this principle, **RhD−ve mothers are now treated prophylactically** with small amounts of avid IgG anti-D at the time of birth of the first child, and this greatly reduces the risk of sensitization. Another success for immunology.

Another example of disease resulting from transplacental passage of maternal antibodies is **neonatal alloimmune thrombocytopenia**. The fall in platelet numbers is greatly ameliorated by high-dose i.v. injections of pooled human IgG, thought by some to involve anti-idiotype networks (cf. p. 443), although the efficacy of Fcγ fragments, anti-RhD and anti-FcγR rather point the finger at blockade of the Fcγ receptors.

Organ transplants

A long-standing allograft which has withstood the first onslaught of the cell-mediated reaction can evoke humoral antibodies in the host directed against surface transplantation antigens on the graft. These may be directly cytotoxic or cause adherence of phagocytic cells or 'nonspecific' attack by K-cells. They may also lead to platelet adherence when they combine with antigens on the surface of the vascular endothelium (figure 17.6, p. 354). Hyperacute rejection is mediated by preformed antibodies in the graft recipient.

Autoimmune type II hypersensitivity reactions

Autoantibodies to the patient's own red cells are produced in **autoimmune hemolytic anemia**. They react at 37°C with epitopes on antigens of the rhesus complex distinct from those which incite transfusion reactions. Red cells coated with these antibodies have a shortened half-life, largely through their adherence to phagocytic cells in the spleen. Similar mechanisms account for the anemia in patients with cold hemagglutinin disease who have monoclonal anti-I after infection with *Mycoplasma pneumoniae*, and in some cases of paroxysmal cold hemoglobinuria associated with the actively lytic Donath–Landsteiner antibodies specific for blood group P. These antibodies are primarily of IgM isotype and only react at temperatures well below 37°C. IgG platelet autoantibodies are responsible for the depletion of platelets in **idiopathic thrombocytopenic purpura**; although the relative contributions of C3b and Fcγ receptors to their clearance by phagocytosis is still a matter of dispute, the persistence of opsonized platelets when Fcγ receptors are blocked (see above) or deficient (in a mouse model) does argue strongly that Fcγ interactions with its receptor are pivotal.

The serums of patients with Hashimoto's thyroiditis contain antibodies which, in the presence of complement, are directly cytotoxic for isolated human thyroid cells in culture. In Goodpasture's syndrome (included here for convenience), antibodies to kidney glomerular basement membrane are present. Biopsies show

(a)

(b)

Figure 16.17. Glomerulonephritis: (a) due to linear deposition of antibody to glomerular basement membrane, here visualized by staining the human kidney biopsy with a fluorescent anti-IgG; and (b) due to deposition of antigen–antibody complexes, which can be seen as discrete masses lining the glomerular basement membrane following immunofluorescent staining with anti-IgG. Similar patterns to these are obtained with a fluorescent anti-C3. (Courtesy of Dr S. Thiru.)

these antibodies, together with complement components, bound to the basement membranes where the action of the full complement system leads to serious damage (figure 16.17). One could also include the stripping of acetylcholine receptors from the muscle endplate by autoantibodies in myasthenia gravis as a further example of type II hypersensitivity.

Type II drug reactions

This is complicated. Drugs may become coupled to body components and thereby undergo conversion from a hapten to a full antigen which will sensitize certain individuals (we don't know which). If IgE antibodies are produced, anaphylactic reactions can result. In some circumstances, particularly with topically applied ointments, cell-mediated hypersensitivity may be induced. In other cases where coupling to serum proteins occurs, the possibility of type III complex-mediated reactions may arise. In the present context, we are concerned with those instances in which the drug appears to form an antigenic complex with the surface of a formed element of the blood and evokes the production of antibodies which are cytotoxic for the cell–drug complex. When the drug is withdrawn, the sensitivity is no longer evident. Examples of this mechanism have been seen in the **hemolytic anemia** sometimes associated with continued administration of chlorpromazine or phenacetin, in the **agranulocytosis** associated with the taking of amidopyrine or of quinidine, and the now classic situation of **thrombocytopenic purpura** which may be produced by sedormid, a sedative of yesteryear. In the latter case, freshly drawn serum from the patient will lyse platelets in the presence, but not in the absence, of sedormid; inactivation of complement by preheating the serum at 56°C for 30 minutes abrogates this effect.

IMMUNE COMPLEX-MEDIATED HYPERSENSITIVITY (TYPE III)

The body may be exposed to an excess of antigen over a protracted period in a number of circumstances: persistent infection with a microbial organism, autoimmunity to self-components and repeated contact with environmental agents. The union of such antigens and antibodies to form a complex within the body may well give rise to acute inflammatory reactions through a variety of mechanisms (figure 16.18). For a start, complexes can stimulate macrophages through their Fcγ-receptors to generate the release of proinflammatory cytokines IL-1 and TNF, reactive oxygen intermediates and nitric oxide (figure 16.18). Complexes which are in-

soluble often cannot be digested after phagocytosis by macrophages and so provide a persistent activating stimulus. If complement is fixed, anaphylatoxins will be released as split products of C3 and C5 and these will cause release of mast cell mediators with vascular permeability changes. The chemotactic factors also produced will lead to an influx of polymorphonuclear leukocytes which begin the phagocytosis of the immune complexes; this in turn results in the extracellular release of the neutrophil granule contents, particularly when the complex is deposited on a basement membrane and cannot be phagocytosed (so-called 'frustrated phagocytosis'). The proteolytic enzymes (including neutral proteinases and collagenase), kinin-forming enzymes, polycationic proteins and reactive oxygen and nitrogen intermediates which are released will of course damage local tissues and intensify the inflammatory responses. Further havoc may be mediated by reactive lysis in which activated C5,6,7 becomes adventitiously attached to the surface of nearby cells and binds C8,9. Intravascular complexes can aggregate platelets with two consequences: they provide yet a further source of vasoactive amines and may also form microthrombi which can lead to local ischemia. (The discerning reader will appreciate the need for the system of inhibitors present in the body.)

The outcome of the formation of immune complexes *in vivo* depends not only on the absolute amounts of antigen and antibody, which determine the intensity of the reaction, but also on their *relative* proportions, which govern the nature of the complexes (cf. figure 6.2, p. 110) and hence their distribution within the body. Between **antibody excess** and **mild antigen excess**, the complexes are rapidly precipitated and tend to be localized to the site of introduction of antigen, whereas in **moderate** to **gross antigen excess**, soluble complexes are formed.

Figure 16.18. Immune complex-mediated (type III) hypersensitivity—underlying pathogenic mechanisms.

Covalent attachment of C3b prevents the Fc–Fc interactions required to form large insoluble aggregates, and these small complexes bind to CR1 complement receptors on the human erythrocyte and are transported to fixed macrophages in the liver where they are safely inactivated. If there are defects in this system, for example deficiencies in classical pathway components, or perhaps if the system is overloaded, then widespread disease involving deposition in the kidneys, joints and skin may result.

Inflammatory lesions due to locally formed complexes

The Arthus reaction

Maurice Arthus found that injection of soluble antigen intradermally into hyperimmunized rabbits with high levels of precipitating antibody produced an erythematous and edematous reaction reaching a peak at 3–8 hours which then usually resolved. The lesion was characterized by an intense infiltration with neutrophils (cf. figure 16.19a and b). The injected antigen precipitates with antibody often within the venule, too fast for the classical complement system to prevent it; subsequently, the complex binds complement and, using fluorescent reagents, antigen, immunoglobulin and complement components can all be demonstrated in this lesion, as illustrated by the inflammatory response to deposits of immune complexes containing

hepatitis B surface antigen in a patient with periarteritis nodosa (figure 16.19c). Anaphylatoxin production, mast cell degranulation, macrophage activation, platelet aggregation and influx of neutrophils all make their contribution. The Arthus reaction can be attenuated by depletion of neutrophils by nitrogen mustard or of complement by anti-C5a; soluble forms of the complement regulatory proteins CD46 (membrane cofactor protein) and CD55 (delay accelerating factor) are also inhibitory.

Reactions to inhaled antigens

Intrapulmonary Arthus-type reactions to exogenous inhaled antigen appear to be responsible for a number of hypersensitivity disorders in humans. The severe respiratory difficulties associated with **farmer's lung** occur within 6–8 hours of exposure to the dust from mouldy hay. The patients are found to be sensitized to thermophilic actinomycetes which grow in the mouldy hay, and extracts of these organisms give precipitin reactions with the subject's serum and Arthus reactions on intradermal injection. Inhalation of bacterial spores present in dust from the hay introduces antigen into the lungs and a complex-mediated hypersensitivity reaction occurs. Similar situations arise in pigeon-fancier's disease, where the antigen is probably serum protein present in the dust from dried feces, in rat handlers sensitized to rat serum proteins excreted in the urine (figure 16.20) and in many other

(a)   (b)   (c)

Figure 16.19. Histology of acute inflammatory reaction in polyarteritis nodosa associated with immune complex formation with hepatitis B surface (HBs) antigen. (a) A vessel showing thrombus (Thr) formation and fibrinoid necrosis (FN) is surrounded by a mixed inflammatory infiltrate, largely polymorphs. (b) High-power view of acute inflammatory response in loose connective tissue of patient with polyarteritis nodosa—polymorphs (PMN) are prominent. (c) Immunofluorescence studies of immune complexes in the renal artery of a patient with chronic hepatitis B infection stained with fluoresceinated antihepatitis B antigen (left) and rhodaminated anti-IgM (right). The presence of both antigen and antibody in the intima and media of the arterial wall indicates the deposition of the complexes at this site. IgG and C3 deposits are also detectable with the same distribution. ((a) and (b) provided by courtesy of Professor N. Woolf; (c) kindly provided by Professor A. Nowoslowski.)

(a)   11.12.72

(b)   27·2·73

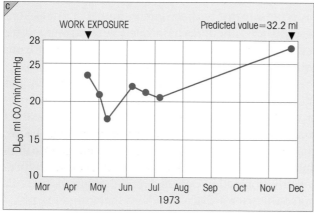

Figure 16.20. Extrinsic allergic alveolitis due to rat serum proteins in a research assistant handling rats (type III hypersensitivity). Typical systemic and pulmonary reactions on inhalation and positive prick tests were elicited by rat serum proteins; precipitins against serum proteins in rat urine were present in the patient's serum. (a) Bilateral micronodular shadowing during acute episodes. (b) Marked clearing within 11 days after cessation of exposure to rats. (c) Temporary fall in pulmonary gas exchange measured by DL_{co} (gas transfer, single breath) following a 3-day exposure to rats at work (arrowed). (From Carroll K.B., Pepys J., Longbottom J.L., Hughes D.T.D. & Benson H.G. (1975) *Clinical Allergy* 5, 443; figures by courtesy of Professor J. Pepys.)

quaintly named cases of **extrinsic allergic alveolitis** resulting from continual inhalation of organic particles, e.g. cheese washer's disease (*Penicillium casei* spores), furrier's lung (fox fur proteins) and maple bark stripper's disease (spores of *Cryptostroma*). Evidence that an immediate anaphylactic type I response may sometimes be of importance for the initiation of an Arthus reaction comes from the study of patients with allergic bronchopulmonary aspergillosis who have high levels of IgE and precipitating IgG antibodies to *Aspergillus* species.

Reactions to internal antigens

Type III reactions are often provoked by the local release of antigen from infectious organisms within the body; for example, living filarial worms, such as *Wuchereria bancrofti*, are relatively harmless, but the dead parasite found in lymphatic vessels initiates an inflammatory reaction thought to be responsible for the obstruction of lymph flow and the ensuing, rather monstrous, elephantiasis. Chemotherapy may cause an abrupt release of microbial antigens in individuals with high antibody levels, producing quite dramatic

Figure 16.21. Erythema nodosum leprosum, forearm. The patient has lepromatous leprosy with superimposed erythema nodosum leprosum. These acutely inflamed nodules were extremely tender and the patient was pyrexial. (Photograph kindly provided by Dr G. Levene.)

immune complex-mediated reactions, such as **erythema nodosum leprosum** in the skin of dapsone-treated lepromatous leprosy patients (figure 16.21) and the Jarisch–Herxheimer reaction in syphilitics on penicillin.

An interesting variant of the Arthus reaction is seen in rheumatoid arthritis where complexes are formed locally in the joint due to the production of self-associating IgG anti-IgG by synovial plasma cells (cf. p. 429).

It has also been recognized that complexes could be generated at a local site by a quite different mechanism involving nonspecific adherence of an antigen to tissue structures followed by the binding of soluble antibody—in other words, the antigen becomes fixed in the tissue *before* not *after* combining with antibody. Although it is not clear to what extent this mechanism operates in patients with immune complex disease, let us describe the experimental observation on which it is based. After injection with bacterial endotoxin, mice release DNA into their circulation which binds specifically to the collagen in the basement membrane of the glomerular capillaries; the endotoxin also polyclonally activates B-cells making anti-DNA which gives rise to antigen–antibody complexes in the kidney.

Disease resulting from circulating complexes

Immune complex glomerulonephritis

The deposition of complexes is a dynamic affair and long-lasting disease is only seen when the antigen is persistent, as in chronic infections and autoimmune diseases. Experimentally, Dixon produced chronic glomerular lesions by repeated administration of foreign proteins to rabbits. Not all animals showed the lesion, and perhaps only those genetically capable of producing low affinity antibody or antibodies to a restricted number of determinants formed soluble complexes in the right size range. The **smallest complexes reach the epithelial side**, but progressively **larger complexes are retained in or on the endothelial side of the glomerular basement membrane** (figure 16.22). They build up as 'lumpy' granules staining for antigen, immunoglobulin and complement (C3) by immunofluorescence (figure 16.17b), and appear as large amorphous masses in the electron microscope (cf. figure 20.5). The inflammatory process damages the basement membrane through engagement of the complexes with effector cells bearing Fcγ receptors, as revealed by the absence of glomerulonephritis despite immune complex deposition in the kidneys of FcγR-deficient New Zealand (B × W) F1 hybrids (a murine model of human systemic lupus erythematosus, SLE; p. 403). Proteinuria results from the leakage of serum proteins through the damaged membrane and serum albumin, being small, appears in the urine even with

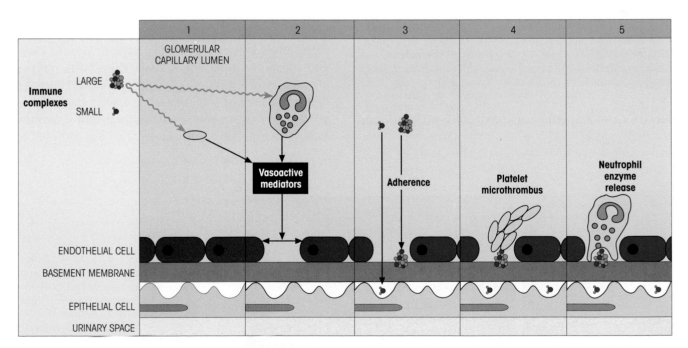

Figure 16.22. Deposition of immune complexes in the kidney glomerulus. (1) Complexes induce release of vasoactive mediators from basophils and platelets which cause (2) separation of endothelial cells. (3) Attachment of larger complexes to exposed basement membrane, with smaller complexes passing through to the epithelial side. (4) Complexes induce platelet aggregation. (5) Chemotactically attracted neutrophils release granule contents in 'frustrated phagocytosis' to damage basement membrane and cause leakage of serum proteins. Complex deposition is favored in the glomerular capillary because it is a major filtration site and has a high hydrodynamic pressure. Deposition is greatly reduced in animals depleted of platelets or treated with vasoactive amine antagonists.

minor degrees of glomerular injury (figure 16.23, lane 3).

Many cases of glomerulonephritis are associated with circulating complexes, and biopsies give a fluorescent staining pattern similar to that of figure 16.17b, which depicts DNA/anti-DNA/complement deposits in the kidney of a patient with SLE (cf. p. 427). Well known is the disease which can follow infection with certain strains of so-called 'nephritogenic' streptococci and the nephrotic syndrome of Nigerian children associated with quartan malaria, where complexes with antigens of the infecting organism have been implicated. Immune complex nephritis can arise in the course of chronic viral infections; for example, mice infected with lymphocytic choriomeningitis virus develop a glomerulonephritis associated with circulating complexes of virus and antibody. This may well represent a model for many cases of glomerulonephritis in humans.

Deposition of immune complexes at other sites

The choroid plexus, being a major filtration site, is also favored for immune complex deposition and this could account for the frequency of central nervous disorders in SLE. Neurologically affected patients tend to have depressed C4 in the cerebrospinal fluid (CSF) and, at post-mortem, SLE patients with neurologic disturbances and high titer anti-DNA were shown to have scattered deposits of immunoglobulin and DNA in the choroid plexus. Subacute sclerosing panencephalitis is associated with a high CSF to serum ratio of measles antibody, and deposits containing Ig and measles Ag may be found in neural tissue.

Vasculitic skin rashes are also characteristic of systemic and discoid lupus erythematosus (figure 16.24a and b), and biopsies of the lesions reveal amorphous deposits of Ig and C3 at the basement membrane of the dermal–epidermal junction (cf. figure 20.6).

Another example of immune complex hypersensitivity is the hemorrhagic shock syndrome found with some frequency in South-East Asia during a second infection with a dengue virus. There are four types of virus, and antibodies to one type produced during a first infection may not neutralize a second strain but rather facilitate its entry into, and replication within, human monocytes by attachment of the complex to

Figure 16.23. Proteinuria demonstrated by electrophoresis. Lane 1: Normal serum as reference. The major band nearest to the cathode is albumin. Lane 2: Normal urine showing a trace of albumin. Lane 3: Glomerular proteinuria showing a major albumin component. Lane 4: Proteinuria resulting from tubular damage with a totally different electrophoretic pattern. Lane 5: Bence-Jones proteinuria representing excreted paraprotein light chains (cf. p. 385). Lane 6: Bence-Jones proteinuria with a trace of the intact paraprotein. Some of the samples have been concentrated. (Electropherograms kindly supplied by T. Heys.)

Figure 16.24. Vasculitic skin rashes due to immune complex deposition. (a) Facial appearance in systemic lupus erythematosus (SLE). Lesions of recent onset are symmetrical, red and edematous. They are often most pronounced on the areas of the face which receive most light exposure, i.e. the upper cheeks and bridge of the nose, and the prominences of the forehead. (b) Vasculitic lesions in SLE. Small purpuric macules are seen.

Fc receptors. The enhanced production of virus leads to immune complex formation and a massive intravascular activation of the classical complement pathway. In some instances drugs such as penicillin become antigenic after conjugation with body proteins and form complexes which mediate hypersensitivity reactions.

It should be said that persistence of circulating complexes does not invariably lead to type III hypersensitivity (e.g. in many cancer patients and in individuals with idiotype–anti-idiotype reactions). Perhaps in these cases the complexes lack the ability to initiate the changes required for complex deposition, but some hold the view that complexes detected in the serum may sometimes be artifacts released from their *in vivo* attachment to the erythrocyte CR1 receptors by the action of factor I during processing of the blood.

Treatment

The avoidance of exogenous inhaled antigens inducing type III reactions is obvious. Elimination of microorganisms associated with immune complex disease by chemotherapy may provoke a further reaction due to copious release of antigen. Suppression of the accessory factors thought to be necessary for the deposition of complexes would seem logical. Disodium cromoglycate, heparin and salicylates are often used, the latter being an effective platelet stabilizer as well as a potent anti-inflammatory agent. Corticosteroids are particularly powerful inhibitors of inflammation and are immunosuppressive. In many cases, particularly those involving autoimmunity, conventional immunosuppressive agents may be justified. Where type III hypersensitivity is thought to arise

from an inadequate immune response, the more aggressive approach of immunopotentiation to boost avidity is being advocated, but that is a path that will be trodden gently.

CELL-MEDIATED (DELAYED-TYPE) HYPERSENSITIVITY (TYPE IV)

This form of hypersensitivity is encountered in many allergic reactions to bacteria, viruses and fungi, in the contact dermatitis resulting from sensitization to certain simple chemicals and in the rejection of transplanted tissues. Perhaps the best known example is the **Mantoux reaction** obtained by injection of tuberculin into the skin of an individual in whom previous infection with the mycobacterium had induced a state of cell-mediated immunity (CMI). The reaction is characterized by erythema and induration (figure 16.25a) which appears only after several hours (hence the term 'delayed') and reaches a maximum at 24–48 hours, thereafter subsiding. Histologically, the earliest phase of the reaction is seen as a perivascular cuffing with mononuclear cells followed by a more extensive exudation of mono- and polymorphonuclear cells. The latter soon migrate out of the lesion leaving behind a predominantly mononuclear cell infiltrate consisting of lymphocytes and cells of the monocyte–macrophage series (figure 16.25b). This contrasts with the essentially 'neutrophil' character of the Arthus reaction (figure 16.19b).

Comparable reactions to soluble proteins are obtained when sensitization is induced by incorporation of the antigen into complete Freund's adjuvant (see p. 192). In some, but not all cases, if animals are primed with antigen alone or in incomplete Freund's adjuvant

 (a) (b) (c)

Figure 16.25. Cell-mediated (type IV) hypersensitivity reactions. (a) Mantoux test showing cell-mediated hypersensitivity reaction to tuberculin, characterized by induration and erythema. (b) Chronic type IV inflammatory lesion in tuberculous lung showing caseous necrosis (CN), epithelioid cells (E), giant cells (G) and mononuclear inflammatory cells (M). (c) Type IV contact hypersensitivity reaction to nickel caused by the clasp of a necklace. ((a) Kindly provided by Professor J. Brostoff and (b) by Professor R. Barnetson; (c) reproduced from the British Society for Immunology teaching slides with permission of the Society and the Dermatology Department, London Hospital.)

(which lacks the mycobacteria), the delayed hypersensitivity state is of shorter duration and the dermal response more transient. This is known as 'Jones–Mote' sensitivity but has recently been termed **cutaneous basophil hypersensitivity** on account of the high proportion of basophils infiltrating the skin lesion.

The cellular basis of type IV hypersensitivity

Unlike the other forms of hypersensitivity which we have discussed, delayed-type reactivity cannot be transferred from a sensitized to a nonsensitized individual with serum antibody; lymphoid cells, in particular the T-lymphocytes, are required. Transfer has been achieved in the human using viable white blood cells and, interestingly, by a low molecular weight material extracted from them (Lawrence's transfer factor). The nature of this substance is, however, a mystery. The extracts contain a variety of factors which appear capable of stimulating precommitted T-cells mediating delayed hypersensitivity, but whether there is also an informational molecule

conferring antigen-specific reactivity is still a highly contentious issue.

It cannot be stressed too often that the hypersensitivity lesion results from an exaggerated interaction between antigen and the *normal* cell-mediated immune mechanisms (cf. p. 185). Following earlier priming, memory T-cells recognize the antigen together with class II *major histocompatibility complex* (MHC) molecules on an antigen-presenting cell and are stimulated into blast cell transformation and proliferation. The stimulated T-cells release a number of cytokines which function as mediators of the ensuing hypersensitivity response, particularly by attracting and activating macrophages if they belong to the Th1 subset, or eosinophils if they are Th2; they also help Tc precursors to become killer cells which can cause damage to virally infected target cells (figure 16.26), the CD8 TCRαβ cytotoxic cells being activated by recognition of MHC class I complexes with processed viral proteins and TCRγδ killers operating through binding to native viral proteins on the surface of the infected cells.

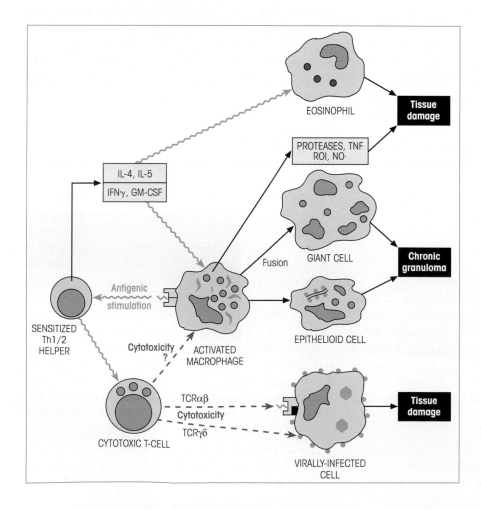

Figure 16.26. The cellular basis of type IV hypersensitivity.

Tissue damage produced by type IV reactions

Infections

The development of a state of cell-mediated hypersensitivity to bacterial products is probably responsible for the lesions associated with bacterial allergy, such as the cavitation, caseation and general toxemia seen in human tuberculosis and the granulomatous skin lesions found in patients with the borderline form of leprosy. When the battle between the replicating bacteria and the body defenses fails to be resolved in favor of the host, persisting antigen provokes a chronic local delayed hypersensitivity reaction. Continual release of cytokines from sensitized T-lymphocytes leads to the accumulation of large numbers of macrophages, many of which give rise to arrays of epithelioid cells, while others fuse to form giant cells. Macrophages bearing bacterial antigen on their surface may become targets for killer T-cells and be destroyed. Further tissue damage will occur as a result of indiscriminate cytotoxicity by lymphokine-activated macrophages (and NK cells?). Morphologically, this combination of cell types with proliferating lymphocytes and fibroblasts associated with areas of fibrosis and necrosis is termed a **chronic granuloma** and represents an attempt by the body to wall off a site of persistent infection (figures 16.25b and 16.26). It should be noted that granulomas can also arise from the persistence of indigestible antigen–antibody complexes or inorganic materials, such as talc, within macrophages, although nonimmunological granulomas may be distinguished by the absence of lymphocytes.

 Crohn's disease is an **inflammatory bowel disease (IBD)** most commonly affecting the distal small intestine, and characterized by transmural inflammation with frequent granulomas but few neutrophils. The study of experimental models suggests that IBD is a dysregulated CD4 Th1-mediated immune response to one or more antigens of the indigenous colonic bacterial flora. Attempts to pin the blame on *Mycobacterium paratuberculosis* have not met with universal acceptance, although the organism can provoke a similar disease in cattle. IBD can be induced in severe combined immunodeficient mice by the transfer of CD45RB^{hi} (naive) CD4 T-cells, but this can be counter-regulated by CD4, CD25, CD45RB^{lo} cells. The aggressor cells belong to the IL-12-driven Th1 population producing TNF and IFNγ, which are highly toxic for enterocytes, whereas the regulators (still not fully characterized as Th3 and/or T-regulatory 1 [TR1] cells) secrete the suppressor cytokines TGFβ and IL-10. Monoclonal anti-TNF is a very effective therapy; probiotic treatment with lactobacilli and *Streptococcus*

salivarius maintains remission in severe colitis, is less Draconian and is easier on the budget (remember the friendly yoghurt adverts). IBD induced by TCRα knockout or by administration of oxazolone presents as a relatively superficial inflammation resembling **ulcerative colitis** that is mediated by IL-4-producing Th2 cells; hence the as yet unsubstantiated observation that ulcerative colitis is a 'Th2 disease'.

The skin rashes in measles and the lesions of herpes simplex may be largely attributed to delayed-type allergic reactions with extensive damage to virally infected cells by Tc cells. By the same token, specific cytotoxic T-cells can have a field-day causing extensive destruction of liver cells infected with hepatitis B virus. Cell-mediated hypersensitivity has also been demonstrated in the fungal diseases candidiasis, dermatomycosis, coccidioidomycosis and histoplasmosis, and in the parasitic disease leishmaniasis.

Sarcoidosis is a disease of unknown etiology affecting lymphoid tissue and involving the formation of chronic granulomas. Evidence for atypical mycobacteria has been obtained, but delayed-type hypersensitivity is depressed and the patients are anergic on skin testing with tuberculin; curiously they give positive responses if cortisone is injected together with the antigen, and it has been suggested that cortisone-sensitive T-suppressors might be responsible for the anergy. The patients develop a granulomatous reaction a few weeks after intradermal injection of spleen extract from another sarcoid patient—the **Kweim reaction**.

Contact dermatitis

The epidermal route of inoculation tends to favor the development of a Th1 response through processing by class II-rich dendritic Langerhans' cells (cf. figure 2.6f) which migrate to the lymph nodes and present antigen to T-lymphocytes. Thus, delayed-type reactions in the skin are often produced by foreign low molecular weight materials capable of binding to peptides within the groove of MHC molecules on the surface of Langerhans' cells, to form new antigens. The reactions are characterized by a mononuclear cell infiltrate peaking at 12–15 hours, accompanied by edema of the epidermis with microvesicle formation (figure 16.27a and b). There is a most unusual twist to this story, however, possibly because the inciting reagent is a reactive hapten. The late mononuclear reaction is entirely dependent upon very early events (1–2 hours) mediated by hapten-specific IgM produced by B-1 cells which, together with complement, activates local vessels to permit T-cell recruitment. Contact hypersensitivity can occur in people who become sensitized while

(a)   (b)

Figure 16.27. Contact sensitivity. (a) Perivascular lymphocytic infiltrates (PL) and blister (Bl) formation characterize a contact sensitivity reaction of the skin. (b) High-power view to show the lymphocytic nature of the infiltrate in a contact hypersensitivity reaction. (Photographs kindly provided by Professor N. Woolf.)

working with chemicals, such as picryl chloride and chromates, or who repeatedly come into contact with the substance urushiol from the poison ivy plant. *p*-Phenylene diamine in certain hair dyes, neomycin in topically applied ointments, and nickel salts formed from articles such as nickel jewellery clasps (figure 16.25c) can provoke similar reactions. T-cell clones specific for nickel salts isolated from the latter group produce a Th1-type profile of cytokines (IFNγ, IL-2) on antigen stimulation (figure 16.9b).

Th2-mediated hypersensitivity

The examples of type IV hypersensitivity we have discussed so far are centered essentially on the Th1 macrophage pathway, but it is now clear that excessive responses by Th2 cells can damage tissues through activation of eosinophils (figure 16.26). As recounted earlier, T-cells synthesizing IL-5 are largely responsible for the sustained influx of eosinophils in asthma and atopic dermatitis (cf. p. 328). They also essentially account for the liver pathology in schistosomiasis which has been attributed to a reaction against soluble enzymes derived from the eggs which lodge in the capillaries (figure 16.28).

Other examples

Delayed hypersensitivity contributes significantly to the prolonged reactions which result from insect bites. The possible implication of allograft rejection by Tc cells as a mechanism for the control of cancer cells is discussed in Chapter 18. In certain organ-specific autoimmune diseases, such as type I diabetes, cell-mediated hypersensitivity reactions undoubtedly provide the major engine for tissue destruction.

The intestinal inflammation in celiac disease, an HLA-DQ2/8-associated enteropathy, is precipitated

Figure 16.28. Th2-mediated response to schistosome egg. Th2-type hypersensitivity lesion of inflammatory cells (M) around a schistosome egg (SE) within the liver parenchyma (LP). (Photograph by courtesy of Professor M. Doenhoff.)

by exposure to dietary wheat gliadin. The disorder involves what is probably a genetically related increased mucosal activity of transglutaminase (the target of anti-endomysium autoantibodies; cf. p. 423). This enzyme deamidates the glutamine residues in gliadin and creates a new T-cell epitope that binds efficiently to DQ2 and is recognized by gut-derived CD4 and γδ T-cells.

Psoriasis involves marked proliferation of epidermal keratinocytes and accelerated incomplete epidermal differentiation. There is inflammation in the skin with pockets of microabscesses containing neutrophils and, in all instances, CD4 cells in the psoriatic dermis and CD8 in the lesional epidermis. A reversal of epidermal dysfunction and a marked reduction in intraepidermal CD8 T-cells were achieved by systemic administration of a fusion protein of IL-2 and fragments of diphtheria toxin, which selectively blocks the growth of activated lymphocytes but not keratinocytes. This shows that the disorder is primarily immunological rather than a dysfunction of keratinocytes which secondarily activate T-cells through, say, TGFβ. The party line now would be that CD8 T-cells attack the skin, activating injury repair programs associated with wound healing, while cytokines act directly as mitogens for epidermal keratinocytes.

STIMULATORY HYPERSENSITIVITY (TYPE V)

Many cells are signaled by agents such as hormones through surface receptors to which they specifically bind the external agent, presumably through complementarity of structure. For example, when thyroid-stimulating hormone (TSH) of pituitary origin binds to the thyroid cell receptors, adenyl cyclase is activated, and the cAMP 'second messenger' which is generated acts to stimulate the thyroid cell. The **thyroid-stimulating antibody** present in the sera of thyrotoxic patients (cf. p. 422) is an autoantibody directed against a site on the TSH receptor which produces the changes required for adenyl cyclase activation. Intriguingly, but not much more at present, there are indications that cimetidine-resistant duodenal ulcer patients might have stimulatory antibodies directed to histamine receptors.

Experimental examples of stimulation by antibodies to cell surface antigens may be cited: the activation of B- and T-lymphocytes by F(ab')₂ fragments directed to their antigen-specific receptors; the production of cell division in thyroid cells by 'growth' autoantibodies; the induction of pinocytosis by antimacrophage serum; and the mitogenic effect of antibodies to sea-urchin eggs. It is worthy of note that, although antibodies to enzymes directed against determinants near to the active site can exert a blocking effect, combination with more distant determinants can sometimes bring about allosteric conformational changes which are associated with a considerable increase in enzymic activity, as has been described for certain variants of penicillinase and β-galactosidase.

'INNATE' HYPERSENSITIVITY REACTIONS

Many infections provoke a **'toxic shock syndrome'** characterized by hypotension, hypoxia, oliguria and microvascular abnormalities and mediated by elements of the innate immune system independently of the operation of acquired immune responses.

Septicemia associated with **Gram-negative bacteria** results in excessive release of TNF, IL-1 and IL-6 through stimulation of macrophages and endothelial cells by the lipopolysaccharide (LPS) endotoxin (cf. figure 1.6). Normally this would enhance host defenses, aiding the recruitment of phagocytes by promoting adherence to endothelium, priming neutrophils for subsequent release of reactive oxygen intermediates, inducing febrile responses (immune responses improve steadily from 33 to 44°C), and so on. Unfortunately, the excess of circulating LPS and the cytokines released by it lead to unwanted pathophysiology at distant sites, such as the **adult respiratory distress syndrome** brought about by an overwhelming invasion of the lung by neutrophils. There is a prolonged pathologically high concentration of nitric oxide but, additionally, LPS can activate the alternative complement pathway, and this may be linked to its ability to induce the release of thromboxane A₂ and prostaglandin from platelets leading to **disseminated intravascular coagulation**.

Whereas the major culprit in Gram-negative sepsis is LPS, **Gram-positive organisms** possess a variety of components which act on host defense elements to initiate septic shock. Thus adherence of *Staphylococcus aureus* to macrophages induces TNFα synthesis, and peptidoglycan-mediated aggregation of platelets by the same organism leads to disseminated intravascular coagulation. The staphylococcal and streptococcal enterotoxins induce toxic shock syndrome by quite different means. By functioning as **superantigens** (cf. p. 103), they react directly with particular T-cell receptor families and give rise to massive cytokine release, including TNF and macrophage migration inhibitory factor (MIF), which is detected in high concentrations in the plasma of patients with septic shock. Various treatments are under investigation. Pentoxifylline blocks TNF production by macrophages. Experimental models of septic shock can be blocked by anti-MIF and by a peptide derived from the natural sequence 150–161 of staphylococcal enterotoxin B, which is part of a domain crucial for T-cell activation.

Germ-line mutations in the extracellular domains of the 55 kDa TNF receptor, TNFRI, define a family of dominantly inherited autoinflammatory syndromes involving unpredictable periodic fever episodes.

The reader's attention has already been drawn to the unusual susceptibility of erythrocytes to lysis in **paroxysmal nocturnal hemoglobinuria** resulting from deficiency in complement control proteins on the red cell surface (see p. 307). Undue C3 consumption is associated with mesangiocapillary glomerulonephritis and partial lipodystrophy in patients with the so-called **C3 nephritic factor**, which appears to be an IgG autoantibody capable of activating the alternative pathway by combining with and stabilizing the C3bBb convertase.

We should include **idiopathic pulmonary fibrosis** in this section. It is a chronic fatal disorder characterized by diffuse fibrosis of the alveolar walls in which local macrophages play a central role. On activation, they produce an early G1 competence growth signal, such as platelet-derived growth factor and fibronectin, and then a late G1 progression growth signal, such as insulin-like growth factor 1. As a result, the fibroblasts multiply and become embedded in a collagen matrix to the respiratory detriment of the host.

The neuropathological hallmarks of Alzheimer's disease are extracellular plaques and intracellular neurofibrillary tangles. One of the constituents of senile plaques is β-amyloid composed of a hydrophobic fragment of amyloid precursor protein (APP). Normally APP is cleaved by an α-secretase into soluble products which cannot form β-amyloid, but members of a family diagnosed with Alzheimer's disease, and having a pathogenic mutation at residues 670–671 of APP, had very low levels of this soluble cleaved form compared with noncarriers. This could also represent a new and promising diagnostic marker.

SUMMARY

• Excessive stimulation of the normal effector mechanisms of the immune system can lead to tissue damage and we speak of hypersensitivity reactions, several types of which can be distinguished.

Anaphylactic hypersensitivity (type I)

• Anaphylaxis involves contraction of smooth muscle and dilatation of capillaries.

• This depends upon the reaction of antigen with specific IgE antibody bound through its Fc to the mast cell high affinity receptor FcεRI.

• Cross-linking and clustering of the IgE receptors activates the Lyn protein tyrosine kinase, recruits other kinases and leads to release from the granules of mediators including histamine, leukotrienes and platelet activating factor, plus eosinophil and neutrophil chemotactic factors and the cytokines IL-3, -4, -5 and GM-CSF.

Atopic allergy

• Atopy stems from an excessive IgE response to extrinsic antigens (allergens) which leads to local anaphylactic reactions at sites of contact with allergen.

• Hay fever and extrinsic asthma represent the most common atopic allergic disorders resulting from exposure to inhaled allergens. Atopic dermatitis is also extremely common.

• Whereas the immediate reaction to extrinsic allergen (maximum at 30 minutes) is due to mast cell triggering, a late phase reaction peaking at 5 hours, involving heavy eosinophil infiltration, is initiated by the activation of alveolar and other macrophages through surface-bound IgE; secreted TNF and IL-1β now act upon epithelial cells and fibroblasts to release powerful eosinophil chemoattractants such as RANTES and eotaxin.

• In asthma, serious prolongation of the response to allergen is caused by T-cells of Th2 type which sustain the recruitment of tissue-damaging eosinophils through the release of IL-5. The soup of powerful bronchoconstrictors, the injurious effect of eosinophil major basic protein and reactive oxygen intermediates and the mucus hypersecretion stimulated by IL-13 and IL-4, all contribute to the drastic airway damage characteristic of chronic asthma.

• Many food allergies involve type I hypersensitivity.

• Strong genetic factors include linkage to the propensity to make the IgE isotype and to genes involving the IL-4/9/13, GM-CSF and CD14 cluster.

• Exposure to certain foods and to Th1-stimulating infections may strongly influence the 'immunostat' setting of the tendency to either Th1 or Th2 responses, the latter increasing the risk of allergy through promotion of IgE synthesis and eosinophil recruitment.

• The offending antigen is identified by intradermal prick tests, giving immediate wheal and erythema reactions, by provocation testing and by RAST.

• Where possible, allergen avoidance is the best treatment.

• A monoclonal antibody directed to the receptor-binding domain of IgE dramatically reduces IgE levels and synthesis, and decreases mast cell responsiveness. Symptomatic treatment involves the use of long-acting β$_2$-agonists and newly developed leukotriene antagonists. Chromones, such as sodium cromoglycate, block chloride channel activity thereby stabilizing mast cells and inhibiting bronchoconstriction. Theophylline, the single most prescribed drug for asthma, is a phosphodiesterase inhibitor which raises intracellular calcium; this causes bronchodilatation and inhibition of IL-5 effects on eosinophils. Chronic asthma is dominated by activated Th2 cells and is treated with topical steroids which display a wide range of anti-inflammatory actions, including the ability to block the production of mediators by

(continued)

stimulated macrophages or Th2 cells. These are supplemented where necessary by long-acting β_2-agonists and theophylline.

• Courses of antigen injection may desensitize by the formation of blocking, or possibly regulatory, IgG antibodies or through T-cell regulation. T-cell epitope peptides may be manipulated to modulate the atopic state.

Antibody-dependent cytotoxic hypersensitivity (type II)
• This involves the death of cells bearing antibody attached to a surface antigen.
• The cells may be taken up by phagocytic cells to which they adhere through their coating of IgG or C3b or lysed by the operation of the full complement system.
• Cells bearing IgG may also be killed by polymorphs and macrophages or by K-cells through an extracellular mechanism (antibody-dependent cellular cytotoxicity).
• Examples are: transfusion reactions, hemolytic disease of the newborn through rhesus incompatibility, antibody-mediated graft destruction, autoimmune reactions directed against the formed elements of the blood and kidney glomerular basement membranes, and hypersensitivity resulting from the coating of erythrocytes or platelets by a drug.

Complex-mediated hypersensitivity (type III)
• This results from the effects of antigen–antibody complexes through (i) activation of complement and attraction of polymorphonuclear leukocytes which release tissue-damaging mediators on contact with the complex, (ii) stimulation of macrophages to release proinflammatory cytokines, and (iii) aggregation of platelets to cause microthrombi and vasoactive amine release.

• Where circulating antibody levels are high, the antigen is precipitated near the site of entry into the body. The reaction in the skin is characterized by polymorph infiltration, edema and erythema maximal at 3–8 hours (Arthus reaction).

• Examples are farmer's lung, pigeon-fancier's disease and pulmonary aspergillosis where inhaled antigens provoke high antibody levels, reactions to an abrupt increase in antigen caused by microbial cell death during chemotherapy for leprosy or syphilis, polyarteritis nodosa linked to complexes with hepatitis B virus and an element of the synovial lesion in rheumatoid arthritis.

• In relative *antigen excess*, soluble complexes are formed which are removed by binding to the CR1 C3b receptors on red cells. If this system is overloaded or if the classical complement components are deficient, the complexes circulate in the free state and are deposited under circumstances of increased vascular permeability at certain preferred sites: the kidney glomerulus, the joints, the skin and the choroid plexus.

• Examples are: glomerulonephritis associated with systemic lupus erythematosus (SLE) or infections with streptococci, malaria and other parasites, neurological dis-

Table 16.3. Comparison of types of hypersensitivity involving acquired responses.

	Anaphylactic (I)	Cytotoxic (II)	Complex-mediated (III)	Cell-mediated (IV)	Stimulatory (V)
Antibody mediating reaction	Homocytotropic Ab Mast-cell binding	Humoral Ab ± CF*	Humoral Ab ± CF*	Receptor on T-lymphocyte	Humoral Ab Non-CF*
Antigen	Usually exogenous (e.g. grass pollen)	Cell surface	Extracellular	Associated with MHC on macrophage or target cell	Cell surface
Response to intradermal antigen: Max. reaction Appearance / Histology	30 min (+ late reaction) Wheal and flare / Degranulated mast cells; edema; (late reaction cellular including eosinophils)	– –	3–8 h Erythema and edema Acute inflammatory reaction; predominant polymorphs	24–48 h Erythema and induration Perivascular inflammation: polymorphs migrate out leaving predominantly mononuclear cells	– –
Transfer sensitivity to normal subject	◄———————— Serum antibody ————————►			Lymphoid cells Transfer factor	Serum antibody
Examples:	Atopic allergy, e.g. hay fever	Hemolytic disease of newborn (Rh)	Complex glomerulonephritis Farmer's lung	Mantoux reaction to TB Granulomatous reaction to TB Contact sensitivity	Thyrotoxicosis

*CF, complement fixation.

(continued p. 348)

turbances in SLE and subacute sclerosing panencephalitis, and hemorrhagic shock in dengue viral infection.

Cell-mediated or delayed-type hypersensitivity (type IV)

• This is based upon the interaction of antigen with primed T-cells and represents tissue damage resulting from inappropriate cell-mediated immunity reactions.

• A number of soluble cytokines including IFNγ are released, which activate macrophages and account for the events that occur in a typical delayed hypersensitivity response such as the Mantoux reaction to tuberculin, that is, the delayed appearance of an indurated and erythematous reaction which reaches a maximum at 24–48 hours and is characterized histologically by infiltration with mononuclear phagocytes and lymphocytes.

• Continuing provocation of delayed hypersensitivity by persisting antigen leads to the formation of chronic granulomas.

• Th2-type cells producing IL-4 and IL-5 can also produce tissue damage through their ability to recruit eosinophils.

• CD8 T-cells are activated by class I major histocompatibility antigens to become directly cytotoxic to target cells bearing the appropriate antigen.

• Examples are: tissue damage occurring in bacterial (tuberculosis, leprosy), viral (measles, herpes), fungal (candidiasis, histoplasmosis) and parasitic (leishmaniasis, schistosomiasis) infections, contact dermatitis from exposure to chromates and poison ivy, insect bites and psoriasis. Inflammatory bowel disease can result from Th1-type reactions to intestinal bacteria or certain foods such as wheat gliadin.

Stimulatory hypersensitivity (type V)

• The antibody reacts with a key surface component such as a hormone receptor and 'switches on' the cell.

• An example is the thyroid hyper-reactivity in Graves' disease due to a thyroid-stimulating autoantibody. Features of these five types of acquired hypersensitivity are compared in table 16.3.

'Innate' hypersensitivity reactions

• Many infections provoke a 'toxic shock syndrome' involving excessive release of TNF, IL-1 and IL-6 and intravascular activation of complement.

• Septic shock associated with Gram-negative bacteria is primarily due to the lipopolysaccharide (LPS) endotoxin.

• Gram-positive organisms cause release of TNF and macrophage migration inhibitory factor (MIF) through direct action on macrophages and stimulation of selected T-cell families by the enterotoxin superantigens. Aggregation of platelets by *S. aureus* induces disseminated intravascular coagulation.

• Aberration of innate mechanisms may underlie idiopathic pulmonary fibrosis and contribute to the β-amyloid plaques in Alzheimer's disease.

See the accompanying website (**www.roitt.com**) for multiple choice questions.

FURTHER READING

Arad G. *et al.* (2000) Superantigen antagonist protects against lethal shock and defines a new domain for T-cell activation. *Nature Medicine* **6**, 414.

Chapel H., Haeney M., Misbah S. & Snowden N. (1999) *Essentials of Clinical Immunology*, 4th edn. Blackwell Science, Oxford. (Very broad account of the diseases involving the immune system. Good illustration by case histories and the laboratory tests available. Also MCQs.)

Coleman J.W. & Blanca M. (1998) Mechanisms of drug allergy. *Immunology Today* **19**, 196.

Holgate S. (ed.) (1999) Allergy and asthma. *Nature* **402** (Suppl.) (Excellent reviews on genetic factors, the role of IgE in the development of asthma, therapeutic strategies, and an especially valuable account of IgE receptor FcεRI signaling.)

Holgate S.T. & Church M.K. (1993) *Allergy*. Gower Medical Publishing, London.

Kinet J.-P. (ed.) (1999) Atopy and other hypersensitivities. *Current Opinion in Immunology* **11**, 603. (A collection of critical reviews on hypersensitivity which appear annually as Issue No. 6 and are highly recommended.)

Molberg O. *et al.* (1998) Tissue transglutaminase selectively modifies gliadin peptides that are recognized by gut-derived T-cells in celiac disease. *Nature Medicine* **4**, 713.

Ravetch J.V. (1998) Uncoupling immune complex formation and kidney damage in autoimmune glomerulonephritis. *Science* **279**, 1052.

Scadding G. (1998) Atopic allergy. In Delves P.J. & Roitt I.M. (eds) *Encyclopedia of Immunology*, 2nd edn, p. 251. Academic Press, London.

Tsuji R.F. *et al.* (1997) Required early complement activation in contact sensitivity with generation of local C5-dependent chemotactic activity, and late T-cell interferon gamma: a possible initiating role of B-cells. *Journal of Experimental Medicine* **186**, 1015.

Wills-Karp M. (1999) Immunologic basis of antigen-induced airway hyperresponsiveness. *Annual Review of Immunology* **17**, 255.

Transplantation

INTRODUCTION

The replacement of diseased organs by a transplant of healthy tissue has long been an objective in medicine but has been frustrated to no mean degree by the uncooperative attempts by the body to reject grafts from other individuals. Before discussing the nature and implications of this rejection phenomenon, it would be helpful to define the terms used for transplants between individuals and species.

Autograft—tissue grafted back on to the original donor.

Isograft—graft between **syngeneic** individuals (i.e. of identical genetic constitution) such as identical twins or mice of the same pure line strain.

Allograft (old term, homograft)—graft between **allogeneic** individuals (i.e. members of the same species but different genetic constitution), e.g. human to human and one mouse strain to another.

Xenograft (heterograft)—graft between **xenogeneic** individuals (i.e. of different species), e.g. pig to human.

It is with the allograft reaction that we have been most concerned, although there is now a serious interest in the use of grafts from other species. The most common allografting procedure is probably blood transfusion where the unfortunate consequences of mismatching are well known. Considerable attention has been paid to the rejection of solid grafts such as skin and the sequence of events is worth describing. In mice, for example, the skin allograft settles down and becomes vascularized within a few days. Between 3 and 9 days the circulation gradually diminishes and there is increasing infiltration of the graft bed with lymphocytes and monocytes but very few plasma cells. Necrosis begins to be visible macroscopically and within a day or so the graft is sloughed completely (figure M17.1.1). **Rejection has all the hallmarks of an immunological response** in that it shows both memory and specificity (Milestone 17.1). Furthermore, the recipient of T-cells from a donor which has already rejected a graft will give accelerated rejection of a further graft of the same type (figure 17.1), showing that the lymphoid cells are primed and retain memory of the first contact with graft antigens.

GENETIC CONTROL OF TRANSPLANTATION ANTIGENS

The specificity of the antigens involved in graft rejection is under genetic control. Genetically identical in-

Milestone 17.1—The Immunological Basis of Graft Rejection

The field of transplantation owes a tremendous debt to Sir Peter Medawar, the outstanding scientist who kick-started and inspired its development. Even at the turn of the century it was an accepted paradigm that grafts between unrelated members of a species would be unceremoniously rejected after a brief initial period of acceptance (figure

Figure M17.1.1. Rejection of CBA skin graft by strain A mouse. (a) Ten days after transplantation; discolored areas caused by destruction of epithelium and drying of the exposed dermis. (b) Thirteen days after transplantation; the scabby surface indicates total destruction of the graft. (Photographs courtesy of Professor L. Brent.)

M17.1.1). That there was an underlying genetic basis for rejection became apparent from Padgett's observations in Kansas City in 1932 that skin allografts between family members tended to survive for longer than those between unrelated individuals and J.B. Brown's critical demonstration in St Louis in 1937 that monozygotic (i.e. genetically identical) twins accepted skin grafts from each other. However, it was not until Medawar's research in the early part of the Second World War, motivated by the need to treat aircrew with appalling burns, that rejection was laid at immunology's door. He showed that a second graft from a given donor was rejected more rapidly and more vigorously than the first and, further, that an unrelated graft was rejected with the kinetics of a first set reaction (figure M17.1.2). This **second set rejection** is characterized by **memory** and **specificity** and thereby bears the hallmarks of an immunological response. This of course was later confirmed by transferring the ability to express a second set reaction with lymphocytes.

The message was clear: to achieve successful transplantation of tissues and organs in the human, it would be necessary to overcome this immunogenetic barrier. Limited success was obtained by Murray at the Peter Bent Brigham Hospital and Hamburger in Paris, who grafted kidneys between dizygotic twins using sublethal X-irradiation. The key breakthrough came when Schwartz and Damashek's report on the immunosuppressive effects of the antimitotic drug 6-mercaptopurine was applied inde-

Figure M17.1.2. Memory and specificity in skin allograft rejection in rabbits. (a) Autografts and allografts from two unrelated donors B and C are applied to the thoracic wall skin of rabbit A which has already rejected a first graft from B (B_1). While the autograft A remains intact, graft C_1 seen for the *first* time undergoes 1st set rejection, whereas a *second* graft from B (B_2) is sloughed off very rapidly. (b) Median survival times of 1st and 2nd set skin allografts showing faster 2nd set rejection. (From Medawar P.B. (1944) The behavior and fate of skin autografts and skin homografts (allografts) in rabbits. *Journal of Anatomy* **78**, 176.)

(continued)

pendently by Calne and Zukowski in 1960 to the prolongation of renal allografts in dogs. This was followed very rapidly by Murray's successful grafting in 1962 of an unrelated cadaveric kidney under the immunosuppressive umbrella of azathioprine, the more effective derivative of 6-mercaptopurine devised by Hutchings and Elion.

This story is studded with Nobel Prize winners and readers of a historical bent will gain further insight into the development of this field and the minds of the scientists who gave medicine this wonderful prize in Terasaki P.I. (ed.) (1991) *History of Transplantation; Thirty-Five Recollections*, UCLA Tissue Typing Laboratory, Los Angeles, CA and, subsequently, Brent L. (1996) *A History of Transplantation Immunology*, Academic Press, London.

Figure 17.1. Graft rejection induces memory which is specific and can be transferred by T-cells. In experiment 1, an A strain recipient of T-cells from another A strain mouse, which had rejected a graft from strain B, will give accelerated (i.e. 2nd set) rejection of a B graft. Experiments 2 and 3 show the specificity of the phenomenon with respect to the genetically unrelated third party strain C.

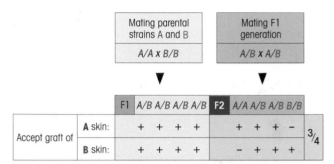

Figure 17.2. Inheritance of genes controlling transplantation antigens. *A* represents a gene expressing the A antigen and *B* the corresponding allelic gene at the same genetic locus. The pure strains are homozygous for *A/A* and *B/B* respectively. Since the genes are codominant, an animal with *A/B* genome will express both antigens, become tolerant to them and therefore accept grafts from either A or B donors. The illustration shows that, for each gene controlling a transplantation antigen specificity, three-quarters of the F2 generation will accept a graft of parental skin. For *n* genes the fraction is $(3/4)^n$. If F1 *A/B* animals are back-crossed with an *A/A* parent, half the progeny will be *A/A* and half *A/B*; only the latter will accept B grafts.

dividuals, such as mice of a pure strain or monozygotic twins, have identical transplantation antigens and grafts can be freely exchanged between them. The Mendelian segregation of the genes controlling these antigens has been revealed by interbreeding experiments between mice of different pure strains. Since these mice breed true within a given strain and always accept grafts from each other, they must be homozygous for the 'transplantation' genes. Consider two such strains A and B with allelic genes differing at one locus. In each case paternal and maternal genes will be identical and they will have a genetic constitution of, say, *A/A* and *B/B* respectively. Crossing strains A and B gives a first familial generation (F1) of constitution *A/B*. Now, all F1 mice accept grafts from either parent showing that they are immunologically tolerant to both A and B due to the fact that the transplantation antigens from each parent are codominantly expressed (figure 4.17). By intercrossing the F1 generation, one would expect an average distribution of genotypes for the F2s as shown in figure 17.2; only one in four would have no *A* genes and would therefore reject an A graft because of lack of tolerance, and one in four would re-

ject B grafts for the same reason. Thus, for each locus, three out of four of the F2 generation will accept parental strain grafts.

In the mouse around 40 such loci have been established but, as we have seen earlier, the complex locus termed H2 (HLA in the human) predominates in the sense that it controls the 'strong' transplantation antigens which provoke intense allograft reactions. We have looked at the structure (cf. figure 4.11) and biology of this **major histocompatibility locus** in some detail in previous chapters (see Milestone 4.2, p. 71). The non-H-2 or 'minor' transplantation antigens, such as the male H-Y, are recognized as processed peptides in association with the *major histocompatibility complex* (MHC) molecules on the cell surface by T-cells but not at all by B-cells. One should not be misled by the term 'minor' into thinking that these antigens do not give rise to serious rejection problems, albeit more slowly than the MHC.

SOME OTHER CONSEQUENCES OF MHC INCOMPATIBILITY

Class II MHC differences produce a mixed lymphocyte reaction (MLR)

When lymphocytes from individuals of different class II haplotype are cultured together, blast cell transformation and mitosis occur (MLR), the T-cells of each population of lymphocytes reacting against MHC class II determinants on the surface of the other population. The responding cells belong predominantly to a population of CD4[+] T-lymphocytes and are stimulated by the class II determinants present mostly on B-cells, macrophages and especially dendritic antigen-presenting cells. Thus, the MLR is inhibited by antisera to class II determinants on the stimulator cells.

The graft-vs-host (g.v.h.) reaction

When competent T-cells are transferred from a donor to a recipient which is incapable of rejecting them, the grafted cells survive and have time to recognize the host antigens and react immunologically against them. Instead of the normal transplantation reaction of host against graft, we have the reverse, the so-called graft-vs-host (g.v.h.) reaction. In the young rodent there can be inhibition of growth (runting), spleen enlargement and hemolytic anemia (due to the production of red cell antibodies). In the human, fever, anemia, weight loss, rash, diarrhea and splenomegaly are observed, with cytokines, especially tumor necrosis factor (TNF), being thought to be the major mediators of pathology. The 'stronger' the transplantation antigen difference, the more severe the reaction. Where donor and recipient differ at HLA or H-2 loci, the consequences can be fatal, although it should be noted that reactions to dominant minor transplantation antigens, or combinations of them, may be equally difficult to control.

Two possible situations leading to g.v.h. reactions are illustrated in figure 17.3. In the human this may arise in immunologically anergic subjects receiving bone marrow grafts, e.g. for combined immunodeficiency (see p. 312), for red cell aplasia after radiation accidents, or as a possible form of cancer therapy. Competent T-cells in blood or present in grafted organs given to immunosuppressed patients may give g.v.h. reactions; so could maternal cells which adventitiously cross the placenta, although in this case there is as yet no evidence of diseases caused by such a mechanism in the human.

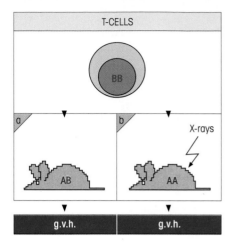

Figure 17.3. Graft-vs-host reaction. When competent T-cells are inoculated into a host incapable of reacting against them, the grafted cells are free to react against the antigens on the host's cells which they recognize as foreign. The ensuing reaction may be fatal. Two of many possible situations are illustrated: (a) the hybrid AB receives cells from one parent (BB) which are tolerated but react against the A antigen on host cells; (b) an X-irradiated AA recipient restored immunologically with BB cells cannot react against the graft and a g.v.h. reaction will result.

MECHANISMS OF GRAFT REJECTION

Lymphocytes can mediate rejection

A great deal of the work on allograft rejection has involved transplants of skin or solid tumors because their fate is relatively easy to follow. In these cases there is little support for the view that humoral antibodies are instrumental in destruction of the graft, although, as we shall see later, this is not necessarily so with transplants of other organs such as the kidney. Whereas passive transfer of *serum* from an animal which has rejected a skin allograft cannot usually accelerate the rejection of a similar graft on the recipient animal, injection of *lymphoid* cells (particularly recirculating small lymphocytes) is effective in shortening graft survival (cf. figure 17.1).

A primary role of lymphoid cells in first set rejection would be consistent with the histology of the early reaction showing infiltration by mononuclear cells with very few polymorphs or plasma cells (figure 17.4). The dramatic effect of neonatal thymectomy on prolonging skin transplants, as mentioned earlier, and the long survival of grafts on children with thymic deficiencies implicate the T-lymphocytes in these reactions. In the chicken, homograft rejection and g.v.h. reactivity are influenced by neonatal thymectomy but not bursectomy. More direct evidence has come from *in vitro* studies showing that T-cells taken from mice rejecting

Figure 17.4. Acute rejection of human renal allograft showing dense cellular infiltration of interstitium by mononuclear cells. (Photograph courtesy of Drs M. Thompson and A. Dorling.)

an allograft could kill target cells bearing the graft antigens *in vitro*. Recent work on the importance of murine and human CD4⁺ cells as effectors has cast some doubt, probably wrongly, on the role of CD8 cytotoxic cells in graft rejection *in vivo*; although sometimes CD4 cells have cytotoxic potential for class II targets, as a rule they are associated with helper activity, in this case particularly for Tc precursors, and with the production of cytokines mediating delayed hypersensitivity reactions. Perhaps they act to encourage access of Tc cells to their targets? We do know that γ-interferon (IFNγ) up-regulates antigen expression on the target graft cell, so increasing its vulnerability to CD8 cytotoxic cells.

The allograft response is powerful

Remember, we defined the MHC by its ability to provoke the most powerful rejection of grafts between members of the same species. This intensity of MHC mismatched rejection is a consequence of the **very high frequency of alloreactive cells** (i.e. cells which react with allografts) **present in normal individuals.** Whereas merely a fraction of a per cent of the normal T-cell population is specific for a given single peptide, upwards of 10% of the T-cells react with alloantigens. This remarkable phenomenon seems to be based largely on the ability of **alloreactive T-cells to recognize allo- (i.e. graft) MHC plus self-peptides** (figure 17.5a). The allogeneic MHC differs from the recipient essentially in the groove residues which contact processed peptide, but much less so in the more conserved helical regions which are recognized by the TCR. Having a different groove structure, the allo-MHC will be able to bind a number of peptides derived from proteins common to donor and host which might be unable to fit the

Figure 17.5. Recognition of graft antigens by alloreactive T-cells. Direct pathway. (a) Polymorphic differences largely affect peptide binding but not T-cell receptor (TCR) contact by the donor MHC. Under these circumstances, the donor MHC molecule will be seen as 'self' by the host T-cells but, unlike the self-MHC, the donor MHC groove on graft antigen-presenting cells will bind large numbers of processed serum and cellular peptides common to graft and recipient to which the responder host T-cells have not been rendered tolerant and which can therefore provoke a reaction in up to 10% of these host T-cells. This provides the intensity of the allograft response. This explanation for the high frequency of alloreactive T-cells is given further credibility by the isolation of individual T-cell clones which react with self- and allo-MHC, each binding a different peptide sequence. (b) Minor polymorphic residue changes in the α-helix may adventitiously allow binding of TCRs to the allo-MHC independently of the associated peptide. Multiple bonds of this nature between the APC and T-cell may give rise to a strong enough interaction to permit T-cell activation. **Indirect pathway.** (c) Polymorphic peptides derived from the graft may be presented by self-MHC on host antigen-presenting cells to an initially small population of T-cells which will expand with time. Regions which differ from self-MHC with respect to polymorphic residues are indicated in blue.

groove in the host MHC and therefore fail to induce self-tolerance. Thus the host T-cells which recognize allo-MHC plus common peptides will not have been eliminated, and will be available to react with the large number of different peptides binding to the allo-groove of the donor antigen-presenting cells (APCs) which migrate to the secondary lymphoid tissue of the graft recipient. In some cases, the polymorphic residues may lie within the regions of the MHC helices which contact TCR directly and, by chance, a **proportion of the T-cell repertoire cross-reacts and binds to the donor MHC with high affinity** (figure 17.5b). Attachment of the T-cell to the APC will be particularly strong since the TCRs will bind to all the donor MHC molecules on the APC, whereas, in the case of normal MHC–peptide recognition, only a small proportion of the MHC grooves will be filled by the specific peptide in question. These **direct pathways of immunization** by the allograft MHC which are usually initiated by the most powerful APC, the dendritic cell, dominate the early sensitization events, since this acute phase of rejection (see below) can be blocked by antibodies to the *allo*-MHC class II.

However, with time, as the donor APCs in the graft are replaced by recipient cells, another rejection mechanism based on an **indirect pathway of sensitization** involving the **presentation of processed allogeneic peptides by host MHC** (figure 17.5c) becomes possible. Although T-cells recognizing peptides derived from polymorphic graft proteins would be expected to be present in low frequency comparable to that observed with any foreign antigen, a graft which has been in place for an extended period will have the time to expand this small population significantly so that later rejection may depend progressively on this indirect pathway. In these circumstances, *anti-recipient* MHC class II can now be shown to prolong renal allografts in rats.

The role of humoral antibody

It has long been recognized that isolated allogeneic cells such as lymphocytes can be destroyed by cytotoxic (type II) reactions involving humoral antibody. However, although earlier experience with skin and solid tumor grafts suggested that they were not readily susceptible to the action of cytotoxic antibodies, it is now clear that this does not hold for all types of organ transplants. Consideration of the different ways in which kidney allografts can be rejected illustrates the point.

Hyperacute rejection within minutes of transplantation, characterized by sludging of red cells and microthrombi in the glomeruli, occurs in individuals with pre-existing humoral antibodies—either due to blood group incompatibility or presensitization to class I MHC through blood transfusion.

Acute early rejection occurring up to 10 days or so after transplantation is characterized by dense cellular infiltration (figure 17.4) and rupture of peritubular capillaries, and appears to be a cell-mediated hypersensitivity reaction mainly involving CD8 cytotoxic attack on graft cells whose MHC antigen expression has been upregulated by γ-interferon.

Acute late rejection, which occurs from 11 days onwards in patients suppressed with prednisolone and azathioprine, may be due to breakthrough of immunosuppression by the immune response, or can be caused by the binding of immunoglobulin (presumably antibody) and complement to the arterioles and glomerular capillaries, where they can be visualized by immunofluorescent techniques. These immunoglobulin deposits on the vessel walls induce platelet aggregation in the glomerular capillaries leading to acute renal shutdown (figure 17.6). The possibility of damage to antibody-coated cells through antibody-dependent cellular cytotoxicity must also be considered.

Insidious and late rejection is associated with subendothelial deposits of immunoglobulin and C3 on the glomerular basement membranes which may sometimes be an expression of an underlying immune complex disorder (originally necessitating the transplant) or possibly of complex formation with soluble antigens derived from the grafted kidney.

The complexity of the action and interaction of cellular and humoral factors in graft rejection is therefore considerable and an attempt to summarize the postulated mechanisms involved is presented in figure 17.7.

There are also circumstances when antibodies may actually *protect* a graft from destruction, a phenomenon termed *enhancement*.

Figure 17.6. Acute late rejection of human renal allograft showing platelet aggregation in a glomerular capillary induced by deposition of antibody on the vessel wall (electron micrograph). gbm, glomerular basement membrane; P, platelet. (Photograph courtesy of Professor K. Porter.)

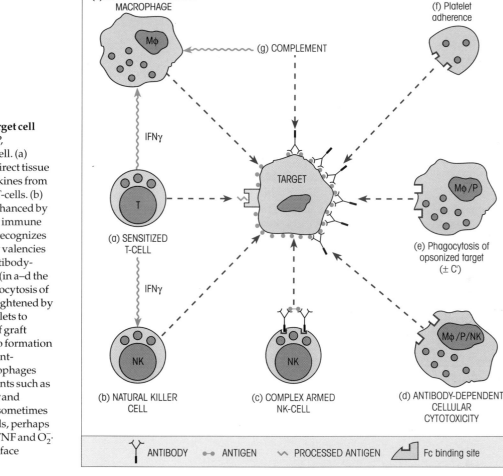

Figure 17.7. Mechanisms of target cell destruction. Mφ, macrophage; P, polymorph; NK, natural killer cell. (a) Direct killing by Tc cells and indirect tissue damage through release of cytokines from delayed-type hypersensitivity T-cells. (b) Killing by NK cells (see p. 18) enhanced by interferon. (c) Specific killing by immune complex-armed NK cell which recognizes the target through free antibody valencies in the complex. (d) Attack by antibody-dependent cellular cytotoxicity (in a–d the killing is extracellular). (e) Phagocytosis of target coated with antibody (heightened by bound C3b). (f) Sticking of platelets to antibody bound to the surface of graft vascular endothelium leading to formation of microthrombi. (g) Complement-mediated cytotoxicity. (h) Macrophages activated nonspecifically by agents such as BCG, endotoxin, poly-I:C, IFNγ and possibly C3b are cytostatic and sometimes cytotoxic for dividing tumor cells, perhaps through extracellular action of TNF and O_2^- radicals generated at the cell surface (see p. 6).

THE PREVENTION OF GRAFT REJECTION

Matching tissue types on graft donor and recipient

Since MHC differences provoke the most vicious rejection of grafts, a prodigious amount of effort has gone into defining these antigen specificities, in an attempt to minimize rejection by matching graft and recipient in much the same way that individuals are cross-matched for blood transfusions (incidentally, the ABO group provides strong transplantation antigens).

HLA tissue typing

HLA alleles are now defined by their gene sequences and individuals can be typed by the *p*olymerase *c*hain *r*eaction (PCR) using discriminating pairs of primers (figure 17.8). Molecules encoded by the class II *HLA-D* loci provoke CD4 T-cell responses, whereas HLA-A, -B and -C products are targets for alloreactive CD8 T-cells.

The polymorphism of the human HLA system

With so many alleles at each locus and so many loci in each individual (figure 17.9), it will readily be appreciated that this gives rise to an exceptional degree of polymorphism which is compounded further by the existence of multiple allotypic forms of the class III MHC complement components C2, C4a, C4b and factor B.

This remarkable polymorphism is of great potential value to the species, since the need for T-cells to recognize their own individual specificities provides a defense against microbial molecular mimicry in which a whole species might be put at risk by its inability to recognize as foreign an organism which generates MHC–peptide complexes similar to self. It is also possible that in some way the existence of a high degree of polymorphism helps to maintain the diversity of antigenic recognition within the lymphoid system of a given species and also ensures heterozygosity (hybrid vigor).

*

▧◁ Conserved sequence
▧◁ Allelic product

Figure 17.8. HLA tissue typing. Identification of HLA alleles depends upon polymerase chain reaction (PCR) amplification using sequence-specific primers. The photograph shows reactions of 96 primer pairs specific for each allele as listed in the protocol given by Bunce M. *et al.* (1995) *Tissue Antigens* **46**, 355. A DNA sample to be typed was added to each PCR mix consisting of a pair of control primers (generating a 796 base pair product from a conserved DRB1 intron sequence) and primers to produce allele-specific products. After DNA amplification, the product was electrophoresed on ethidium bromide prestained gel and visualized by ultraviolet light. All lanes contain a band corresponding to the control product, while positive reactions are those lanes containing an additional allele-specific band of predetermined size. This sample has the HLA type: A*2501,2601–04; B*1401/02,1801/02; Cw*0802,1203; DRB1*1501–05,0701; DRB4*0101–03; DRB5*0101/02/0201/02; DQB1*0201/02,0602. *This lane contains a DNA base pair ladder. The advantages of the method are correct assignment of homozygosity, higher resolution and improved accuracy. (Photograph kindly supplied by Dr D. Briggs.)

HLA-LOCUS	HLA TISSUE TYPE (ALLELIC FORMS)	♂ PARENTS ♀
DP	DP1–6	
DQ	DQ2,4,5,6,7,8,9	
DR	DR1,4,7,8,9,10,11/12(5),13/14(6),15/16(2),17/18(3)	
B	B7,8,13,15,18,27,35,37–42,44,46–65,73,78	
A	A1,2,3,11,23–26,29–34,36,43,66,68,69,74	
C	Cw1–8	

ⓐ ⓑ　ⓒ ⓓ

ⓐⓒ　ⓐⓓ　ⓑⓒ　ⓑⓓ

CHILDREN'S HAPLOTYPES

Figure 17.9. Polymorphic HLA specificities and their inheritance. The complex lies on chromosome 6, the DP locus being closest to the centromere. The numbers at the A and B loci do not overlap. The nomenclature for the DR alleles is set out in Bodmer J.G. *et al.* (1994) *Tissue Antigens* **44**, 1. DR11/12(5) shows that the 'old pre-Bodmer' nomenclature DR5 can now be split by DNA analysis into two new specificities, DR11 and DR12. This list includes the most common alleles but is not complete! Since there are several possible alleles at each locus, the probability of a random pair of subjects from the general population having identical HLA specificities is very low. However, there is a 1:4 chance that two siblings will be identical in this respect because each group of specificities on a single chromosome forms a haplotype which will be inherited *en bloc*, giving four possible combinations of paternal and maternal chromosomes. Parent and offspring can only be identical (1:2 chance) if the mother and father have one haplotype in common.

The value of matching tissue types

Improvements in operative techniques and the use of drugs such as cyclosporin A have greatly diminished the effects of mismatching HLA specificities on solid graft survival but, nevertheless, most transplanters favor a reasonable degree of matching (see figure 17.17). The consensus is that matching at the DR loci is of greater benefit than at the B loci, which in turn are of more relevance to graft survival than the A loci. In addition, the need for cross-matching to detect pre-sensitized recipients is now taken very seriously. Bone marrow grafts, however, require a high degree of compatibility and the greater accuracy of DNA typing methods can be most helpful in this respect.

Because of the many thousands of different HLA phenotypes possible (figure 17.9), it is usual to work with a large pool of potential recipients on a continental basis (Eurotransplant), so that when graft material becomes available the best possible match can be made. The position will be improved when the pool of available organs can be increased through the development of long-term tissue storage banks, but techniques are not good enough for this at present, except in the case of bone marrow cells which can be kept viable even after freezing and thawing. With a paired organ such as the kidney, living donors may be used; siblings provide the best chance of a good match (cf. figure 17.9). However, the use of living donors poses difficult ethical problems and there has been encouraging progress in the use of cadaver material. There is active interest in the possibility of using animal organs (see below) or mechanical substitutes, while some are even trying to prevent the disease in the first place!

Agents producing general immunosuppression

Graft rejection can be held at bay by the use of agents which nonspecifically interfere with the induction or expression of the immune response (figure 17.10). Because these agents are nonspecific, patients on immunosuppressive therapy tend to be susceptible

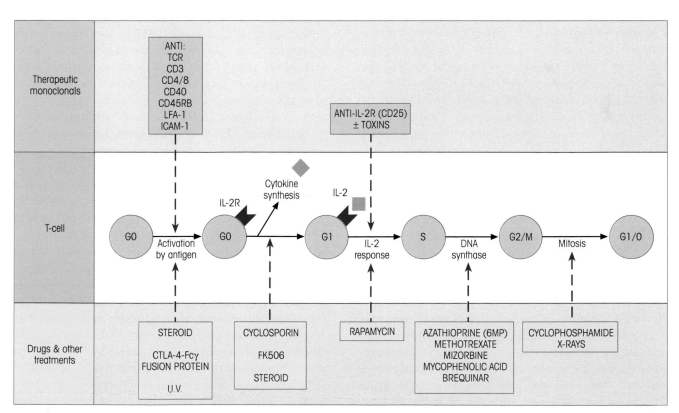

Figure 17.10. Immunosuppressive agents used to control graft rejection. The new name for FK506 is tacrolimus. Mycophenolic acid, a purine analog produced by metabolism of mycophenolate mofetil, is a powerful new immunosuppressant undergoing early trials which inhibits proliferation but also suppresses expression of CD25, -71, -154 (CD40L) and CD28. Another potent drug is deoxyspergualin which interferes with lymphocyte function in an, as yet, ill-understood manner. Leflunomide effectively blocks T-dependent and -independent antibody synthesis *in vivo* by inhibiting dihydroorotate dehydrogenase, an enzyme required for *de novo* synthesis of uridine 5'-PO$_4$. Simultaneous treatment with agents acting at sequential stages in development of the rejection response would be expected to lead to strong synergy and this is clearly seen with cyclosporin A and rapamycin.

to infections; they are also more prone to develop lymphoreticular cancers, particularly those of viral etiology.

Targeting lymphoid populations

Anti-CD3 monoclonals are in widespread use as anti-T-cell reagents to reverse acute graft rejection. The potential therapeutic benefits though have been constrained by their immunogenicity and their propensity to activate a severe cytokine release syndrome involving complex 'flu-like' symptoms. These problems can be circumvented by 'humanizing' the antibody (see p. 123) and by mutating position 297 to prevent glycosylation and consequently binding to Fc receptors and to complement. An IgM monoclonal to conserved regions on the TCR now available seems to provoke fewer untoward reactions than conventional anti-CD3.

The IL-2 receptor α chain (CD25), expressed by activated but not resting T-cells, represents another exploitable target. A humanized version of a murine monoclonal anti-IL-2Rα, dubbed daclizumab (a name seemingly derived from a Harry Potter story), had a longer half-life and of course reduced immunogenicity. When used to supplement standard baseline immunosuppression consisting of cyclosporin plus corticosteroids, acute rejection episodes at 6 months in recipients of cadaveric kidney grafts occurred in only 28% as compared with 47% in the placebo controls. The results were sufficiently encouraging for the FDA to provide market clearance for the use of daclizumab in the prevention of acute kidney transplant rejection. Following the relative ease of engraftment of allogeneic bone marrow in patients with a deficiency of the 'adhesin' molecule LFA-1 (see p. 306), attention is now turning to the use of anti-LFA-1 as an immunosuppressant for such grafts.

Immunosuppressive drugs

The development of an immunological response requires the active proliferation of a relatively small number of antigen-sensitive lymphocytes to give a population of sensitized cells large enough to be effective. Many of the immunosuppressive drugs now employed were first used in cancer chemotherapy because of their toxicity to dividing cells. Aside from the complications of blanket immunosuppression mentioned above, these antimitotic drugs are especially toxic for cells of the bone marrow and small intestine and must therefore be used with great care.

A commonly used drug in this field is **azathioprine**

which has a preferential effect on T-cell-mediated reactions. It is broken down in the body first to 6-mercaptopurine and then converted to the active agent, the ribotide. Because of the similarity in shape, this competes with inosinic acid for enzymes concerned with the synthesis of guanylic and adenylic acids; it also inhibits the synthesis of 5-phosphoribosylamine, a precursor of inosinic acid, by a feedback mechanism. The net result is inhibition of nucleic acid synthesis. Another drug, **methotrexate**, through its action as a folic acid antagonist also inhibits synthesis of nucleic acid. The N-mustard derivative **cyclophosphamide** probably attacks DNA by alkylation and cross-linking, so preventing correct duplication during cell division. These agents appear to exert their damaging effects on cells during mitosis and, for this reason, are most powerful when administered after presentation of antigen at a time when the antigen-sensitive cells are dividing.

An exciting group of fungal metabolites is having a dramatic effect in human transplantation and in the therapy of immunological disorders through its ability to target T-cells. **Cyclosporin A** (CsA), a neutral hydrophobic cyclical peptide containing 11 amino acids which is extremely insoluble, selectively blocks the transcription of IL-2 in activated T-cells. Resting cells which carry the vital memory for immunity to microbial infections are spared and there is little toxicity for dividing cells in gut and bone marrow. Some studies also point to an 'exquisite' sensitivity of dendritic APCs to the drug. Another T-cell-specific immunosuppressive drug, **FK506**, isolated from a species of *Streptomyces*, also blocks cytokine production. The latest addition to the stable is **rapamycin**, a product of the fungus *Streptomyces hygroscopicus*, which is a macrolide like FK506, but in contrast acts to block signals induced by combination of IL-2 with its receptor.

We now have greater insight into the mode of action of these drugs (figure 17.11). Both CsA and FK506 complex with different specific binding proteins termed **immunophilins** (cyclophilin and FK-binding protein respectively), which for obscure reasons have peptidyl–prolyl isomerase activity; these complexes then interact with and inhibit the calcium- and calmodulin-dependent phosphatase, calcineurin A, which is responsible for producing the transcription factors for IL-2, apoptosis and exocytosis in activated T-cells. Transcription of IL-10 is spared suggesting that switching from Th1 to Th2 responses may be a consequence. Although rapamycin also binds to the FK-binding protein, the complex has a quite different biological activity in that it blocks the IL-2-induced activation of the p70 S6 kinase which phosphorylates ribosomal S6 prior to cell proliferation.

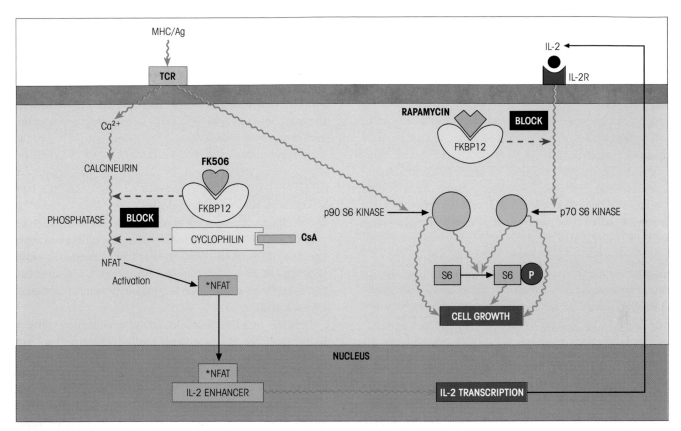

Figure 17.11. The mode of action of cyclosporin, FK506 and rapamycin. The complexes of CsA with cyclophilin and of FK506 with FKBP12 (one of a family of FK506-binding proteins) bind to and inactivate the phosphatase calcineurin responsible for activating nuclear factor of activated T-cells (NFAT) (and possibly OAP and Oct-1; cf. p. 168), which is a transcription factor for IL-2 synthesis. Transfection with calcineurin decreases the inhibitory powers of CsA and FK506. On binding to cyclophilin, CsA undergoes an awesome conformational change enabling it to exteriorize hydrophobic side-chains to form a patch which can bind calcineurin, rather like double-sided tape. Aminodextran derivatized with approximately 10 molecules of CsA agglutinated T-cells and, although it cannot penetrate the lymphocytes, it inhibited phorbol ester-induced IL-2 synthesis, suggesting a reaction with cyclophilin on the cell membrane rather than in the cytoplasm. The rapamycin–FKBP12 complex blocks the activation of p70 S6 kinase by transduced IL-2 signals, thereby inhibiting cell growth.

Cyclosporin now has a proven place as first-line therapy in the prophylaxis and treatment of transplant rejection. Figure 17.12 gives an example of its use in kidney transplantation, but it has also been evaluated in a wide range of disorders where T-cell-mediated hypersensitivity reactions are suspected. Indeed, the benefits of cyclosporin in diseases such as idiopathic nephrotic syndrome, type 1 insulin-dependent diabetes, Behçet's syndrome, active Crohn's disease, aplastic anemia, severe corticosteroid-dependent asthma and psoriasis have been interpreted to suggest or confirm a pathogenic role for the immune system. However, effects not only on Langerhans' dendritic cells but also on the proliferation of normal and transformed keratinocytes *in vitro* may contribute to the favorable outcome in psoriasis. A rapid onset of benefit and relapse when treatment is stopped are common features of cyclosporin therapy.

There are, of course, side-effects. It has to be used at doses below those causing renal fibrosis due to stimulation of TGFβ production by several cell types. There is also some cause for concern that cyclosporin may make patients susceptible to EB virus-induced lymphomas since the drug inhibits T-cells which control EB virus transformation of B-cells *in vitro*; however, the latest results suggest that the incidence of lymphoma is relatively low in comparison with that reported for allografted patients on conventional immunosuppressive therapy. Although not itself carcinogenic, cyclosporin can promote tumor progression, probably through its effect on TGFβ.

FK506 is greatly superior to CsA on a molar basis *in vitro* but is not substantially more effective when used in kidney grafting; however, its tropism for liver could be exploited. Because they act at different stages in the activation of the T-cell, CsA and rapamycin show a most impressive degree of synergy which allows the two drugs to be used at considerably lower dose levels

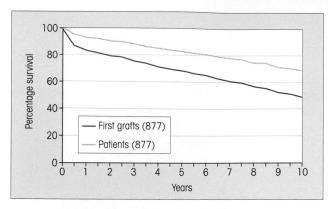

Figure 17.12. Actuarial survival of primary cadaveric kidney grafts in 877 patients treated at the Oxford Transplant Centre with triple therapy. **Cyclosporin**: 10 mg/kg/day orally given as a single dose (first dose given before surgery) and reduced according to whole-blood trough levels (200–400 ng/ml in first 3 months and then maintained at 100–200 ng/ml). **Azathioprine**: 100 mg/day orally; reduced if leukocyte count < 5000. **Prednisolone**: 20 mg/day given in divided doses orally and reduced to a maintenance dose of 10 mg/day by 6 months. The initial dose is reduced to 15 mg/day in patients of less than 60 kg body weight. In patients with stable renal function at 1 year, prednisolone is discontinued over a period of some months. (Data kindly provided by Professor Peter J. Morris.)

with correspondingly less likelihood of side-effects (figure 17.10). Another possible synergistic partner for cyclosporin is fludarabine which, unlike cyclosporin, blocks signaling by STAT-1, an intracellular intermediate activated by interferons and important for cell-mediated immunity. Combination therapies may also include azodicarbonamide which blocks the calcium flux associated with CD3 activation and the drugs mycophenolic acid and leflunomide which limit the availability of DNA precursors.

Steroids such as prednisolone intervene at many points in the immune response, affecting lymphocyte recirculation and the generation of cytotoxic effector cells, for example; in addition, their outstanding anti-inflammatory potency rests on features such as inhibition of neutrophil adherence to vascular endothelium in an inflammatory area and suppression of monocyte/macrophage functions such as microbicidal activity and response to cytokines. Corticosteroids form complexes with intracellular receptors which then bind to regulatory genes and block transcription of TNF, IFNγ, IL-1, -2, -3, -6 and MHC class II, i.e. they block expression of cytokines from both lymphocytes and macrophages, whereas cyclosporin has its main action on the former.

In parentheses, the immunophilins may be involved in other cellular functions, such as the regulation of the N-methyl-D-aspartate subtype of neural glutamate receptors and the augmentation of neuronal process ex-

tension by growth-associated protein-43, leading to the propositions that FK506 could be clinically employed in stroke patients and in the treatment of nerve degeneration. A close association of FKBP12 with the surface receptor for transforming growth factor-β (TGFβ) has also been revealed. With good fortune these drugs will take us down some very unexpected and intriguing pathways.

Strategies for antigen-specific depression of allograft reactivity

If the disadvantages of blanket immunosuppression are to be avoided, we must aim at knocking out only the reactivity of the host to the antigens of the graft, leaving the remainder of the immunological apparatus intact — in other words, the induction of **antigen-specific tolerance**.

It turns out that bone marrow represents a privileged source of tolerogenic alloantigens, and the production of stable lymphohematopoietic mixed chimerism by bone marrow engraftment is proving to be a potent means of inducing robust specific transplantation tolerance to solid organs across major MHC mismatches. However, successful allogeneic bone marrow transplantation in immunocompetent adults normally requires cytoablative treatment of recipients with irradiation or cytotoxic drugs and this has tended to restrict its use to malignant conditions. A most encouraging recent study has now shown the feasibility of inducing long-lasting tolerance not only to bone marrow cells but also to fully MHC-mismatched skin grafts in naive recipients receiving high-dose bone marrow transplantation and costimulatory blockade by single injections of monoclonal anti-CD154 (CD40L) plus a CTLA-4-Ig fusion protein (figure 17.13). A persistent hematopoietic macrochimerism is achieved with a significant proportion of donor-type lymphocytes in the thymus indicating intrathymic deletion of donor-reactive T-cells.

While this protocol permits long-term engraftment of bone marrow and solid organs, it seems that direct blockade with just anti-CD154 and CTLA-4-Ig is sufficient to induce tolerance to solid organ grafts. Stimulation of alloreactive T-cells by the graft in the presence of costimulatory blockade leads to apoptosis, a process promoted by rapamycin which improves the tolerant state. Bcl-X$_L$ (cf. figure 11.5, p. 203) prevents both T-cell apoptosis and tolerance induction by this treatment revealing the importance of apoptotic T-cell deletion for the establishment of antigen-specific unresponsiveness. In a further twist to the tale, the apoptotic T-cells 'reach from beyond the grave' by producing IL-10, so

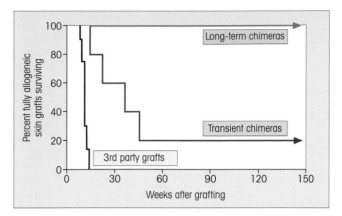

Figure 17.13. Induction of tolerance and macrochimerism by fully allogeneic bone marrow transplantation plus costimulatory blockade. B6 mice received bone marrow cells from the fully allogeneic B10.A strain with injections of anti-CD154 (CD40L) and the CTLA-4-Ig fusion protein which blocks B7–CD28 interactions (CTLA is a T-cell receptor for B7 which downregulates T-cell activation; cf. pp. 165 and 170). Eight mice showing long-term persistence of multilineage donor cells (macrochimerism) were fully tolerant to B10.A skin grafts. Five mice with transient chimerism showed moderate prolongation of skin graft survival relative to unrelated 3rd party grafts. (Data taken from Wekerle T. *et al.* (2000) *Nature Medicine* **6**, 464, with permission.)

Figure 17.14. Induction of allograft tolerance by nondepleting anti-CD4 plus anti-CD8. Tolerance to skin grafts from donors with multiple minor transplantation antigen mismatches was achieved by concurrent injection of IgG2a monoclonal antibodies to CD4 and CD8 which do not induce cell depletion (green arrow). The maintenance of tolerance depends upon the continued presence of antigen which enables the unresponsive cells to interact with newly arising immunocompetent cells on the surface of the same antigen-presenting cells and render them unresponsive through an infectious tolerance mechanism (cf. figures 12.9 and 20.24). Whether the mechanism involves 'infectious anergy', direct suppression, 'immune deviation' of potentially aggressive Th1 cells by suppressor Th2, downregulation of the antigen-presenting cell, or all four in various combinations, is unresolved. Loss of tolerance on depletion of CD4 but not CD8 cells (red arrows) shows that active tolerance is maintained by the CD4 subset. (Figure synthesized from data kindly provided by Dr S.P. Cobbold and Professor H. Waldmann.)

that their phagocytosis along with antigen leads to the presentation of the antigen in a tolerogenic form which maintains tolerance through the production of immunoregulatory cells.

Despite the role of the *mature* dendritic cell as the champion stimulator of resting T-cells, the dendritic cell *precursors* may present antigen in the absence of B7 costimulators and, by mechanisms echoing those described above in the costimulatory blockade experiments, would appear to have a powerful potential for tolerance induction. This concept is of particular relevance to the specific unresponsiveness generated by grafts of liver, which being a hematopoietic organ, continually exports large numbers of these immature dendritic cells.

Nondepleting anti-CD4 and -8 monoclonals, by depriving T-cells of fully activating signals, can render them anergic when they engage antigen through their specific receptors. These anergic cells can induce unresponsiveness in newly recruited T-cells ('infectious tolerance', p. 233) and so establish specific and indefinite acceptance of mouse skin grafts across class I or multiple minor transplantation antigen barriers (figure 17.14). It should be noted that skin allografts provide the most difficult challenge for tolerance induction, and transplants of organs such as the heart, which are less fastidious than skin, require less aggressive immunotherapy.

Given the wide variety of different peptide epitopes presented by the graft MHC, full-frontal attack on the alloreactive T-cells by administration of tolerogenic peptides represents quite a challenge, and the strategy of using costimulatory blockade with the antigens being provided by the graft itself looks to be a more promising route.

IS XENOGRAFTING A PRACTICAL PROPOSITION?

Because the supply of donor human organs for transplantation lags seriously behind the demand, a widespread interest in the feasibility of using animal organs is emerging. Pigs are more favored than primates as donors both on the grounds of ethical acceptability and the hazards of zoonoses. The first hurdle to be overcome is **hyperacute rejection** due to xenoreactive natural antibodies in the host. Humans lack α-1,3-galactosyl transferase and galactose α-1,3-galactose and therefore develop antibodies to this epitope which is present on many common bacteria and expressed abundantly on the xenogeneic vascular endothelium. The natural antibodies bind to the endothelium and activate complement in the absence of regulators of the

Figure 17.15. Strategies for avoiding complement-mediated hyperacute rejection of a xenograft caused by reaction of natural antigalactose antibodies with Galα-1,3-Gal on the surface of the pig graft cells. Heart xenografts from transgenic pigs expressing the human complement regulatory proteins decay accelerating factor (DAF) or CD59 functioned for prolonged periods in baboons. Transfection of pig cells with α-1,2-fucosyl transferase converted the terminal sugars into the blood group H and rendered the cells resistant to lysis by the antigalactose. Other strategies involve transfection with genes encoding an α-galactosidase or intracellular recombinant scFv reacting with α-1,3-galactosyl transferase.

human complement system, such as decay accelerating factor, CD59 and MCP (cf. figure 15.2), precipitating the hyperacute rejection phenomenon. Novel genetic engineering strategies for the solution of this problem are outlined in figure 17.15.

The next crisis is **acute vascular rejection** occurring within 6 days as antibodies produced by Th2 cells react with the xenoantigens on donor epithelium. In contrast with the response to allografts, IL-12 and IFNγ actually inhibit acute vascular rejection and, over the long term, IFNγ may protect the graft by promoting the formation of NO· which prevents constriction of blood vessels. Brequinar sodium (figure 17.10), an inhibitor of pyrimidine biosynthesis and suppressor of both B- and T-cell-mediated responses, has been evaluated for efficacy, but induction of tolerance would clearly be more desirable although tricky.

Even when the immunological problems are overcome, it remains to be seen whether the xenograft will be compatible with human life over a prolonged period, latent pig viruses being an obvious worry.

TISSUE ENGINEERING

The ideal would be to create the tissue for a **graft entirely from cells of the recipient**, i.e. an autograft, which would eliminate the need for immunosuppression. Science fiction? Probably not. We will steadily accumulate the knowledge concerning the various growth factors required to guide relatively undifferentiated stem cells into the desired mature form under culture conditions *in vitro*. In many instances, it is proving possible to isolate stem cells from various adult or-

gans, but the most exciting development has come from cloning 'Dolly' the sheep. This has revealed the feasibility of taking the nucleus from a differentiated adult cell and reprograming it into an embryonic state responsive to early growth factors, which can be selected to determine its future destiny as an islet, brain or liver cell or what have you (figure 17.16).

CLINICAL EXPERIENCE IN GRAFTING

Privileged sites

Corneal grafts survive without the need for immunosuppression. Because they are avascular they tend not to sensitize the recipient. This privileged protection is boosted by the local production of immunosuppressive factors such as TGFβ, IL-1Ra, limited expression of MHC and the strategic presence of FasL which can induce apoptosis in infiltrating lymphocytes. Nonetheless, they do become cloudy if the individual has been *presensitized*. Grafts of **cartilage** are successful in the same way but an additional factor is the protection afforded the chondrocytes by the matrix. With bone and artery it doesn't really matter if the grafts die because they can still provide a framework for host cells to colonize.

Kidney grafts

Thousands of kidneys have been transplanted and with improvement in patient management there is a high survival rate. In the long term (5 years or more), the desirability of reasonable matching at

Figure 17.16. Anticipated production of autologous grafts by tissue engineering. Undifferentiated cells are obtained directly from the patient either as stem cells (if available) or by transplanting the nuclei of mature cells into enucleated embryonic cells. They are cultured in a biodegradable matrix with appropriate growth factors to provide a tissue populated with differentiated cells which can function as an autologous graft.

Figure 17.17. First cadaveric kidney graft survival in Europe for the period January 1993 to December 1997 ($n = 12\,584$) on the basis of mismatches for HLA-A, -B and -DR. There is a significant influence of matching, $p < 0.001$, for both sets of data. (Data kindly supplied by Drs Guido Persijn and Jacqueline Smits of the Eurotransplant International Foundation.)

the HLA-A, -B and -D loci becomes apparent (figure 17.17).

Patients are partially immunosuppressed at the time of transplantation because uremia causes a degree of immunological anergy. The combination of azathioprine and prednisolone was commonly employed in the long-term management of kidney grafts, but is now supplemented by cyclosporin A in the so-called **triple therapy** (figure 17.12). One hopes that the synergy between cyclosporin and rapamycin, and possibly other immunosuppressants, will lead to the emergence of powerful new therapeutic regimens. If kidney function is poor during a rejection crisis, renal dialysis can be used. As mentioned above, there is active interest in the possibility of xenografting. When transplantation is performed because of immune complex-induced glomerulonephritis, the immunosuppressive treatment used may help to prevent a similar lesion developing in the grafted kidney. Patients with glomerular basement membrane antibodies (e.g. Goodpasture's syndrome) are likely to destroy their renal transplants unless first treated with plasmapheresis and immunosuppressive drugs.

Heart transplants

The overall 1-year survival figure for heart transplants has moved up to near the 80% mark (figure 17.18), helped considerably by the introduction of cyclosporin A therapy. Its nephrotoxicity is a drawback, although the analog cyclosporin G is better in this respect, and synergic combination therapy with rapamycin should reduce this side-effect markedly. Full HLA matching is of course not practical, but single DR mismatches gave 90% survival at 3 years compared with a figure of 65% for two DR mismatches. Aside from the rejection problem, it is likely that the number of patients who would benefit from cardiac replacement is much greater than the number dying with adequately healthy hearts. More attention will have to be given to the possibility of xenogeneic grafts and mechanical substitutes.

One interesting nugget. The immune response to adenoviral vectors can induce inflammation and loss of gene expression in transfected tissues, except for cardiac isografts which remain free of inflammation. This suggests a novel way of introducing an immuno-

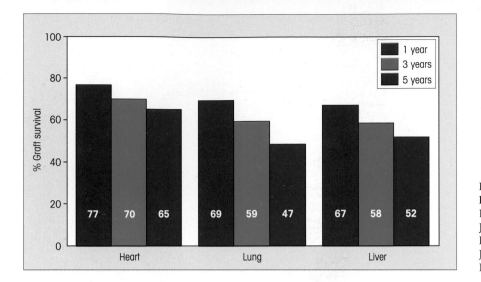

Figure 17.18. Graft survival rates for first heart, liver and lung transplantations in Eurotransplant performed between January 1992 and December 1993. (Data kindly supplied by Drs Guido Persijn and Jacqueline Smits, Eurotransplant International Foundation.)

suppressant such as TGFβ, which can be produced in high concentrations within the milieu of a cardiac graft without invoking systemic side-effects.

Liver transplants

Survival rates for orthotopic liver grafts are not quite as high as those achieved with heart transplants (figure 17.18). The hepatotrophic capacity of FK506 is an added bonus which makes it the preferred drug for liver transplantation. Rejection crises are dealt with by high-dose steroids and, if this proves ineffective, anti-lymphocyte globulin. The use of a totally synthetic colloidal hydroxyethyl starch solution, containing lactobionate as a substitute for chloride, allows livers to be preserved for 24 hours or more and has revolutionized the logistics of liver transplantation. To improve the prognosis of patients with primary hepatic or bile duct malignancies, which were considered to be inoperable, transplantation of organ clusters with liver as the central organ has been designed, e.g. liver and pancreas, or liver, pancreas, stomach and small bowel or even colon. Nonetheless, the outcome is not very favorable in that up to three-quarters of the patients transplanted for hepatic cancer have recurrence of their tumor within 1 year. For the future we must look forward to the creation of autologous liver from adult cells when tissue engineering techniques have been developed sufficiently.

Experience with liver grafting between pigs revealed an unexpected finding. Many of the animals retained the grafted organs in a healthy state for many months without any form of immunosuppression and enjoyed a state of unresponsiveness to grafts of skin or kidney from the same donor. True tolerance is induced by the donor-type intrahepatic hematopoietic stem cells and immature dendritic cells (see above) and possibly also by the liver parenchyma itself, known to produce copious amounts of soluble MHC class I.

Work is in progress on the transfer of isolated hepatocytes attached to collagen-coated microcarriers injected i.p. for the correction of isolated deficiencies such as albumin synthesis. This attractive approach has much wider application as a general vehicle for gene therapy.

Bone marrow grafting

Patients with certain immunodeficiency disorders and aplastic anemia are obvious candidates for treatment with **bone marrow stem cells** with their potential to differentiate into all the formed elements of the blood; so, too, are acute leukemia patients treated radically with intensive chemotherapy and possibly whole-body irradiation in attempts to eradicate the neoplastic cells, as will be discussed in the next chapter.

Bone marrow contains not only hematopoietic but also mesenchymal stem cells which can give rise to cartilage, tendons and bone; after expansion in culture by a factor of 5–10 times, they provide an excellent treatment for children with osteogenesis imperfecta, a genetic disorder in which the osteoblasts produce defective type I collagen with resulting osteopenia and severe bony deformities. Good results are being obtained with stem cell transplantation *in utero* for inherited blood disorders using populations from paternal bone marrow enriched for the stem cell marker, CD34. From the practical standpoint, it has been recognized that cord blood contains sufficient hematopoietic stem cells for bone marrow replacement, but what is even more convenient is to enhance the number of CD34-positive progenitor cells in relatively small volumes of peripheral blood by recombinant stem cell factor, IL-1β, IL-3, IL-6 and erythropoietin in the presence of stromal cells or fibronectin monolayers *ex vivo* prior to transplantation. It is encouraging also that both colony-stimulating factors G-CSF and GM-CSF greatly accelerate the return of myeloid cells after lethal doses of myelotoxic agents preceding autologous bone marrow transplantation; there are fewer infections, less use of i.v. antibodies and earlier discharge from hospital. They also accelerate the engraftment of allogeneic bone marrow without exacerbating g.v.h. disease.

Graft-vs-host disease is a major problem in bone marrow grafting

G.v.h. disease resulting from the recognition of recipient antigens by allogeneic T-cells in the bone marrow inoculum represents a serious, sometimes fatal, complication, and the incidence of g.v.h. disease is reduced if T-cells in the grafted marrow are first depleted with a cytotoxic cocktail of anti-T-cell monoclonals. Unexpectedly, complete purging of the T-cells leads to an alarmingly high incidence of graft failure, apparently due to the loss of relatively rare facilitating cells expressing TCR, CD3, CD8 and a previously unknown 33 kDa cell surface glycoprotein, FCp33. How these and other facilitating cells, such as CD8+ dendritic cells, work is, to put it mildly, unknown.

It is fondly hoped that successful engraftment and avoidance of g.v.h. reactions will be achieved in the clinic—in the not too distant future(?)—by strategies such as those involving allogeneic marrow transplantation under costimulatory blockade without cytoablative treatment of graft or recipient, as described earlier (figure 17.13). Until then, successful results are more likely with highly compatible donors, particularly if fatal g.v.h. reactions are to be avoided, and here siblings offer the best chance of finding a matched donor (figure 17.9). Undoubtedly, non-HLA minor transplantation antigens are important and are more difficult to match. Acute g.v.h. disease occurring within the first 100 days following infusion of allogeneic marrow primarily affects the skin, liver and gastrointestinal tract. Antibodies to TNF or IL-1R block mortality. Current therapy uses cyclosporin with prednisolone, but inclusion of methotrexate in this regimen is said to improve efficacy. Chronic g.v.h. disease (i.e. later than 100 days) has a relatively good prognosis if limited to skin and liver, but if multiple organs are involved, clinically resembling progressive systemic sclerosis, the outcome is poor. Patients are treated with cyclosporin and prednisolone, but recently thalidomide has been found to be very helpful because of its anti-TNF effect. The pathogenesis is not straightforward and chronic disease could arise by a curious mechanism involving the sneaking through of autoreactive T-cells, which fail to be deleted in the thymus possibly because of thymic damage due to pre- or post-transplant therapy, e.g. associated viral infection, irradiation or even cyclosporin itself. It may be significant that cyclosporin inhibits the programed cell death of immature thymocytes which occurs on activation by anti-CD3, and it is known that an autologous 'g.v.h.' reaction supervenes on termination of prolonged cyclosporin administration to young irradiated rats which had received syngeneic bone marrow.

Other organs

It is to be expected that improvement in techniques of control of the rejection process will encourage transplantation in several other areas—not in cases of endocrine disorders such as Hashimoto's disease (cf. p. 397) where exogenous replacement therapy is convenient, but, for example, in diabetes where the number of transplants recorded is rising rapidly and the current success rate is around 40%, although major problems still are inadequate output of insulin by the grafted islets and an adequate supply of tissue. Considerable advances have been made in very substantially expanding the number of islet cells which can be derived from pancreatic duct precursors, while monkey islets may not prove to be a bad bet in that they have low surface MHC and are nonvascularized, so avoiding the presentation of the dangerous Gal.Gal epitope (cf. p. 361) which is enriched on vascular endothelium in some marked species. *In vivo* transfection of hepatocytes with an adenoviral vector encoding the homeoprotein PDX-1, which is a glucose-dependent transactivator of the insulin gene, induced them to make insulin in diabetic mice—very impressive, lots of potential, but early days yet. The 5-year survival rate of 47% for lung transplants is improving but is still less than satisfactory. One also looks forward to the day when the successful transplantation of skin for lethal burns becomes more commonplace.

Reports are coming in of an experimental foray into the grafting of **neural tissues**. Mutant mice with degenerate cerebellar Purkinje cells, which mimic the human condition cerebellar ataxia, can be restored by engraftment of donor cerebellar cells at the appropriate sites; these express insulin-like growth factor-1 (IGF-1), migrate to form a layer in lieu of the missing cells, induce sprouting in host neurons and become synaptically integrated. Clinical trials with transplantation of human embryonic dopamine neurons to reverse the neurological deficit in Parkinson's disease have been severely hampered by the excessive death of the grafted cells. The hypothesis that this was due to oxidative stress led to a study showing that grafted neurons from transgenic mice overexpressing Cu/Zn superoxide dismutase (cf. p. 6) had a greatly increased survival rate. Another candidate is Huntington's chorea which has been tracked down to a mutation producing a protein with an expanded polymorphic glutamine repeat, toxic to spiny striatal neurons. Embryonic striatal allografts, producing the nontoxic wild-type protein, survive for a prolonged period, become integrated into the host brain and induce functional alleviation of motor deficits, all in the absence of immunosuppression. To date, the need to use embryonic tissue has been a bugbear, but the recent identification of neurogenic precursor cells from the adult human hippocampus may give a glimpse of the Promised Land.

Cryopreservation of sperm is a successful strategy in the management of adult cancer sufferers to protect the sperm from mutagenic cancer treatment. This is not available to prepubertal boys, but an alternative for them is cryopreservation of their spermatogonial stem cells for reintroduction post-treatment, since the Sertoli cells which support differentiation into mature spermatozoa will function normally. As knowledge from the human genome sequence accumulates, there is a potential for identifying and correcting genetic defects in the spermatogonia before their reintroduction, but ethical committees fight shy of this sort of 'Frankenstein' tinkering. More acceptably, in cases of male infertility due to dysfunctional Sertoli cells, it should be possible to develop mature spermatids by culture of the spermatogonia with Sertoli cells derived from a normal individual.

Work proceeds apace to produce a successful prosthetic vascular graft which would remain patent as a blood conduit, prevent thrombosis of the blood in low flow or adverse states and control anastomotic cellular hyperplasia with overgrowth of smooth muscle cells and matrix production. This has proved difficult to achieve, but there are encouraging attempts to engineer a composite vascular graft in which microvessel endothelial cells present in a small sample of subcutaneous abdominal wall fat, obtained by the relatively simple cosmetic liposuction technique, grow as an antithrombotic endothelial layer to line the surface of an expanded polytetrafluoroethylene tube. Expect development in this field, particularly for the replacement of arteries.

ASSOCIATION OF HLA TYPE WITH DISEASE

Linkage disequilibrium and disease susceptibility

An impressive body of data is accumulating which links specific HLAs with particular disease states in the human (table 17.1) and even more striking relationships may be uncovered as the complexity of the HLA-D region is unraveled. The relationships are influenced by **linkage disequilibrium**, a state where closely linked genes on a chromosome tend to remain associated rather than undergo genetic randomization in a given population, so that the frequency of a pair of alleles occurring together is greater than the product of the individual gene frequencies (figure 17.19a). This could result from natural selection favoring a particular haplotype or from insufficient time elapsing since the first appearance of closely located alleles to allow them to

Table 17.1. Association of HLA with disease. (Data mainly from Ryder *et al.*, see legend to figure 17.19, and Thorsby E. (1995) *The Immunologist* **3**, 51.)

DISEASE	HLA ALLELE	RELATIVE RISK
a Class II associated		
Hashimoto's disease	DR11	3.2
Primary myxedema	DR17(*3)	5.7
Thyrotoxicosis (Graves')	DR17(*3)	3.7
Insulin-dependent diabetes	DQ8	14
	DQ2/8	20
	DQ6	0.2
Addison's disease (adrenal)	DR17(*3)	6.3
Goodpasture's syndrome	*DR2	13.1
Rheumatoid arthritis	DR4	5.8
Juvenile rheumatoid arthritis	DR8	8.1
Sjögren's syndrome	DR17(*3)	9.7
Chronic active hepatitis (autoimmune)	DR17(*3)	13.9
Multiple sclerosis	*DR2,*DQ6	12
Narcolepsy	DQ6	38
Dermatitis herpetiformis	DR17(*3)	56.4
Celiac disease	DQ2	250
Tuberculoid leprosy	*DR2	8.1
b Class I, HLA-B27 associated		
Ankylosing spondylitis	B27	87.4
Reiter's disease	B27	37.0
Post-salmonella arthritis	B27	29.7
Post-shigella arthritis	B27	20.7
Post-yersinia arthritis	B27	17.6
Post-gonococcal arthritis	B27	14.0
Uveitis	B27	14.6
Amyloidosis in rheumatoid arthritis	B27	8.2
c Other class I associations		
Subacute thyroiditis	B35	13.7
Psoriasis vulgaris	Cw6	13.3
Idiopathic hemochromatosis	A3	8.2
Myasthenia gravis	B8	4.4

*DR specificities relate to 'old nomenclature', figure 17.9.

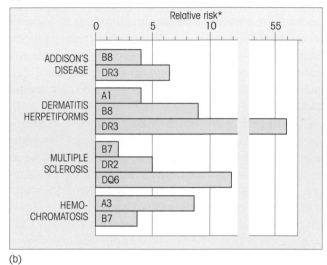

| | GENE FREQUENCY % | | |
| HLA GENES | SINGLE GENE | PAIRED GENES | |
		EXPECTED	OBSERVED
A1	16		
B8	10	1.6	8.8
A3	13		
B7	10	1.3	2.8

(a)

(b)

Figure 17.19. Linkage disequilibrium and the association between HLA and disease. (a) Two examples of linkage disequilibrium. The expected frequency for a pair of genes is the product of each individual gene frequency. B8 and DR3 (old nomenclature; figure 17.9) are in linkage disequilibrium as are B7 and DR2 (old nomenclature); thus the haplotypes A1, B8, DR3 and A3, B7, DR2 are relatively common. (b) Influence of linkage disequilibrium on disease association. *Relative risk = the increased chance of contracting the disease for individuals bearing the antigen relative to those lacking it. (Data from Ryder L.P., Andersen E. & Svejgaard A. (1979) HLA and Disease Registry 1979. *Tissue Antigens* supplement.)

become randomly distributed throughout the population. Be that as it may, a significant association between a disease and a given HLA specificity does not imply that we have identified the disease susceptibility gene, because we might find an even better correlation with another HLA gene in linkage disequilibrium with the first. To take an example: in multiple sclerosis, an association with the B7 allele was first established but, when patients were typed for the D locus, a much stronger correlation with DR2 emerged (figure 17.19b). The initial correlation with B7 resulted from linkage disequilibrium between B7 and DR2. We still cannot be sure that DR2 itself is the disease susceptibility gene since, carrying the argument a stage further, we cannot exclude the possibility of finding an even greater association with another closely linked gene, and indeed recent studies reveal an even tighter relationship to

DQB1*0602. However, in those instances where two susceptibility genes encoding α and β chains synergize *and* are in the *trans* configuration (i.e. on different chromosomes), linkage disequilibrium is less likely to be the explanation.

Ethnic studies may help by making available recombination events which alter haplotypes and permit the identification of susceptibility determinants outside their normal context. Thus, the DQα (DQA1*0201) linked to DR7 on the Caucasian haplotype has a neutral effect on diabetes susceptibility but, in the black population, DR7 is associated with a high-risk DQα (DQA1*0301) and now becomes a susceptibility haplotype.

Association with immunological diseases

With odd exceptions such as idiopathic hemochromatosis and congenital adrenal hyperplasia resulting from a 21-hydroxylase deficiency, which only gain membership of this august club through linkage disequilibrium, HLA-linked diseases are intimately bound up with immunological processes. By and large, the HLA-D-related disorders are autoimmune with a tendency for *DR3* or linked genes to be associated with organ-specific diseases. It has been suggested that HLAs might affect the susceptibility of a cell to viral attachment or infection, thereby influencing the development of autoimmunity to associated surface components. Inevitably though, because class II genes tend to dominate these relationships, the temptation is to think in terms of immune response genes controlling the nature of the reaction to the relevant autoantigen or to whatever might be a causative agent, perhaps through an ability to bind certain antigenic peptides. A given HLA-D allele may permit the binding of foreign peptides and cross-reacting self-epitopes, or may itself contribute the self-epitope since *processed* MHC molecules appear abundantly on the cell surface. The modern MHC–peptide tetramer technology (cf. p.138) or the alternative peptide/MHC–Ig dimer reagents should be useful for the detection of sensitized T-cells in these patients and for tracking down the identity of the relevant epitopes; diagnostic applications would follow.

Insulin-dependent diabetes mellitus is associated with DQ8 (DQA1*0301, DQB1*0302) and DQ2 (DQA1*0501, DQB1*0201), but the strongest susceptibility is seen in the **DQ2/8 heterozygote** arguing in favor of a role for the *trans*-encoded DQ molecule(s) in these individuals, most probably DQ(α1*0301, β1*0201). The fact that two genes are necessary to determine the strongest susceptibility, and the universality of this finding in all populations studied, implies that the DQ molecules themselves, not other molecules in linkage disequilibrium, are primarily involved in disease susceptibility. Possession of some subtypes of DQ6 gives a dominantly protective effect (table 17.1; relative risk 0.2). Thus the degree of HLA-associated predisposition to type 1 diabetes will be a composite of the effects of the particular combination of *cis*- or *trans*-encoded DQ molecules. To get down to the molecular level, different polymorphic amino acids at residues DQα52 and DQβ57 have a powerful influence on disease susceptibility.

DR4 and, to a lesser extent, DR1 are risk factors for **rheumatoid arthritis** in white Caucasians. Analysis of DR4 subgroups, and of other ethnic populations where the influence of DR4 is minimal, has identified a particular linear T-cell sequence from residues 67–74 as the disease susceptibility element, and the variations observed are based on sharing of this sequence with other HLA-DR specificities, which presumably arose from the recombination and gene conversion events responsible for MHC polymorphism (table 17.2). This stretch of amino acids is highly polymorphic and forms pockets 4 and 7 of the peptide-binding cleft. There are striking differences between the sets of peptides bound by DR subtypes associated with rheumatoid arthritis and those that are not; notably, differences involve the amino acid charge at residues 4 or 5 of the peptide sequence bound to the cleft. Analysis of the peptides bound spontaneously to the DR molecules from patients could yield an important clue to pathogenesis. As in diabetes, the DR2 allele is under-represented and DR2-positive patients have less severe disease, implying that a DR2-linked gene might be protective in some way (through interaction with a heat-shock protein maybe?).

The association with HLA in **ankylosing spondylitis** is quite remarkable; up to 95% of patients are of B27 phenotype as compared with around 5% in controls. The incidence of B27 is also markedly raised in other conditions when accompanied by sacroiliitis, e.g. Reiter's disease, acute anterior uveitis, psoriasis and other forms of infective sacroiliitis, such as *Yersinia*, gonococcal and *Salmonella* arthritis. The extraordinarily close association with B27 and the development of a somewhat similar disease in rodents made transgenic for the *B27* gene speak for the B27 molecule itself as a central pathogenic factor. There are nine subtypes of B27 encoded by the B*2701–2708 alleles, all of which are associated with ankylosing spondylitis and have a 'B' pocket in their cleft which is very exclusive with respect to binding the arginine side-chain. The hunt should be on for a nonapeptide with an arginine at residue 2. The involvement of infective agents may provide a clue. The cross-reaction of B27 with *Klebsiella pneumoniae* nitrogenase reported by Ebringer and colleagues is certainly provocative in this respect. One suggestion is that a bacterial peptide may cross-react with a B27-derived sequence and provoke an autoreactive T-cell response.

Deficiencies in C4 and C2, which are MHC class III molecules, clearly predispose to the development of **immune complex disease** (see p. 308), and so it would be expected that the inheritance of null genes or alleles coding for the less active complement allotypes would increase the risk of rheumatological disorders and add yet further complexity to the correlations between HLA types and disease.

Table 17.2. Shared sequences on the DRβ1 α-helix in different haplotypes confer susceptibility to rheumatoid arthritis. (Data from Bell J.I. & McMichael A.J. (1993) In Lachmann P.J., Peters D.K., Rosen F.S. & Walport M.J. (eds) *Clinical Aspects of Immunology*, p. 748. Blackwell Scientific Publications, Oxford.)

	HLA-DR SPECIFICITY	DRβ1 GENE	HLA-DRβ RESIDUES IN THE THIRD ALLELIC HYPERVARIABLE REGION									
			66				70				74	
Susceptible to RA	DR1	*0101	Asp	Leu	Leu	Glu	Gln	Arg	Arg	Ala	Ala	Val
	DR4	*0404	–	–	–	–	–	–	–	–	–	–
	DR4	*0405	–	–	–	–	–	–	–	–	–	–
	DR4	*0401	–	–	–	–	–	Lys	–	–	–	–
	DR10	*1001	–	–	–	–	Arg	–	–	–	–	–
Not susceptible to RA	DR4	*0402	–	Ile	–	–	Asp	Glu	–	–	–	–
	DR4	*0407	–	–	–	–	–	–	–	–	Glu	–
	DR7	*0701	–	Ile	–	–	Asp	–	–	Gly	Gln	–
Nucleotide sequences	DR1	*0101	GAC	CTC	CTG	GAG	CAG	AGG	CGG	GCC	GCG	GTG
	DR4	*0401	---	---	---	---	---	-A-	---	---	---	---

Last, it is worthy of note that the relationship of MHC to disease resistance and vaccine efficacy in farm animals is beginning to preoccupy veterinary scientists; it is known, for instance, that susceptibility to Marek's disease in White Leghorn chickens is associated with distinct MHC haplotypes.

REPRODUCTIVE IMMUNOLOGY

The fetus is a potential allograft

A further consequence of polymorphism in an outbred population is that mother and fetus will almost certainly have different MHCs. Some examples of selection for heterozygotes (where maternally and paternally derived haplotypes are different) over homozygotes (both fetal haplotypes identical with the mother's) in viviparous animals suggest that this is beneficial. Likewise, the placentas of F1 offspring are larger than normal when mothers are preimmunized to the paternal H2 haplotype and smaller when mothers are tolerant to these antigens.

The threat posed to the fetus as a potential graft due to the possession of paternal transplantation antigens so intrigued Lewis Thomas that he was moved to suggest that rejection of the fetus might initiate parturition, although it would be difficult to account for the normal birth of female offspring to pure-strain mating pairs where fetus and mother would have identical histocompatibility antigens without further postulating a placenta-specific surface antigen.

Nonetheless, in the human hemochorial placenta, maternal blood with immunocompetent lymphocytes does circulate in contact with the fetal trophoblast and we have to explain how the fetus avoids allograft rejection, despite the development of an immunological response in a proportion of mothers as evidenced by the appearance of anti-HLA antibodies and cytotoxic lymphocytes. In fact, prior sensitization with a skin graft fails to affect a pregnancy, showing that trophoblast cells are immunologically protected; indeed, they are resistant to most cytotoxic mechanisms although susceptible to IL-2-activated NK cells. Some of the many speculations which have been aired on this subject are summarized in figure 17.20.

Undoubtedly, the most important factor is the well-documented lack of both conventional class I and class II MHC antigens on the placental villous trophoblast which protects the fetus from allogeneic attack. These fundamental changes in the regulation of MHC genes also lead to the unique expression of the nonclassical HLA-G protein on the extravillous cytotrophoblast. This may protect the trophoblast from killing by uter-

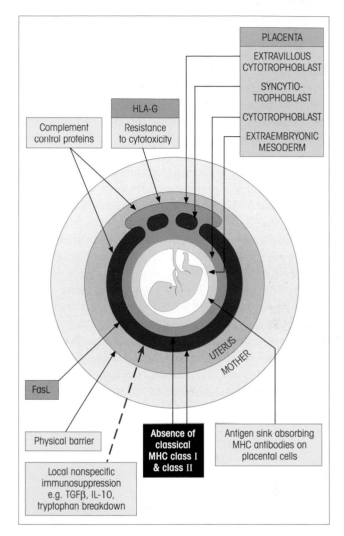

Figure 17.20. Mechanisms postulated to account for the survival of the fetus as an allograft in the mother.

ine endometrial large granular lymphocytes which are an NK cell subset, since HLA-null lymphoblastoid cells transfected with HLA-G are resistant to NK lysis. This would be consistent with the 'missing self hypothesis' which postulates that MHC class I inhibits a positive signal from a potential target to the NK cell. On the other hand, the placenta is vulnerable to IL-2-activated uterine NK cells, which may therefore fine tune overaggressive invasion by the trophoblast early in pregnancy and may control the normal development of the blastocyst in the decidualized uterus, in contrast with the excessive trophoblast proliferation and tissue destruction produced by transfer of blastocysts to mouse kidney.

Maternal IgG antipaternal MHC is found in 20% of first pregnancies and this figure rises to 75–80% in multiparous women. Some of these antibodies cross-react with HLA-G, but the vulnerability of the trophoblast cells to complement is blocked by the presence on their surface of the control proteins which inactivate C3 convertase (cf. p. 307).

Cytokines seem to have a complex role in post-implantation pregnancy given the production of growth factors such as CSF-1 and GM-CSF, which have a trophic influence on the placenta, and of transforming growth factor-β (TGFβ), which could help to damp down any activation of NK cells by potentially abortive events such as intrauterine exposure to lipopolysaccharide (LPS) or to interferons. The placenta itself produces IL-10, the importance of which was revealed by IL-10 'knockout' experiments (cf. p. 142) which caused runting of the fetus compared with its littermate controls—incidentally this is a slick demonstration that IL-10 is synthesized by the embryo rather than the trophoblast.

Other factors which may protect the fetus are the presence of Fas-ligand at the trophoblast maternal–fetal interface, and the suppression of T-cell activity through tryptophan degradation brought about by the catabolic enzyme indoleamine 2,3-dioxygenase present in trophoblast cells and macrophages.

Fertility can be controlled immunologically

Notwithstanding the complacent attitudes of some members of the chattering classes, informed opinion recognizes the enormity of the problems posed by the world population explosion. That being so, a rich variety of strategic approaches are being followed, one of which involves the targeting of key hormones (figure 17.21a) by the production of neutralizing autoantibodies.

Immunization, actually autoimmunization, with diphtheria toxoid-linked **luteinizing hormone releasing hormone** (LHRH), which regulates gonadotropin synthesis, impairs fertility in male animals and causes a marked atrophy of the prostate accompanied by a devastating fall in testosterone levels—immunological castration no less. The therapy may have a role in androgen-dependent prostatic carcinoma, while in postpartum women it should prevent ovulation and prolong lactational amenorrhea without adverse effects. Internal image anti-idiotype $Ab_{2\beta}$ (cf. p. 208) has been raised against monoclonal antiprogesterone and shown to provoke **progesterone neutralizing antibodies** in experimental animals.

Figure 17.21. Immunological contraception. (a) Target hormones. (b) Purely diagrammatic representation of human chorionic gonadotropin (hCG) showing epitopes specific for hCG (green) and structures similar if not identical to luteinizing hormone (LH) (dark red). (c) β-hCG mutant in which the hCG-specific epitopes have been preserved but epitopes shared with LH lost. As a candidate vaccine this should avoid the problem of inducing antibodies cross-reacting with LH. (d) Structure of β-hCG showing some of the residues altered (magenta, yellow and cyan) to produce epitope-loss mutants, fulfilling the criteria in (c). (Reproduced from Jackson A.M. *et al.* (1996) *Journal of Reproductive Immunology* **31**, 21, with permission from Elsevier Science, Ireland Ltd.)

Most attention has focused on a human vaccine based on **human chorionic gonadotropin** (hCG) which is made by the preimplantation blastocyst and is essential for the establishment of early pregnancy (figure 17.21a); it is also the antigen assayed in the urine tests for pregnancy which cause so much pleasure or consternation as the case may be. The α chain of hCG is common to *f*ollicle-*s*timulating *h*ormone (FSH), *t*hyroid-*s*timulating *h*ormone (TSH) and LH while the β-subunit shows around 80% homology with LH (figure 17.21b). Clearly immunization with whole hCG would elicit some exceedingly unwelcome reactions and two vaccines try to avoid them wholly or in part. Both couple the antigen to tetanus or diphtheria toxoid carriers. The WHO vaccine uses the 37-amino acid C-terminal peptide (CTP) which is wholly specific for hCG but not

exciting as an immunogen. The Indian vaccine combines β-hCG with ovine α chain. This evokes much better antibody responses, and in Phase 2 clinical trials only one pregnancy was observed in 1224 cycles when neutralizing antibodies were above a certain level. Despite strong cross-reactions with LH there was said to be no disturbance of ovulation or loss of libido. As contraceptive cover while antibodies were rising, cell-mediated hypersensitivity was induced by local intrauterine implantation of purified extracts from Neem, an ancient Indian tree. As antibody levels fall, fertility is regained. Long-term maintenance of adequate antibody titers should be possible with biodegradable microspheres or a recombinant *Salmonella* construct incorporating the *β-hCG* gene.

SUMMARY

Graft rejection is an immunological reaction

- It shows specificity, the second set response is brisk, it is mediated by lymphocytes and antibodies specific for the graft are formed.

Genetic control of transplantation antigens

- In each vertebrate species there is a *m*ajor *h*istocompatibility *c*omplex (MHC) which is responsible for provoking the most intense graft reactions.
- Parental MHC antigens are codominantly expressed on cell surfaces.

Other consequences of MHC incompatibility

- Class II MHC molecules provoke a mixed lymphocyte reaction of proliferation and blast transformation when genetically dissimilar lymphocytes interact.
- Class II differences are largely responsible for the reaction of tolerated grafted lymphocytes against host antigen (graft-vs-host (g.v.h.) reaction).
- Siblings have a 1:4 chance of identity with respect to MHC.

Mechanisms of graft rejection

- Preformed antibodies cause hyperacute rejection within minutes.
- CD8 lymphocytes play a major role in the acute early rejection of first set responses.
- The strength of allograft rejection is due to the surprisingly large number of allospecific precursor cells. These derive mainly from the variety of T-cells which recognize

allo-MHC plus self-peptides plus a small number which directly recognize the allo-MHC molecule itself (the direct pathway); later rejection increasingly involves allogeneic peptides presented by self-MHC (the indirect pathway).
- Acute late rejection of organ grafts from 11 days onwards is caused by Ig and C binding to graft vessels.
- Insidious and late rejection may be due to immune complex deposition or breakthrough against immunosuppression.

Prevention of graft rejection

- This can be minimized by cross-matching donor and graft for ABO and MHC tissue types. Individual MHC antigens are typed by the PCR using discriminating primer pairs.
- Rejection can be blocked by agents producing general immunosuppression such as antimitotic drugs (e.g. azathioprine), anti-inflammatory steroids and antilymphocyte monoclonals. Cyclosporin A, FK506 and rapamycin represent exciting groups of T-cell-specific drugs; complexes of cyclosporin and FK506, with their cellular ligands, block calcineurin, a phosphatase which activates the IL-2 transcription factor NFAT, while rapamycin complexes with the FK-binding protein to block kinases involved in cell proliferation.
- Antigen-specific depression through tolerance induction can be achieved with injection of allogeneic bone marrow with costimulatory blockade by anti-CD154 (CD40L) plus a CTLA-4-Ig fusion protein. Dendritic cell precursors

(continued p. 372)

can also induce tolerance through antigen presentation in the absence of B7 costimulators.

Tissue engineering

• A distinct goal is to create autografts from stem cells or embryonically reprogramed adult nuclei differentiating in culture under the influence of specified growth factors.

Xenografting

• Strategies are being developed to prevent hyperacute rejection of pig grafts in humans due to reaction of natural antibodies in the host with galactose epitopes on pig cells and acute vascular rejection by acquired antibodies produced by the xenogeneic antibody response.

Clinical experience in grafting

• Cornea and cartilage grafts are avascular, produce local immunosuppressive factors and are comparatively well tolerated.

• Kidney grafting gives excellent results and has been the most widespread, although immunosuppression must normally be continuous.

• High success rates are also being achieved with heart and liver transplants particularly helped by the use of cyclosporin. Lung and pancreatic β-cell grafts are less successful.

• Bone marrow grafts for immunodeficiency and aplastic anemia are accepted from matched siblings, but it is difficult to avoid g.v.h. disease with allogeneic marrow without first purging CD8 T-cells in the graft or preferably by inducing tolerance using costimulatory blockade. Recombinant G-CSF and GM-CSF accelerate the return of myeloid cells after grafting.

• Experimental studies on transplantation of neural tissue and the production of prosthetic vascular grafts have been described.

Association of HLA type with disease

• HLA specificities are often associated with particular diseases, e.g. HLA-B27 with ankylosing spondylitis, B8

with myasthenia gravis, DR17 with Sjögren's syndrome, DR4 with rheumatoid arthritis, DQ2 and 8 with insulin-dependent diabetes mellitus and DR2, DQ6 with multiple sclerosis.

• The association may be related to an ability to bind particular antigenic peptides or to cross-react with certain infectious agents.

The fetus as an allograft

• Differences between MHC of mother and fetus may be beneficial to the fetus but as a potential graft it must be protected against transplantation attack by the mother.

• A major defense mechanism is the lack of classical class I and II MHC antigens on syncytiotrophoblast and cytotrophoblast which form the outer layers of the placenta.

• The extravillous cytotrophoblast expresses a nonclassical nonpolymorphic MHC class I protein, HLA-G, which may act to inhibit cytotoxicity by maternal NK cells.

• Syncytio- and cytotrophoblasts bear surface complement regulatory proteins which break down C3 convertase and so block any complement-mediated damage.

• Local production of IL-10 and TGFβ, tryptophan degradation and the presence of FasL may suppress unwanted reactions.

Immunological contraception

• Autoimmunization against hormones such as LHRH and hCG, which play a key role in reproduction, can block fertility.

• The C-terminal peptide of β-hCG and a complex of human β-hCG with sheep α chain have been used in human trials. If antibody titers are sufficiently high, prevention of pregnancy is close to 100% in the latter case. As antibody levels fall, fertility is regained.

See the accompanying website (**www.roitt.com**) for multiple choice questions.

FURTHER READING

Austen K.F., Burakoff S.J., Rosen F.S. & Strom T.B. (eds) (1996) *Therapeutic Immunology*. Blackwell Science, Oxford.

Bodmer J.G., Marsh S.G., Albert E.D. *et al.* (1994) Nomenclature for factors of the HLA system. *Tissue Antigens* **44**, 1.

Borel J.F. *et al.* (1996) *In vivo* pharmacological effects of cyclosporin and some analogues. *Advances in Pharmacology* **35**, 115. (An in-depth review of the field by the discoverer of cyclosporin and his colleagues.)

Daar A.S. (Chairman) (1999) Animal-to-human organ transplants—a solution or a new problem? (An in-depth round table discussion.) *Bulletin of the World Health Organization* **77**, 54.

Friend P.J. *et al.* (1999) Phase I study of an engineered aglycosylated humanized CD3 antibody in renal transplantation rejection. *Transplantation* **68**, 1632.

Gurdon J.B. & Colman A. (1999) The future of cloning. *Nature* **402**, 743.

Kahn A. (2000) Converting hepatocytes to β-cells—a new approach for diabetes? *Nature Medicine* **6**, 505.

Mellor A.L. & Munn D.H. (2000) Immunology at the maternal–fetal interface: lessons for T-cell tolerance and suppression. *Annual Review of Immunology* **18**, 367.

Morris P.J. (ed.) (2000) *Kidney Transplantation: Principles and Practice,* 5th edn. W.B. Saunders Company, Philadelphia.

Murphy W.J. & Blazar B.R. (1999) New strategies for preventing graft-versus-host disease. *Current Opinion in Immunology* **11**, 509.

Pazmanty L., Mandelboim O., Vales-Gomes M. *et al.* (1996) Protection from natural killer cell-mediated lysis by HLA-G expression on target cells. *Science* **274**, 792.

Thorsby E. (1995) HLA-associated disease susceptibility. *The Immunologist* **3**, 51.

Transplantation (2001) *Current Opinion in Immunology.* (Critical reviews of high quality appearing annually.)

Vince G.S. & Johnson P.M. (1996) Reproductive immunology: conception, contraception, and the consequences. *The Immunologist* **4**, 172.

Wilson S.E. & Aston R. (1994) Overview: recent developments in macrolide immunosuppressants. *Expert Opinion on Therapeutic Patents* **4**, 1445. (Academics should be aware of the enormous amount of data in the patent literature.)

Tumor immunology

INTRODUCTION

For as long as we can recollect, immunologists have wanted to believe that they would be the chosen ones to knock the stuffing out of the cancer problem. The fortunes of tumor immunology have fluctuated widely, flavor of the month at one time, a subject fit only for no-hopers at another. It looks as though its time has come at last.

The ability to reject transplants of tissue may be traced back a long way down the evolutionary tree—back even as far as the annelid worms. Long before the studies on the involvement of self-*m*ajor *h*istocompatibility *c*omplex (MHC) in immunological responses, Lewis Thomas suggested that the allograft rejection mechanism represented a means by which the body's cells could be kept under **immunological surveillance** so that altered cells with a neoplastic potential could be identified and summarily eliminated. For this to operate, cancer cells must display some new discriminating surface structure which can be recognized by the immune system.

CHANGES ON THE SURFACE OF TUMOR CELLS (figure 18.1)

Virally controlled antigens

A substantial minority of tumors arise through infection with **oncogenic viruses**, Epstein–Barr virus (EBV) in lymphomas, *h*uman *T*-cell *l*eukemia *v*irus-1 (HTLV-1) in leukemia and papilloma virus in cervical cancers. After infection, the viruses express genes homologous with cellular oncogenes which encode factors affecting growth and cell division. Failure to control these genes therefore leads to potentially malignant transformation. Virally derived peptides associated with surface MHC on the surface of the tumor cell behave as powerful transplantation antigens which generate haplotype-specific cytotoxic T-cells (Tc). All tumors induced by a given virus should carry the same surface antigen, irrespective of their cellular origin, so that immunization with any one of these tumors would confer resistance to subsequent challenge with the others provided that there were no artful mutations by the virus (Milestone 18.1). Unfortunately, viruses are not innately friendly.

Milestone 18.1 —Tumors Can Induce Immune Responses

The first convincing evidence for tumor-associated antigens came from the work of Prehn and Main who demonstrated quite clearly that **chemically induced cancers** can induce immune responses to themselves but not to other tumors produced by the same carcinogen (figure M18.1.1a). Tumors induced by **oncogenic viruses** are different in that processed viral peptides are present on the surface of all neoplastic cells bearing the viral genome so that Tc cells raised to one tumor will cross-react with all others produced by the same virus (figure M18.1.1b).

Dramatic advances were made by Boon and colleagues. First, they showed that random mutagenesis of transplantable tumors, i.e. tumors which can be passaged with-

in a pure mouse strain without provoking rejection, can give rise to mutant progeny with strong transplantation antigens. As a result they could not be grown in syngeneic animals with a normal immune system; accordingly they were referred to as **tum–** variants. Boon's team developed a powerful technology (cf. figure 18.2) which enabled them to use Tc clones specific for the tum– variant to screen cosmid clones for the mutant gene. These two breakthroughs, the recognition that mutation in tumors can generate strong transplantation reactions, and the development of the technique for identifying the relevant antigens with Tc cells, heralded really profound developments in tumor immunology and put it firmly on the map as a key area for cancer research.

Figure M18.1.1. The specificity of immunity induced by tumors. (a) A chemically induced tumor MCA-1 can induce resistance to an implant of itself but not to a tumor produced in a syngeneic mouse by the same carcinogen. Thus each tumor has an individual antigen, now thought to be a processed mutant endogenous protein complexed with a heat-shock protein. More recent data suggest that, if immunized animals are challenged with much lower numbers of tumor cells, a greater degree of cross-protection between tumors may be observed, which has been ascribed to a 44 kDa oncofetal antigen, possibly an immature version of a laminin receptor protein. (b) Tumors produced by a given oncogenic virus immunize against tumors produced in syngeneic mice by the same but not other viruses. Thus tumors produced by an oncogenic virus share a common antigen.

Expression of normally silent genes

The dysregulated uncontrolled cell division of the cancer cell creates a milieu in which the products of normally silent genes may be expressed. Sometimes these encode differentiation antigens normally associated with an earlier fetal stage. Thus tumors derived from the same cell type are often found to express such **oncofetal antigens** which are also present on embryonic cells. Examples would be α-fetoprotein in hepatic carcinoma and carcinoembryonic antigen (CEA) in cancer of the intestine. Certain monoclonal antibodies also react with tumors of neural crest origin and fetal melanocytes. Another monoclonal antibody defines the SSEA-1 antigen found on a variety of human tumors and early mouse embryos but absent from adult cells with the exception of human granulocytes and monocytes.

But the exciting quantum leap forward stems from the original observation that cytosolic viral nucleoprotein could provide a target for Tc cells by appearing on the cell surface as a processed peptide associated with MHC class I (cf. p. 94). This established the general principle that the intracellular proteins which are not destined to be positioned in the surface plasma membrane can still signal their presence to T-cells in the outer world by the processed peptide–MHC mecha-

nism. Cytotoxic T-cells specific for tumor cells, obtained from mixed cultures of peripheral blood cells with tumor, can be used to establish the identity of the antigen employing the strategy described in figure 18.2. By something of a *tour de force* a gene encoding a melanoma antigen, MAGE-1, was identified. It belongs to a family of 12 genes, six of which are expressed in a significant proportion of melanomas as well as

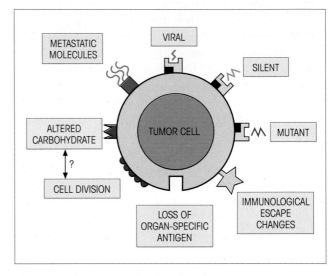

Figure 18.1. Tumor-associated surface changes.

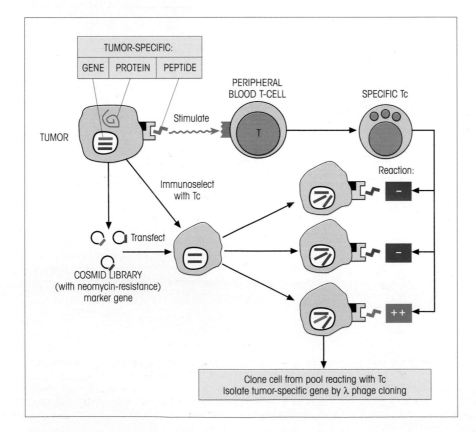

Figure 18.2. Identification of tumor-specific gene using tumor-specific cytotoxic T-cell (Tc) clones derived from mixed tumor–lymphocyte culture. A cosmid library incorporating the tumor DNA is transfected into an antigen-negative cell line derived from the wild-type tumor by immunoselection with the Tc. Small pools of transfected cells are tested against the Tc. A positive pool is cloned by limiting dilution and the tumor-specific gene (*MAGE-1*) cloned from the antigen-positive well(s). (Based on van der Bruggen P. *et al.* (1991) *Science* **254**, 1643. Copyright © 1991 by the AAAS.) The original **MAGE-1** belongs to a family of 12 genes. Further melanoma-specific genes, including *MART-1*, *gp100* and *tyrosinase*, have been discovered.

head and neck tumors, nonsmall cell lung cancers and bladder carcinomas. MAGE-1 is *not* expressed in normal tissues except for germ-line cells in testis and gives rise to antigenic T-cell epitopes which, in the light of the absence of class I MHC on the testis cells, must be considered tumor-specific. This exciting research reveals the tumor-specific antigen as an expression of a normally silent gene.

Mutant antigens

The seminal work on tum– mutants (see Milestone 18.1) has persuaded us that single point mutations in oncogenes can account for the large diversity of antigens found on carcinogen-induced tumors. The specific immunity provoked by chemically induced tumors can be elicited by **heat-shock protein** 70 (hsp70) and hsp90 isolated from the tumor cells, but their immunogenicity is lost when the associated low molecular weight peptides are removed. These peptides could, however, stimulate the specific CD8 cytotoxic T-cell clones generated by the tumors, and three possible mechanisms have been advanced to account for the enhancement of tumor immune responses by

hsps. First, they can act as 'danger' signals by activating antigen-presenting cells. Second, necrotic tumor cells expressing the hsps can transfer hsp–peptide complexes to host antigen-presenting cells where they can cross-prime cytotoxic CD8 T-cells through the MHC class I endogenous presentation pathway. And last, the hsps may influence the capacity of the tumor cell itself to process and present endogenous mutated and, of course, 'silent' antigens as targets for specific T-cells (figure 18.3).

There is considerable evidence for the production of mutated peptides in human tumors. The gene encoding the p53 cell cycle inhibitor is a hotspot for mutation in cancer and hsp70/p53 peptide complexes have been isolated from human breast tumors. The oncogenic human *ras* genes differ from their normal counterparts by point mutations usually leading to single amino acid substitutions in positions 12, 13 or 61. Such mutations have been recorded in 40% of human colorectal cancers and their preneoplastic lesions, in more than 90% of pancreatic carcinomas, in acute myelogenous leukemia and in preleukemic syndromes. The mutated ras peptide can induce proliferative T-cell lines *in vitro*. Tumors induced by UV light produce

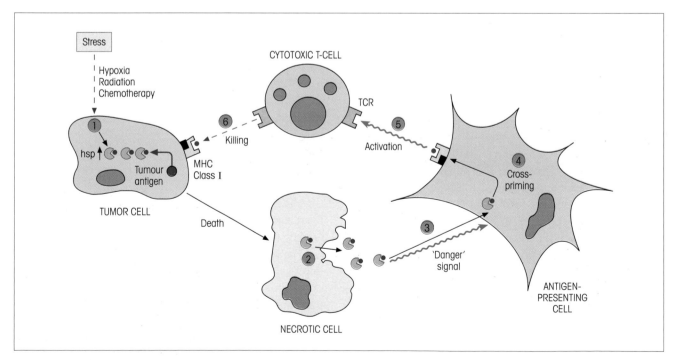

Figure 18.3. The role of heat-shock proteins (hsps) in tumor immunogenicity. (1) Stress factors upregulate hsps which can form complexes with processed tumor antigen and increase surface presentation of antigenic peptide by MHC class I. (2) They can also lead to necrosis and release of hsp–peptide complexes, which (3) can act as stimulatory danger signals to dendritic antigen-presenting cells and penetrate the cytoplasm, where (4) they can enter the MHC class I processing pathway by so-called cross-priming. (5) CD8 resting T-cells become activated and (6) kill the tumor cells. (Based on Wells A.D. & Malkowsky M. (2000) *Immunology Today* **21**, 129.)

individual Tc cells not reacting with other tumors or normal cells and it would be surprising if this were not a further example of tumor-specific mutant peptide antigenicity.

Changes in carbohydrate structure

The chaotic internal control of metabolism within neoplastic cells often leads to the presentation of abnormal surface carbohydrate structures. Sometimes one sees blocked synthesis, e.g. deletion of blood group A. In other cases there may be enhanced synthesis of structures absent in progenitor cells: thus some gastrointestinal cancers express the Lewis Le^a antigen in individuals who are $Le(a^-,b^-)$ and others produce extended chains bearing dimeric Le^a or $Le(a,b)$.

Abnormal mucin synthesis can have immunological consequences. Consider the mucins of pancreatic and breast tissue. These consist of a polypeptide core of 20-amino acid tandem repeats with truly abundant O-linked carbohydrate chains. A monoclonal antibody SM-3 directed to the core polypeptide reacts poorly with normal tissue where the epitope is masked by glycosylation, but well with breast and pancreatic carcinomas possessing shorter and fewer O-linked chains. Tc cells specific for tumor mucins are not MHC restricted and the slightly heretical suggestion has been made that the T-cell receptors (TCRs) are binding multivalently to closely spaced SM-3 epitopes on unprocessed mucins; alternatively, and closer to the party line, recognition is by $\gamma\delta$ cells.

Changes on the surface of cycling cells

In some instances it is possible that the changes which occur in the carbohydrate moiety of tumor surface membrane glycoproteins are a natural consequence of cell division. For example, Thomas found that the density of surface sugar determinants cross-reacting with blood group H fell as murine mastocytoma cells moved into the G1 phase of the division cycle, while, reciprocally, group B determinants increased. Surface components binding the lectin, wheat-germ agglutinin are poorly represented on resting T- and B-cells but, within 24 hours of stimulation by lymphocyte polyclonal activators and before DNA synthesis begins, high concentrations of lectin-binding sites appear on the surface.

Unusual events may be observed in active **cells associated with tumor growth** and spread as distinct from the tumors themselves. For example, the 95 kDa surface glycoprotein, F19, is expressed in the **reactive stromal fibroblasts** in more than 90% of carcinomas of the colon, breast, lung and pancreas, making them a novel target for immunological attack since normal adult tissues and benign epithelial tumors express zero or very low levels. In like vein, the highly sialylated cell surface glycoprotein endosialin (FB5) is present in the newly generated vasculature of a significant proportion of malignant tumors but not in blood vessels of normal tissues.

Molecules related to metastatic potential

Changes in surface carbohydrates can have a dramatic effect on malignancy. For example, colonic cancers expressing sialyl Le^x have a poor prognosis and higher propensity to metastasize. Lung cancer patients whose tumors showed deletion of blood group A had a much worse prognosis than those with continuous A; the finding that patients expressing $H/Le^y/Le^b$ also had a poorer prognosis than antigen-negative subjects is consistent with this observation.

The role of **CD44** (HERMES/Pgp-1) in cell trafficking, based on its interaction with vascular endothelium, has afforded it some prominence in the facilitation of metastatic spread. CD44 occurs in several isoforms with a varying number of exons between the transmembrane and common N-terminus. Normal epithelium expresses the CD44H isoform with hyaluran-binding domains, but lacking the intervening v1–v10 exons; expression of certain of these exons on tumors is indicative of a growth advantage, since they are present with higher frequency on more advanced cancers. Stable transfection of a nonmetastatic tumor with a CD44 cDNA clone encompassing exons v6 and v7 induced the ability to form metastatic tumors—a most striking effect. Further, injection of a monoclonal anti-CD44 v6 prevented the formation of lymph node metastases. Exons v6 and v10 have now been shown to bind blood group H and chondroitin 4-sulfate, respectively, and the latest hypothesis is that these carbohydrates can bind to CD44H on endothelium and thence homotypically to each other so generating a metastatic nidus.

Changes have quite frequently been observed in the expression of class I MHC molecules. For example, oncogenic transformation of cells infected with adenovirus 12 is associated with highly reduced class I as a consequence of very low levels of TAP-1 and -2 mRNA. Mutation frequently leads to diminished or absent class I expression linked in most cases to increased metastatic potential, presumably reflecting decreased vulnerability to T-cells but not NK cells. In breast cancer, for example, around 60% of metastatic tumors lack class I.

SPONTANEOUS IMMUNE RESPONSES TO TUMORS

Immune surveillance against strongly immunogenic tumors

When present, many of these antigens can provoke immune responses in experimental animals which lead to resistance against tumor growth, but they vary tremendously in their efficiency. Powerful antigens associated with tumors induced by oncogenic viruses or ultraviolet light generate strong resistance, while the transplantation antigens on chemically induced tumors (Milestone 18.1) are weaker and somewhat variable; disappointingly, tumors which arise spontaneously in animals produce little or no response. The **immune surveillance theory** would predict that there should be more tumors in individuals whose adaptive immune systems are suppressed. This undoubtedly seems to be the case for **strongly immunogenic tumors**. There is a considerable increase in skin cancer in immunosuppressed patients living in high sunshine regions north of Brisbane and, in general, transplant patients on immunosuppressive drugs are unduly susceptible to skin cancers, largely associated with papilloma virus, and EBV-positive lymphomas. The EBV-related Burkitt's lymphomas crop up with undue frequency in regions infested with malarial infection, known to compromise the efficacy of the immune system. Likewise, the lymphomas which arise in children with T-cell deficiency linked to Wiskott–Aldrich syndrome or ataxia telangiectasia express *EBV* genes; they show unusually restricted expression of EBV latent proteins which are the major potential target epitopes for immune recognition, while cellular adhesion molecules, such as *i*ntercellular *a*dhesion *m*olecule-1 (ICAM-1) and *l*ymphocyte *f*unction-*a*ssociated molecule-3 (LFA-3), which mediate conjugate formation with Tc cells, cannot be detected on their surface (figure 18.4). Knowing that most normal individuals have highly efficient EBV-specific Tc cells, this must be telling us that only by downregulating appropriate surface molecules can the lymphoma cells escape even the limited T-cell surveillance operating in these patients.

As might be predicted, tumors are positively brimming with various **immunological escape mechanisms** (figure 18.4) and thus they resemble successful infections. Downregulation of HLA class I to make the tumor a less attractive target for cytolytic T-cells is a favorite ploy. We have already referred to this as a common feature of breast cancer metastases, and this is true also of cervical carcinoma where, prognostical-

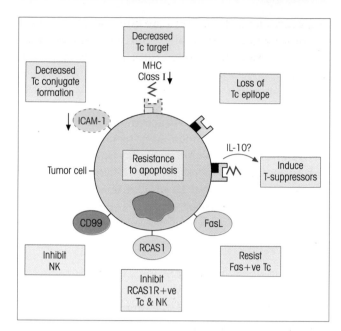

Figure 18.4. Tumor escape mechanisms.

ly, loss of HLA-B44 in premalignant lesions is an indicator of tumor progression. Loss of tumor antigen epitopes represents another escape mechanism and mutations in an oncogenic virus itself can increase its tumorigenic potential. Thus the frequent association of a high-risk variant of human papilloma virus with cervical tumors in HLA-B7 individuals is attributed to the loss of a T-cell epitope which would otherwise generate a protective B7-mediated cytolytic response. Tumors can also decrease their vulnerability to cytotoxic T-cell attack by expression of surface FasL (cf. p. 19) and a growth inhibitory molecule, RCAS1, which react with T-cells bearing their corresponding receptors and stop them in their tracks. It should also be borne in mind that the internal defects in apoptosis which favor the emergence of a tumor clone will, in addition, make them more difficult to kill by cytotoxic T-cells. In a way, it is comforting to draw the conclusion that the existence of these 'Houdini' mechanisms is evidence for a selective pressure being exerted by the adaptive immune system.

Cancers which express neoantigens of **low immunogenicity** do not come creeping out of the woodwork when patients are radically immunosuppressed and, although T-cell responses can often be rescued from tumor-infiltrating lymphocytes or relatively high numbers of tumor-specific CD8 T-cells may be detected by the peptide–HLA tetramer technique in peripheral blood, they may be functionally deficient due perhaps to suppression by local IL-10 and TGFβ. Mutation of p53 and its overexpression are very common events in human cancer and are often associated with the production of antibodies; but while these could prove to have a diagnostic utility, it is most unlikely that they are of benefit to the patient, the current view being that *cell-mediated* responses are crucial to the attack against internal antigens expressed in solid tumors. Reluctantly, one has to accept the view that, with tumors of weak immunogenicity, we are dealing with low-key reactions which clearly play little role in curbing the neoplastic process. That is not to say that these 'weak' antigens cannot be exploited for therapeutic purposes as we shall soon see.

A role for innate immunity?

Perhaps in speaking of immunity to tumors, one too readily thinks only in terms of acquired responses, whereas it is now accepted that innate mechanisms are of significance. Macrophages which often infiltrate a tumor mass can destroy tumor cells in tissue culture through the copious production of reactive oxygen intermediates (ROIs) and tumor necrosis factor (TNF) when activated by a diversity of factors, bacterial lipopolysaccharide, double-stranded RNA, T-cell γ-interferon (IFNγ), and so forth.

There is an uncommon flurry of serious interest in **natural killer (NK)** cells. It is generally accepted that they subserve a function as the earliest cellular effector mechanism against dissemination of blood-borne metastases. Let's look at the evidence. Patients with advanced metastatic disease often have abnormal NK activity and low levels appear to predict subsequent metastases. In experimental animals, removal of NK cells from mice with surgically resected B16 melanoma resulted in uncontrolled metastatic disease and death. Acute ethanol intoxication in rats boosted the number of metastases from an NK-sensitive tumor 10-fold, but had no effect on an NK-resistant cancer, hinting at a possible underlying cause for the association between alcoholism, infectious disease and malignancies. (Those who enjoy the odd Bacchanalian splurge should not be too upset—be comforted by the beneficial effect in heart disease, but no excesses please!) Powerful evidence implicating these cells in protection against cancer is provided by beige mice which congenitally lack NK cells. They die with spontaneous tumors earlier than their nondeficient +/bg littermates, and the incidence of radiation-induced leukemia is reduced by prior injection of cloned isogeneic NK cells which could be suppressing preleukemic cells. Note, however, that tumors induced chemically or with murine leukemia virus were handled normally.

Resting NK cells are spontaneously cytolytic for certain, but by no means all, tumor targets; cells activated by IL-2 and possibly by IL-12 and -18 display a wider lethality. As described earlier in Chapter 4, recognition of the surface structures on the target cell involves various activating and inhibitory receptors, but it is important to re-emphasize that recognition of class I imparts a **negative inactivating** signal to the NK cell. Conversely, this implies that downregulation of MHC class I, which tumors employ as a strategy to escape Tc cells (figure 18.4), would make them **more susceptible to NK attack**. The tumor cells can fight back by expressing CD99, which downregulates NK CD16, and the growth inhibitor RCAS1, which induces apoptosis in NK as well as in Tc cells (figure 18.4). It is not clear whether surface FasL, which can repel attack by the Fas-positive cytolytic T-cells, is also effective against NK cells, but the relative resistance of tumor cells to apoptosis must be innately protective.

Divisions are surfacing in the NK ranks. The NK cells, which remarkably constitute up to 50% of the liver-associated lymphocytes in humans, have a higher level of expression of IL-2 receptor and adhesion molecules such as integrins compared with NK cells in peripheral blood. They are precursors of a subset of activated adherent NK cells (A-NK) which adhere rapidly to solid surfaces under the influence of IL-2 and are distinguished from their nonadherent counterparts by their superiority in entering solid tumors and in prolonging survival following adoptive transfer with IL-2 into animal models of tumor growth or metastasis. The nonadherent NK variety are better at killing antibody-coated cancer cells through antibody-dependent cellular cytotoxicity (ADCC), mediated by their CD16 FcγRIII receptor.

Be kind to your NK cells. Really late nights which involve major curtailment of slow-wave sleep lead to drastic falls in NK cells and levels of IL-2, quite apart from bleary eyes.

UNREGULATED DEVELOPMENT GIVES RISE TO LYMPHOPROLIFERATIVE DISORDERS

We should now turn our attention to the manner in which cells involved in immune responses themselves may undergo malignant transformation, giving rise to leukemia, lymphoma or myeloma characterized by uncontrolled proliferation. An obvious example is the subset of adult human T-cell leukemia associated with **HTLV-1** (human T-cell leukemia virus type 1). After infection of the T-cell, the viral tax protein, which is constitutively expressed, stimulates transcription of

IL-2, IL-2R, etc., leading to vigorous proliferation; however, only if there is a subsequent chromosome abnormality (see below) does malignant transformation take place.

Deregulation of protooncogenes is a characteristic feature of many lymphocytic tumors

The realization that viral oncogenes are almost certainly derived from normal host genes concerned in the regulation of cellular proliferation has led to the identification of many of these so-called protooncogenes. One of them, c-*myc*, appears to be of crucial importance for entry of the lymphocyte, and probably many other cells, from the resting G0 stage to the cell cycle, while shutdown of c-*myc* expression is linked to exit from the cycle and return to G0. Thus deregulation of c-*myc* expression will prevent cells from leaving the cycle and consign them to a fate of continuous replication. This is just what is seen in many of the neoplastic B-lymphoproliferative disorders, where the malignant cells express high levels of c-myc protein usually associated with a reciprocal chromosomal translocation involving the c-*myc* locus. For example, Burkitt's lymphoma is a B-cell neoplasia with a relatively high incidence among African children in whom there is an association with the EBV; in most cases studied, the c-*myc* gene, located on chromosome 8 band q24, is joined by a reciprocal translocation event to the μ heavy chain gene on chromosome 14 band q32 (figure 18.5). It is suggested that the normal mechanisms which downregulate c-*myc* can no longer work on the translocated gene and so the cell is held in the cycling mode. Less frequently, c-*myc* translocates to the site of the κ (chromosome 2) or λ (chromosome 22) loci.

Chromosome translocations are common in lymphoproliferative disorders

Most lymphomas and leukemias have visible chromosome abnormalities bound up with translocations to B-cell immunoglobulin or T-cell receptor gene loci but not necessarily involving c-*myc*. A reciprocal translocation between the μ chain gene on chromosome 14 and the *bcl*-2 oncogene on chromosome 18 has been identified in almost all follicular B-cell lymphomas, and another between the T-cell gene on chromosome 14 (q11) and another presumed oncogene on chromosome 11 in a *T*-cell *acute lymphoblastic leukemia* (TALL).

Lymphomagenesis is a multistep process. The lack of proliferative control engendered by deregulation of c-*myc* and other similar events induced by chromosomal translocations is permissive for the vulnerability to induction of neoplasia, but is not in itself sufficient to bring about malignant transformation. Thus, transgenic mice harboring a c-*myc* gene driven by the μ heavy chain enhancer (E_μ-*myc* mice) have hyperplastic expansions of the pre-B-cell population in the bone marrow and spleen during the preneoplastic period and yet do not develop tumors until 6–8 weeks of age; and then they are monoclonal not polyclonal, suggesting that a random second event is required before autonomy is achieved. Indeed, if the E_μ-*myc* transgenic mice are now infected with viruses carrying the v-*raf* oncogene, they rapidly develop lymphomas. It is generally thought that, whereas factors like c-myc can make a cell competent for mitosis, it is only the additional upregulation of **cell cycle progression genes** like *fos*, *jun* and *myb* or the loss of **cell cycle suppressor gene products** like p53 which allow cell division to occur. Deregulation of two such events may synergize in the process of malignant transformation and the associated unfettered cell proliferation.

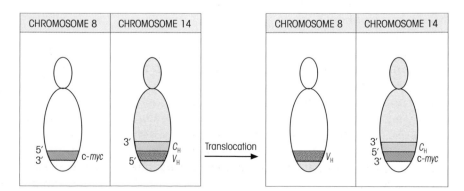

Figure 18.5. Translocation of the c-*myc* gene to the μ chain locus in Burkitt's lymphoma.

Transgenic mice with a susceptibility to the development of cancer may be exploited to supplement the Ames' test for potential carcinogens. Conversely, mice with disrupted *p53* which develop tumors very smartly are ideal for studying treatments which might impede tumorigenesis. The protective effect of caloric restriction on neoplastic change was admirably confirmed in this system.

Different lymphoid malignancies show maturation arrest at characteristic stages in differentiation

Lymphoid cells at almost any stage in their differentiation or maturation may become malignant and proliferate to form a clone of cells which are virtually 'frozen' at a particular developmental stage because of defects in maturation. The malignant cells bear the markers one would expect of normal lymphocytes reaching the stage at which maturation had been arrested. Thus, chronic lymphocytic leukemia cells resemble mature B-cells in expressing surface class II and Ig, albeit of a single idiotype in a given patient. Using monoclonal antibodies directed against the terminal deoxynucleotidyl transferase (see figure 18.7a), class II MHC, Ig and specific antigens on cortical thymocytes, mature T-cells and non-T, non-B acute lymphoblastic leukemia cells, it has been possible to classify the lymphoid malignancies in terms of the phenotype of the equivalent normal cell (figure 18.6).

Susceptibility to malignant transformation is high in lymphocytes at an early stage in ontogeny. If we look at Burkitt's lymphoma, the EBV-induced translocation of the c-*myc* to bring it under control of the *IgH* gene complex is most likely to occur at the pro-B-cell stage, since the chromatin structure of the Ig locus opens up for transcription as signaled by the appearance of sterile C$_\mu$ transcripts. Furthermore, the cell is likely to escape immunological recognition because, in its undifferentiated resting form, it has downregulated its EBV-encoded antigens and MHC class I polymorphic specificities, and the adhesion molecules LFA-1, LFA-3 and ICAM-1, as mentioned above.

At one time it was thought that maturation arrest occurred at the stage when the cell first became malignant, but we now know that the tumor cells can be forced into differentiation by agents such as phorbol myristate acetate, and the current view is that cells may undergo a few differentiation steps after malignant transformation before coming to a halt. The demonstration of a myeloma protein idiotype on the cytoplasmic μ chains of pre-B-cells in the same patient certainly favors the idea that the malignant event had occurred

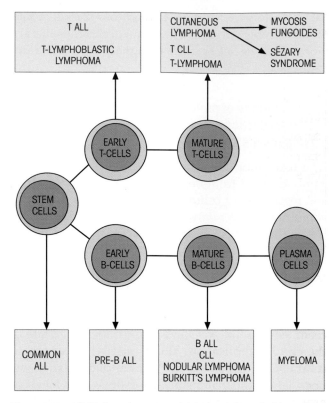

Figure 18.6. Cellular phenotype of human lymphoid malignancies. ALL, acute lymphoblastic leukemia; CLL, chronic lymphocytic leukemia. (After Greaves M.F. & Janossy G, personal communication.)

in a pre-B-cell whose progeny formed the plasma cell tumor. However, an alternative explanation could be transfection of normal pre-B-cells by an oncogene complex from the myeloma cells, possibly through a viral vector. With the exciting discovery of retroviruses associated with certain human T-cell leukemias, this is an interesting possibility.

Immunohistological diagnosis of lymphoid neoplasias

With the availability of a range of monoclonal antibodies and improvements in immuno-enzymatic technology, great strides have been made in exploiting, for diagnostic purposes, the fact that malignant lymphoid cells display the markers of the normal lymphocytes which are their counterparts.

Leukemias

This point can be made rather well if one looks at the markers used to distinguish between the various types of leukemia (table 18.1). Whereas T ALL and B ALL

Table 18.1. Classification of lymphocytic leukemia by immuno-enzymatic staining.

Lymphocyte marker	Common ALL	Pre-B ALL	B-cell ALL	T-cell ALL	Chronic lymphocytic leukemia
*CALLA (CDIO)	+	+	−	−	−
Cytoplasmic μ	−	+	−	−	−
Surface μ	−	−	+	−	+
Surface κ or λ	−	−	+	−	+
Pan-B	−	+	+	−	+
TdT	+	+	−	+	−
CD5	−	−	−	+	+
CD2	−	−	−	+	−
HLA-DR	+	+	+	−	+

*Antigen-specific for lymphoid precursor cells and pre-B-cells.

cases have a poor prognosis, the patients positive for the common acute lymphoblastic leukemia antigen (CALLA; figure 18.7b), which includes most childhood leukemias, belong to a prognostically favorable group, many of whom are curable with standard therapeutic combinations of vincristine, prednisolone and L-asparaginase. Bone marrow transplantation may help in the management of patients with recurrent ALL provided that a remission can first be achieved. Expression of the lymphoid lineage markers CD2 and CD19 on leukemic blasts is an indication of good prognosis in adults with the disease.

Chronic lymphocytic leukemia is uncommon in people under 50 years and is usually relatively benign, although the 10–20% of patients with a circulating monoclonal Ig have a bad prognosis. Excessive numbers of CLL small lymphocytes are found in the blood (figure 18.7c–e) and, being derived from a single clone, they can be stained only with anti-κ or anti-λ (table 18.1). Their weak expression of CD5 strongly suggests that they may be derived from the equivalent of the B-1 cell population, especially since they can be encouraged to make the IgM polyspecific autoantibodies typical of this subset, if pushed by phorbol ester stimulation.

Lymphomas

The extensive use of markers has greatly helped in the diagnosis of non-Hodgkin's lymphomas. In the first place, the sometimes difficult distinction between a lymphoproliferative condition and carcinoma can be made with ease by using monoclonal antibodies to the leukocyte common antigen (CD45), which will react with all lymphoid cells whether in paraffin or cryostat sections, and antibodies to cytokeratin which recognize most carcinomas (figure 18.7f). Second, the cell of origin of the lymphoma can be ascertained by panels of monoclonals which differentiate the cellular elements which form normal lymphoid tissue.

The majority of non-Hodgkin's lymphomas are of B-cell origin and the feature which gives the game away to the diagnostic immunohistologist is the synthesis of monotypic Ig, i.e. of one light chain only (figure 18.7g); in contrast, the population of cells at a site of reactive B-cell hyperplasia will stain for both κ and λ chains (figure 18.7h).

Follicle center cell lymphomas (figure 18.7g) imitating the reactive germinal center account for over 50% of the B-lymphomas. They exhibit monotypic surface Ig, and the larger centrocytes and centroblasts which make up two-thirds of the cases contain cytoplasmic Ig. They stain for MHC class II and weakly for CALLA. Morphologically similar cells make up tumors variously labeled as 'mantle zone lymphoma' or 'small cleaved cell lymphoma' but differ from follicle center cells in positive surface staining for IgM *and* IgD and CD5, and negativity for CALLA. Burkitt's lymphoma lymphoblastoid cells (figure 18.7i) exhibit the common ALL antigen and surface IgM.

The overall prognosis for patients with non-Hodgkin's lymphoma is poor, even though improved by combined chemotherapy. Transplanted patients are 35 times more likely to develop lymphoma than normals, and there are indications that this cannot necessarily be attributed to the long-term immunosuppression.

Hodgkin's disease attacks the gross architecture of lymphoid tissue and is characterized by the binucleate giant cells known as Reed–Sternberg cells (figure 18.7j) which appear to have a germinal center B-cell lineage. Therapy depends upon the stage of the disease; patients with disease localized to lymphoid tissue above the diaphragm respond well to radiotherapy, while those with more widespread disease are treated more aggressively.

Plasma cell dyscrasias

Multiple myeloma

This is defined as a malignant proliferation of a clone of plasma cells in the bone marrow secreting a monoclonal Ig. The myeloma or 'M' component in serum is recognized as a tight band on paper electrophoresis (figure 18.8) as all molecules in the clone are of course identical and have the same mobility. Since Ig-

Figure 18.7. (*Opposite*) **Immunodiagnosis of lymphoproliferative disorders.** (a) Cytocentrifuged blast cells from a case of acute lymphoblastic leukemia stained by anti-terminal deoxynucleotidyl transferase (TdT) using an immuno-alkaline phosphatase method (cells treated first with mouse monoclonal anti-TdT, then anti-mouse Ig and finally with an immune complex of mouse anti-alkaline phosphatase+alkaline phosphatase before developing the enzymatic reddish-purple color reaction). Many strongly stained blast cells are seen together with unlabeled normal marrow cells. (b) Immuno-alkaline phosphatase staining of bone marrow cells from a case of acute lymphoblastic leukemia, using monoclonal antibody specific for the common acute lymphoblastic leukemia antigen (anti-CALLA; antibody J5). The majority of cells are strongly labeled. Two nonreactive cells are indicated by arrows. (c, d, e) Immuno-alkaline phosphatase labeling of blood smears from a case of chronic lymphocytic leukemia with three monoclonal antibodies (anti-HLA-DR, anti-CD3 antigen and anti-CD1 antigen): (c) HLA-DR antigen is present on all the leukemic cells seen, but absent from a polymorph (arrowed); (d) three normal T-cells are labeled for the CD3 antigen, but the leukemic cells are negative; (e) CD1 antigen is strongly expressed on two normal lymphocytes (arrowed), but also weakly expressed on the chronic lymphocytic leukemia (CLL) cells. This pattern is typical of CLL. (f) A case of gastric carcinoma (stained at the bottom using anticytokeratin, Ke) with a heavy lymphocytic infiltrate (top, stained with antileukocyte common antigen, LC). (g) Diffuse follicle center type B-cell lymphoma showing λ light chain restriction; compare with (h) a reactive lymph node staining for both κ and λ light chains. (i) Burkitt's lymphoma showing 'starry sky' appearance. (j) Hodgkin's disease showing mixed cellularity and characteristic binucleate Reed–Sternberg cell with massive prominent nucleoli in the center of the figure. (k) Birefringent amyloid deposits in kidney glomeruli visualized by Congo Red staining under polarized light. (l) A case of malignant lymphoma associated with macroglobulinemia, showing lymphoplasmacytoid cells stained by the brown immunoperoxidase reaction for cytoplasmic IgM.
((a)–(e) Very kindly provided by Professor D. Mason, and (f)–(l) by Professor P. Isaacson.)

Figure 18.8. Myeloma paraprotein demonstrated by gel electrophoresis of serum. Lane 1, normal; lane 2, γ-paraprotein; lane 3, near β-paraprotein; lane 4, fibrinogen band in the γ region of a *plasma* sample; lane 5, normal serum; lane 6, immunoglobulin deficiency (low γ); lane 7, nephrotic syndrome (raised α₂-macroglobulin, low albumin and Igs); lane 8, hemolysed sample (raised hemoglobin/haptoglobin in α₂ region); lane 9, polyclonal increase in Igs (e.g. infection, autoimmune disease); lane 10, normal serum. (Gel kindly provided by Mr A. Heys.)

secreting cells produce an excess of light chains, free light chains are present in the plasma of multiple myeloma patients, can be recognized in the urine as Bence-Jones protein (cf. figure 16.23) and give rise to amyloid deposits (see below). The characteristic 'punched out' osteolytic lesions in bones are thought to be due to the release of osteoclastic factors such as IL-6 by the abnormal plasma cells in the marrow. If untreated, the disease is rapidly progressive. With chemotherapy, the mean survival time from diagnosis is now about 5 years.

'M' bands have been found in the sera of a number of individuals who have no clinical signs of myeloma; the comparative rarity with which invasive multiple myeloma develops in these people and the constant level of the monoclonal protein over a period of years suggest the presence of benign tumors of the lymphocyte–plasma cell series.

Amyloid. Between 10% and 20% of patients with myeloma develop widespread amyloid deposits which contain the variable region of the myeloma light chain. Being identical, the variable region fragments polymerize and form the characteristic amyloid fibrils which are recognizable by their birefringence on staining with Congo Red (figure 18.7k). Other components in amyloid have not yet been characterized. The fibrils are relatively resistant to digestion and accumulate in the ground substance of connective tissue where they can lead to pathological changes in the kidneys, heart and brain. Amyloid can also be formed secondarily to chronic inflammatory conditions such as rheumatoid arthritis and familial Mediterranean fever, but in this case involves the polymerization of a unique substance, Amyloid A (AA), a protein derived from the N-terminal part of a serum precursor (SAA) of molecular weight 90 kDa. SAA behaves as an acute phase protein in that its concentration increases rapidly in response to tissue injury or inflammation. Levels rise with age and the minority of individuals with high values are those most likely to develop amyloid.

Waldenström's macroglobulinemia

This disorder is produced by the unregulated proliferation of cells of an intermediate appearance called lymphoplasmacytoid cells which secrete a monoclonal IgM, the Waldenström macroglobulin (figure 18.7l). Remarkably, many of the monoclonal proteins have autoantibody activity, anti-DNA, anti-IgG (rheumatoid factor), and so on. It has been suggested that, like the CLL cells, they are of the B-1 lineage which secrete 'natural' antibodies (cf. p. 236). Since the IgM is secreted in large amounts and is confined to the intravascular compartment, there is a marked rise in serum viscosity, the consequences of which can be temporarily mitigated by vigorous plasmapheresis. The disease runs a fairly benign course and the prognosis is quite good, although the appearance of lymphoplasmacytoid tumor cells in the blood is an ominous sign.

Heavy chain disease

Heavy chain disease is a rare condition in which quantities of abnormal heavy chains are excreted in the urine—γ chains in association with malignant lymphoma and α chains in cases of abdominal lymphoma with diffuse lymphoplasmacytic infiltration of the small intestine. The amino acid sequences of the N-terminal regions of these heavy chains are normal, but they have a deletion extending from part of the variable domain through most of the $C_H 1$ region so that they lack the structure required to form cross-links to the light chains. One idea is that the defect arises through faulty coupling of V- and C-region genes (cf. p. 42).

Immunodeficiency secondary to lymphoproliferative disorders

Immunodeficiency is a common feature in patients with lymphoid malignancies. The reasons for this are still obscure, but it seems as though the malignant cells interfere with the development of the corresponding normal cells, almost as though they were producing some cell-specific chalone (inhibitor) or transfecting suppressor factor. Thus, in multiple myeloma, the levels of normal B-cells and of nonmyeloma Ig may be grossly depressed and the patients may be susceptible to infection with pyogenic bacteria.

APPROACHES TO CANCER IMMUNOTHERAPY

Although immune surveillance seems to operate only against strongly immunogenic tumors, the exciting new information on the antigenicity of mutant and previously silent proteins, and the changes in carbohydrate structures, should be of tremendous encouragement to any red-blooded investigator with an eye to develop new immunotherapies for cancer which exploit the already impressive range of antigens currently available (table 18.2).

On one point all are agreed: if immunotherapy is to succeed, it is essential that the tumor load should first be reduced by surgery, irradiation or chemotherapy,

Table 18.2. Potential tumor antigens for immunotherapy. (Reproduced with permission from Fong L. & Engleman E.G. (2000) Dendritic cells in cancer immunotherapy. *Annual Review of Immunology* 18, 245.)

Antigen	Malignancy
Tumour specific	
Immunoglobulin V-region	B-cell non-Hodgkin's lymphoma, multiple myeloma
TCR V-region	T-cell non-Hodgkin's lymphoma
Mutant p21/ras	Pancreatic, colon, lung cancer
Mutany p53	Colorectal, lung, bladder, head and neck cancer
Developmental	
p210/bcr-abl fusion product	Chronic myelogenous leukemia, acute lymphoblastic leukemia
MART-1/Melan A	Melanoma
MAGE-1, MAGE-3	Melanoma, colorectal, lung, gastric cancers
GAGE family	Melanoma
Telomerase	Various
Viral	
Human papilloma virus	Cervical, penile cancer
Epstein–Barr virus	Burkitt's lymphoma, nasopharyngeal carcinoma, post-transplant lymphoproliferative disorders
Tissue specific	
Tyrosinase	Melanoma
gp100	Melanoma
Prostatic acid phosphatase	Prostate cancer
Prostate-specific antigen	Prostate cancer
Prostate-specific membrane antigen	Prostate cancer
Thyroglobulin	Thyroid cancer
α-fetoprotein	Liver cancer
Overexpressed	
Her-2/*neu*	Breast and lung cancers
Carcinoembryonic antigen	Colorectal, lung, breast cancer
Muc-1	Colorectal, pancreatic, ovarian, lung cancer

since not only is it unreasonable to expect the immune system to cope with a large tumor mass, but considerable amounts of antigen released by shedding would tend to prevent the generation of any significant response in some cases due to the stimulation of T-suppressors. This leaves the small secondary deposits as the proper target for immunotherapy.

Antigen-independent cytokine therapy

Sporadic successes have greeted the use of components of the immune system for antigen-independent therapy.

Interleukin treatment

On activation by IL-2 or IL-12, NK cells are capable of killing a variety of fresh tumor cells *in vitro* and, on the basis of studies on mice with mammary glands carrying the HER-2/*neu* oncogene, it would not be unreasonable to conduct a trial of systematic IL-12 treatment in cancer patients with minimum residual disease in an attempt to prevent recurrence and to inhibit incipient metastases.

Interferon therapy

In trials using IFNα and IFNβ, a 10–15% objective response rate was seen in patients with renal carcinoma, melanoma and myeloma, an approximate 20% response rate among patients with Kaposi's sarcoma, about 40% positive responders in patients with various lymphomas and a remarkable response rate of 80–90% among patients with hairy cell leukemia and mycosis fungoides.

With regard to the mechanisms of the antitumor effects, in certain tumors IFNs may serve primarily as antiproliferative agents; in others, the activation of NK cells and macrophages may be important, while augmenting the expression of class I MHC molecules may make the tumors more susceptible to control by immune effector mechanisms. In some circumstances the antiviral effect could be contributory.

For diseases like renal cell cancer and hairy cell leukemia, IFNs have induced responses in a significantly higher proportion of patients than have conventional therapies. However, in the wider setting, most investigators consider that their role will be in combination therapy, e.g. with active immunotherapy or with various chemotherapeutic agents where synergistic action has been observed in murine tumor systems. IFNα and β synergize with IFNγ and the latter synergizes with TNF. IFNα acts as a radiation sensitizer and its ability to increase the expression of estrogen receptors on cultured breast cancer cells suggests the possibility of combining IFN with anti-estrogens in this disease.

Colony-stimulating factors

Normal cell development proceeds from an immature stem cell with the capacity for unlimited self-renewal, through committed progenitors, to the final lineage-specific differentiated cells with little or no potential for self-renewal. Therapy aimed at inducing tumor cell differentiation is founded on the idea that the induction of cell maturation decreases and possibly abrogates the capacity of the malignant clone to divide. Along these lines, GM-CSF has been shown to enhance the differentiation, decrease the self-renewal capacity and suppress the leukemogenicity of murine myeloid leukemias. Recombinant human products are now undergoing trials.

It is over 100 years since the physician Coley gave his name to the mixture of microbial products termed **Coley's toxin**. This concoction certainly livens up the innate immune system and does produce remission in a minority of patients. The suggestion has been made that these beneficial effects are due to the release of TNF since the vascular endothelium of tumors is unduly susceptible to damage by this cytokine and hemorrhagic necrosis is readily induced. It is questionable whether the critical levels of TNF are reached in the human since these would be very toxic, although one study involving perfusion of an isolated limb with TNF, IFNγ and melphalan provoked lesions in the tumor endothelium without affecting the normal vasculature. Opinion is coming round to the view that the Coley phenomenon may be linked more to boosting a pre-existing weak antitumor immunity.

Exploitation of cell-mediated immune responses

The current dogma is that T-cells rather than antibodies are capable of savaging solid tumors, particularly those expressing processed intracellular antigens on their surface, and, since the majority are MHC class II negative, it looks as though we are aiming at essentially CD8 cytotoxic T-cell responses, although CD4 T-cells can be involved in protective reactions against tumor-associated vasculature.

Virally induced tumors

Based on the not unreasonable belief that certain forms of cancer (e.g. lymphoma) are caused by oncogenic viruses, attempts are being made to isolate the virus and prepare a suitable vaccine from it. In fact, large-scale protection of chickens against the development of Marek's disease lymphoma has been successfully achieved by vaccination with another herpes virus native to turkeys. In human Burkitt's lymphoma, work is in progress to develop a vaccine to exploit the ability of Tc cells to target **EBV-related antigens** on the cells of all Burkitt's tumors. It may be an advantage to treat the patient at the same time with cytokines to upregulate the expression of ICAM-1, LFA-3 and possibly of the virus itself.

Immunization with whole tumor cells

This has the advantage that we do not necessarily have to know the identity of the antigen concerned. The disadvantage is that the majority of tumors are weakly immunogenic, and do not present antigen effectively and so cannot overcome the **barrier to activation of resting T-cells**. Remember, the surface MHC–peptide complex on its own is not enough; costimulation with molecules such as B7.1 and B7.2 and possibly certain cytokines is required to push the G0 T-cell into active proliferation and differentiation. Once we get to this stage, however, **the activated T-cell no longer requires the accessory costimulation** to react with its target, for which it has a greatly increased avidity due to upregulation of accessory binding molecules such as CD2 and LFA-1 (cf. p. 165; figure 18.9). The system works! Vaccination with B7-transfected murine melanoma generated CD8⁺ cytolytic effectors which protected against subsequent tumor challenge; in other words, transfection enabled the melanoma cells to present their own antigens efficiently, while the untransfected cells were vulnerable targets for the cytotoxic T-cells so produced. A further telling observation was that an irradiated nonimmunogenic melanoma line which had been transfected with a retroviral vector carrying the *GM-CSF* gene stimulated potent and specific antitumor immunity, almost certainly by enhancing the differentiation and activation of host antigen-presenting cells. A less sophisticated but more convenient approach ultimately utilizing similar mechanisms involves the administration of the irradiated melanoma cells together with BCG which, by generating a plethora of inflammatory cytokines, increases the efficiency of presentation of tumor antigens derived from necrotic cells. In a large-scale study of over 1500 patients, 26% of vaccinees were alive at 5 years compared with only 6% of those treated with the best available conventional therapy. It would be exciting to suppose that in the future we might expose a tumor surgically and then transfect it *in situ* by firing gold particles (cf. p. 302) bearing appropriate gene constructs such as B7, IFNγ (to upregulate MHC class I and II), GM-CSF, IL-2, and so on (figure 18.9). There is a real risk of inducing autoimmune responses to cryptic epitopes (cf. p. 407) shared with other normal tissues which the prudent investigator will not overlook.

Therapy with subunit vaccines

The variety of potential protein targets so far identified (table 18.2) has spawned a considerable investment in clinical therapeutic trials using peptides as vaccines. Because of the pioneering work in characterizing melanoma-specific antigens, this tumor has been the focus of numerous studies which exploit to the full the academic background to modern immunology. Encouraging results in terms of clinical benefit, linked to the generation of cytolytic T-cells (CTLs), have been obtained following vaccination with peptides complexed with heat-shock proteins or modified at class I anchor residues to improve MHC binding. The inclusion of accessory factors, such as IL-2 or GM-CSF, and **CTLA-4 blockade** can be crucial for success. Poten-

Figure 18.9. Immunotherapy by transfection with costimulatory molecules. The tumor can only stimulate the resting T-cell with the costimulatory help of B7-1 and -2 and/or cytokines such as GM-CSF, γ-interferon and various interleukins, IL-2, -4 and -7. CTLA-4 blockade enhances immunogenicity. Alternatively, the T-cell can be stimulated directly by tumor antigens presented by dendritic cells (DCs) which can themselves be activated by cross-linking their surface CD40 with antibody (see below). Once activated, the T-cell with upregulated accessory molecules can now attack the original tumor lacking costimulators.

tially tolerogenic peptide vaccines can be converted into strong primers for CTL responses by triggering CD40 with a cross-linking antibody which can substitute for T-cell help in the direct activation of CTLs (figure 18.10). Anti-CD40 treatment alone was also shown to partially protect mice bearing *CD40-negative* lymphoma cells, an effect attributed to the activation of endogenous dendritic antigen-presenting cells (cf. figure 18.9).

The unique **idiotype** on monoclonal B-cell tumors is a mouth-watering target for immunotherapy. Although one might expect the unique sequences in the hypervariable CDR loops to be the obvious candidates, one study has revealed that peptides derived from the **immunoglobulin framework** function as commonly expressed CTL epitopes. The advantage here is that one does not have to synthesize an individual idiotype peptide for each patient, while mutations in the idiotypic determinant, which would allow the tumor to escape from the immune response, are far less likely to occur with a framework peptide. Whether this approach will prove ultimately preferable to those employing scFv vaccines cannot be predicted at present. A DNA construct of a tumor scFv fused to a pathogen-derived sequence from tetanus toxin gave excellent protective immunity against a mouse myeloma; there was no surface Ig on the tumor cells and protection must have been afforded through targeting of processed idiotype complexed with MHC by CD4 and CD8 cells.

Anticipating a more widespread use of naked DNA for immunotherapy, immunogenicity has been enhanced by making the vaccine **self-replicating** using a construct with a gene encoding RNA replicase from Semliki Forest virus. The improved efficacy correlated with caspase-dependent apoptotic death of transfected cells which facilitated their uptake by dendritic cells. Concurrent IL-12 proved to be a potent accessory adjuvant. These alphavirus replicon-based RNA vaccines are noninfectious and reversion cannot occur because the constructs lack structural protein genes; further, since they do not go through a DNA intermediate, there is little chance of genomic integration.

The sheer power of the **dendritic antigen-presenting cell (DC)** for the initiation of T-cell responses has been the focus of an ever-burgeoning series of immunotherapeutic strategies which have elicited tumor-specific protective immune responses via injection of isolated DC loaded with tumor lysates or tumor antigens or peptides derived from them. Considerable success has been achieved in animal models and increasingly with human patients (figure 18.11). The copious numbers of DCs needed for each patient's individual therapy are obtained by expansion of CD34-positive precursors in bone marrow by culture with GM-CSF, IL-4 and TNF, and sometimes with extra goodies such as stem cell factor (SCF) and Fms-like tyrosine kinase 3 (Flt3)-ligand. CD14-positive monocytes from peripheral blood are easier to access, and generate DC in the presence of GM-CSF plus IL-4; however, they need additional maturation with TNFα which increases cost and the chance of bacterial contamination. Another approach is to expand the DCs *in vivo* by administration of Flt3-ligand. The circulating blood DCs increase in number 10–30-fold and can be harvested by leukophoresis.

Some general points may be made. First, where peptides are used to load the DC, sequences which bind strongly to a given MHC class I haplotype must be identified; sequences will vary between patients with different haplotypes and they may not include potential CD4 helper epitopes. Recombinant proteins will overcome most of these difficulties, and a mixture should be even better since it should recruit more CTLs and be more able to 'ride out' any new tumor antigen mutations. However, proteins taken up by DCs are relatively inefficient at 'cross-priming' CD8 CTLs through the class I processing pathway, although several tactics are being explored to circumvent this problem: they include conjugation to an HIV-tat 'transporter' peptide which increases class I presentation

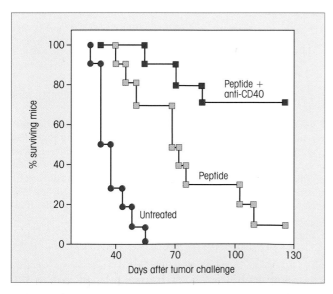

Figure 18.10. CD40 ligation enhances the protective effect of a peptide vaccine against a pre-existing tumor. Six days after injection of human papilloma virus-16 (HPV16)-transformed syngeneic cells, mice were immunized with the HPV16-E7 peptide in incomplete Freund's adjuvant with or without an anti-CD40 monoclonal, or left untreated. (Data from Diehl L. *et al.* (1999) *Nature Medicine* **5**, 774, reproduced with permission.)

(a)   (b)

Figure 18.11. Clinical response to autologous vaccine utilizing dendritic cells pulsed with idiotype from a B-cell lymphoma. Computed tomography scan through patient's chest (a) prevaccine and (b) 10 months after completion of three vaccine treatments. The arrow in (a) points to a paracardiac mass. All sites of disease had resolved and the patient remained in remission 24 months after beginning treatment. (Photography kindly supplied by Professor R. Levy from the article by Hsu F.J. *et al.* (1996) *Nature Medicine* **2**, 52; reproduced by kind permission of Nature America Inc.)

100-fold and transfection with RNA and recombinant vectors such as fowlpox. Second, the procedure is cumbersome and costly but, if it becomes common, it will be streamlined and, anyway, the costs must be set against the expenses of conventional therapy and the immeasurable benefit to the patient. Third, why does the administration of small numbers of antigen-pulsed DCs induce specific T-cell responses and tumor regression in patients in whom both the antigen and DCs are already plentiful? The suggestion has been made that DCs in or near malignant tissues may be defective, perhaps due to vascular endothelium growth factor (VEGF) or IL-10 secretion by the tumor. It will certainly be interesting to see whether direct treatment of patients with Flt3-ligand plus accessory cytokines or intratumoral transfection with MIP-3α (CCL20) (cf. p. 187), which attracts immature DCs, can initiate an antitumor response through maturation and activation of endogenous DCs.

Treatment of leukemia

Radical cytoablative treatment of leukemia patients using radiochemotherapy will destroy bone marrow stem cells. These can be removed prior to treatment, purged of any leukemic cells with cytotoxic antibodies, and reinfused subsequently to 'rescue' the patient (figure 18.12). However, not all leukemic cells are eliminated by this treatment, and a more effective strategy is transplantation of *allogeneic* bone marrow from reasonably MHC-compatible donors which exerts an important, albeit not completely understood, graft-vs-leukemia effect. Purging the bone marrow of T-cells to prevent graft-vs-host (g.v.h.) disease, which is a seri-

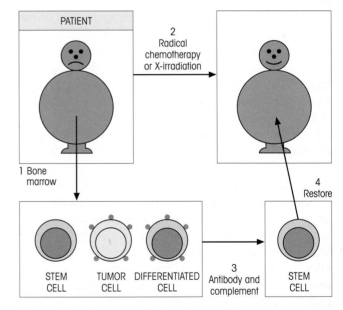

Figure 18.12. Treatment of leukemias by autologous bone marrow rescue. By using cytotoxic antibodies to a differentiation antigen (●) present on leukemic cells and even on other normal differentiated cells, but absent from stem cells, it is possible to obtain a tumor-free population of the latter which can be used to restore hematopoietic function in patients subsequently treated radically to destroy the leukemic cells. Another angle is positive selection of stem cells utilizing the CD34 marker.

ous complication of such transplants, would at the same time remove the prized antileukemic activity. A dilemma. 'Suicide gene therapy' could provide a solution as illustrated in figure 18.13. Stem cells from the T-cell-purged allogeneic bone marrow are given together with donor T-cells transfected with herpes simplex virus thymidine kinase. The T-cells provide

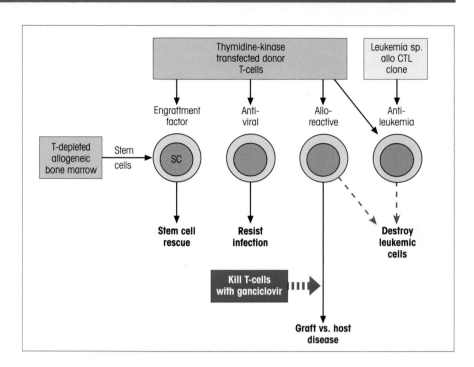

Figure 18.13. Treatment of leukemia with allogeneic bone marrow transfer. T-depleted allogeneic marrow provides the stem cells to 'rescue' the patient treated with cytoablative therapy. T-cells from the donor, transfected with thymidine kinase (TK), help engraftment, provide protection against infection and eliminate residual tumor cells by a graft-vs-leukemia effect. The alloreactive cells eventually produce graft-vs-host disease and can be eliminated by administration of ganciclovir. This is converted by the TK into a nucleoside analog which ultimately becomes toxic for dividing cells. The alternative shown is to destroy leukemic cells by supplementing purged allogeneic marrow with a leukemia peptide-specific CTL clone produced in third party T-cells. (Based on articles by Cohen J.L., Boyer O. & Klatzmann D. (1999) *Immunology Today* **20**, 172; and Stauss H.J. (1999) *Immunology Today* **20**, 180.)

factors which facilitate engraftment, defense against viral infection and the graft-vs-leukemia action at a time when the recipient patient will have a low tumor burden. With time, as graft-vs-host disease develops, the dividing aggressor donor T-cells can be switched off by administration of ganciclovir through the mechanism explained in the legend to figure 18.13.

An alternative which avoids g.v.h. disease altogether is to inject the purged bone marrow together with an allogeneic cytotoxic T-cell clone specific for a leukemia-associated peptide presented by the MHC allele of the prospective recipient patient. This usually works because the residues on the MHC helices which contact the T-cell receptor are relatively conserved (unlike those within the groove), so that the allo-T-cells can recognize the MHC–peptide complex from the leukemia. Potential targets are cyclin-D1 and mdm-2 which are overexpressed in tumor cells and, in leukemic cells in particular, the transcription factors WT-1 and GATA1 and the differentiation antigens myeloperoxidase and CD68, which are expressed exclusively in hematopoietic cells and are likely to have established tolerance in the patient but not in the allogeneic CTL donor (who will have been exposed to different processed peptides) (cf. p. 353). A rather masterful development would be to transfect the recipient with the genes encoding the T-cell receptor of the allo-CTL clone. Again, looking to the future, transfection of T-cells *in vitro* with a humanized scFv–Fcγ–transmembrane segment–CD3ζ construct

has been shown to render them cytotoxic for cells expressing the surface antigen.

Therapy with monoclonal antibodies

The strategies

Antibodies reacting with antigens on the surface of tumor cells can protect the host by complement-mediated opsonization and lysis (modified by host complement regulatory proteins) and through recruitment of macrophage and NK ADCC function by engagement of FcγRIII receptors, although for macrophages this is partially countered by inhibitory FcγRII signals. These FcR-bearing cells serve not only as cytotoxic effectors but also as multivalent surfaces which hyper-cross-link antibody-coated target cells so providing, in many cases, a transmembrane signal which leads to apoptosis or premature exit from the cell cycle. This effect appears to sensitize neoplastic cells to irradiation and DNA-damaging chemotherapy and holds out the exciting prospect of novel synergistic treatments whose efficacy may be enhanced by the increased immunogenicity of the dying cells.

Immunologists have long been bemused by the idea of eliminating tumor cells by specific antibody linked to a killer molecule and there is a truly impressive array of ingenious initiatives. It is axiomatic that multimeric fragments bind much more avidly than monomeric fragments due principally to the lower off-rates (cf. p. 87), and that constructs in the 60–120 kDa range are optimal for targeting solid tumors—too large and penetration is difficult, too small and kidney secretion is excessively fast. Monovalent fragments include Fv, scFv selected by antigen from phage libraries (cf. p. 124) and V_H domains based on the large CDR loops of the camels and llamas. For polymers we have bivalent and bispecific (think about the difference) diabodies (cf. p. 125), trivalent and trispecific triabodies, even tetrabodies, and Fabs have been linked into dimers or trimers.

Radioimmunotherapy, using isotopes such as ^{90}Y, ^{111}In or ^{131}I linked to antibody, delivers doses of radiation to tumor tissue which would be impossibly toxic with external beam sources. Results are even better when used in synergy with chemotherapy. Immunotoxins represent another class of magic bullet in which the toxin of plant or bacterial origin is attached to an antibody or growth factor; after binding to the cell surface, the toxin is internalized and kills the cell by catalytic inhibition of protein synthesis. Along the same lines, internalizing a photosensitizer renders the cells vulnerable to photodynamic therapy. Delivery of anticancer drugs by attachment to antibodies would seem to be an obvious goal, but a more sophisticated strategy involves the grand sounding antibody-directed enzyme-prodrug therapy (ADEPT). After injection of the prodrug, each antibody–enzyme conjugate attached to its cell target produces a large number of small toxic molecules which can diffuse into the tumor mass and also give a bystander effect on adjacent tumor cells even if they express only low levels of antigen. Aminopeptidase which acts on 2-L-pyroglutamyl methotrexate to liberate methotrexate is one of the conjugates used.

Clinical results

Useful responses to unmodified monoclonal antibodies have been chalked up. These include anti-Her-2 (an epidermal growth factor receptor also known as erbB2 and neu) for metastatic breast cancer, anti-CD52 (Campath-1H) for a range of hematological tumors and 17-1A for colorectal cancer.

^{131}I-labeled anti-CD20 kills B-cell lymphomas by ADCC and by signaling-induced apoptosis, acting in synergy with DNA damage due to γ-radiation, with perhaps a contribution from enhanced tumor immunogenicity. Therapy with this agent has been spectacularly successful; in one long-term trial, injection of the radiolabeled anti-CD20 into lymphoma patients prepared by myeloablation with stem cell rescue gave major responses in 86% with remissions lasting from 27 to 87 months. Likewise, radionuclide conjugates of a humanized anti-CD33 score very highly in myeloid leukemia and can root out large tumor burdens. Trials of ^{90}Y-anti-MUC-1 in ovarian cancer provide further encouragement for the intrepid immunotherapists.

Attack on the tumor blood supply

For solid tumors, the focus is upon two main targets. The first would be **minimal residual micrometastases in the bone marrow** which occur in one-third to one-half of patients with epithelial cancer after curative radical treatment of the primary lesion. The second would be the **reactive tissue evoked by the malignant process**, such as stromal fibroblasts expressing the F19 glycoprotein and newly formed blood vessels.

Tumors generally cannot grow beyond the size of 1 mm in diameter without the support of blood vessels and, because the tumor is new tissue, its blood vessels will also have to be new. These vessels form through the process known as **angiogenesis**, the sprouting of new blood vessels from existing ones, but they are biochemically and structurally different from normal resting blood vessels and so provide differential targets for therapeutic monoclonal antibodies, even though the cancer cells themselves in a solid tumor are less vulnerable to antibodies directed to specific antigens on their surface. Thus, receptors for VEGF and Eph, oncofetal fibronectin, matrix metalloproteases MMP-2 and MMP-9 and the pericyte markers aminopeptidase A and the NG2 proteoglycan are all highly and selectively expressed in vasculature undergoing angiogenesis.

A noteworthy maneuver, which is unexpectedly successful, is to identify peptides which home specifically to the endothelial cells of certain tumors by injecting peptide phage libraries *in vivo*. One of the panel of peptide motifs which has emerged from this probing strategy includes RGD in the cyclic peptide CDCRGD-CFC, a selective binder of the $\alpha_V\beta_3$- and $\alpha_V\beta_5$-integrins known to be upregulated in angiogenic tumor endothelial cells. For therapeutic exploitation, these peptides can be linked to appropriate drugs, such as doxorubicin, or a pro-apoptotic peptide. Overall, there are undoubtedly a substantial number of targets for the 'magic bullets'.

IMMUNODIAGNOSIS OF SOLID TUMORS

Circulating and cellular tumor markers

Analysis of blood for the oncofetal antigens, α-fetoprotein in hepatoma and carcinoembryonic antigen in tumors of the colon, has provided valuable diagnostic information, but enthusiasm has been slightly curtailed by the knowledge that there is a high incidence of so-called 'false positives'. Reappearance of these proteins after surgical removal of the primary is strongly indicative of fresh tumor growth. A hefty increase in the ratio of free to bound prostate-specific antigen (PSA) in the blood may signal cancer of the prostate. The GM1 monosialoganglioside has been demonstrated in the blood of 96% of patients with pancreatic carcinoma and 64% of patients with colorectal carcinomas, as against 2% in normal subjects.

Identification of the cell type by monoclonal antibodies is of value for the diagnosis and treatment of an increasing number of tumors, including the lymphoproliferative disorders as discussed earlier (see p. 382).

Table 18.3. Detection of bone marrow micrometastases by staining for epithelial cytokeratin in colorectal cancer patients. (From data of Schlimok G. *et al.* (1990) *Journal of Clinical Oncology* 8, 831.)

Dukes' Stage		Positive reaction with mAb CK2 for cytokeratin in bone marrow aspirate	
		No. patients	% Positive
A	Limited to mucosa	3	0
B	Extending into muscularis propria	58	14
C	Involving local nodes	62	34
D	With distant metastatic spread	33	39

Tumor imaging *in vivo*

The same principles which govern the localization of monoclonal antibodies for tumor therapy apply equally to imaging. Maximizing the binding to tumor relative to normal tissue and surrounding fluids is the name of the game. For example, the use of a bifunctional antibody which targets the tumor and an isotope chelator can be followed 24–120 hours later with the chelate-containing radionuclide which allows clearance of uncombined antibody.

The Thomson–Friedenreich (T) antigen (Galβ1-3-GalNAcα-O-Ser), expressed in the mucins of various types of epithelial cancer, has proved to be a highly successful target for antibody imaging. So has the F19 glycoprotein associated with proliferating fibroblasts in the stroma of many carcinomas, as presumably the many antigens associated with tumor angiogenesis will prove to be.

Detection of micrometastases in bone marrow

Because of the difficulty in detecting individual tumor cells in distant organs, the diagnosis of early disseminated cancer has not been possible, and attempts to identify earlier stages and to monitor the immunotherapy of early disease have been hindered. A major advance was made when micrometastases were demonstrated by immunocytochemistry in the bone marrow of patients with colorectal cancer and were related to more widespread disease (table 18.3) and a high relapse rate. The method involves scanning pelvic crest bone marrow aspirates taken at surgery for epithelial cells by staining for cytokeratin (cf. figure 18.7f) and proliferation markers such as the Ki67 nuclear antigen and receptors for transferrin and epidermal growth factor. Detection of micrometastases in the marrow of patients with small cell lung carcinoma also predicted early relapse.

SUMMARY

Changes on the surface of tumor cells

• Processed peptides derived from oncogenic viruses are powerful MHC-associated transplantation antigens.

• Some tumors express genes which are silent in normal tissues: sometimes they have been expressed previously in embryonic life (oncofetal antigens).

• Many tumors express weak antigens associated with point mutations in oncogenes such as *ras* and *p53*. Peptides presented by heat-shock proteins 70 and 90 represent the unique chemically induced tumor antigens. The surface Ig on chronic lymphocytic leukemia (CLL) cells is a unique tumor-specific antigen.

• Dysregulation of tumor cells frequently causes structural abnormalities in surface carbohydrate structures.

• Some surface changes are a consequence of cell division *per se*.

(*continued p. 394*)

- The v6 and v10 exons of CD44 are intimately involved with metastatic potential. Loss of blood group A determinants leads to a poor prognosis.

Immune response to tumors

- T-cells generally mount effective surveillance against tumors associated with oncogenic viruses or UV induction which are strongly immunogenic.
- More weakly immunogenic tumors are not controlled by T-cell surveillance, although sometimes low-grade responses are evoked.
- NK cells probably play a role in containing tumor growth and metastases. They can attack MHC class I-negative tumor cells because the class I molecule imparts a negative inactivation signal to NK cells. The A-NK subset, which expresses high levels of adhesion molecules, is more cytolytic for fresh tumor cells.
- Tumors utilize a variety of mechanisms to escape host immune responses.

Unregulated development gives rise to lymphoproliferative disorders

- Deregulation of the c-*myc* protooncogene is a characteristic feature of many B-cell tumors.
- Chromosome translocations are common.
- Lymphoid malignancies show maturation arrest at characteristic stages in differentiation.
- The surface markers of leukemias and lymphomas identified by monoclonal antibodies are important aids in diagnosis. Most non-Hodgkin's lymphomas are of B-cell origin, are associated with EBV and express a monoclonal surface Ig.
- Multiple myeloma represents a malignant proliferation of a single clone of plasma cells producing a single 'M' band on electrophoresis. 10–20% have widespread amyloid deposits containing the variable region of the myeloma light chain.
- Waldenström's macroglobulinemia is produced by unregulated proliferation of a clone producing monoclonal IgM causing a marked rise in serum viscosity.
- Malignant lymphoid cells produce secondary immunodeficiency by suppressing differentiation of the corresponding normal lineage.

Approaches to cancer immunotherapy

- Immunotherapy is only likely to work after a tumor mass has been debulked.
- Innate immune mechanisms can be harnessed. Systemic IL-12 may be effective against minimal residual disease. IFNγ and β are very effective in the T-cell disorders, hairy cell leukemia and mycosis fungoides, less so but still

significant in Kaposi's sarcoma and various lymphomas; they may be used in synergy with other therapies. GM-CSF enhances proliferation and decreases leukemogenicity of murine myeloid leukemias.
- Cancer vaccines based on oncogenic viral proteins can be expected.
- Weakly immunogenic tumors provoke effective anticancer responses if given with an adjuvant, such as BCG, or if transfected with costimulatory molecules, such as B7 and cytokines IFNγ, IL-2, -4 and -7. CD8 CTLs are favored for the attack on solid tumors.
- A variety of potential protein targets have been identified and intense effort is being expended in the investigation of peptides as subunit vaccines. Their immunogenicity can be enhanced by complexing with heat-shock proteins and by accessory factors such as GM-CSF, CTLA-4 blockade and anti-CD40 stimulation.
- Naked DNA and self-replicating RNA vaccines are strong candidates.
- Powerful immunogens have been created by pulsing dendritic antigen-presenting cells with peptides from melanoma antigens and framework regions of CLL Ig.
- A graft-vs-leukemia effect is achieved by allogeneic CTLs or by allogeneic bone marrow transplantation with measures to limit graft-vs-host disease.
- Monoclonal antibodies conjugated to toxins or radionuclides can target tumor cells or antigens on new blood vessels or the reactive stromal fibroblasts associated with malignancy. Encouraging, even impressive, therapeutic results have been obtained with antibodies to CD20 in B-cell lymphoma, CD33 in myeloid leukemia, anti-MUC-1 in ovarian cancer and c-erbB2 overexpressed on breast cancers. Bifunctional antibodies can bring effectors such as NK and Tc close to the tumor target.

Immunodiagnosis of solid tumors

- Many circulating tumor markers are diagnostic, e.g. α-fetoprotein in hepatic carcinoma and carcinoembryonic antigen in colorectal carcinoma.
- Monoclonal antibody to tumor surfaces can provide a basis for imaging. Certain tumor mucins, the F19 glycoprotein on reactive stromal fibroblasts and VEGF on new blood vessels around the tumor are good targets.
- Detection of micrometastases in bone marrow by immunocytochemistry provides valuable information on prognosis and the efficacy of new therapies.

See the accompanying website (**www.roitt.com**) for multiple choice questions.

FURTHER READING

Begent R.H.J. *et al.* (1996) Clinical evidence of efficient tumor targeting based on single-chain Fv antibody selected from a combinatorial library. *Nature Medicine* **2**, 979.

Blachere N.E. et al. (1997) Heat shock protein–peptide complexes, reconstituted in vitro, elicit peptide-specific cytotoxic T-lymphocyte responses and tumor immunity. (Strategy initiated by P.K. Srivastava.) *Journal of Experimental Medicine* **186**, 1315.

Cancer (2001) *Current Opinion in Immunology* **13**(5). (Critical overviews of the whole field appearing annually, which are well-worth reading.)

Castellino F. *et al.* (2000) Receptor-mediated uptake of antigen/heat shock protein complexes (by antigen-presenting cells) results in MHC class I antigen presentation via two distinct processing pathways (TAP/proteasome and endosomal). *Journal of Experimental Medicine* **191**, 1957.

Fong L. & Engleman E.G. (2000) Dendritic cells in cancer immunotherapy. *Annual Review of Immunology* **18**, 245.

Forbes I.J. & Leong A.S.-Y. (1987) *Essential Oncology of the Lymphocyte.* Springer-Verlag, Berlin.

Leonard R.C.F., Duncan L.W. & Hay F.G. (1990) Immunocytological detection of residual marrow disease at clinical remission predicts metastatic relapse in small cell lung cancer. *Cancer Research* **50**, 6545.

Mannel D., Murray C., Risau W. & Clauss M. (1996) Tumor necrosis: factors and principles. *Immunology Today* **17**, 254.

Morton D.L. & Barth A. (1996) Vaccine therapy for malignant melanoma. *CA: A Cancer Journal for Clinicians* **46**, 225.

Ruoslahti E. & Rajotte D. (2000) An address system in the vasculature of normal tissues and tumors. *Annual Review of Immunology* **18**, 813.

Stein H. & Mason D.Y. (1985) Immunological analysis of tissue sections in diagnosis of lymphoma. In A.V. Hoffbrand (ed.) *Recent Advances in Haematology*, Vol. 4, p. 127. Churchill Livingstone, Edinburgh.

Van Elsas A., Hurwitz A.A. & Allison J.P. (1999) Combination immunotherapy of B16 melanoma using anti-CTLA-4 and GM-CSF-producing vaccines induces rejection of s.c. and metastatic tumors accompanied by autoimmune depigmentation. *Journal of Experimental Medicine* **190**, 355.

Van Ginderachter J.A. *et al.* (2000) B7-1, IFN-γ and anti-CTLA-4 co-operate to prevent T-cell tolerization during immunotherapy against a murine T-lymphoma. *Journal of Cancer* **87**, 539.

Autoimmune diseases
1 — Scope and etiology

INTRODUCTION

The monumental repertoire of the adaptive immune system has evolved to allow it to recognize and ensnare virtually any shaped microbial molecules, either at present in existence or yet to come, and in so doing, has been unable to avoid the generation of lymphocytes which react with the body's own constituents. This is abundantly so for T-cells which actually depend upon a degree of self-recognition for positive selection to operate during their development within the thymus gland (p. 228). We have already discussed the mechanisms which exist to prevent these self-components from provoking an adaptive immune response but, as with all machinery, there is always a chance that these systems might break down, and the older the individual, the greater the chance of this happening. Notwithstanding the IgM low affinity **autoantibodies** (i.e. antibodies capable of reacting with 'self'-components) produced by CD5$^+$ B-cells as part of the 'natural' antibody spectrum which we will discuss later, we are here concerned more with autoimmune phenomena which appear in relation to certain defined human diseases. Ideally, we wish to apply the term '**autoimmune disease**' to those cases where it can be shown that the **autoimmune process contributes to the pathogenesis of the disease** rather than situations where apparently harmless autoantibodies are formed following tissue damage, e.g. heart antibodies appearing after a myocardial infarction. Yet the role of autoimmunity in many disorders is still not clearly defined, and it is as a matter of convenience that we will refer to all maladies firmly associated with autoantibody formation as 'autoimmune diseases', except where it can be shown that the immunological phenomena are purely secondary findings.

THE SCOPE OF AUTOIMMUNE DISEASES

The spectrum of autoimmune diseases

These disorders may be looked upon as forming a spectrum. At one end we have '**organ-specific diseases**' with organ-specific autoantibodies. **Hashimoto's disease** of the thyroid is an example: there is a specific lesion in the thyroid involving infiltration by mononuclear cells (lymphocytes, macrophages and plasma cells), destruction of follicular cells and germinal center formation, accompanied by the production of circulating antibodies with absolute specificity for certain thyroid constituents (Milestone 19.1).

Milestone 19.1 — The Discovery of Thyroid Autoimmunity

Although Dacie's studies on red cell autoantibodies in certain forms of hemolytic anemia were amongst the earliest to implicate autoimmunity in the pathogenesis of disease, a direct link to disorders affecting whole organs was not established until 1956 when three major papers on thyroid autoimmunity appeared.

In an attempt to confirm Paul Ehrlich's concept of 'horror autotoxicus'—the body's dread of making antibodies to self—Rose and Witebsky immunized rabbits with rabbit thyroid extract in complete Freund's adjuvant. To what one might hazard was Witebsky's dismay and Rose's delight, this procedure resulted in the production of thyroid autoantibodies and chronic inflammatory destruction of the thyroid gland architecture (figure M19.1.1a and b).

Having noted the fall in serum γ-globulin which followed removal of the goiter in Hashimoto's thyroiditis and the similarity of the histology (figure M19.1.1c) to that of Rose and Witebsky's rabbits, Roitt, Doniach and Campbell tested the hypothesis that the plasma cells in the gland might be making an autoantibody to a thyroid component, so causing the tissue damage and chronic inflammatory response. Sure enough, the sera of the first patients tested had precipitating antibodies to an autoantigen in

(a)

(b)

(c)

Figure M19.1.1. Experimental autoallergic thyroiditis. (a) The follicular architecture of the normal thyroid. (b) Thyroiditis produced by immunization with rat thyroid extract in complete Freund's adjuvant; the invading chronic inflammatory cells have destroyed the follicular structure. (Based on the experiments of Rose N.R. & Witebsky E. (1956) Studies on organ specificity. V. Changes in the thyroid gland of rabbits following active immunization with rabbit thyroid extracts. *Journal of Immunology* **76**, 417.) (c) Similarity of lesions in spontaneous human autoimmune disease to those induced in the experimental model. Other features of Hashimoto's disease such as the eosinophilic metaplasia of acinar cells (Askenazy cells) and local lymphoid follicles are not seen in this experimental model, although the latter occur in the spontaneous thyroiditis of Obese strain chickens.

(continued p. 398)

Figure M19.1.2. Thyroid autoantibodies in the serum of a patient with Hashimoto's disease demonstrated by precipitation in agar. Test serum is incorporated in agar in the bottom of the tube; the middle layer contains agar only, while the autoantigen is present in the top layer. As serum antibody and thyroid autoantigen diffuse towards each other, they form a zone of opaque precipitate in the middle layer. Saline and kidney extract controls are negative. (Based on Roitt I.M., Doniach D., Campbell P.N. & Hudson R.V. (1956) Autoantibodies in Hashimoto's disease. *Lancet* **ii**, 820.)

Figure M19.1.3. The long-acting thyroid stimulator in Graves' disease. Injection of TSH causes a rapid release of ^{131}I from the prelabeled animal thyroid in contrast to the prolonged release which follows injection of serum from a thyrotoxic patient. (Based on Adams D.D. & Purves H.D. (1956) Abnormal responses in the assay of thyrotrophin. *Proceedings of the University of Otago Medical School* **34**, 11.)

normal thyroid extracts which was soon identified as thyroglobulin (figure M19.1.2).

In far off New Zealand (depending on your geographical location!), Adams and Purves, in seeking a circulating factor which might be responsible for the hyperthyroidism of Graves' thyrotoxicosis, injected patient's serum into guinea-pigs whose thyroids had been prelabeled with ^{131}I, and followed the release of radiolabeled material from the gland with time. Whereas the natural pituitary thyroid-stimulating hormone (TSH) produced a peak in serum radioactivity some 4 hours or so after injection of the test animal, serum from thyrotoxic patients had a prolonged stimulatory effect (figure M19.1.3). The so-called *long-acting thyroid stimulator* (LATS) was ultimately shown to be an IgG mimicking TSH through its reaction with the TSH receptor but differing in its time-course of action, largely due to its longer half-life in the circulation.

Moving towards the center of the spectrum are those disorders where the lesion tends to be localized to a single organ but the antibodies are nonorgan-specific. A typical example would be **primary biliary cirrhosis** where the small bile ductule is the main target of inflammatory cell infiltration but the serum antibodies present—mainly mitochondrial—are not liver-specific.

At the other end of the spectrum are the '**nonorganspecific or systemic autoimmune diseases**' broadly belonging to the class of rheumatological disorders, exemplified by **systemic lupus erythematosus (SLE)**, where both lesions and autoantibodies are not confined to any one organ. Pathological changes are widespread and are primarily lesions of connective tissue with fibrinoid necrosis. They are seen in the skin (the 'lupus' butterfly rash on the face is characteristic),

kidney glomeruli, joints, serous membranes and blood vessels. In addition, the formed elements of the blood are often affected. A bizarre collection of autoantibodies is found, some of which react with the DNA and other nuclear constituents of all cells in the body.

An attempt to fit the major diseases considered to be associated with autoimmunity into this spectrum is shown in table 19.1.

Autoantibodies in human disease

At this stage in the discussion it may be of value to have a more precise account of the major autoantibodies detected in the different diseases to provide a framework for reference. Table 19.2 documents a list of these antibodies and the methods employed in their detection. The notes accompanying the table amplify specific

Table 19.1. Spectrum of autoimmune diseases.

ORGAN SPECIFIC

Hashimoto's thyroiditis
Primary myxedema
Graves' disease
Pernicious anemia
Autoimmune atrophic gastritis
Addison's disease
Premature menopause (few cases)
Male infertility (few cases)
Myasthenia gravis
Insulin-dependent diabetes mellitus
Goodpasture's syndrome
Pemphigus vulgaris
Pemphigoid
Sympathetic ophthalmia
Phacogenic uveitis
Multiple sclerosis
Autoimmune hemolytic anemia
Idiopathic thrombocytopenic purpura
Idiopathic leukopenia
Primary biliary cirrhosis
Active chronic hepatitis HBs−ve
Ulcerative colitis
Sjögren's syndrome
Rheumatoid arthritis
Scleroderma
Wegener's granulomatosis
Poly/dermatomyositis
Discoid lupus erythematosus
Systemic lupus erythematosus (SLE)

NONORGAN SPECIFIC

points, while some of the tests are illustrated in figures 19.1, 6.9, 6.10 and 7.3. As antigens are characterized and become available in purified form, the convenient ELISA is becoming a dominant technique.

Overlap of autoimmune disorders

There is a tendency for more than one autoimmune disorder to occur in the same individual and when this happens the association is often between diseases within the same region of the autoimmune spectrum (cf. table 19.1). Thus patients with autoimmune thyroiditis (Hashimoto's disease or primary myxedema) have a much higher incidence of pernicious anemia than would be expected in a random population matched for age and sex (10% as against 0.2%). Conversely, both thyroiditis and Graves' disease are diagnosed in pernicious anemia patients with an unexpectedly high frequency. Other associations are seen between Addison's disease and autoimmune thyroid disease and occur in the rare cases of juveniles with pernicious anemia and polyendocrinopathy which includes Addison's disease, hypoparathyroidism, diabetes and thyroiditis.

There is an even greater overlap in serological findings. Thirty per cent of patients with autoimmune thyroid disease have concomitant parietal cell antibodies in their serum. Conversely, thyroid antibodies have been demonstrated in up to 50% of pernicious anemia patients. It should be stressed that these are not cross-reacting antibodies. The thyroid-specific antibodies will not react with stomach and vice versa. When a serum reacts with both organs it means that two populations of antibodies are present, one with specificity for thyroid and the other for stomach.

At the nonorgan-specific end of the spectrum, systemic autoimmune disease such as SLE is clinically associated with rheumatoid arthritis and several other disorders which are themselves uncommon: hemolytic anemia, idiopathic leukopenia and thrombocytopenic purpura, dermatomyositis and Sjögren's syndrome. Antinuclear antibodies and antiglobulin (rheumatoid) factors are a general feature.

Sjögren's syndrome occupies an interesting position (table 19.3); aside from the clinical and serological features associated with systemic disease mentioned above, characteristics of an organ-specific disorder are evident. Antibodies reacting with salivary ducts are demonstrable and there is an abnormally high incidence of thyroid autoantibodies; histologically the affected lacrimal and salivary glands reveal changes of a similar nature to those seen in Hashimoto's disease, namely a replacement of the glandular elements by patchy lymphocytic and plasma cell granulomatous tissue. Associations between diseases at the two ends of the spectrum have been reported, but, as might be predicted from the serological data (table 19.3), they are not common.

Patients with organ-specific disorders are slightly more prone to develop cancer in the affected organ, whereas generalized lymphoreticular neoplasia shows up with uncommon frequency in nonorgan-specific disease.

Animal models of autoimmune disease

Both spontaneous and induced animal models have given tremendous insights into the nature of human autoimmune disease and, to assist our discussions, we felt it would be helpful to list them (table 19.4).

NATURE AND NURTURE

Genetic factors in autoimmune disease

Autoimmune phenomena tend to aggregate in certain families. For example, the first degree relatives (sibs, parents and children) of patients with Hashimoto's disease show a high incidence of thyroid autoantibodies (figure 19.2) and of overt and subclinical thyroiditis.

Table 19.2. Autoantibodies in human disease.

DISEASE	ANTIGEN	DETECTION OF IMMUNOLOGICAL REACTIVITY
Hashimoto's thyroiditis	Thyroglobulin	Precipitins; passive hemagglutination; ELISA
Primary myxedema	Thyroid peroxidase: Cytoplasmic	IFT on unfixed thyroid; passive hemagglutination; ELISA
	Cell surface	IFT on viable thyroid cells; C'-mediated cytotoxicity
Graves' disease	Cell surface TSH receptors	Bioassay–stimulation of mouse thyroid *in vivo*; blocking combination TSH with receptors; stimulation adenyl cyclase
	'Growth' receptors	Induction of cell division in thyroid fragments
Pernicious anemia	Intrinsic factor	Neutralization; blocking combination with vit-B_{12}; binding to intrinsic factor-B_{12} by coprecipitation
	Parietal cell H^+–K^+ ATPase	IFT on unfixed gastric mucosa
Addison's disease	Cytoplasm adrenal cells (17α-/21-hydroxylase)	IFT on unfixed adrenal cortex
Premature onset of menopause[1]	Cytoplasm steroid-producing cells	IFT on adrenal and interstitial cells of ovary and testis
Male infertility (some)[2]	Spermatozoa	Sperm agglutination in ejaculate
Insulin-dependent diabetes[3]	Cytoplasm of islet cells	IFT on unfixed human pancreas
	Insulin, GAD and ICA512	ELISA
Type B insulin resistance with acanthosis nigricans	Insulin receptor	Block hormone binding to receptor
Atopic allergy (some)	β-Adrenergic receptor	Blocking radioassay with hydroxybenzylpindolol
Myasthenia gravis	Skeletal and heart muscle	IFT on skeletal muscle
	Acetylcholine receptor	Blocking or binding radioassay with α-bungarotoxin
Lambert–Eaton syndrome	Ca^{2+} channels in nerve endings	IgG produces neuromuscular defects in mice
Multiple sclerosis[4]	Brain incl. MBP	MBP-reactive T-cells
Goodpasture's syndrome	Glomerular and lung basement membrane	Linear staining by IFT of kidney biopsy with fluorescent anti-IgG
		Radioimmunoassay with purified Ag; ELISA
Pemphigus vulgaris	Desmosomes between prickle cells in epidermis (cadherin)	IFT on skin
Pemphigoid	Basement membrane	IFT on skin
Phacogenic uveitis	Lens	Passive hemagglutination
Sympathetic ophthalmia	Uvea	(Delayed skin reaction to uveal extract)
Autoimmune hemolytic anemia[5]	Erythrocytes	Coombs' antiglobulin test
Idiopathic thrombocytopenic purpura	Platelets	Shortened platelet survival *in vivo*
Primary biliary cirrhosis	Mitochondria (pyruvate dehydrogenase)	IFT on mitochondria-rich cells (e.g. distal tubules of kidney)
Active chronic hepatitis (HBV & HCV −ve)	Smooth muscle/nuclear lamins/nuclei	IFT (e.g. on gastric mucosa)
	Kidney/liver microsomes (cyt P450)	IFT (kidney)
Ulcerative colitis	Colon 'lipopolysaccharide'	IFT; passive hemagglutination (cytotoxic action of lymphocytes on colon cells)
	Colon epithelial cell surface protein	ADCC on colon cancer cell line
		Ab data in this disease not universally accepted
Sjögren's syndrome[6]	SS-A(Ro) SS-B(La)	IFT; gel precipitation; ELISA
	Ducts/mitochondria/nuclei/thyroid	IFT
	IgG	Antiglobulin (rheumatoid factor) tests
Rheumatoid arthritis[7]	IgG	Antiglobulin test; latex agglutination; sheep red cell agglutination test (SCAT; commercial product, RAHA test) and ELISA; agalacto-glycoform
	Collagen	Passive hemagglutination
Discoid lupus erythematosus	Nuclear/IgG	IFT/antiglobulin test
Scleroderma[8]	Nuclear/IgG/centromere	IFT
	Nuclear/IgG/Scl-70	IFT; countercurrent electrophoresis; ELISA
Dermatomyositis[9]	Nuclear/IgG/Jo-1	IFT; countercurrent electrophoresis; ELISA
Mixed connective tissue disease[10]	Extractable nuclear	IFT; countercurrent electrophoresis; ELISA
Systemic lupus erythematosus	DNA[11]	ELISA; IFT on Crithidia
	snRNP (Sm & ribonucleoprotein)	IFT; gel precipitation techniques; ELISA
	Nucleoprotein	IFT
	Array of other Ag including formed elements of blood/IgG	
	Cardiolipin/β2-glycoprotein1	Radioimmunoassay
Wegener's granulomatosis	Neutrophil cytoplasm (ANCA; myeloperoxidase/serine proteinase)[12]	IFT on alcohol fixed polymorphs; ELISA

IFT, immunofluorescent test (cf. figure 7.3); ELISA, enzyme-linked immunosorbent assay (cf. figure 6.10).

Table 19.3. Organ-specific and nonorgan-specific serological interrelationships in human disease.

DISEASE	% POSITIVE REACTIONS FOR ANTIBODIES TO:			
	THYROID*	STOMACH*	NUCLEI*	IgG†
Hashimoto's thyroiditis	99.9	32	8	2
Pernicious anemia	55	89	11	
Sjögren's syndrome	45	14	56	75
Rheumatoid arthritis	11	16	50	75
SLE	2	2	99	35
Controls‡	0–15	0–16	0–19	2–5

*Immunofluorescence test.
†Rheumatoid factor classical tests.
‡Incidence increases with age and females > males.

Parallel studies have disclosed similar relationships in the families of pernicious anemia patients, in that gastric parietal cell antibodies are prevalent in the relatives who are wont to develop achlorhydria and atrophic gastritis. Turning to SLE, disturbances of immunoglobulin synthesis and a susceptibility to develop 'connective tissue diseases' have been reported, but there are some conflicting accounts still not resolved.

These familial relationships could be ascribed to environmental factors such as infective microorganisms, but there is powerful evidence that important genetic components must be involved. The data on **twins** is unequivocal. When thyrotoxicosis or insulin-dependent diabetes mellitus (IDDM) occurs in twins, there is a far greater concordance rate (i.e. both twins affected) in identical than in nonidentical twins. Second, we have already noted that lines of animals have been bred which spontaneously develop autoimmune disease (table 19.4). In other words, **the autoimmunity is genetically programed**. There is an Obese line of chickens with autoimmune thyroiditis, the Nonobese diabetic (NOD) mouse modeling human IDDM and the New Zealand Black (NZB) strain succumbing to autoimmune hemolytic anemia. The hybrid of NZB with another strain, the New Zealand White

Notes to table 19.2

1 Antibodies occur in the minority of patients with associated Addison's disease of the adrenal and are directed to the 17α/21-hydroxylase, the cholesterol side-chain cleavage enzyme and a 51 kDa gonadal antigen.

2 Only a small percentage show agglutinins. Spermatozoa may be agglutinated head to head, tail to tail or joined through their midpiece. Seen also in a small percentage of infertile women.

3 Most if not all insulin-dependent diabetics have islet cell antibodies at some stage during the first year of onset but these tend to decline progressively. In contrast, islet cell antibodies in diabetic patients with an associated autoimmune polyendocrinopathy persist for many years. GAD (glutamic acid decarboxylase) Ab also occur in Stiff man syndrome. ICA512 is a protein tyrosine kinase.

4 MBP, myelin basic protein.

5 The Coombs' test involves the demonstration of bound antibody on the washed red cell by agglutination with an antiglobulin (cf. figure 16.16). Erythrocyte autoantibodies, which bind well over the temperature range 0–37°C ('warm' Ab), are mostly IgG; approximately 60% of cases are primary, the remainder being associated with other autoimmune disorders, e.g. SLE and ulcerative colitis. 'Cold' Ab, which react best over the range 0–20°C, are mostly IgM, and red cells coated with this Ab can often be agglutinated by anticomplement serum; approximately half are primary, the others being associated with *Mycoplasma pneumoniae* infection or generalized neoplastic disease of the lymphoreticular tissues.

6 Antibodies specifically reacting with the epithelium of salivary gland excretory ducts are demonstrable by immunofluorescence in over half the cases of secondary Sjögren's associated with RA or SLE. SS-A and SS-B antibodies give a speckled nuclear fluorescence pattern.

7 The main antiglobulin factors react with the Fc portion of IgG which is usually adsorbed on to latex particles (human IgG) or present in an antigen–antibody complex (sheep red cells coated with a subagglutinating dose of rabbit antibody). In the ELISA test, rabbit IgG is bound to a plastic tube, patient's serum added and the antiglobulin bound assessed by subsequent binding of labeled anti-human IgG or IgM (cf. figure 6.10). Rheumatoid factors specific for human IgG can be detected by this test using human Fcγ to coat the tubes and labeled anti-human Fdγ (the portion of the heavy chain in the Fab fragment) or IgM for the final stage.

8 In scleroderma (progressive systemic sclerosis) antinucleolar antibodies are frequently found. Scl-70 is topoisomerase 1.

9 Jo-1 is histidine tRNA synthetase.

10 This syndrome combines features of scleroderma, RA, SLE and dermatomyositis. The antigens are extractable from the nucleus and give a speckled fluorescence pattern.

11 Antibodies to single- or double-stranded DNA are assayed by a DNA-coated tube test.

12 Component of primary granule, probably serine proteinase III, gives cytoplasmic staining. In periarteritis nodosa, antibodies to myeloperoxidase give perinuclear staining in alcohol-fixed polymorphonuclear neutrophils (PMNs). Some sera react with azurocidin, a potent antibiotic. ANCA (antineutrophil cytoplasmic antibody) directed against bactericidal/permeability increasing protein is a marker for inflammatory bowel disease and primary sclerosing cholangitis.

Figure 19.1. Fluorescent antibody studies in autoimmune diseases. (a) Thyroid peroxidase (thyroid microsomal) antibodies staining cytoplasm of acinar cells. (b) Human thyroid sections stained for MHC class II: *left*—normal thyroid with unstained follicular cells and an isolated strongly MHC class II-positive dendritic cell; *right*—Graves' disease (thyrotoxic) thyroid with abundant cytoplasmic MHC class II indicative of active synthesis. (c) Fluorescence of cells in the pancreatic islets of Langerhans' stained with serum from insulin-dependent diabetic. (d) The same, showing cells stained simultaneously for somatostatin (the yellow cells are stained with rhodamine anti-somatostatin and fluorescein anti-human IgG which localizes the patient's bound autoantibody). (e) Serum of patient with Addison's disease staining cytoplasm of monkey adrenal granulosa cells. (f) Fluorescence of distal tubular cells of the kidney after reaction with mitochondrial autoantibodies. (g) Diffuse nuclear staining on a thyroid section obtained with nucleoprotein antibodies from a SLE patient. (h) Serum of a scleroderma patient staining the nucleoli of SV40-transformed human keratinocytes (K14) in monolayer culture. ((a), (c), (d), (e), (f) and (g) kindly provided by Prof. F. Bottazzo; (b) by Professor R. Pujol-Borrell; and (h) by Dr F.T. Wojnarowska.)

Table 19.4. Spontaneous and induced animal models of autoimmune disease.

		MODEL	AUTOIMMUNE DISEASE
ORGAN-SPECIFIC	SPONTANEOUS	Nonobese diabetic (NOD) mouse; BB rat NOD.H2^{h4} congenic Obese strain (OS) chicken; Buffalo rat	Insulin-dependent diabetes *Thyroiditis Thyroiditis

	INDUCED	**Complete Freund's adjuvant (CFA) incorporating brain
		  CFA incorporating thyroid, adrenal, sperm, type II
		  collagen, ACh-R, retinal S1 protein or g.b.m.
		Mouse bearing IFNγ-insulin promoter transgene
		Cross reaction: heterologous with autologous r.b.c.
		             Coxsackie B with myosin
		Thymectomy in 2–4 day old mice
		Neonatal thymectomy + X-irradiation in rats
		HgCl$_2$ in rats
			Autoimmune encephalomyelitis
			Destruction of cell/tissue bearing relevant antigen
			
			Diabetes
			Anemia
			Myocarditis
			Widespread organ-specific
			Thyroiditis
			'Goodpasture's'

SYSTEMIC	SPONTANEOUS	New Zealand Black (NZB) mouse strain NZB x W, BXSB p21 Knockout mouse MRL/*lpr* Motheaten mouse strain	Autoimmune hemolytic anemia SLE SLE SLE, arthritis Widespread fatal systemic disease
	INDUCED	Parent bone marrow into F1 mice CFA incorporating anti-DNA idiotype CFA incorporating TB hsp	G.v.h., pseudo SLE SLE Adjuvant arthritis

*Fed high iodine diet.

**Antigen emulsified in water/oil mixture containing killed tubercle bacilli or derivative.

ACh-R, acetyl choline receptor; r.b.c., erythrocytes; g.b.m., glomerular basement membrane.

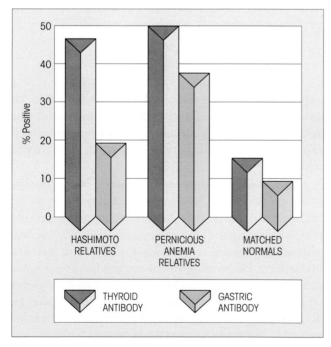

Figure 19.2. The high incidence of thyroid and gastric autoantibodies in the first degree relatives of patients with Hashimoto's disease or pernicious anemia. Note the overlap of gastric and thyroid autoimmunity and the higher incidence of gastric autoantibodies in pernicious anemia relatives. In general, titers were much higher in patients than in controls. (Data from Doniach D. & Roitt I.M. (1964) *Seminars in Haematology* **1**, 313.)

(B×W hybrid), actually develops antinuclear antibodies including anti-dsDNA and a fatal immune complex-induced glomerulonephritis, key features of human SLE.

These diseases are **genetically complex**. Genome-wide searches for mapping the genetic intervals containing genes for predisposition to disease by linkage to the many thousand microsatellite markers (polymorphic variable numbers of tandem repeats, VNTR) have so far identified 20 such regions for IDDM in NOD mice and some 25 for murine SLE.

Generally speaking, a genetic predisposition to sustained inflammatory responses and loss of tolerance to self are major contributory factors. Dominant amongst the genetic associations with autoimmune diseases is **linkage to the major histocompatibility complex (MHC)**; of the many examples, we may recall the increased risk of IDDM for DQ8 individuals, and the higher incidence of DR3 in Addison's disease and of DR4 in rheumatoid arthritis (table 17.1, p. 366). Figure 19.3 shows a multiplex family with IDDM in which the disease is closely linked to a particular HLA haplotype. Another pointer to the central role of class II structure in determining T-cell responsiveness to self derives from the inability of the NOD mouse to develop pancreatic autoimmunity when just a single amino acid residue in the α-helix of the H-2 β chain is altered by

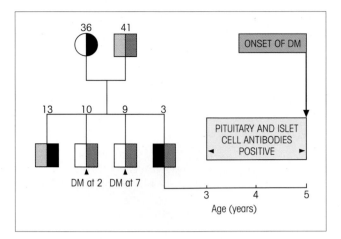

Figure 19.3. HLA haplotype linkage and onset of insulin-dependent diabetes (DM). Haplotypes: □ A3, B14, DR6; ■ A3, B7, DR4; ▨ A28, B51, DR4; and ▨ A2, B62, C3, DR4. Disease is linked to possession of the A2, B62, C3, DR4 haplotype. The 3-year-old brother had complement-fixing antibodies to the islet cell surface for 2 years before developing frank diabetes indicative of the lengthy pathological process preceding disease. (Data provided by Prof. G.F. Bottazzo.)

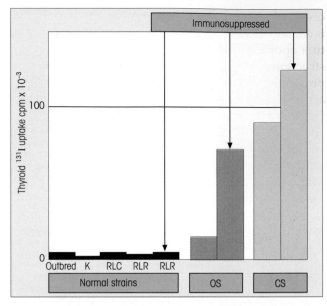

Figure 19.4. Abnormality in the Obese strain (OS) chicken thyroid. [131]I uptake in (OS) chickens and the related Cornell strain (CS) from which they were derived, compared with normal strains. Endogenous TSH production was suppressed by administration of thyroxine so that one was measuring TSH-independent ^{131}I uptake. Immune suppression showed that the abnormally high uptake was not due to immunological stimulation. (From Sundick R.S., Bagchi N., Livezey M.D., Brown T.R. & Mack R.E. (1979) Abnormal thyroid regulation in chickens with autoimmune thyroiditis. *Endocrinology* (*Baltimore*) **105**, 493.)

introduction of a transgene. The close relationship to MHC is not altogether unexpected given that, as we shall see, autoimmune diseases are T-cell dependent and most T-cell responses are MHC restricted.

Amongst the plethora of non-MHC-linked loci may be genes responsible for the editorial control of re-arranged Ig variable region genes encoding high avidity anti-DNA. Others may control the pattern of cytokine secretion affecting the milieu in early SLE which permits polyclonal B-cell activation, or influence the balance of Th1/Th2 subsets which could enhance susceptibility to IDDM or lead to resistance in otherwise predisposed subjects. Mice lacking the *p21* gene, which is a cell cycle regulator in the immune system, develop antibodies to dsDNA and other features of SLE. The gene maps within a recently defined MHC susceptibility locus with strong evidence for disease linkage. A mutation in the *IL-2* gene not affecting its functional ability to produce proliferation may be a candidate for *Idd-3* contributing to spontaneous diabetes in the NOD mouse and for *Aod-2* controlling autoimmune ovarian dysgenesis provoked by neonatal thymectomy. Polymorphism at a candidate locus identified in more than one autoimmune disease is interesting, a good example being *CTLA-4*, recently linked to IDDM and Graves' disease. CTLA-4 mediates antigen-specific apoptosis capable of clonally deleting previously activated T-cells, and other 'apoptotic genes' such as *Fas*, *FasL* and *Bcl-2* are all involved in different autoimmune disorders. With so many cells dying

naturally from apoptosis, it is clearly desirable for them to be immunologically inert, a state that may be achieved by the activation of transglutaminase which causes protein cross-linking and increased phagocytic removal.

Appropriate breeding experiments disclose that the genes predisposing to aggressive autoimmunity, on the one hand, are distinct from those which determine which autoantigens are involved, on the other. The '**autoimmunity genes**' contribute the common element underlying the overlaps in autoantibodies and disease discussed above, although within this group the genes which predispose to organ-specific disease must be different from those in nonorgan-specific disorders (as judged by the minimal overlap between them).

Evidence for '**autoantigen and tissue selection**' genes derives not only from breeding experiments with NZB×W mice showing separate control of red cell and nuclear antibodies, but also from genetic analysis of Obese chickens which has delineated an influence of the MHC, abnormalities in regulatory T-cell control *and* a defect in the thyroid gland expressed as an abnormally high uptake of [131]I (figure 19.4). Unlike normal thyroid cells, Hashimoto thyrocytes in culture display Fas molecules on their surface and, since FasL is constitutively expressed, this leads of course to mutual apoptotic homicidal death. However, since destruction of the gland during the course of disease is a prolonged process, it seems likely that, *in vivo*, this catastrophic scenario may be tempered by anti-apoptotic factors such as bcl-2. In the family studies described above (figure 19.2), there must be additional genes which are organ-related, in that relatives of patients with pernicious anemia are more prone to gastric autoimmunity than are members of Hashimoto kindreds. Further to this point, analysis has mapped the *IDDM-2* diabetes susceptibility gene to a VNTR lying 5′ to the insulin gene, which affects the transcriptional activity for insulin production and influences the level of thymic expression of insulin during a critical period in the development of self-tolerance. Susceptible strains have a low level of *thymic* but a high level of *pancreatic* insulin mRNA compared with their resistant counterparts which could foster the insulin autoreac-

tivity often seen in the early stages of IDDM. (Yes, quite unexpectedly, it does look as though mRNA for a number of 'organ-specific' antigens can be detected in the fetal thymus!)

Unraveling complex polygenic conditions is a very tough assignment. If we may take murine SLE as archetypal, genetic analysis of the predisposition to disease is most compatible with a threshold liability model requiring additive, or epistatic, contributions of multiple susceptibility genes probably linked to different stages of disease pathogenesis (figure 19.5).

Hormonal influences in autoimmunity

There is a general trend for autoimmune disease to occur far more frequently in women than in men (figure 19.6) probably due, in essence, to differences in hormonal patterns. There is a suggestion that higher estrogen levels are found in patients and administration of male hormones to mice with SLE reduces the severity of disease. Pregnancy is often associated with amelioration of disease severity, particularly in rheumatoid arthritis (RA), and there is sometimes a striking relapse after giving birth, a time at which there are drastic changes in hormones such as prolactin, not forgetting the loss of the placenta. We should also note the frequent development of postpartum hypothyroidism in women with pre-existing thyroid autoimmunity.

In Chapter 11, we dwelt on the importance of the neuroendocrine immune feedback encompassing the cytokine–hypothalamic–pituitary–adrenal control circuit. Abnormalities in this feedback loop have now been revealed in several autoimmune disorders. Patients with mild RA have lower corticosteroid levels than normals or patients with

Figure 19.5. Possible stages in development of SLE in susceptible individuals. Genes or gene products are in red. A variety of genes are involved in end-organ targeting. Epistatic interactions between *SLE 1* and *3*, derived from the NZW strain, produce severe lupus when introduced together into an otherwise resistant B6 strain as a double congenic, even though neither alone causes severe disease. The NZW strain itself, which contains both genes, is resistant to disease because it has a genetic suppressor region, four of which have been identified in various murine lupus strains.

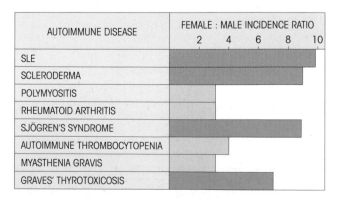

Figure 19.6. Increased incidence of autoimmune disease in females.

osteoarthritis or osteomyelitis despite the presence of inflammation. Moreover, RA patients undergoing surgery manifest grossly inadequate cortisol secretion in the face of high levels of plasma IL-1 and IL-6 (figure 19.7), a phenomenon now attributed to defective hypothalamic control. The OS chicken, several strains of lupus mice and the Lewis rat, which is abnormally susceptible to the induction of autoimmunity, all show blunted IL-1-induced corticosteroid responses. Both T- and B-cells from NOD mice survive for abnormally long periods in culture and their thymocytes are relatively resistant to corticosteroid-induced apoptosis. This would imply that the feedback cycle is not operating at the lymphocyte level and could cause dysregulated immune function; the ability of IL-1 in-

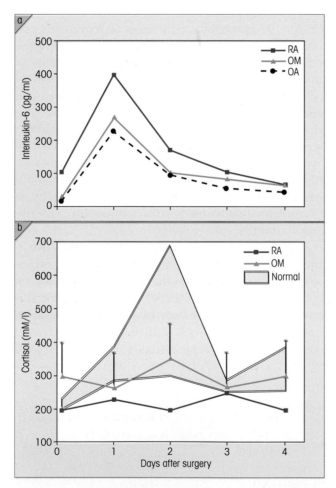

Figure 19.7. Failure of feedback control of cortisol production in rheumatoid arthritis (RA). After surgery (a) RA patients have even higher levels of plasma IL-6 than osteoarthritis (OA) and osteomyelitis (OM) controls. Nonetheless, (b) they have profoundly deficient production of cortisol which is evidence of faulty feedback control. (Data kindly provided by Professor G. Panayi from Chikanza I.C. *et al.* (1992) Defective hypothalamic response to immune and inflammatory stimuli in patients with rheumatoid arthritis. *Arthritis and Rheumatism* **35**, 1281, with permission from the publishers.)

jections to delay the onset of diabetes would accord with this view.

Does the environment contribute?

Twin studies

Although the 50% concordance rate for the development of the autoimmune disease insulin-dependent diabetes mellitus (IDDM) in identical twins is considerably higher than that in dizygotic twins and suggests a strong genetic element, there is still 50% unaccounted for. This is not necessarily all due to environment, since although monozygotic twins have identical germ-line immunoglobulin and T-cell receptor (TCR) genes, the processes of diversification of receptors and of internal anti-idiotype interactions are so complex that the resulting receptor repertoires will be extremely variable and unlikely to be identical. Nonetheless, a later study on concordance rates for IDDM in monozygotic twins gave the extraordinarily high figure of 70% if they were DR3/DR4 heterozygotes, but only 40% if they were not. Thus, in the same disease, the genetic element can be almost completely dominant or be a significant but minor factor in determining the outcome. As we turn to the nonorgan-specific diseases, such as SLE, we find an even lower genetic contribution with a concordance rate of only 23% in same-sex monozygotic twins, compared with 9% in same-sex dizygotic twins. There are also many examples where clinically unaffected relatives of patients with SLE have a higher incidence of nuclear autoantibodies if they are household contacts than if they live apart from the proband. However, within a given home, the spouse is less likely to develop autoantibodies than blood relatives. Summing up, in some disorders the major factors are genetic, whereas in others environmental influences seem to dominate.

Nonmicrobial factors

What environmental agents can we identify? Diet could be one—fish oils containing long-chain, highly polyunsaturated ω-3 fatty acids are reputed to be beneficial for patients with RA; someone must know whether rheumatologists in Greenland are underworked! Sunshine is an undisputed trigger of the skin lesions in SLE. Exposure to organic solvents can initiate the basement membrane autoimmunity which results in Goodpasture's syndrome—witness the high incidence of this disease in HLA-DR2 individuals who work in dry-cleaning shops or siphon petrol from other people's petrol tanks. A more contrived situation is the production of a similar disease in Brown Norway rats by the injection of mercuric chloride, but it makes its point, and there are several drug-induced diseases such as SLE, myasthenia gravis, autoimmune hemolytic anemia, and so on.

Microbes

Of course everyone's favorite environmental agent has to be an infectious microorganism and we do have some clear-cut examples of autoimmune disease following infection, usually in genetically predisposed individuals: acute rheumatic fever follows group A streptococcal pharyngitis in 2–3% of patients with a hereditary susceptibility and B3 coxsackie virus produces autoimmune myositis in certain mouse strains.

In most cases of human chronic autoimmune disease, the problem is the long latency period which makes it difficult to track down the initiating event (cf. figure 19.3) and, secondly, viable organisms usually cannot be isolated from the affected tissues.

Some groups are focusing down on **very slow-growing forms of mycobacteria** which are exceedingly difficult to culture but appear to be associated with various hypersensitivity states. *M. paratuberculosis* is linked with Jöhne's disease, a chronic granulomatous intestinal infection of cattle similar to Crohn's disease. Genetic probes have identified mycobacterial sequences in sarcoidosis. The granulomatous Takayasu arthritis is often accompanied by very powerful responses to TB. Whipple's disease associated with arthralgias and skin changes evolves so slowly that it can often take 10 years for the diagnosis to be made and, although organisms can be identified in macrophages at electron microscopy level, none can so far be cultivated. There has been a breakthrough in the HLA-B27-related **reactive arthritis** provoked by infection with *Chlamydia*, *Yersinia* or *Salmonella*, in that T-cell responses to bacterial fragments or perhaps to cross-reacting self-epitopes present in affected joints can now be demonstrated years after the primary infection. These studies and the ability of EB virus and *Chlamydia* DNA probes to hybridize to a not insignificant proportion of synovial tissues from rheumatoid arthritis patients raises important questions regarding the cellular localization and molecular status of the 'microbial' nucleic acid in these cells.

Given the possibility that we may ultimately identify persistent microorganisms in some disorders, we then have to re-examine the question of whether the hypersensitivity lesions are driven by the microbe or by self-antigen, i.e. are we dealing with a microbially triggered autoimmune disease or autoimmune phenomena secondarily superimposed on an underlying microbial hypersensitivity? Perhaps both circumstances occur. Certainly we know that cross-reactions with microbial components can initiate autoimmunity (see p. 412), and recently it has been shown that infection with the helminth *Nippostrongylus brasiliensis* can break tolerance to an unrelated staphylococcal superantigen; perhaps infections of this nature can stimulate such a welter of cytokines as to nonplus and maybe activate anergic, potentially autoreactive T-cells. They can also act as superantigens in bringing about the polyclonal stimulation of certain TCR Vβ families. Further complexity is injected by the knowledge that environmental microbes may sometimes **protect** against spontaneous autoimmune disease; the incidence of diabetes is greatly increased if NOD mice are kept in specific pathogen-free conditions, while Sendai virus inhibits the development of arthritis in the MRL/*lpr* strain. The extraordinary variation in incidence of diabetes in NOD colonies bred in a wide variety of different animal houses (figure 19.8) testifies to the dramatic influence of environmental flora on the expression of autoimmune disease.

AUTOREACTIVITY COMES NATURALLY

Tolerance mechanisms do not destroy all self-reactive lymphocytes. Processing of an autoantigen will lead to certain (dominant) peptides being preferentially expressed on *a*ntigen-*p*resenting *c*ells (APCs) while others (cryptic) only appear in the MHC groove in very low concentrations which, although capable of expanding their cognate T-cells in the context of thymic positive selection (cf. p. 228), may nonetheless fail to provide a sufficiently powerful signal for negative selection of these cells. As a consequence, autoreactive T-cells specific for **cryptic epitopes** will survive in the repertoire which will therefore be biased towards weak self-reactivity.

Because conventional B-2 cells are less susceptible than T-cells to tolerization by low concentrations of circulating autoantigens such as thyroglobulin (figure 12.16), autoreactive B-cells specific for such antigens will circulate albeit unaccompanied by their cognate helper T-cells (figure 12.17). The reader will also recall the B-1 cell population, which starts off early in life by forming a network connected by germ-line idiotypes. The cells are stimulated, presumably by T-independent type 2 idiotypic interactions, to produce so-called **'natural antibodies'**, a term applied to those serum antibodies thought to be present before external antigen challenge and therefore arising independently of conventional antigen stimulation. These are

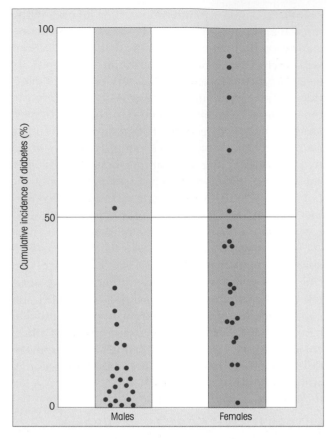

Figure 19.8. The incidence of spontaneous diabetes in geographically dispersed colonies of NOD mice at 20 weeks of age. Each point represents a single colony. The extreme spread of values is not attributable to genetic drift to any significant extent. The lower incidence in males is particularly evident. (Data adapted from Pozzilli P., Signore A., Williams A.J.K. & Beales P.E. (1993) NOD mouse colonies around the world. *Immunology Today* **14**, 193.)

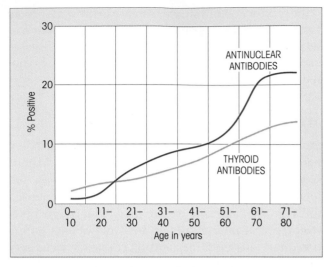

Figure 19.9. Incidence of autoantibodies in the general population. A serum was considered positive for thyroid antibodies if it reacted at a dilution of 1:10 in the tanned red cell test or neat in the immunofluorescent test, and positive for antinuclear antibodies if it reacted at a dilution of 1:4 by immunofluorescence. The class of antibody was not determined in these studies.

germ-line antibodies, mostly IgM, although a proportion belong to the IgG and IgA classes. They include a basic set of autoantibodies with low affinity reactivity for multiple specificities and cross-reactivity with common bacterial antigens usually of a carbohydrate nature. One can see this as a strategy which ensures that preliminary excitation of cells by these internal network interactions will provide bacterial protection, especially since the polymeric nature of the carbohydrate antigens ensures that the IgM antibodies, even though of low affinity, can bind with high avidity to the microbes.

Other functions for these natural antibodies have been proposed which are not mutually exclusive: Grabar viewed them as transporting agents responsible for scavenging effete body components. Others envisage a homeostatic role in which they actually prevent stimulation of autoreactive cells in the conventional B-2 cell population either by masking autoanti-

gen epitopes or by overall idiotype regulation. The latter view receives some encouragement from a report that the IgM fraction of normal serum can block binding of autologous IgG F(ab')$_2$ fragments to a range of autoantigens. These natural autoantibodies presumably make a contribution to the so-called 'nonspecific' Ig binding of otherwise normal sera to test autoantigens, but slightly stronger reactions are evident in a small proportion of younger people and the incidence increases with age (figure 19.9). Although not associated with clinically apparent tissue damage, it should be noted that, in the case of the thyroid and stomach at least, biopsy has linked the presence of raised titers of antibody, especially of the IgG class, with minor thyroiditis or gastritis lesions (as the case may be), and postmortem examination has identified 10% of clinically normal middle-aged women with significant but limited degrees of lymphadenoid change in the thyroid, similar in essence to that characteristic of Hashimoto's disease.

As enthusiasts for symmetry and order might have predicted, there appears to be an analogous T-cell population, of phenotype CD3$^+$ CD4$^-$8$^-$ bearing the B-cell marker B220, containing large internally activated cells which react strongly with self-T-cells and are expanded in early life. It is possible that they connect to the CD5$^+$ B-cell network through idiotype interactions with cells of this lineage present in the thymus. The reader may be surprised to learn that, in generating T-cell lines, it is not an uncommon experience to isolate

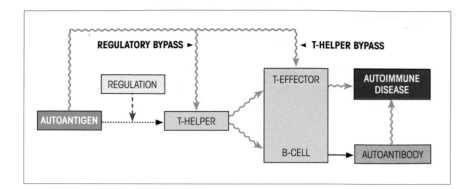

Figure 19.11. Autoimmunity arises through bypass of the control of autoreactivity. The constraints on the stimulation of self-reactive helper T-cells by autoantigen can be circumvented either through bypassing the helper cell or by disturbance of the regulatory mechanisms.

normally unresponsive because of clonal deletion, clonal anergy, T-suppression or inadequate autoantigen presentation. Immediately, one could conceive of an *abnormal* degree of responsiveness to self-antigens as a result of relatively low intrathymic expression of a particular molecule (cf. p. 405). Abnormalities in the signaling pathways affecting the thresholds for positive and negative selection in the thymus would also affect subsequent responsiveness to peripheral autoantigens. So might defects in apoptotic cell death. It would be interesting to know whether the innate resistance of the NZB mouse to tolerization by a protein antigen such as bovine serum albumin can be nailed to one of these causes or whether it is a consequence of defects in regulatory cells (see below).

AUTOIMMUNITY CAN ARISE THROUGH BYPASS OF T-HELPERS

Provision of new carrier determinant

Allison and Weigle argued independently that, if autoreactive T-cells are tolerized and thereby unable to collaborate with B-cells to generate autoantibodies (figures 19.12a and 19.15), provision of new carrier determinants to which no self-tolerance had been established would bypass this mechanism and lead to autoantibody production (figures 19.12b and 19.15).

1 *Modification of the autoantigen*

A new carrier could arise through some modification to the molecule, for example by defects in synthesis or by an abnormality in lysosomal processing yielding a split product exposing some new groupings (figure 19.12b.1). Aside from the possibility of post-translational modifications, such as subtle changes in glycosylation patterns as seen in the low galactosylation of the Fcγ sugar chains in rheumatoid arthritis, many studies on spontaneous autoimmune disease

have failed to reveal an abnormality in the antigen. Remember the experiment in which neonatal thyroidectomized Obese strain chickens make autoantibodies if injected with thyroglobulin prepared from *normal* chickens, suggesting that the immunological response rather than the antigen is abnormal. Nonetheless, there may be defects in the iodine metabolism of the gland itself in this strain (figure 19.4), and recent work has shown that the severity of thyroiditis is ameliorated when the birds are put on a low iodine diet.

Modification can also be achieved through combination with a drug (figure 19.12b.3). The autoimmune hemolytic anemia associated with the administration of α-methyldopa might be attributable to modification of the red cell surface in such a way as to provide a carrier for stimulating B-cells which recognize the rhesus antigen. This is normally regarded as a 'weak' antigen and would be less likely to induce B-cell tolerance than the 'stronger' antigens present on the erythrocyte. Isoniazid may produce arthritis associated with nuclear antibodies and, unlike most other cases of drug-induced autoimmunity, synthesis of these antibodies is said to continue after cessation of drug therapy. A high proportion of patients on continued treatment with procainamide develop nuclear antibodies and 40% present with clinical signs of SLE. Myasthenia gravis and symptoms of pemphigus have been described in some patients on penicillamine. It is not clear in every case whether the drug provides carrier help through direct modification of the autoantigen or of some independent molecule concerned in associative recognition.

2 *Cross-reactions with B-cell epitopes*

Many examples are known in which potential human autoantigenic B-cell epitopes are present on a microbial exogenous cross-reacting antigen which provides the new carrier that provokes autoantibody formation (figure 19.12b.2). The mechanism is spelt out in more

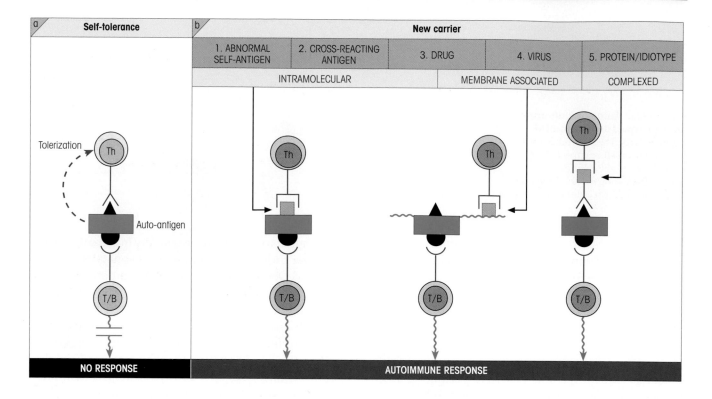

Figure 19.12. T-helper bypass through new carrier epitope (■) generates autoimmunity. For simplicity, processing for MHC association has been omitted from the diagram, but is elaborated in figure 19.13. (a) The pivotal autoreactive T-helper is unresponsive either through tolerance or inability to see a cryptic epitope. (b) Different mechanisms providing a new carrier epitope.

detail in figure 19.13a. Two low molecular weight envelope proteins of *Yersinia enterolytica* share epitopes with the extracellular domain of the human thyroid-stimulating hormone (TSH) receptor; in rheumatic fever, antibodies produced to the *Streptococcus* also react with heart, and the sera of 50% of children with the disease who develop Sydenham's chorea give neuronal immunofluorescent staining which can be absorbed out with streptococcal membranes. Colon antibodies present in ulcerative colitis have been found to cross-react with *Escherichia coli* 014. There is also some evidence for the view that antigens common to *Trypanosoma cruzi* and cardiac muscle and peripheral nervous system provoke some of the immunopathological lesions seen in Chagas' disease.

3 *Molecular mimicry of T-cell epitopes*

The drawback with the Allison–Weigle model of cross-reaction of B-cell epitopes and the provision of a new T-cell carrier is that, once the cross-reacting agent is

eliminated from the body, and with it the T-cell epitope, the only way that the autoimmunity can be sustained is for the activated B-cell to capture circulating autoantigen and, after processing, present it to the T-helper (figure 19.13c). This is not possible for **cell-associated antigens** but their special link with T-cell recognition puts them in a totally different ballpark. In this case, if an infecting agent mimics an autoantigen by producing a **cross-reacting T-cell epitope**, the resulting T-cell autoimmunity could theoretically persist even after elimination of the infection. The autoantigen will normally be presented to the resting autoreactive T-cell as a **cryptic epitope** and by definition will be unable to provide an activating signal. The cross-reacting infectious agent will provide abundant antigen on professional APCs which can prime the T-cell and upregulate its adhesion molecules so that it now has the **avidity** to bind to and be persistently activated by the cryptic self-epitope presented on the target tissue cell provided that it is associated with the appropriate MHC molecule (figure 19.13b). Remember the transgenic cytotoxic T-cells (Tc) which could only destroy the pancreatic β-cells bearing a viral transgene when they were **primed** by a real viral infection (cf. figure 12.10). Recall also the tumor cells that could only be recognized by primed not resting T-cells (cf. figure 18.9). Theoretically, the resting T-cell could also be primed in a nonantigen-specific manner by a microbial **superantigen**.

Figure 19.13. Mechanisms of microbial induction of autoimmunity and epitope spread. (This is a complex mouthful but digestion is recommended because these ideas are crucial. The more faint-hearted may require an ice-pack and persistence, but following the numbers should help.) (a) A microbial antigen bearing an epitope Y which cross-reacts with self and a foreign T-cell epitope X is (1) processed by an antigen-presenting cell, (2) activates the T-helper which (3) recognizes the processed X after capture by an anti-Y B-cell and (4) stimulates the B-cell to secrete anti-Y autoantibody. (b) The *activated* anti-X T-helper, as distinct from the *resting* cell, may recognize and be stimulated by a cross-reacting cryptic T-cell epitope expressed by a tissue cell. This will maintain the autoimmune response even after elimination of the microbe, because of the persistence of the self-epitope. The tissue expressing the epitope will also be a target for immunological attack. Note also that a T-helper primed nonspecifically by a polyclonal super-antigen activator could also fulfil the same function of responding to a cryptic epitope. (c) If the autoantigen is soluble or capable of uptake and processing after capture by the activated autoreactive B-cell (1) (either from (a) or through nonspecific polyclonal activation), a new epitope can be presented on the B-cell class II which now stimulates an autoreactive (anti-Z) T-helper (2) which can now sustain an autoimmune response entirely through autoantigen stimulation (3). It can also produce epitope spread within the same molecule through helping a B-cell which captures the autoantigen through a new epitope W (4). It can also permit epitope spread to another component in an intermolecular complex such as nucleosomal histone–DNA or idiotype-positive (Id+) anti-DNA–DNA which is 'piggy-backed' into the B-cell (5) which presents processed antigen to the T-helper (6) in the cases cited, specific for histone or Id, respectively. *Denotes activation.

Although we have ascribed the dominant role of MHC alleles as risk factors for autoimmune diseases to their ability to present key antigenic epitopes to autoreactive T-cells, they might also operate in a quite distinct way. We may recollect that, during intrathymic ontogeny, T-cells are positively selected by weak interaction with self-peptides complexed with MHC. Now since around **50% of the class II peptides are MHC de-rived** (figure 5.22), then the mature T-cells leaving the thymus will have been selected with a strong bias to weak recognition of self-MHC peptides presented by class II. There must therefore be a major pool of self-reactive T-cells vulnerable to stimulation by exogenously derived cross-reacting epitopes which mimic these MHC peptides. Just so. The critical sequence QKRAAVDTY of the rheumatoid arthritis susceptibility allele HLA-DRB1*0401 (table 17.2) is closely similar to the QKRAAYDQY of the dnaJ heat-shock protein of *E. coli*, and this peptide presented by DQ causes proliferation of synovial T-cells from RA patients. In fact, a large number of microbial peptide sequences with varying degrees of homology with human proteins have been identified (table 19.5), although it should be emphasized at this stage that they only provide clues for further study. The mere existence of a homology is no certainty that infection with that organism will necessarily lead to autoimmunity because everything depends on several contingencies, including the manner in which the proteins are processed by the APCs, and we cannot predict, as yet, which peptides will be presented and in what concentration.

4 'Piggy-back' T-cell epitopes and epitope spread

One membrane component may provide help for the immune response to another (associative recognition). In the context of autoimmunity, a new helper determinant may arise through drug modification as mentioned above, or through the insertion of viral antigen into the membrane of an infected cell (cf. figure 19.12b.4). That this can promote a reaction to a pre-existing cell component is clear from the studies in which infection of a tumor with influenza virus elicited resistance to uninfected tumor cells. The appearance of cold agglutinins often with blood group I specificity after *Mycoplasma pneumoniae* infection could have a similar explanation. In a comparable fashion, T-cell help can be provided for a molecule such as DNA, which cannot itself form a T-cell epitope, by complexing with a T-dependent carrier, in this example a histone, or an anti-DNA idiotype to which T-cells were sensitized. For this mechanism to work, the helper component must still be physically attached to the fragment bearing the B-cell epitope. When this is recognized by the B-cell receptor, the helper component will be 'piggy-backed' into the B-cell, processed and presented as an epitope for recognition by T-cells (figure 19.13c). By the same token, the autoimmune response can spread to other epitopes on the same molecule.

Idiotype bypass mechanisms

We have argued the evidence for internal regulated idiotype networks involving self-reactivity at some length. This raises the possibility of involving autoreactive lymphocytes with responses to exogenous agents through idiotype network connections, particularly since some autoimmune diseases are characterized by major cross-reactive idiotypes.

Thus, knowing that T-helpers with specificity for the idiotype on a lymphocyte receptor can be instrumental in the stimulation of that cell, it is conceivable that an environmental agent such as a parasite or virus, which triggered antibody carrying a public idiotype (cross-reactive idiotype, CRI), which happened to be shared with the receptor of an autoreactive T- or B-cell, could provoke an autoimmune response (figure 19.14b). Similarly, if it is correct that the germ-line idiotypes on autoantibodies generate a whole range of anti-idiotypes which mediate the response to exogenous antigens, then, by the same token, it is conceivable that antibodies produced in response to an infection may react with the corresponding idiotype on the autoreactive lymphocyte (figure 19.14a). For example, a hybridoma from a myasthenia gravis patient secreted an anti-Id to an acetylcholine receptor autoantibody; this anti-Id was found to react with the bacterial product 1,3-dextran. Finally, it is possible for Id network interactions to allow a viral infection to give rise to autoantibodies reacting with the viral receptor (figure 19.14c). Since viruses all bind to specific complementary receptors on the cells they infect, this sequence of events may have serious consequences; we note for example that β-adrenergic receptors are the surface targets for certain reoviruses and that rabies virus binds to the acetylcholine receptor.

Polyclonal activation

Microbes often display adjuvant properties through their possession of polyclonal lymphocyte activators such as bacterial endotoxins, which act by providing nonspecific inductive signals that bypass the need for specific T-cell help, either by stimulation of CD8 T-cells through upregulation of dendritic cell CD40 or by direct interaction with B-cell mitogen receptors (cf.

Table 19.5. Molecular mimicry: homologies between microbes and body components as potential cross-reacting T-cell epitopes.

Microbial molecule	Body component
Bacteria:	
Arthritogenic *Shigella flexneri*	HLA-B27
Klebsiella nitrogenase	HLA-B27
Proteus mirabilis urease	HLA-DR4
Mycobact. tuberculosis 65 kDa hsp	Joint (adjuvant arthritis)
E.coli DNAJ hsp	RA shared DRB1 T-cell epitope
Viruses:	
Coxsackie B	Myocardium
Coxsackie B	Glutamic acid decarboxylase
EBV gp110	RA shared DRB1 T-cell epitope
HBV octamer	Myelin basic protein
HSV glycoprotein	Acetylcholine receptor
Measles hemagglutinin	T-cell subset
Retroviral gag p32	U-1 RNA

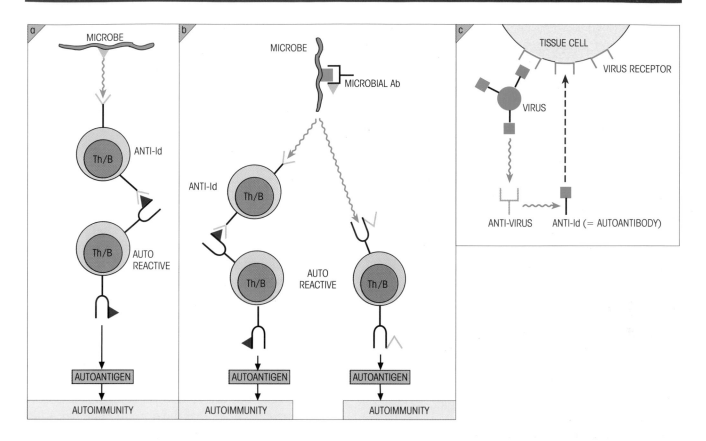

Figure 19.14. Idiotypic mechanisms leading to autoimmunity. (a) Microbial antigen cross-reacts with autoreactive lymphocyte Id. (b) Microbial antibodies either share Ids with or are anti-Id to autoreactive lymphocytes. (c) Anti-virus generates anti-Id which is autoantibody to viral receptor (Plotz).

p. 171). This can occur by direct interaction with the B-lymphocyte or indirectly through stimulating the secretion of nonspecific factors from T-cells or macrophages. The variety of autoantibodies detected in cases with infectious mononucleosis must surely be attributable to the polyclonal activation of B-cells by the Epstein–Barr (EB) virus. They are seen also in lepromatous leprosy where the abundance of mycobacteria reproduces some of the features of Freund's adjuvant. However, unlike the usual situation in human autoimmune disease, these autoantibodies tend to be IgM and, normally, do not persist when the microbial components are cleared from the body. It is likely that the reactions largely involve B-1 cells. Curiously, lymphocytes from many patients with SLE and from mice with spontaneous lupus produce abnormally large amounts of IgM when cultured *in vitro* as if they were under polyclonal activation. Nevertheless, it is difficult to see how a pan-specific polyclonal activation could give rise to the patterns of autoantibodies characteristic of the different autoimmune disorders without the operation of some antigen-directing factor. We have already hinted at scenarios in which polyclonally activated B- or T-cells might contribute to a sustained autoimmune response (see legend to figure 19.13b and c).

AUTOIMMUNITY CAN ARISE THROUGH BYPASS OF REGULATORY MECHANISMS

Regulatory cells try to damp down autoimmunity

It should be emphasized that these T-helper bypass mechanisms for the induction of autoimmunity do not by themselves ensure the continuation of the response, since normal animals have been shown to be capable of damping down autoantibody production through regulatory T-cell interactions as, for example, in the case of red cell autoantibodies induced in mice by injection of rat erythrocytes (figure 19.15). When regulatory T-cell activity is impaired by low doses of cyclophosphamide, or if strains like the SJL which have prematurely aging regulators are used, induced autoimmunity is prolonged and more severe. Yet another example is the protection against autoimmune diabetes and thyroiditis which develops in irradiated adult thymectomized rats by injection of CD4+,

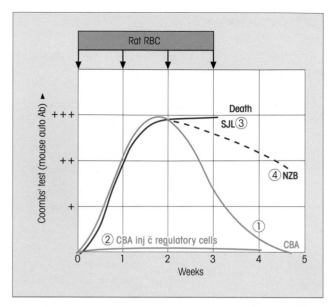

Figure 19.15. Regulation of self-reactivity. When CBA strain mice (1) are injected with rat red cells, autoantibodies are produced by this cross-reacting antigen (see p. 413) which coat the host erythrocytes and are detected by the Coombs' antiglobulin test (see p. 334). Despite repeated injections of rat erythrocytes, the autoantibody response is switched off by the expansion of CD4 mouse red cell-specific regulatory cells which do not affect antibody production to the heterologous erythrocyte determinants. When these regulatory cells are injected into naïve CBA mice (2), rat red cells cannot induce autoantibodies. The SJL strain (3), in which suppressor activity declines rapidly with age, is unable to regulate the autoimmune response and develops particularly severe disease. The response is also prolonged in the autoimmune NZB strain (4). (Based on data of Cooke A. & Hutchings P., e.g. *Immunology* 1984, **51**, 489.)

CD45RB^{lo}, RT6$^+$ T-cells from a normal donor. This phenotype (Tr1) is characteristic of the mucosal regulatory cells which mediate oral tolerance; they produce IL-10 on activation and promote the differentiation of T-cells that secrete TGFβ and skew responses towards the Th2-type pole. This notion accords with the finding that the generation of regulatory cells which modulate susceptibility can be influenced by gut flora: Fisher rats raised in a pathogen-free facility are susceptible to adjuvant arthritis (table 19.4) unless moved to conventional surroundings, although this resistance is lost if they are fed the antibiotic, neomycin. Furthermore, resistance can be transferred to susceptible rats by spleen cells stimulated *in vitro* with C-terminal determinants of mycobacterial hsp65. This ties up with suppression of diabetes in NOD mice by injection of a peptide from mammalian hsp. Yet another player in the field is the NK1 T-cell which is deficient in NOD mice, but can prevent the development of diabetes if transferred from F1(Balb/c×NOD) donors. From quite a different tack, small numbers of an encephalitogenic T-cell clone **vaccinated** normal recipients against the patho-

genic consequences of a subsequent higher dose, hinting strongly at anti-idiotypic control. The interrelationships between this panoply of antigen-, idiotype-, hsp- and possibly nonspecific regulators (figure 19.16) need sorting.

Neonatal thymectomy deletes potential self-regulators

We are surely nodding our grudging assent to the idea that, in general, manipulations which reduce regulatory T-cells encourage the development of autoantibodies. Even so, the effect of thymectomy within a narrow window of 2–4 days after birth in the mouse is quite startling in that it gives rise to widespread organ-specific autoimmune disease affecting mainly the stomach, thyroid, ovary, prostate and sperm; circulating antibodies are frequently detected and deposits of Ig and complement are often seen around the basement membranes. Spleen cells from intact adult males, but not females, injected into these 3-day thymectomized mice can prevent the development of prostatitis, although both are able to prevent gastritis, from which one concludes that the normal male has additional suppressor T-cells specific for prostate and activated by prostate antigens. We have alluded earlier to the evidence for intrathymic expression of mRNA for a whole set of nominally organ-specific antigens such as insulin, thyroglobulin and myelin basic protein. These are expressed in rare large medullary cells often at the center of lymphocyte rosettes, presumably guiding the formation of potential organ-specific suppressive regulators between days 2 and 4, the time at which thymectomy upsets the balance between autoreactive and suppressor cells.

If neonatal thymectomy really does greatly deplete the T-suppressor population, the early induction or exacerbation of spontaneous autoimmune states in susceptible animals—autoimmune hemolytic anemia in NZB mice and thyroiditis in Obese strain chickens and Buffalo rats—is not entirely unexpected.

Defects in regulation contribute to spontaneous autoimmunity

Such would be the conclusion from the demonstration that transfer of disease from splenocytes of recently diabetic NOD mice into NOD–SCID congenics could be inhibited by the CD4, CD45RB^{lo} (memory) splenic subset of young, nondiabetic animals. Along the same lines, it was shown long ago that Coombs' positivity (i.e. the state in which circulating red cells are coated with autoantibody) can be transferred with the spleen cells of a Coombs'-positive NZB mouse to a *young, neg-*

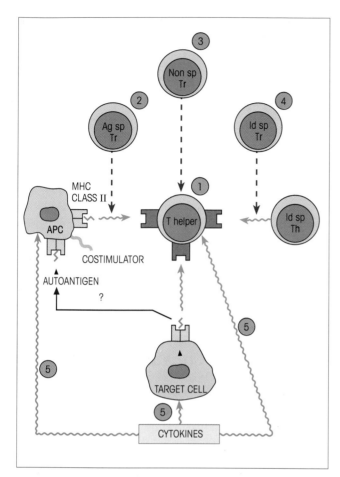

Figure 19.16. Bypass of regulatory mechanisms leads to triggering of autoreactive T-helper cells through defects in (1) tolerizability or ability to respond to or induce T-regulators (Tr), or (2) expression of antigen-specific, (3) hsp and other nonspecific or (4) idiotype-specific T-regulators, or (5) through imbalance of the cytokine network, producing derepression of class II genes with inappropriate cellular expression of class II and presentation of antigen on target cell, stimulation of APC, and possible activation of anergic T-helper. The beneficial effect of pooled whole Ig in certain human autoimmune diseases, such as idiopathic thrombocytopenic purpura, and of T-cell vaccination in experimental autoimmune encephalomyelitis (EAE) and adjuvant arthritis in rats lends weight to the idea of idiotype control mechanisms. Evidence for a regulatory CD4 subset comes from studies reporting inflammatory infiltrates in liver, lung, stomach, thyroid and pancreas in athymic rats reconstituted with CD45RB^{hi}/CD4 T-cells but not with unfractionated or CD45RB^{lo} CD4 cells (presumably the regulators).

ative mouse of the same strain, but the continued production of red cell antibodies is short lived unless the recipient's T-cells are first depleted by pretreatment with antilymphocyte serum.

A progressive loss of regulatory cells with age may account for the inability of the NZB mouse to normalize the experimental induction of red cell autoimmunity (figure 19.15) and for the increasing resistance to the induction of tolerance to soluble proteins in elderly NZB mice, apparently associated with a sudden fall in the plasma concentration of the thymic peptide thymulin before the onset of disease (note: thymulin is said to inhibit the autoreactive response of spleen cells to syngeneic fibroblasts in culture).

Do abnormalities in apoptotic mechanisms contribute to these regulatory defects? T- and B-cells of NOD mice are resistant to apoptosis, as are lymphocytes of the MRL/*lpr* lupus mouse strain which has a *fas* gene mutation. This mutation produces the characteristic lymphoproliferation, and possibly failure to limit the expansion of self-reactive T- and B-cell clones by apoptosis. The *gld* lupus model complements this situation with mutations in the *fas ligand*.

Peripheral T-cell responses are seriously controlled by dendritic cells. The subset of phenotype CD11c$^+$/b$^-$/8α^+ favors Th1 cells, while that of CD11c$^+$/b$^+$/8α^- promotes Th2 responses. IL-4 prevents maturation of dendritic cells, and subsequent interaction of these immature cells with cognate T-cells results in peripheral tolerization. CD30/CD30L signaling is important for peripheral deletion of self-reactive T-cells; thus, deletion of pancreatic islet reactive CD8 T-cells failed to occur in CD30 knockout mice and these cells were highly aggressive, as few as 150 provoking diabetes in adoptive recipients. The numbers of dendritic cells in humans at risk for diabetes and in NOD mice are grossly reduced, which would accord with a critical role in preventing disease by promoting autoregulatory responses. Another curious feature is that macrophages from diabetic patients and relatives with the susceptible HLA haplotype constitutively express high levels of the COX-2 enzyme responsible for the synthesis of prostanoids. Something interesting is simmering here and should break surface soon.

We have previously drawn attention to the distinctive properties of the B-1 population with respect to its propensity to synthesize IgM autoantibodies and its possible intimate relationship to the setting up of the regulatory idiotype network (cf. p. 207), and one must seriously entertain the hypothesis that unregulated activity by these cells could be responsible for certain autoimmune disorders. The pitifully named motheaten strain is heavily into autoimmunity, and the mice make masses of anti-DNA and anti-polymorphs and die with intense pneumonitis, often before they have tasted the fruits of life. They exhibit reduced catalytic activity of their protein tyrosine phosphatase 1C due to mutation. Their IgM levels rise to a staggering 25–50 times normal and—this is quite bizarre—their B-cells are nearly all CD5$^+$, i.e. B-1. This population is also raised in the NZB mouse and largely accounts for the production of the IgM autoantibodies in this strain. Now here is a persuasive experiment. When transgenes encoding an NZB red cell autoantibody were introduced into normal mice, no B-2 cells were present and 50% developed autoimmune disease. Intraperitoneal injection of erythrocytes deleted the B-1 cells and prevented disease. This tells us that the NZB hemolytic anemia is due to red blood cell autoantibodies produced by B-1 cells, that this population is only tolerized properly when the antigen gains access to the peritoneum where they develop, and that some (around 50%), but not all, animals can control the autoreactive clones. Whether B-1 cells escape regulatory control and undergo an unrestrained isotype switch to the pathogenic IgG antibodies responsible for disease in other models, such as the NZB×W mouse, is still a question on which the jury's verdict is awaited, although depletion of B-1 lymphocytes greatly reduces the immune complex glomerulonephritis. The IdD-23 idiotype characteristic of natural autoantibodies has been identified on a monoclonal IgG anti-DNA—but one idiotype doesn't make a summer, if we can misquote a well-known saying!

In humans, a high proportion of B-1 cells make IgM rheumatoid factors (anti-Fcγ) and anti-DNA using germ-line genes. In rheumatoid arthritis patients, although there are increased numbers of circulating B-1 cells, the polyclonal rheumatoid factors synthesized do not, by and large, bear the public idiotypes of this subset. SLE could be different because the 16/6 public idiotype associated with germ-line genes encoding anti-DNA is found on a significant fraction of the IgG anti-DNA in patients' serums. Gene sequencing may be required to establish the relationship between B-1 cells and IgG autoantibody synthesis.

Aside from the defective IL-1/6–hypothalamic feedback loop giving rise to low corticosteroid levels in rheumatoid arthritis described earlier (cf. figure 19.7), less is known of regulatory circuits in humans, although there is increasing evidence that nonspecific T-suppressor function in SLE may be poorly regulated. B-lymphocytes from patients with active disease secrete larger amounts of Ig when cultured *in vitro* than normal B-cells. Concanavalin-A-induced nonspecific suppressors are reduced or absent and T-cells with Fcγ receptors, which suppress pokeweed mitogen-stimulated lymphocytes, are low, the defect being greater the more active the disease. The production of thymulin and of IL-2 is also depressed in these patients. A significant proportion of clinically unaffected close relatives also demonstrate abnormally low levels of nonspecific suppressors, indicating that the deficit in SLE patients is not a consequence of the illness or its treatment and that additional factors must be implicated in the causation of disease.

In any case, it is difficult to account for the antigenic specificity of different autoimmune disorders on the basis of a generalized depression of nonspecific suppressors *alone*, without invoking defects in either antigen- or idiotype-specific suppressor T-cells. There is, however, a further possibility which has aroused much interest.

Upregulation of T-cell interaction molecules

The majority of organ-specific autoantigens normally appear on the surface of the cells of the target organ in the context of class I but not class II MHC molecules. As such they cannot communicate with T-helpers and are therefore immunologically silent. Pujol-Borrell, Bottazzo and colleagues reasoned that, if the class II genes were somehow derepressed and class II molecules were now synthesized, they would endow the surface molecules with potential autoantigenicity (figure 19.16). Indeed, they have been able to show that human thyroid cells in tissue culture can be persuaded to express HLA-DR (class II) molecules on their surface after stimulation with γ-interferon (IFNγ), and, further, that the cytoplasm of epithelial cells from the glands of patients with Graves' disease (thyrotoxicosis) stains strongly with anti-HLA-DR reagents, indicating active synthesis of class II polypeptide chains (figure 19.1b). Inappropriate class II expression has also been reported on the bile ductules in primary biliary cirrhosis and on endothelial cells and some β-cells in the diabetic pancreas both in the human and in the BB rat model.

Whether adventitious expression of class II on these cells through activation by something like virally induced IFN is responsible for *initiating* the autoimmune process by priming autoreactive T-helpers, or whether reaction with *already activated* T-cells induces class II by release of IFNγ and makes the cell a more attractive target for provoking subsequent tissue damage, is still an unresolved issue. However, transfection of mice with the class II *H-2A* genes linked to the insulin promoter led to expression of class II on the β-islet cells of the pancreas but did *not* induce autoimmunity. Lack of B7 costimulatory molecules seems to be responsible for the failure of these class II-positive β-cells to activate naive T-cells, a job which may have to be left to the professional dendritic APCs.

Cytokine imbalance may induce autoimmunity

In contrast, transfection with the *IFNγ* gene on the insulin promoter under the same circumstances produced a local inflammatory reaction in the pancreas with aberrant expression of class II *and* diabetes; this must have been a result of autoimmunity since a normal pancreas grafted into the same animal suffered a similar fate. This implies that unregulated cytokine production producing a local inflammatory reaction can initiate autoimmunity, probably by enhancing the presentation of islet antigen by recruiting and activating dendritic cells, by increasing the concentration of processed intracellular autoantigen available to them, and by increasing their avidity for naive T-cells through upregulation of adhesion molecules; perhaps previously anergic cells may be made responsive to antigen (figure 19.16). Once primed, the T-cells can now interact with the islet β-cells which will be displaying increased amounts of class II and adhesion molecules for T-cells on their surface.

This all seems very straightforward but, although other proinflammatory cytokines, IL-12 and TNF as well as IFNγ, can promote the induction of organ-specific autoimmune disease at an early time by priming pathogenic Th1 responses, late expression of the same cytokines can drive the terminal differentiation and death of autoreactive T-cells. Thus we can in fact correct some spontaneous models of autoimmune disease by the injection of cytokines: IL-1 cures the diabetes of NOD mice, *t*umor *n*ecrosis *f*actor (TNF) prevents the onset of SLE symptoms in NZB×W hybrids and *t*ransforming *g*rowth *f*actor-*β1* (TGFβ1) is known to protect against collagen arthritis and relapsing *e*xperimental *a*utoimmune *e*ncephalomyelitis (EAE). The pleiotropic effects of the cytokines on different cell types involved at different stages in these diseases, and their positive and negative networking interactions with each other, add some uncertainty to the analysis and prediction of these complex events.

AUTOIMMUNE DISORDERS ARE MULTIFACTORIAL

We must come back to this. Undoubtedly, the autoimmune diseases have a multifactorial etiology combining polygenic traits and environmental influences. Many of the defects we have discussed, individually not necessarily uncommon, may contribute in various combinations to different disorders. No one gene is sufficient or required for disease onset and in any individual, disease susceptibility, presentation in terms of target organ severity and prognosis reflect additive or epistatic effects of several fortuitously inherited alleles, many of which may be shared with other autoimmune diseases. Even in a disease-prone strain of mice expressing an identical array of susceptibility genes, the proportion of animals developing autoimmune pathology (penetrance) increases with age and suggests that the expression of these complex traits requires an internal stochastic or environmental triggering of events, the probability of which increases with time. Thus, superimposed upon a genetically complex susceptibility, we might be dealing with some aging process affecting the thymus or the lymphoid stem cells and their internal control of self-reactivity. Sex hormones and defective pituitary–adrenal feedback loops may contribute. Now throw into this melange a panoply of dietary and other environmental factors, particularly microbial agents, which could have a variety of effects on the target organs, the lymphoid system and the cytokine network.

SUMMARY

The immune system balances precariously between effective responses to environmental antigens and regulatory control of an array of potentially suicidal responses to self-molecules.

The scope of autoimmune diseases
• Autoimmunity is associated with certain diseases which form a spectrum. At one pole, exemplified by Hashimoto's thyroiditis, the autoantibodies and the lesions are **organ-specific** with the organ acting as the target for autoimmune attack; at the other pole are the **nonorgan-specific** or **systemic autoimmune diseases**, such as SLE, where the autoantibodies have widespread reactivity and the lesions resemble those of serum sickness relating to deposition of circulating immune complexes.

• There is a tendency for organ-specific disorders such as thyroiditis and pernicious anemia to overlap in given individuals, while overlap of rheumatological disorders is greater than expected by chance.

• There are a number of models of organ-specific and systemic autoimmune diseases which occur spontaneously (e.g. nonobese diabetic mice or NZB×W hybrids with SLE) or can be induced experimentally (e.g. thyroiditis by thyroglobulin in complete Freund's adjuvant (CFA) and

(*continued p. 420*)

perhaps SLE by immunization with Id⁺ anti-DNA monoclonal in CFA).

Genetic and environmental influences
• Multifactorial genetic factors increase predisposition to autoimmune disease: these include HLA tissue type, the predisposition to aggressive autoimmunity and the selection of potential autoantigens.
• Females have a far higher incidence of autoimmunity than males, perhaps due to hormonal influences.
• Feedback control of lymphocytes through the cytokine–hypothalamus–pituitary–adrenal loop may be defective as shown for rheumatoid arthritis.
• Twin studies indicate a strong environmental influence in many disorders; both microbial and nonmicrobial factors have been suspected.

Autoreactivity comes naturally
• B-1 cells form a pool of mutually stimulating cells spontaneously producing 'natural antibodies' which interact idiotypically and frequently show multispecific autoreactivity.
• The immune system appears to have a set of T-cells directed to a limited number of dominant autoantigens which are tightly controlled.

Is autoimmunity driven by antigen?
• In spontaneous models of diabetes and thyroiditis, removal of antigen prevents autoimmunity.
• The development of high affinity mutated antibodies and immune responses to clusters of anatomically related antigens strongly imply B-cell selection of autoantigen.
• T-cell specificities in systemic autoimmunity are unknown but may be anti-idiotype.
• Autoantigens are, for the most part, accessible to circulating lymphocytes which normally include autoreactive T- and B-cells. Dominant autoantigens will induce tolerance but T-cells specific for peptides presented at low concentrations (cryptic epitopes) will be potentially autoreactive.

The T-helper is pivotal for control
• It is assumed that the key to the system is the control of autoreactive T-helper cells which are normally unresponsive because of clonal deletion, clonal anergy, T-suppression or inadequate autoantigen processing.

Autoimmunity can arise through bypass of T-helpers
• Abnormal modification of the autoantigen, cross-reaction with exogenous antigens or 'piggy-back' recognition of T-helper epitopes can provide new carrier determinants and epitope spread.
• T-helpers could also be bypassed by idiotype network interactions with cross-reactions between public idiotypes on autoantibodies and microbial antibodies or microbes themselves, or by antibodies formed to antiviral idiotypes which behaved as internal images of the virus and reacted with the cell surface viral receptor.
• Finally, B-cells and T-cells can be stimulated directly by polyclonal activators such as EB virus or superantigens.

Autoimmunity can arise through bypass of regulatory mechanisms
• T-helper bypass alone may be insufficient to *maintain* autoimmunity and it is generally considered that, in addition, a defect in cells which normally regulate autoimmunity is required.
• This could occur through an inability of the central T-helper cell to be tolerized or to respond to or induce T-suppressors.
• It could also arise through defects in antigen-specific, idiotype-specific and hsp and perhaps other nonspecific T-suppressor systems.
• Another possibility would be the derepression of class II genes giving rise to inappropriate cellular expression of class II so breaking the 'silence' between cellular autoantigen and autoreactive T-inducer.
• This would make the cell a target for activated T-cells but, without costimulators such as B7, perhaps only professional APCs could prime the resting autoreactive T-cell.
• Cytokine imbalance provides the circumstances for this to occur although the situation may be very complex.

Autoimmune disorders are multifactorial
• Given the polygenic predisposition, these changes could come about by some spontaneous internal dysregulation related perhaps to aging, and/or through environmental factors, particularly microbes, which could act in an uncomfortably large number of different ways.

See the accompanying website (**www.roitt.com**) for multiple choice questions.

FURTHER READING
Suggestions for further reading are given at the end of Chapter 20.

Autoimmune diseases
2 —Pathogenesis, diagnosis and treatment

INTRODUCTION

We should now look at the evidence which helps to uncover the mechanisms by which autoimmunity, however it arises, plays a **primary pathogenic role** in the production of tissue lesions within the group of diseases labeled as 'autoimmune'.

PATHOGENIC EFFECTS OF HUMORAL AUTOANTIBODY

Blood cells

The erythrocyte antibodies play a dominant role in the destruction of red cells in **autoimmune hemolytic anemia**. Normal red cells coated with autoantibody eluted from Coombs' positive erythrocytes (cf. figure 16.16) have a shortened half-life after reinjection into the normal subject, essentially as a result of their adherence to Fcγ receptors on phagocytic cells in the spleen. Remember also that B-1 cells in a mouse bearing a transgene encoding the New Zealand Black (NZB) mouse red cell autoantibody cause hemolytic disease (cf. p. 418). To put the case for B-1 cells beyond all reasonable doubt, any manipulation of NZB mice which elimi-

nates these cells, such as intraperitoneal injection of water, treatment with anti-interleukin (IL)-10 or introduction of the *xid* gene, prevents the development of hemolytic anemia.

Some children with immunodeficiency associated with very low white cell counts have a serum lymphocytotoxic factor which requires complement for its activity. Lymphopenia occurring in patients with systemic lupus erythematosus (SLE) and rheumatoid arthritis (RA) may also be a direct result of antibody, since nonagglutinating antibodies coating the white cells have been reported in such cases.

Platelet antibodies are apparently responsible for **idiopathic thrombocytopenic purpura** (ITP). IgG from a patient's serum when given to a normal individual causes a depression of platelet counts and the active principle can be absorbed out with platelets. The transient neonatal thrombocytopenia which may be seen in infants of mothers with ITP is explicable in terms of transplacental passage of IgG antibodies to the child.

The primary **antiphospholipid syndrome** is characterized by recurrent venous and arterial thromboembotic phenomena, recurrent fetal loss, thrombocytopenia and cardiolipin antibodies. Passive transfer of such antibodies into mice is fairly devastating,

Figure 20.1. Neonatal thyrotoxicosis. (a) The autoantibodies which stimulate the thyroid through the TSH receptors are IgG and cross the placenta. (b) The thyrotoxic mother therefore gives birth to a baby with thyroid hyperactivity which spontaneously resolves as the mother's IgG is catabolized. (Photograph courtesy of Professor A. MacGregor.)

resulting in lower fecundity rates and recurrent fetal loss. The effect seems to be mediated through reaction of the autoantibodies with a complex of cardiolipin and β_2-glycoprotein 1 which inhibits triggering of the coagulation cascade. The placental trophoblast is a primary target of these antibodies since the villous cytotrophoblast is one of the few cell types which externalizes phosphatidyl serine during development.

Surface receptors

Thyroid

Under certain circumstances antibodies to the surface of a cell may stimulate rather than destroy (cf. 'stimulating hypersensitivity'; Chapter 16). This would seem to be the case in **Graves' disease** (thyrotoxicosis or Basedow's disease) where a direct link with autoimmunity came with the discovery by Adams and Purves of thyroid-stimulating activity in the serum of these patients (Milestone 19.1), ultimately shown to be due to the presence of antibodies to TSH receptors (TSH-Rs), which seem to act in the same manner as TSH itself (cf. p. 345). Both operate through the adenyl cyclase system as indicated by the potentiating effect of theophylline, and both produce similar changes in ultrastructural morphology in the thyroid cell, but it is one of Nature's 'passive transfer experiments' which links TSH-R antibodies most directly with the pathogenesis of Graves' disease. When thyroid-stimulating antibodies (TSAbs) from a thyrotoxic mother cross the placenta, they cause the production of neonatal hyperthyroidism (figure 20.1), which resolves after a few weeks as the maternal IgG is catabolized.

There is a good correlation between the titer of TSAb and the severity of hyperthyroidism. Because TSAbs act independently of the pituitary–thyroid axis, iodine uptake by the gland is unaffected by the administration of thyroxine or tri-iodothyronine, whereas normally this would cause feedback inhibition and suppression of uptake; this forms the basis of an important diagnostic test for thyrotoxicosis.

There is reason to believe that enlargement of the thyroid in this disorder is due to the action of antibodies which react with a 'growth' receptor and directly stimulate cell division as distinct from metabolic hyperactivity. In contrast, sera from patients with **primary myxedema** (atrophic thyroiditis) contain antibodies capable of blocking the stimulation of growth by TSH, thereby preventing the regeneration of follicles which is a feature of the enlarged **Hashimoto goiter**. Graves' disease is often associated with exophthalmos which might be due to cross-reaction of antibodies to a 64 kDa membrane protein present on both thyroid and eye muscle.

Muscle and nerve

The transient muscle weakness seen in a proportion of babies born to mothers with **myasthenia gravis** calls to mind neonatal thrombocytopenia and hyperthyroidism and would certainly be compatible with the transplacental passage of an IgG capable of inhibiting neuromuscular transmission. Strong support for this view is afforded by the consistent finding of antibodies to muscle acetylcholine receptors (ACh-Rs) in myasthenics and the depletion of these receptors within the motor endplates. In addition, myasthenic symptoms can be induced in animals by injection of monoclonal antibodies to ACh-R or by active immunization with the purified receptors themselves. Nonetheless, the majority of babies with myasthenic mothers do not display muscle disease and it may be that they are protecting themselves through production of antibodies directed to idiotypes on the maternal autoantibodies.

Many myasthenics develop thymomas bearing molecules which cross-react with ACh-R although structurally not belonging to that gene family. It must be on the cards that molecular mimicry based on comparable peptide sequences may prime autoreactive T-cells which then drive genuine anti-ACh-R responses. An association with ACh-R polymorphism hints at some contribution to risk from the autoantigen.

Neuromuscular defects can also be elicited in mice injected with serum from patients with the **Lambert–Eaton** syndrome containing antibodies to presynaptic calcium channels. Autoantibodies to sodium channels which cross-react with *Campylobacter* bacilli have been identified in **Guillain–Barré syndrome**, a self-resolving peripheral polyneuritis. Rather more wayout is **Rasmussen's encephalitis**, a childhood disease of relentless and intractable focal seizures with an inflammatory histopathology in the brain; these patients have antibodies which act as agonists and kill kainic acid-responsive neurons through overstimulation of type 3 glutamine receptors. Would one uncover yet more phenomena of this kind in other neurological disorders if the search was widened and intensified?

Stomach

The underlying histopathological lesion in **pernicious anemia** is an atrophic gastritis in which a chronic inflammatory mononuclear invasion is associated with degeneration of secretory glands and failure to produce gastric acid. The development of achlorhydria is almost certainly accelerated by the inhibitory action of antibodies to the gastric proton pump, an H^+,K^+-dependent ATPase located in the membranes of the secretory canaliculi, and possibly also the gastrin receptors.

The idea that some cases of gastric ulcer may result from the stimulation of acid secretion by activation through antibodies to histamine receptors is appealing and we still await the further work required to establish its validity.

Other cellular receptors

Some patients with **atopic allergy** have serum blocking antibodies to β-adrenergic receptors and these may represent just one of many different types of factor which could alter the baseline sensitivity of mast cells and make the individual more at risk for the development of disease. The flip side of the coin is revealed in the cardiomyopathy of Chagas' disease where antibodies to these receptors act as agonists and increase the heart rate. Antibodies which block insulin receptors are a rare exotic species found in patients with acanthosis nigricans (type B) and ataxia telangiectasia associated with insulin resistance.

Other tissues

Gut

Some patients with **autoimmune atrophic gastritis** diagnosed by achlorhydria and parietal cell antibodies (see above and table 19.2) just meander on year after year without developing the vitamin B_{12} deficiency which precipitates **pernicious anemia**. It is probable that autoallergic destruction is roughly balanced by regeneration of mucosal cells, an explanation which could account for the observation that high doses of steroids may restore gastric function in certain patients with pernicious anemia. However, the balance would be upset were the patient now to produce antibodies to intrinsic factor in the lumen of the gastrointestinal tract; these would neutralize the small amount of intrinsic factor still available and the body would move into negative balance for B_{12}. The symptoms of B_{12} deficiency, pernicious anemia and sometimes subacute degeneration of the cord, would then appear some considerable time later as the liver stores became exhausted (figure 20.2).

The normally acquired tolerance to dietary proteins seems to break down in **celiac disease** where T-cell sensitivity to wheat gluten in the small intestine can be demonstrated. Since gluten can bind strongly to the extracellular matrix protein, endomysium, one could hypothesize that uptake of the complex by IgA B-cells specific for endomysium would 'piggy-back' the gluten into the B-cell for processing and presentation on MHC class II to gluten-specific T-helpers (cf. figure 19.13). Stimulation of the B-cell would now follow with secretion of the IgA endomysial antibodies which are exclusive to patients with celiac disease. Together with the increased expression of Fcα receptors in the lamina propria and evidence of complement and eosinophil activation, it is conceivable that antibody-mediated mechanisms could be pathogenic.

Skin

An antibody pathogenesis for **pemphigus vulgaris** is favored by the recognition of a 130 kDa autoantigen on stratified squamous epithelial cells which is a member of the cadherin family of Ca^{2+}-dependent adhesion molecules. Likewise, antibodies to desmoglein 1 probably mediate the blistering of the epidermis in **pemphigus foliaceus**.

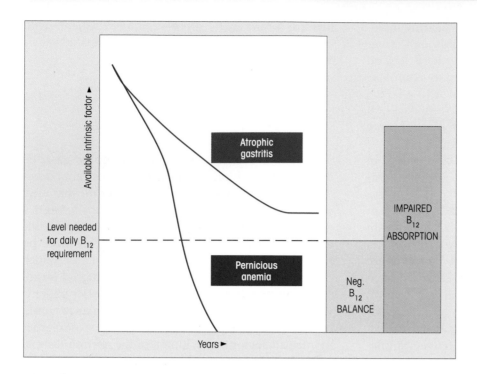

Figure 20.2. Pathogenesis of pernicious anemia. Patients with long-standing atrophic gastritis having parietal cell but no intrinsic factor antibodies do not go into negative B_{12} balance. Pernicious anemia develops when intrinsic factor antibodies become superimposed upon the atrophic gastritis. (After Doniach D. & Roitt I.M. (1964) *Seminars in Hematology* **I**, 313.)

Sperm

In some **infertile males**, agglutinating antibodies cause aggregation of the spermatozoa and interfere with their penetration into the cervical mucus.

Glomerular basement membrane (g.b.m.)

With immunological kidney disease, the experimental models preceded the finding of parallel lesions in the human. Injection of cross-reacting heterologous g.b.m. preparations in complete Freund's adjuvant produces glomerulonephritis in sheep and other experimental animals. Antibodies to g.b.m. can be picked up by immunofluorescent staining of biopsies from nephritic animals with anti-IgG. The antibodies are largely, if not completely, absorbed out by the kidney *in vivo* but they appear in the serum on nephrectomy and can passively transfer the disease to another animal of the same species.

An entirely analogous situation occurs in humans in certain cases of glomerulonephritis, particularly those associated with lung hemorrhage (**Goodpasture's syndrome**). Kidney biopsy from the patient shows *linear* deposition of IgG and C3 along the basement membrane of the glomerular capillaries (figure 16.17a). After nephrectomy, g.b.m. antibodies can be detected in the serum. Lerner and his colleagues eluted the g.b.m. antibody from a diseased kidney and injected it into a squirrel monkey. The antibody rapidly fixed to the g.b.m. of the recipient animal and produced a fatal nephritis (figure 20.3). It is hard to escape the conclusion that the lesion in the human was the direct result of attack on the g.b.m. by these complement-fixing antibodies. The lung changes in Goodpasture's syndrome are attributable to cross-reaction with some of the g.b.m. antibodies.

Curiously, mercuric chloride produces anti-g.b.m. glomerulonephritis in Brown Norway rats and, *pari passu*, as the disease remits, there is an upsurge in anti-idiotype suppressors. Nonsusceptible strains produce suppressors rather promptly.

Heart

Neonatal lupus erythematosus is the most common cause of permanent **congenital complete heart block**. Almost all cases have been associated with high maternal titers of anti-La/SS-B or anti-Ro/SS-A. The mother's heart is unaffected. The key observation was that anti-Ro bound to neonatal rather than adult cardiac tissue and altered the transmembrane action potential by inhibiting repolarization (figure 20.4). IgG anti-Ro reaches the fetal circulation by transplacental passage but, although maternal and fetal hearts are exposed to the autoantibody, only the latter is affected. Anti-

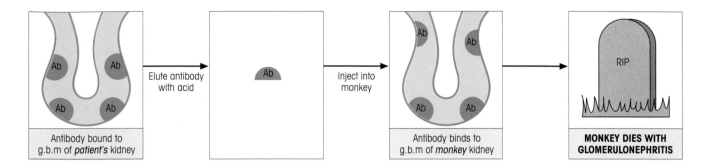

Figure 20.3. Passive transfer of glomerulonephritis to a squirrel monkey by injection of antiglomerular basement membrane (anti-g.b.m.) antibodies isolated by acid elution from the kidney of a patient with Goodpasture's syndrome. (After Lerner R.A., Glascock R.J. & Dixon F.J. (1967) *Journal of Experimental Medicine* **126**, 989.)

La/SS-A also binds to affected fetal hearts reacting with laminin in the basement membrane.

PATHOGENIC EFFECTS OF COMPLEXES WITH AUTOANTIGENS

Systemic lupus erythematosus (SLE)

Where autoantibodies are formed against soluble components to which they have continual access, complexes may be formed which can give rise to lesions similar to those occurring in serum sickness, especially when defects in the early classical complement components prevent effective clearance. Thus, although homozygous complement deficiency is a rare cause of SLE (cf. figure 16.24), the archetypal immune complex disorder, it represents the most powerful disease susceptibility genotype so far identified; more than 80% of cases with homozygous C1q and C4 deficiency have SLE. Up to one-half of the patients carry autoantibodies to the collagenous portion of C1q, but in truth there are a rich variety of different autoantigens in lupus (cf. table 19.2), some of them constituents of the nucleosome (cf. figure 19.1g), with the most pathomnemonic being **double-stranded DNA** (dsDNA). Anti-dsDNA is enriched in cryoglobulins and acid eluates of renal tissue from patients with lupus nephritis where it can be identified, presumably in complexes containing complement, by immunofluorescent staining of kidney biopsies from patients with evidence of renal dysfunction. The staining pattern with a fluorescent anti-IgG or anti-C3 is punctate or 'lumpy-bumpy' as once described (figure 16.17b), in marked contrast with the linear pattern caused by the g.b.m. antibodies

in Goodpasture's syndrome (figure 16.17a; p. 335). The complexes grow in size to become large aggregates visible in the electron microscope as amorphous humps on both sides of the g.b.m. (figure 20.5). During the active phase of the disease, serum complement levels fall as components are affected by immune aggregates in the kidney and circulation. Deposition of complexes is widespread as the name implies and, although 40% of patients *eventually* develop kidney lesions, the corresponding figures for organ involvement are 98% for skin (figure 20.6), 98% for joints/muscle, 64% for lung, 60% for blood, 60% for brain and 20% for heart.

Spontaneous production of anti-dsDNA is also a dominant feature of the animal models of SLE, NZB× W, MRL/*lpr*, BXSB and the *p21* single gene knockout mice, which involve fatal immune complex disease. Cationic anti-DNA, with arginines strategically positioned in locations of paratopic significance, emerges strongly as the disease progresses. The high affinity and IgG class of these antibodies, and the amelioration of symptoms and reduction of renal glomerular immune complexes by treatment of NZB×W mice with DNase I or anti-CD4, provide convincing evidence for a T-dependent antigen-driven complex-mediated pathology. But since DNA itself is not a thymus-dependent antigen and the SLE autoantibodies include a cluster directed to the physically linked antigens constituting the nucleosome, one might envisage a 'piggy-back' mechanism of the type portrayed in figure 19.13. Knowing that nucleosome 'blebs' appear on the surface of apoptotic cells and that a spontaneous expansion of nucleosome-specific T-cell populations precedes the clinical onset of SLE, a likely scenario would involve the internalization of nucleosome material captured on the surface receptors of anti-DNA B-cells, presentation of processed histone peptide–MHC class II complex to the histone-specific T-helper cells, and clonal proliferation of DNA antibody-forming cells (figure 20.7). Complexes of anti-DNA with circulating nucleosome material are demonstrable, and

Figure 20.4. Anti-Ro affects conduction in neonatal but not adult heart. (a) Action potential of neonatal NZW rabbit cardiac fiber before and 20 minutes after superfusion with serum containing anti-Ro/SS-A; the repolarization phase of the action potential is reduced by 30%. (b) The same with an adult cardiac fiber showing only 5% reduction. (Reproduced from Alexander E. *et al.* (1992) *Arthritis and Rheumatism* **35**, 176.) Anti-La/SS-B can be eluted from the fetal cardiac tissue of infants with congenital heart block. It reacts with fetal but not adult laminin in the basement membrane. Autoantibodies to the endogenous retroviral envelope protein (ERV-3) appear during pregnancy and disappear after delivery, except in women with autoimmune diseases where they persist, the highest levels being found in women with a history of congenital heart block children.

Figure 20.5. Renal biopsy of an SLE patient with severe immune complex glomerulonephritis and proteinuria. Electron micrograph showing irregular thickening of glomerular capillary walls by subepithelial complexes (a) and subendothelial complexes (b). The mesangial region shows abundant (probably phagocytosed) complexes. (Courtesy of Dr A. Leatham.)

Figure 20.6. The 'lupus band' in SLE. *Left*—section of skin showing slight thickening of the dermo-epidermal junction with underlying scattered inflammatory cells and a major inflammatory focus in the deeper layers. Low power H & E. *Right*—green fluorescent staining of a skin biopsy at higher power showing deposition of complexes containing IgG (anti-C3 gives the same picture) on the basement membrane at the dermo-epidermal junction. (Kindly provided by Professor D. Isenberg.)

these will bind through the histone (and presumably cationic anti-DNA) to extracellular heparan sulfate where they can accumulate and damage end-organ targets such as the kidney glomerulus.

There is yet another 'piggy-back' pathway. The possible involvement of idiotypes was mooted in the last chapter by reference to experiments in which immunization of mice with human monoclonal antinuclear antibodies gave rise to the production of new antibodies of similar idiotype and specificity—in biblical terms, 'antibody begets antibody'. Suppose a major public idiotype network is kicked into action by a microbial infection (cf. figure 19.14); for example, the 16/6 idiotype on a human anti-DNA circulating as a natural autoantibody is also carried on a germ-line antibody to *Klebsiella*. A T-helper cell recognizing

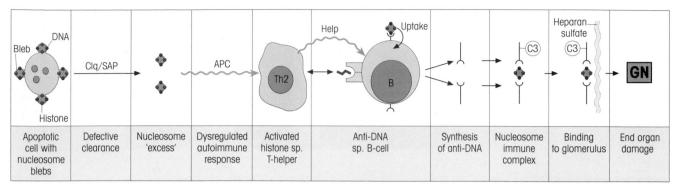

Figure 20.7. Conceivable pathogenetic pathway leading to end-organ damage in SLE. Nucleosomes derived from apoptotic cells can stimulate anti-DNA production by a 'piggy-back' mechanism in susceptible hosts. The resulting complexes bind to heparan sulfate in the glomerular basement membrane where they induce glo-merulonephritis. The high incidence of lupus in Clq deficient individuals and the susceptibility of lupus patients to skin rashes on exposure to UV in sunlight, which induces apoptosis in skin cells, are well known. SAP, serum amyloid precursor; APC, antigen-presenting cell; GN, glomerulonephritis.

processed 16/6 Id could stimulate anti-DNA B-cells which had captured a complex of DNA with the Id-positive natural autoantibody (cf. figure 19.13 and p. 208).

Rheumatoid arthritis

Morphological evidence for immunological activity

The joint changes in RA are in essence produced by the **malign growth of the synovial cells** as a pannus overlaying and destroying cartilage and bone (figure 20.8a–f). The synovial membrane which surrounds and maintains the joint space becomes intensely cellular as a result of considerable immunological hyper-reactivity, as evidenced by large numbers of T-cells, mostly CD4, in various stages of activation, usually associated with dendritic cells and macrophages (figure 20.8l); clumps of plasma cells are frequently observed and sometimes even secondary follicles with germinal centers are present as though the synovium had become an active lymph node (figure 20.8g–i). Indeed, it has been estimated that the synthesis of immunoglobulins by the synovial tissue ranks with that of a stimulated lymph node. There is widespread expression of surface HLA-DR (class II); T- and B-cells, dendritic and synovial lining cells and macrophages are all positive, indicative of some pretty lively action (figure 20.8k). The thesis is that this fiery immunological reactivity provides an intense stimulus to the synovial lining cells which undergo a Dr Jekyll to Mr Hyde transformation into the invasive pannus which brings about joint erosion through the release of destructive mediators.

IgG autosensitization and immune complex formation

Autoantibodies to the IgG Fc region (see figure 20.10a), known as **antiglobulins** or **rheumatoid factors**, are the hallmark of the disease, being demonstrable in virtually all patients with RA. The majority have IgM antiglobulins which react in the classical latex and sheep cell agglutination tests (table 19.2; note 7), and both they and the 'seronegative' patients who fail to react in these tests can be shown to have elevated levels of **IgG antiglobulins** detectable by solid-phase immunoassay (cf. p. 429; figure 20.9).

If, therefore, autosensitization to IgG is an almost universal feature of the disease, one might expect plasma cells in the synovium to be synthesizing antiglobulins. In fact 10–20% bind fluoresceinated IgG, either in the form of heat-aggregated material (figure 20.8j) or immune complexes (rheumatoid factor is a low affinity antibody and good binding is only seen when multivalent IgG is used as antigen). We must take into account a strange and unique feature of IgG antiglobulins; because they are both antigen and antibody at the same time, they are capable of **self-association** (figure 20.10b) and this hides the majority of free antiglobulin valencies. Cleverly realizing that destruction of the Fc regions by pepsin would liberate these hidden binding sites, Munthe and Natvig observed that a greater percentage of the plasma cells in the synovium displayed an anti-IgG specificity following treatment with this enzyme.

IgG aggregates, presumably products of these plasma cells, can be regularly detected in the synovial tissues and in the joint fluid where they give rise to typical acute inflammatory reactions with fluid exudates.

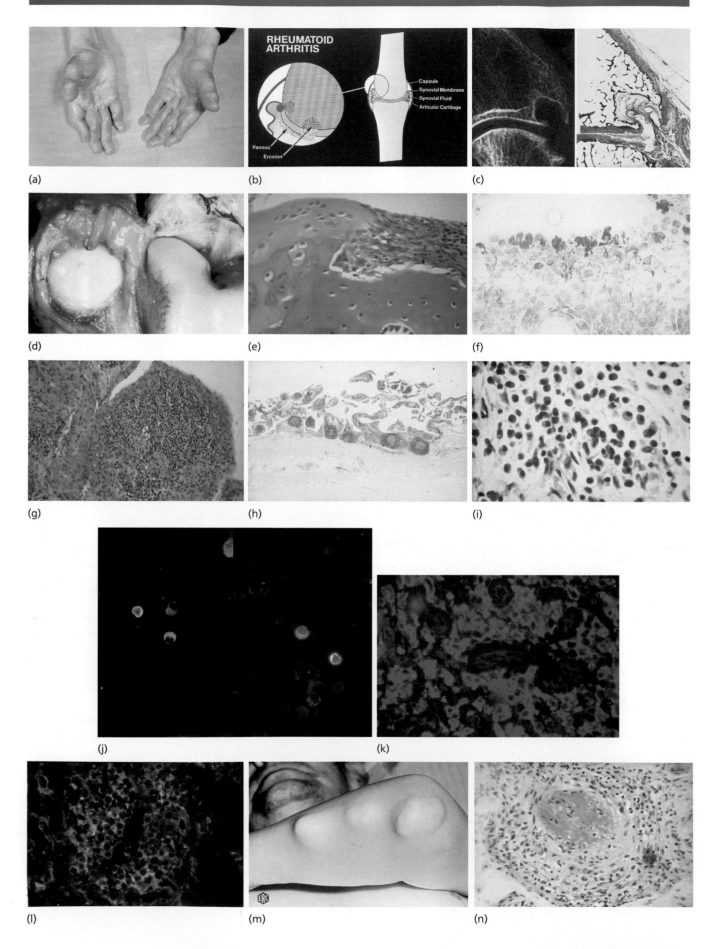

(a)

(b)

(c)

(d)

(e)

(f)

(g)

(h)

(i)

(j)

(k)

(l)

(m)

(n)

Analysis shows them to consist almost exclusively of immunoglobulins and complement, while a major proportion of the IgG is present as self-associated antiglobulin as shown by binding to an Fcγ immunosorbent after treatment with pepsin.

Abnormal patterns of IgG glycosylation

The two C_H2 domains in the Fc region are held apart (cf. p. 48) by two asparagine-linked sugars of the general structure shown in figure 20.11a and the terminal galactose lies in a special 'lectin-like' pocket (figure 20.11b). Some chains end in *N*-acetylglucosamine and lack the terminal galactose sugars. What is extraordinary is that the percentage of sugars completely lacking galactose in the IgG of both juvenile and adult RA patients is nearly always higher than in the controls and can be as high as 60%. This abnormal glycosylation could have four possible consequences.

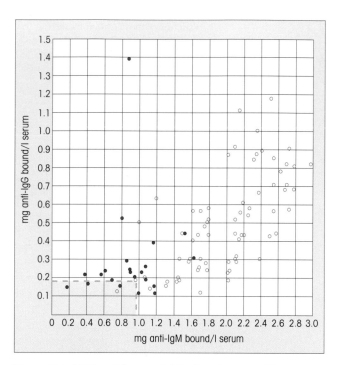

Figure 20.9. IgM and IgG antiglobulins determined by tube radioassay in patients with seropositive (open circles) and seronegative (filled circles) rheumatoid arthritis. The dashed lines indicate the 95% confidence limits (mean ± 2 SD) of the normal group. (From Nineham L., Hay F.C. & Roitt I.M. (1976) *Journal of Clinical Pathology* **29**, 1121.)

Figure 20.10. Self-associated complexes of IgG antiglobulins. Although of relatively low affinity, the strength of binding is boosted by the 'bonus effect' of the mutual attachment and, furthermore, such complexes in the joint may be stabilized by IgM antiglobulin and C1q which have polyvalent binding sites for IgG. Degradation of the Fc regions by pepsin releases the 'hidden' binding sites involved in the self-association. X-ray analysis of a complex of IgG Fc with two Fab fragments, isolated from a monoclonal IgM rheumatoid factor derived from an RA patient, showed binding of the Fab paratopes using the outer rather than the inner residues of the conventional antigen combining site CDRs; this suggests a novel form of cross-reactivity by allowing simultaneous binding to another antigen. (Sutton B. *et al.* (2000) *Immunology Today* **21**, 177.)

Figure 20.8. (*Opposite*) **Rheumatoid arthritis (RA).** (a) Hands of a patient with chronic RA showing classical swan-neck deformities. (b) Diagrammatic representation of a diarthrodial joint showing bone and cartilagenous erosions beneath the synovial membrane-derived pannus. (c) Proximal interphalangeal joint depicting marked bony erosion and marginal erosion of the cartilage. (d) Early pannus of granulation tissue growing over the patella. (e) Histology of pannus showing clear erosion of bone and cartilage at the cellular margin. (f) Histology of the pannus stained for macrophage nonspecific esterase; note long, stained dendritic processes. (g) Chronic inflammatory cells in the deeper layers of the synovium in RA. (h) A hypervillous synovium revealing well-formed secondary follicles with germinal centers (relatively rare occurrence). (i) A high power view of an area of diseased synovium showing collections of classical plasma cells. (j) Plasma cells isolated from a patient's synovial tissue stained simultaneously for IgM (with fluorescein-labeled F(ab')$_2$ anti-μ) and rheumatoid factor (with rhodamine-labeled aggregated Fcγ). Two of the four IgM-positive plasma cells appear to be synthesizing rheumatoid factors. (k) Rheumatoid synovium showing large numbers of cells stained by anti-HLA-DR (anti-class II). (l) Rheumatoid synovium showing class II-positive accessory cells (green) in intimate contact with CD4⁺ T-cells (orange). (m) Large rheumatoid nodules on the forearm. (n) Granulomatous appearance of the rheumatoid nodule with central necrotic area surrounded by epithelioid cells, macrophages and scattered lymphocytes. Plasma cells making rheumatoid factor are often demonstrable and the lesion probably represents a response to the formation of insoluble anti-IgG complexes. (Kindly given by (a) Dr D. Isenberg; (c), (d), (e), (g), (h) and (i) Dr L.E. Glynn; (f) Professor J. Edwards; (j) Professors P. Youinou and P. Lydyard; and (k) and (l) Professor G. Janossy.)

Figure 20.11. The Fc sugars and their role in bridging the two C$_H$2 domains of IgG. (a) Typical structure of each N-linked sugar. Some chains lack one (G1) or both terminal galactoses (agalacto-IgG; G0). (b) Structure of the C$_H$2 regions and the association between the terminal galactose on the 1,6 arm and the protein surface. The 1,3 arms, one of which must lack galactose, bridge the two domains. GlcNAc, N-acetylglucosamine; Man, mannose; Gal, galactose; Fuc, fucose.

1 The Fc may have increased autoantigenicity.

2 Self-associated IgG complexes (figure 20.10b) would be held together more strongly if the terminal galactose on the Fab sugar of one IgG fits into the lectin site on C$_H$2 left vacant by the lack of galactose on the Fc sugar.

3 The interaction with inflammatory mediators may be enhanced (figure 20.12). The exposure of N-acetylglucosamine in the agalacto-IgG glycoform allows recognition of immune complexes by mannose-binding protein with activation of the classical complement pathway (cf. p. 17) and stimulation of macrophages through binding of TNF. This increased inflammatory potency is clearly seen in the superiority of agalacto-anticollagen over its normally glycosylated counterpart in the production of collagen arthritis through synergy with cell-mediated immunity (see figure 20.13).

4 The interaction with Fcγ receptors on certain effector cells may be considerably modified as, for example, in defective feedback control of autoantibody production.

It is well established that pregnant women with RA have a remission of their disease as they approach term, but an exacerbation postpartum; as the arthritis remits, the agalacto-IgG values fall but, as the disease worsens after birth, agalacto-IgG becomes abnormal again suggesting intimate involvement with the disease process. Long-term studies in closed communities of Pima Indians, who have an unusually high incidence of RA, have shown that changes in IgG galactose provide an early marker of future clinical

Figure 20.12. Enhancement of inflammation by complexes containing agalacto-IgG. Mannose-binding protein combines with the exposed N-acetylglucosamine (GlcNAc) and through MASP (mannose-binding protein-associated serine protease) (cf. p. 17) activates classical complement pathway C2. TNF is a lectin which also binds GlcNAc and so stimulates macrophages at the surface of the complex. The IL-6 released further promotes agalacto-IgG synthesis by B-cells.

disease and we know they can be of **prognostic value** in patients with early RA.

The production of tissue damage

As explained in the legend to figure 20.10, the complexes can be stabilized by the multivalent Fcγ-binding

Figure 20.13. Induction of chronic arthritis by passive transfer of agalacto-IgG. Two injections of heat-denatured collagen type II in CFA (complete Freund's adjuvant) induce delayed sensitivity but no antibody or arthritis. Subsequent i.v. injection of murine monoclonal IgG anti-native collagen produced a moderate arthritis appearing after 20 days, whereas agalacto-IgG obtained by treatment of the IgG with β-galactosidase very rapidly produced a more severe arthritis. PBS, phosphate-buffered saline. (From Rademacher T.W., Williams P.J. & Dwek R.A. (1994) *Proceedings of the National Academy of Sciences of the United States of America* **91**, 6123, with permission of the National Academy of Sciences, Washington DC.)

molecules, IgM rheumatoid factor and C1q, and when present in the joint space they may initiate an Arthus reaction leading to an influx of polymorphs with which they react to release *reactive oxygen intermedi-ates* (ROIs) and lysosomal enzymes. These include neutral proteinases and collagenase which can **damage the articular cartilage** by breaking down proteo-glycans and collagen fibrils. More damage results if the complexes are adherent to the cartilage, since the polymorph binds but is unable to internalize them ('frustrated phagocytosis'); as a result, the lysosomal hydrolases are released extracellularly into the space between the cell and the cartilage where they are protected from enzyme inhibitors such as α_2-macroglobulin. We have already drawn attention to the enhanced inflammatory potency of complexes containing agalacto-IgG.

The aggregates may also stimulate the macrophage-like cells of the synovial lining, either directly through their surface receptors or indirectly through phagocy-tosis and resistance to intracellular digestion. At this point we should acknowledge that the release of cy-tokines such as TNF and GM-CSF from activated T-cells provides further potent macrophage stimulation.

The activated synovial cells grow out as a malign pannus (cover) over the cartilage (figure 20.8d) and, at

the margin of this advancing granulation tissue, break-down can be seen (figure 20.8e), almost certainly as a result of the release of enzymes, ROIs and especially of IL-1, 6 and TNF. Activated macrophages also secrete plasminogen activator and the plasmin formed as a consequence activates a latent collagenase produced by synovial cells. Sensitization to partially degraded collagen may occur and this could lead secondarily to amplification of the lesion. The secreted products of the stimulated macrophage can activate chondrocytes to exacerbate **cartilage breakdown**, and osteoclasts to bring about **bone resorption** which is a further compli-cation of severe disease (figure 20.8c). Subcutaneous nodules are granulomas (figure 20.8m and n) possibly formed through local production of insolubilized self-associating antiglobulins.

The contribution of these immune complexes to the pathogenesis of RA is built into the overview pre-sented in figure 20.14, where it will be seen that a role for the T-cells must by no means be overlooked and will be discussed in the following section.

T-CELL-MEDIATED HYPERSENSITIVITY AS A PATHOGENIC FACTOR IN AUTOIMMUNE DISEASE

Rheumatoid arthritis again

The chronically inflamed synovium is densely crowd-ed with activated T-cells and their critical role in the disease process is emphasized by the beneficial effects of cyclosporin and anti-CD4 treatments, and by the increased risk of disease associated with the 'shared epitope' sequences Q(R)K(R)RAA from residues 70–74 on the DRβ chain of DR1 and certain DR4 alleles (cf. table 17.2). High levels of IL-15 within the synovial membrane can recruit and activate T-cells whose secre-tion of cytokines and ability to induce macrophage synthesis of TNF and further IL-15 will drive pannus development powerfully with consequent erosion of cartilage and bone (figure 20.14). Chondrocytes them-selves may also be disease targets.

Just as in SLE, the antigenic specificity of these T-cells is still unknown. An appealing clue has come from the finding that the QKRAA shared epitope sequence, which lies within a polymorphic region of HLA-DR4/1 subtypes, is also present in the dnaJ heat-shock proteins from *E. coli*, *Lactobacillus lactis* and *Brucella ovis*, as well as the Epstein–Barr virus gp110 protein. This already provides an opportunity for priming of T-cells with autoreactive specificity for a processed peptide containing QKRAA presented by another HLA molecule, as discussed previously

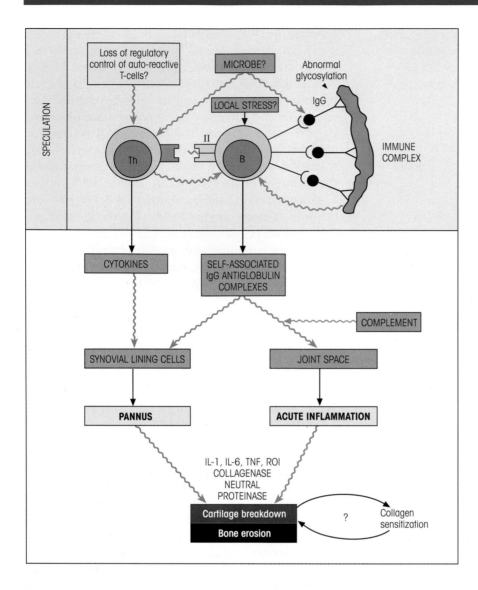

Figure 20.14. Immune pathogenesis of rheumatoid arthritis and speculation on the induction of autoimmunity. The defective pituitary–adrenal regulatory control on cell-mediated immunity in these patients was described in Chapter 19. The identity of the peptide(s) associated with the class II molecule is unknown. There are numerous opportunities for cross-reactions between the DRβ 'shared epitope' and various microbial heat-shock proteins. It has been reported that synovial fluid T-cells of juvenile rheumatoid arthritis patients respond strongly to human heat-shock protein 60, whereas those of adult rheumatoid arthritis patients do not. Recent data (Matsumoto *et al.* (1999) *Science* **286**, 1732) accord with the view that there must be some feature of the joint which makes it particularly sensitive to immune responses, maybe especially immune complexes, involving ubiquitous antigens.

(p. 414). The plot deepens with the realization that QKRAA binds to a second *E. coli* heat-shock protein dnaK and that HLA-DR containing the QKRAA sequence binds the *self* analogue of dnaK, namely hsp73, which targets selected proteins to lysosomes for processing. What this all means remains to be resolved but note the involvement of the hsp family yet again. Suspicion of previous microbial encounters is engendered by the discovery by PCR amplification of nucleotide sequences characteristic of *Mycoplasma fermentans*, *Chlamydia* and Epstein–Barr virus in a substantial proportion of synovial tissues removed from RA patients. Further work on the intracellular location, molecular status and possible expression of this material is awaited with interest.

The antigenic history of **reactive arthritis** is more amenable to study since it is triggered by an infection either of the urogenital tract by *Chlamydia trachomatis*

or of the enteric tract with *Yersinia*, *Salmonella*, *Shigella* or *Campylobacter*. The synovial tissue in reactive arthritis remarkably still retains antigenic descendants or memorials of the initiating bacteria many years after infection which can drive local T-cells. All the microbes are either obligate or facultative intracellular bacteria and so may escape the immune system by hiding inside cells, probably aided by high local production of IL-4. However, we may be dealing with molecular mimicry. Natural infection with *Salmonella typhimurium* generates CD8 cytotoxic T-cells which recognize an immunodominant epitope of the GroEL molecule presented by the class Ib Qa-1 and cross-react with a peptide from mouse hsp60, so permitting a reaction with stressed macrophages. HLA-B27 individuals are particularly at risk and the importance of the microbial component is emphasized by experiments on mice bearing the B27 transgene; if reared in a germ-free environment, lesions are restricted to the skin, but in the microbiological wilderness of the normal animal house, the skin, gut and joints are all affected. Why, as in RA, are the joints targeted and what does B27 do? Only one in 300 of the T-cells in the reactive arthritis synovium is CD8 and therefore class I restricted. It could be that a cross-reactive B27 sequence functions as a cryptic epitope perpetuating a gentle microbial stimulus with an amplifying autoimmune response.

Two experimentally induced models of arthritis are heavily dependent on T-cells. **Adjuvant arthritis** resulting from immunization of rats with complete Freund's adjuvant (CFA) only can be transferred to naive recipients with a T-cell clone specific for the mycobacterial heat-shock protein hsp60. The **collagen arthritis** model involves injection of type II collagen in complete Freund's, but here a synergy between cell-mediated hypersensitivity and antibody seems to operate: sensitization with denatured collagen in CFA-induced T-cell-mediated immunity but no arthritis unless the mice were also given IgG from animals primed with *native* collagen (figure 20.13).

Spontaneous models of arthritis are hard to come by. Up to 30% of MRL/*lpr* mice have arthritic lesions but this incidence varies with the animal house. If animals harbor Sendai virus, they are protected from arthritis; what is that telling us? To complete the circle, they also have raised levels of agalacto-IgG.

Before leaving the subject, one should not overlook the curious behavior of fibroblasts isolated from synovial tissue in established rheumatoid arthritis. In culture, they secrete collagenase which would contribute to cartilage breakdown, but more ominously they proliferate spontaneously due to unrestrained control of the cell cycle by cyclin-dependent kinases 4 and 6 and their respective D-cyclins. This implies that they would be refractory to conventional therapies and might be a cause of apparently intractable disease.

Organ-specific endocrine disease

To make a fairly sweeping statement, inflammatory organ-specific diseases are generally linked to T-helper-1 (Th1) responses. Clones producing EAE or transferring diabetes from NOD mice produce IL-2 and γ-interferon (IFNγ), while in collagen arthritis IL-12 can be substituted for the mycobacteria in the complete Freund's adjuvant. On the other hand, Th2 CD4s are responsible for the polyclonal activation in murine lupus, the glomerulonephritis and necrotizing vasculitis induced in Brown Norway rats by mercuric chloride, and the chronic autoimmunity generated during graft-vs-host disease. We will see that Th2 re-

sponses can downregulate destructive Th1 cells. Last, the Th1/Th2 polarization is not apparent in diseases such as myasthenia gravis, Graves' thyrotoxicosis, Sjögren's syndrome and primary biliary cirrhosis.

Autoimmune thyroiditis

The inflammatory infiltrate in autoimmune thyroiditis is usually essentially mononuclear in character (see figure M19.1.1c) and, although not an infallible guide, this has been taken as an expression of T-cell-mediated hypersensitivity. Firm evidence for a direct participation of T-lymphocytes has yet to be provided, although the demonstration of class II molecules on patients' thyrocytes and the presence of antigen-specific Th1 cells in the thyroid would accord with an involvement of these cells.

We must turn to the animal models for further evidence albeit indirect. Draconian stamping out of T-cells in the Obese strain chicken by neonatal thymectomy, and repeated injection of anti-T-cell serum, prevented the spontaneous development of atrophic autoimmune thyroiditis. It is also of interest to note that, at the target cell level, the threshold for induction of MHC class II on OS thyrocytes by IFNγ is far lower than that reported for normal thyroid cells, further reinforcing the notion that a thyroid abnormality is a contributory factor to the susceptibility phenotype. The other model, in which thyroiditis is induced by thyroglobulin in complete Freund's adjuvant (see figure M19.1.1b), can be transferred to naive histocompatible recipients with CD4$^+$ T-cell clones specific for peptides containing thyroxine established from immunized animals. The cells infiltrate between the thyroid follicles and probably kill the epithelial cells by a combination of locally released IFNγ and TNF. We see now that there is considerable diversity in the autoimmune response to the thyroid leading to tissue destruction, metabolic stimulation, growth promotion or mitotic inhibition which in different combinations account for the variety of forms in which autoimmune thyroid disease presents (figure 20.15).

Insulin-dependent diabetes mellitus (IDDM)

Just as in autoimmune thyroiditis, IDDM involves chronic inflammatory infiltration and destruction of the specific tissue, in this case the insulin-producing β-cells of the pancreatic islets of Langerhans. The delay in onset of disease achieved by early treatment with cyclosporin, at levels which have little effect on antibody production, points an accusing finger at effector T-cells as the agents of destruction, since this drug tar-

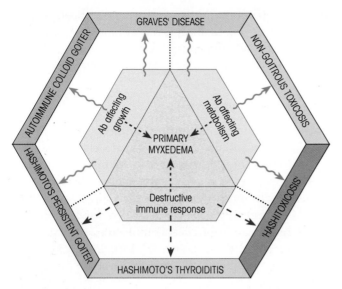

Figure 20.15. Relationship of different autoallergic responses to the circular spectrum of autoimmune thyroid diseases. Responses involving thyroglobulin and the thyroid peroxidase (microsomal) surface microvillous antigen lead to tissue destruction, whereas autoantibodies to TSH (and other ?) receptors can stimulate or block metabolic activity or thyroid cell division. 'Hashitoxicosis' is the down-to-earth term used by our Scots colleagues to describe a gland showing Hashimoto's thyroiditis and thyrotoxicosis simultaneously. (Courtesy of Professors D. Doniach and G.F. Bottazzo.)

gets T-cell cytokine synthesis so specifically. *In vitro* T-cell responses to islet cell antigens including glutamic acid decarboxylase (GAD) directly reflect the risk of progression to clinical IDDM. The strength of the risk factors associated with certain HLA-DQ alleles also has a strong whiff of T-cell action although, quite mysteriously, monocytes (and dendritic APCs?) constitutively expressing cyclooxygenase-2 (COX-2), the inducible enzyme responsible for the synthesis of prostaglandin E_2 and other prostanoids, were present in relatives (of IDDM patients) bearing these alleles and in the patients themselves.

To obtain further insight into the cellular siege and destruction of the islet β-cells, one has to turn to the **Nonobese diabetic (NOD) mouse** which spontaneously develops diabetic disease closely resembling human IDDM in its range of autoimmune responses and the association of islet breakdown with a chronic infiltration by T-cells and macrophages (figure 20.16). T-cells infiltrating the islets in diabetic mice had a Th1-type cytokine profile and could transfer disease to NOD recipients congenic for the severe combined immunodeficiency (*SCID*) mutation. The CD4/CD45RB[lo] memory subset of splenocytes from

young nondiabetic NOD mice inhibited this transfer, but the same subset from older diabetic mice had lost its regulatory power and had become pathogenic. This change to a Th1-type response coincided with the onset of diabetes and is consistent with the observation that IL-12, which favors Th1 responses, exacerbates disease. Just as in the human disease, MHC class II alleles hold a pivotal controlling position and introduction of a transgene, in which residues at position 56 or 57 of the H-2Aβ chain are altered, drastically inhibits the development of diabetes. One of the non-MHC susceptibility loci in NOD mapped to the *IL-1R* and *Bcg* genes on chromosome 1 was associated with natural resistance to infection by intracellular parasites. As a result, the NOD mouse is resistant to *Mycobacterium avium*, but after recovery from infection the onset of diabetes is prevented. That responses to hsp60 may be involved is implied by reports that a 24-amino acid peptide from this protein is the target of diabetogenic T-cells in both patients and the NOD mouse, and treatment with this peptide or with a NOD peptide-specific Th1 clone downregulates spontaneous disease. Cohen has interpreted this as a result of dysregulation of the 'immunological homunculus' (cf. p. 208) and notes that the level of a particular idiotype associated with a TCR CDR3 consistently falls prior to the onset of diabetes, while mice reared under germ-free conditions which might inhibit the development of a natural idiotype network are more susceptible to IDDM. Time will test the validity of this hypothesis. Notwithstanding this evidence relating to hsp and idiotypes, in the final analysis, one has to take into account the following: up to 50% of the infiltrating T-cells isolated from pre-diabetic NOD islets are insulin-specific and can transfer disease to young NOD mice; GAD-specific T-cells can also be recovered and are also diabetogenic; and tolerance to either insulin or GAD prevents the onset of disease. Presumably the latter can be accommodated by an organ-related bystander tolerance mechanism described below (p. 445). Overall, the data seem to be consistent with the necessity for two pathogenic pathways, one dependent on hsp and the other on an organ-specific response, operating either synergistically or serially, to achieve the final destruction of the pancreatic β-cells.

GAD in the central and peripheral nervous system produces γ-aminobutyric acid (GABA), a major inhibitory neurotransmitter, from glutamine. Autoantibodies to GAD are seen not only in early diabetes, but also in **Stiff man syndrome** (sounds like a cue for a Western) where the GABA-ergic pathways controlling motor neuron activity are defective. The antibodies cannot be pathogenic because GAD is present on the

(a)

(b)

(c)

(d)

Figure 20.16. Destruction of pancreatic islet β-cells by infiltrating T-cells in the Nonobese diabetic (NOD) mouse. (a) Normal intact islet. (b) Early peri-islet infiltration. (c) Penetration of the islet by infiltrating T-cells. (d) Almost complete destruction of insulin-producing cells with replacement by invading T-cells. Insulin stained by rhodamine-conjugated antibodies and T-cells by fluoresceinated anti-CD3. (Data reproduced from Quartey-Papafio R., Lund T., Cooke A. *et al.* (1995) *Journal of Immunology* **154**, 5567; photographs kindly provided by Dr Jenny Phillips.)

inner surface of the plasma membrane, but T-cells could be. How the brain as distinct from the pancreatic islet could be specifically targeted is a conundrum but 30% of patients do develop IDDM.

Multiple sclerosis (MS)

The idea that MS could be an autoimmune disease has for long been predicated on the morphological resemblance to *experimental autoimmune encephalomyelitis* (EAE), a demyelinating disease leading to motor paralysis (figure 20.17) produced by immunization with myelin, usually *myelin basic protein* (MBP) in complete Freund's. T-cell clones specific for MBP belong to restricted TCR Vβ families. They will transfer disease but this can be exacerbated by injection of a monoclonal antibody to Theiler's virus, a murine encephalomyelitis virus, cross-reacting with an epitope on myelin and oligodendrocytes. Presum-

ably the T-cell incites a local inflammation affecting the endothelial cells at the blood–brain barrier which opens the gate for antibody to penetrate the brain tissue.

How much of this is relevant to human disease? First, the serologically determined Caucasian DR2 phenotype (DRB1*1501, DQA1*0102, DQB1*0602) is strongly associated with susceptibility to MS. At least 37% of activated T-cells responsive to IL-2/4 in cerebrospinal fluid were specific for myelin components, compared with a figure of 5% for subjects with other neurological disturbances. A Leu.Arg.Gly. amino acid sequence motif found in around 40% of TCR Vβ5.2 N(D)N rearrangements in T-cells from MS lesions was present in a Vβ5.2 clone from an MS patient cytotoxic towards targets containing the MBP 89–106 peptide and in encephalitogenic rat T-cells specific for MBP peptide 87–99. One is greatly encouraged to continue with attempts to induce tolerance.

(a)

(b)

(c)

(d)

Figure 20.17. Experimental autoimmune encephalomyelitis (EAE), a demyelinating model for multiple sclerosis induced by immunization with brain antigens in complete Freund's adjuvant (CFA). (a) Early lesion of EAE in the rat at 9 days after immunization with rat spinal cord homogenate in CFA. The lesion in brain white matter, which is probably a few hours old, shows perivenous infiltration of lymphocytes and monocytes (a pure mononuclear inflammation) with cells invading the nervous parenchyma. Myelin is not stained. (b) Lumbar spinal cord of rat with chronic EAE after immunization with myelin proteolipid protein. Large demyelinating lesions in dorsal columns, in both left (large) and right (small) columns, as well as on lower left. Also gray matter involved with ongoing inflammation, in particular affecting left dorsal horn. Normal myelin is stained brown. (c) Chronic relapsing EAE in guinea-pig. Large demyelinated plaques in brain white matter (arrows) closely similar to plaques of multiple sclerosis. (d) Acute EAE in cat with optic nerve involvement. (Legend and slides provided by Dr B. Waksman; (b) originally from Dr Trotter, (c) from Drs Lassmann and Wisniewski and (d) from Dr Patterson.)

Psoriasis

Given the evidence for T-cell-mediated pathogenesis (p. 344), the isolation of clones specific for group A β-hemolytic streptococci from guttate skin lesions has fostered the thought that pathology is initiated by exotoxin (i.e. superantigen) recruited T-cells and is maintained by specific cells reacting both with streptococcal M protein and a cryptic skin epitope, possibly a keratin variant presented by cytokine-activated keratinocytes. There is extensive sequence homology between M proteins and type I keratin.

SOME OTHER SYSTEMIC VASCULAR DISORDERS WITH IMMUNOPATHOLOGICAL COMPONENTS

The characteristic feature of **Wegener's granulomatosis** is a necrotizing granulomatous vasculitis. Although the antibodies to proteinase III (antineutrophil cytoplasmic antibodies (cANCA); figure 20.18 and table 19.2) characteristic of this disease are directed to an intracellular antigen associated with the primary granules of the polymorph, recent studies reveal a possible mechanism by which they might induce

Figure 20.18. Antineutrophil cytoplasmic antibodies (ANCA). *Left*—cytoplasmic cANCA (cf. table 12.2) diffuse staining specific for proteinase III in Wegener's granulomatosis; *right*—perinuclear p-ANCA staining by myeloperoxidase antibodies in periarteritis nodosa. Fixed neutrophils are treated first with patient's serum then fluorescein-conjugated anti-human Ig. (Kindly provided by Dr G. Cambridge.)

vasculitic lesions. Cytokine priming of polymorphs causes translocation of proteinase III to the cell surface, whereupon reaction with the autoantibody activates the cell causing degranulation and generation of *reactive oxygen intermediates* (ROIs). A possible scenario might go something like this: tumor necrosis factor (TNF) induced by infection could activate endothelial cells to secrete interleukins IL-1 and IL-8 which attract neutrophils, upregulate their lymphocyte function associated molecule-1 (LFA-1) adhesion molecules, and prime them for reaction with the proteinase III antibody. Endothelial cell injury would then be a consequence of the release of superoxide anion and other ROIs. Other authors have laid claim to endothelial membrane antibodies which upregulate adhesion molecules and increase secretion of IL-6 and 8 and MCP-1. Anti-ANCA idiotypes are demonstrable in the IgM fraction of serum from patients in remission and their removal uncovers underlying IgG ANCA activity.

A giant cell arteritis of large- and medium-sized arteries, involving mainly CD8+ T-cells and macrophages, characterizes the pathology of **temporal arteritis**. The antigen is elusive but the disease is strongly associated with HLA-DR4 and is exquisitely sensitive to high-dose steroids.

Systemic sclerosis, also known as **scleroderma**, is a generalized disease of connective tissue with increased deposition of collagen and other matrix components, causing extensive fibrotic destruction of the skin and internal organs centered around small arteries and microvasculature, eventually producing capillary occlusion. To put it mildly, the pathogenesis is poorly understood, but the high frequency of positive results for centromere, nucleolar and topoisomerase-1 (Scl-70) autoantibodies and rheumatoid factors betokens some major intrusion by autoimmune elements, and there is multisystem infiltration by CD8+ T-cells secreting mainly TGFβ and IL-6. So far, the only clues pointing to early etiological factors have come from animal models of scleroderma. So-called 'tight skin' mice have a mutation in the fibrilin-1 gene coding for an extracellular matrix protein which might be responsible for activating T-cells. Another model, the UCD 200 chicken, reveals endothelial cell apoptosis as a very early event, speculatively due to ADCC mediated by endothelial cell antibodies; mononuclear cell infiltration occurred later with fibrosis as the hallmark of late disease. Anyway, in human scleroderma, TGFβ secreted by T-cells would stimulate dermal fibroblasts to overproduce collagen and, ultimately, just like the synovial fibroblasts in RA, they acquire a semi-autonomy making the disease very difficult to treat.

Atherosclerotic plaques are focal lesions of large elastic and muscular arteries producing intimal thickening and are composed of a subendothelial fibrous cap of collagen and matrix-rich connective tissue, lipid-filled macrophages, proliferating smooth muscle cells and some CD4 T-lymphocytes. Rupture of a plaque leads to thrombosis. The mood is swinging towards the idea that autoimmunity may initiate or exacerbate the process of plasma lipid deposition and plaque formation. The two lead candidate antigens are heat-shock protein 60 (hsp60) and the low density lipoprotein (LDL), apoprotein B, which is the main carrier of cholesterol.

The indicative evidence is as follows (figure 20.19). Immunization with mycobacterial hsp65 elicits atherosclerotic lesions at classical predilection sites subject to major hemodynamic stress, and a cholesterol-rich diet makes them worse. Antibodies are produced which are said to react with heat- or TNF-stressed endothelial cells, implying that hsps are somehow implicated. Furthermore, such endothelial provocation and activation of the macrophages by contact with LDL generate oxidative free radicals, which convert lecithin within the LDL to lysolecithin which is chemoattractant and cytotoxic, and polyunsaturated fatty acids to alkenals which react with the lysine residues of apoprotein B making it 'tasty' for the macrophage scavenger receptors and, perhaps, autoantigenic. Pointing the finger at these oxidative processes as keys to atherogenesis receives support from the epidemiological data on an inverse correlation between coronary heart disease in patients and

Figure 20.19. Expression of heat-shock protein 60 in an early human arteriosclerotic lesion. Frozen, unfixed, 4 μm thick section of a fatty streak (=early lesion) of a human carotid artery stained in indirect immunofluorescence with a monoclonal antibody to heat-shock protein 60 and a fluorescein-labeled second antibody. A strong reaction with endothelial cells as well as cells infiltrating the intima, including foam cells, is evident. (Original magnification × 400.) (Photograph kindly provided by Professor G. Wick.)

dietary intake of antioxidants, and the observation that the induction of atherosclerotic fatty streaks by high cholesterol diets in rabbits can be prevented by the antioxidant probucol, despite its lack of influence on plasma cholesterol levels. Yet another piece in the jigsaw: β_2-glycoprotein-1, which figures prominently in the antiphospholipid syndrome (cf. p. 421), is also abundantly present in atherosclerotic lesions. Clarification is awaited.

DIAGNOSTIC VALUE OF AUTOANTIBODY TESTS

Serum autoantibodies frequently provide valuable diagnostic markers. The most useful routine test is screening of the serum by immunofluorescence on a frozen section prepared from a composite block of un-fixed human thyroid and stomach, and rat kidney and liver. This is supplemented by agglutination tests for rheumatoid factors and for thyroglobulin, thyroid peroxidase and red cell antibodies and by ELISA for antibodies to intrinsic factor, DNA, IgG, extractable nuclear antigens, and so on (see table 19.2). The salient information is summarized in table 20.1. ELISAs are taking over and tests with purified gene-cloned antigens arranged in minispot arrays will one day supplant the need for immunofluorescence which is time-consuming and more skilled.

The tests will also prove of value in screening for people at risk, e.g. relatives of patients with autoimmune diseases such as diabetes, thyroiditis patients for

gastric autoimmunity and vice versa, and ultimately the general population if the sociological consequences are fully understood and acceptable.

The development of easily performed commercial ELISPOT (cf. p. 140) assay kits for monitoring the production of individual cytokines by peripheral blood T-cells incubated with specific antigens will be greatly welcomed.

TREATMENT OF AUTOIMMUNE DISORDERS

Control at the target organ level

The majority of approaches to treatment, not unnaturally, involve manipulation of immunological responses (figure 20.20). However, in many organ-specific diseases, metabolic control is usually sufficient, e.g. thyroxine replacement in primary myxedema, insulin in juvenile diabetes, vitamin B_{12} in pernicious anemia, antithyroid drugs for Graves' disease, and so forth. Anticholinesterase drugs are commonly used for long-term therapy in myasthenia gravis; thymectomy is of benefit in most cases and it is conceivable that the gland contains acetylcholine (ACh) receptors in a particularly immunogenic form (? associated with HLA class II expression).

It is worth recording that maintenance therapy to replace the loss of an organ-specific molecule, such as insulin in IDDM, might have the effect of subduing metabolic activity and reducing expression of the target antigen. Help should be on the way for patients with burnt-out pancreatic β-cells. Xenografts of genetically engineered fetal or neonatal pig islets (cf. figure 17.15) are under study, and other good news is that stem cells contained within ductal structures of the adult pancreas can be differentiated in culture to provide a 10 000-fold increase in the number of available islets per organ, although any recurrence of immunologically mediated damage would need to be dealt with. Perhaps transfection of the grafted cells with TGFβ might provide an appropriately suppressive microenvironment. A slightly cheeky but novel approach to the repair of damaged target organs is to target a nonpathogenic specific T-cell clone expressing a transgenic growth factor to the inflamed area. Thus, a nonaggressive Th2 clone, specific for the proteolipid (PLP) brain antigen, delivered a platelet-derived growth factor (PDGF-A) transgene to the inflamed brain of an animal with EAE; contact with antigen stimulated the clone and the secreted growth factor induced proliferation of the oligodendrocyte progenitor cells involved in remyelination. This would be a highly customized therapy only suitable for the well-

Table 20.1. Autoimmunity tests and diagnosis.

DISEASE	ANTIBODY	COMMENT
Hashimoto's thyroiditis	Thyroid	Distinction from colloid goiter, thyroid cancer and subacute thyroiditis Thyroidectomy usually unnecessary in Hashimoto goiter
Primary myxedema	Thyroid	Tests +ve in 99% of cases. If suspected hypothyroidism assess 'thyroid reserve' by TRH stimulation test
Thyrotoxicosis	Thyroid	High titers of cytoplasmic Ab indicate active thyroiditis and tendency to post-operative myxedema: anti-thyroid drugs are the treatment of choice although HLA-B8 patients have high chance of relapse
Pernicious anemia	Stomach	Help in diagnosis of latent PA, in differential diagnosis of non-autoimmune megaloblastic anemia and in suspected subacute combined degeneration of the cord
Insulin-dependent diabetes mellitus (IDDM)	Pancreas	Insulin Ab early in disease. GAD Ab standard test for IDDM. Two or more autoAb seen in 80% of new onset children or prediabetic relatives but not in controls
Idiopathic adrenal atrophy	Adrenal	Distinction from tuberculous form
Myasthenia gravis	Muscle ACh receptor	When positive suggests associated thymoma (more likely if HLA-B12), positive in >80%
Pemphigus vulgaris and pemphigoid	Skin	Different fluorescent patterns in the two diseases
Autoimmune hemolytic anemia	Erythrocyte (Coombs' test)	Distinction from other forms of anemia
Sjögren's syndrome	Salivary duct cells, SS-A, SS-B	
Primary biliary cirrhosis	Mitochondrial	Distinction from other forms of obstructive jaundice where test rarely +ve Recognize subgroup within cryptogenic cirrhosis related to PBC with +ve mitochondrial Ab
Active chronic hepatitis	Smooth muscle anti-nuclear and 20% mitochondrial	Smooth muscle Ab distinguish from SLE Type 1 classical in women with Ab to nuclei, smooth muscle, actin and asialoglycoprotein receptor (these Ab disappear on remission indicating reduction in steroids) Type 2 in girls and young women with anti-LKM-1 (cyt P450)
Rheumatoid arthritis	Antiglobulin, e.g. SCAT and latex fixation Antiglobulin + raised agalacto-Ig Perinuclear	High titer indicative of bad prognosis Prognosis of rheumatoid arthritis V.sp. for early RA. Dominant residue citrulline (post-translational modification of arginine)
SLE	High titer antinuclear, DNA Phospholipid	DNA antibodies present in active phase Ab to double-stranded DNA characteristic; high affinity complement-fixing Ab give kidney damage, low affinity CNS lesions Thrombosis, recurrent fetal loss and thrombocytopenia
Scleroderma	Nucleolar + centromere Scl-70	Characteristic of the disease
Wegener's granulomatosis	Neutrophil cytoplasm	Antiserine protease closely associated with disease; treatment urgent

heeled, but a cheaper gambit is to inject a plasmid DNA coding for Fas ligand in liposomes directly into the organ under attack. This manipulation, carried out in an experimental autoimmune thyroiditis model, induced persisting expression of FasL on thyroid follicular cells and total abrogation of antithyroglobulin cytotoxic T-lymphocytes.

The reader may recall the spontaneous proliferation of RA synovial fibroblasts when placed in culture. These cells undergo irreversible cell cycle arrest if subjected to γ-irradiation, which induces the synthesis of the p16^{INK4a} senescence protein. This is a tumor suppressor which blocks the stable association of cyclin-dependent kinases 4 and 6 with their respective D-cyclins and inhibits their ability to mastermind the passage of cells into the G1 phase of the cell growth cycle. Injection of the RA fibroblasts with a recombinant adenovirus encoding the *p16^{INK4a}* gene halted their growth and reduced synovial cell hyperplasia in the adjuvant arthritis model. If focus on expression of

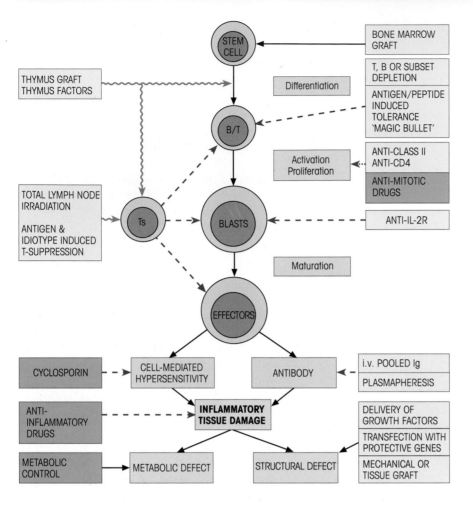

Figure 20.20. The treatment of autoimmune disease. Current conventional treatments are in dark orange; some feasible approaches are given in lighter orange boxes. (In the case of a live graft, bottom right, the immunosuppressive therapy used may protect the tissue from the autoimmune damage which affected the organ being replaced.)

this gene fosters a new therapeutic approach to RA, it might also find utility in other disorders such as atherosclerosis, scleroderma and possibly late stage asthma. Conceivably, the benefit of adding methotrexate to anti-TNF therapy in RA (see below) might be partly attributable to an effect on fibroblast proliferation.

Based on the possibility that multiple sclerosis is virally driven, patients have been treated with IFNβ; relapse rates were reduced by a third in relapsing–remitting disease, but there was only a modest effect on progressive disease. Note, however, that IFNβ influences some T-cell functions in addition to its effect on viral proliferation.

Anti-inflammatory drugs

Patients with severe myasthenic symptoms respond well to high doses of steroids and the same is true for serious cases of other autoimmune disorders, such as SLE and immune complex nephritis, where the drug helps to suppress the inflammatory lesions.

In RA, steroids are very effective, but the recognition of a defective pituitary–adrenal feedback loop in these patients has inspired a novel approach aiming to restore normal corticosteroid levels by a depot of methylprednisolone (Depomedrone) which delivers a low daily dose—the earlier in the disease the better. This treatment accelerates the induction of remission and decreases the side-effects of second-line agents such as gold salts. Selectins and adhesion molecules on endothelial cells and leukocyte integrins appear to be downregulated and this would seriously impede the influx of inflammatory cells into the joint. Anti-inflammatory drugs such as salicylates, innumerable synthetic prostaglandin inhibitors and metalloproteinase poisons are widely used. The so-called second-line drugs, sulfasalazine, penicillamine, gold salts and antimalarials such as chloroquine, all find an important place in therapy but their mode of action is unknown.

Treatment with antibodies to adhesion molecules such as CD44 effectively blocks experimental arthritis but there are considerable practical and economic problems in adapting to human disease. Therapeutic blocking of other mediators directly concerned in immunological tissue damage will be feasible as cytokine and complement antagonists become available. Neutralizing TNF with a humanized monoclonal antibody is most effective in the short term, so revealing the pathogenetic role of this cytokine. Most significantly, synergistic administration with methotrexate does seem to offer more lasting benefit (figure 20.21).

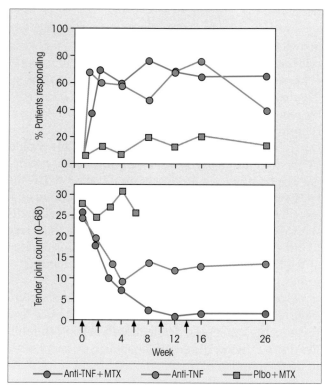

Figure 20.21. Synergy of anti-TNF and methotrexate in the treatment of rheumatoid arthritis. Top panel: Duration of response to therapy as defined by 20% Paulus criteria at three doses of monoclonal chimeric anti-TNF (infliximab) with and without methotrexate (MTX) and placebo (Plbo) plus MTX. Results shown are the proportion (%) of patients responding at weeks 1, 2, 4, 8, 12, 16 and 26. The Paulus response is achieved by 20% improvement in four out of six of the following: tender joint and swollen joint scores, duration of morning stiffness, erythrocyte sedimentation rate and a two grade improvement in the patient's and observer's assessment of disease severity. Lower panel: Serial measurements (median values) of the tender joint count, before (day 0), during (weeks 1–14) and after (weeks 14–26) treatment. Results are included only up to the point at which ≥50% of patients remained in the trial (up to week 6 for the placebo plus MTX group). Arrows indicate the timing of infusions of infliximab at weeks 0, 2, 6, 10 and 14. Methotrexate was given weekly and virtually eradicated the production of antibodies to the human chimeric antibody. (Data kindly provided by Professors R.N. Maini, M. Feldmann *et al.*, see Maini R.N. *et al.* (1998) reproduced with permission from Lippincott, Williams & Wilkins, MD, USA, *Arthritis and Rheumatism* **41**, 1552.)

Transfection of synovial cells with the natural IL-1 receptor antagonist IL-1Ra may turn out to be a useful long-term strategy.

Immunosuppressive drugs

In a sense, because it blocks cytokine secretion by T-cells, cyclosporin is an anti-inflammatory drug and, since cytokines like IL-2 are also obligatory for lymphocyte proliferation, cyclosporin is also an antimitotic drug. It is of proven efficacy in uveitis, early type I diabetes, nephrotic syndrome and psoriasis and of moderate efficacy in idiopathic thrombocytopenic purpura, SLE, polymyositis, Crohn's disease, primary biliary cirrhosis and myasthenia gravis. In a double-blind randomized control trial, cyclosporin demonstrated significant though not complete disease suppression over 12 months in a group of previously refractory rheumatoid arthritis (RA) patients. Unfortunately, high toxic doses were used but the synergy with rapamycin is a strong indication for a trial of combined therapy. Leflunomide is a promising new agent for treatment of RA. Its active metabolite inhibits *de novo* rUMP synthesis leading to G1 arrest of cycling lymphocytes.

While awaiting more selective therapy, conventional nonspecific antimitotic agents such as azathioprine, cyclophosphamide and methotrexate, usually in combination with steroids, have been used effectively in SLE, RA, chronic active hepatitis and autoimmune hemolytic anemia for example. High-dose i.v. cyclophosphamide plus adrenocorticotropic hormone (ACTH) or total lymph node irradiation through its effect on the peripheral immune system either slowed or stopped the advance of disease in approximately two-thirds of progressive multiple sclerosis (MS) patients for 1–2 years, a strong indication that the disease is mediated by immune mechanisms. This is further supported by the unfortunate finding that IFNγ exacerbates disease in the majority. Pulsing MS patients with the antileukocyte humanized monoclonal Campath-1H (anti-CD52) produced a brutal and surprisingly persistent reduction in T-cell numbers. Over a 2-year period virtually no new lesions were detected, although in half the patients there was progression of pre-existing lesions. A startling 33% developed Graves' disease (wow!), although this disturbing statistic was not a feature of many other disorders, including RA, where Campath-1H has been used.

It is true that the EAE animal model can be countered by some very diverse manipulations: the antidepressant, roliprim, suppresses cytokine production, a non-hypocalcemic derivative of vitamin D_3 potently blocks

IL-12 secretion, type IV phosphodiesterase inhibitors suppress Th1 cells and blockade of non-*N*-methyl-D-aspartate (NMDA) receptors ameliorates the neurological sequelae. The problem is that, as it is so difficult to carry out clinical trials in MS, few if any of these approaches are likely to see the light of day.

Immunological control strategies

Cellular manipulation

It should one day be practical to correct any relevant defects in stem cells or in thymus processing by gene therapy, bone marrow or thymus grafting or perhaps, in the latter case, by thymic hormones. Many centers are trying out autologous stem cell transplantation following hemato-immunoablation by cytotoxic drugs in severe cases of autoimmune disease. Around two-thirds of a series of difficult cases of SLE, scleroderma, juvenile and adult RA and so on, stabilized or improved. Transplant-related mortality risk at 2 years was $8\pm6\%$, comparable to that seen with cancer patients.

If defects in programed cell death in antigen-activated T-cells contribute in any way to the development of certain autoimmune diseases, bisindolyl-maleimide, which potentiates weak and moderate apoptotic signals, might be therapeutic.

Because T-cell signaling is so pivotal, it is the target for many strategies (figure 20.22). Injection of monoclonal anti-MHC class II and anti-CD4 successfully fends off lupus in spontaneous mouse models, and it is relevant to record the preliminary clinical observations that injection of immunoglobulins eluted from placentas, and shown to contain anti-allo-class II, significantly ameliorates the symptoms of RA. Immunization with a cyclic peptide from a polymorphic region of the β chain of the Nonobese diabetic (NOD) class II molecule protected a large proportion of the mice from disease. It is unclear whether the mechanism involves a block on MHC antigen presentation or relates to the MHC mimicry hypothesis (cf. p. 413).

Some take the anti-IL-2 receptor approach to deplete activated T-cells (figure 20.22 (1)), but we would like to refer back to our discussion of the long-lasting effect of *nondepleting* anti-CD4 for the induction of tolerance (figure 20.22 (2) and (3)), particularly when reinforced by repeated exposure to antigen (cf. p. 361). Antigen reinforcement of course is an obvious continuing feature in autoimmune disease, so that anti-CD4 should be ideal as a therapy in disorders where the natural 'switch-off' tolerogenic signals are still accepted by the CD4 cells. Ongoing trials in RA still look promising. Excellent remissions have been recorded in patients with Wegener's granulomatosis who were refractory to normal treatment, following sequential injection of anti-CD52 (Campath-1H) and nondepleting anti-CD4 monoclonals.

We can manage perfectly well in life without a complete set of our TCR *Vβ* genes; after all, wild mice, and presumably ourselves, delete large tracts of Vβ families during thymic differentiation and it does not seem to do them much harm. So, the argument runs, if the autoimmune T-cell clones specific for the autoantigen in a given disease happen to be restricted to membership of a particular Vβ family, we could delete all members of that family *in vivo* with the appropriate antiserum and yet not make irreparable holes in the host's defenses (figure 20.22 (6)). In PL mice immunized with the N-terminal peptide of myelin basic protein, anti-Vβ8 eliminated experimental autoallergic encephalitis almost entirely, so the strategy can work. Not so good with SJL mice which respond to peptide 89–101 with 50% of the T-cells using Vβ17 receptors; in this case, anti-Vβ17 did not block disease. Clearly, until we have a wider knowledge of the extent of Vβ restriction for each antigen and also for each individual, we must suspend judgment on the general feasibility of the strategy.

Now, if one takes the view that rheumatoid factor immune complexes are major players in the patho-

Figure 20.22. Strategic options for therapy based on T-cell targeting.

genesis of the RA joint lesions, logic suggests the radical approach of B-cell ablation with monoclonal anti-CD20 as used in the treatment of B-cell leukemia. Results to date are provocatively encouraging.

Manipulation of regulatory mediators

We can correct some spontaneous models of autoimmune disease by injection of cytokines: IL-1 cures the diabetes of NOD mice; TNF prevents the onset of SLE symptoms in NZB×W hybrids; and transforming growth factor-β1 (TGFβ1) is known to protect against collagen arthritis and relapsing EAE. We have already reminded ourselves of the maintenance doses of steroids to restore the defective adrenal feedback control on leukocytes in RA.

If we now take it as almost gospel that the Th1 subset is pathogenic in solid organ-specific disease, attempts to switch the phenotype to Th2 should be beneficial. On the assumption that IL-4 or IL-10 can effect this switch, then treatment of an autoimmune individual with these cytokines should defuse the Th1 cells, as was indeed observed in an EAE model. The exacerbation of Th1-mediated disease by IL-12 raises the possibility that the highly avid dimer of one of the IL-2 receptor chains might be a potent inhibitor. However, with the exception of steroids in RA, there is quite a gap between therapy in experimental animals and its application to human disease. Our earlier suggestion of transfection of the target organ with a protective cytokine like TGFβ (figure 20.22 (8)) may prove to be a good bet (visions of firing a biolistic gun at islets pretransplantation?).

Idiotype control with antibody

The powerful immunosuppressive action of anti-idiotype antibodies has led to much rumination on the feasibility of controlling autoantibody production by provoking appropriate interactions within the immune network. We have focused previously on the intimate network interactions between hormone receptors, hormones and their respective antibodies (cf. p. 209) and it might be that the autoimmune disorders involving these receptors are especially amenable to idiotype control. There is a growing realization that, in general, more fundamental suppression can be achieved by utilizing the internal elements of the idiotype network rather than anti-idiotype reagents raised in other species. Thus, xenogeneic anti-idiotypes have only won transient and partial improvement in the spontaneous thyroiditis of the Buffalo rat and the autoimmune lupus of NZB×W mice, presumably due to compensation by idiotype-negative clones. On the other hand, much more profound changes have been achieved by treatment with monoclonal autoantibodies (idiotypes) derived from the autoimmune strain in question. Thus, prior administration without adjuvant of two peptides taken from the CDRs of a pathogenic murine 16/6 Id$^+$ anti-DNA monoclonal was reported to inhibit the induction of SLE by immunization with the intact monoclonal in CFA.

Curiously, **intravenous injection of Ig pooled from many normal donors** is of positive benefit in a number of autoimmune blood diseases, recurrent abortions associated with cardiolipin antibodies, juvenile dermatomyositis and patients with autoantibodies to procoagulant factor VIII. The latter has been studied in some detail and the inhibitory effects of F(ab')$_2$ fractions from the normal Ig pool suggest that we are dealing with anti-idiotypic reactions; it is as though the normal pool was re-establishing a properly controlled network. These are intriguing observations which deserve serious consideration, although to some extent their use is marred by expense.

Vaccination with T-cell idiotypes

It is possible to protect animals against the induction of experimental allergic encephalomyelitis by immunization with an attenuated T-cell clone specific for myelin basic protein (MBP). This must be mediated by the induction of suppressor T-cells specific for the effector cell receptor idiotype. Confirmation has come from experiments showing that the encephalitis can be prevented if mice are first immunized with a synthetic peptide from the Vβ chain of the encephalitogenic clone; this procedure generates CD8 T-cells specific for the receptor peptide presented by class I MHC, and which transfer protection against induction of encephalitis.

This gambit (figure 20.22 (5)) has now been played in human disease. A TCR peptide vaccine embodying the Vβ5.2 sequence expressed in MS plaques and on T-cells specific for MBP was used to treat MS patients in a double-blind trial (10 μg weekly for 4 weeks and then monthly for 10 months). Lack of response to vaccination was associated with increased response to MBP and clinical progression, but successful vaccination boosted the frequency of TCR peptide-specific T-cells, reduced the frequency of MBP-specific cells and prevented clinical progression without side-effects. The reactive cells were predominantly Th2-like and directly inhibited MBP-specific Th1 responses, primarily through release of IL-10 and probably through an anti-idiotypic regulatory network. Although many of the

T-cells in the lesions would not belong to the Vβ5.2 family, they could be switched off by organ-related bystander tolerance (see figure 20.22).

T-cell vaccination has been used to protect against the spontaneous development of diabetes in NOD mice and the production of arthritis following sensitization with type II collagen. It has also proved possible to switch off Freund adjuvant-induced arthritis with an attenuated clone of T-cells generated in response to the 65 kDa mycobacterial heat-shock protein. This adjuvant model has been looked at in depth (I. Cohen). Perversely, the earliest T-cell responses preceding the adjuvant-induced arthritis were antigen-specific suppression and anti-idiotypic reactivity; responses to the antigen itself emerged a few days before the appearance of clinical arthritis. T-cell vaccination accelerated the kinetics of the antigen response, abolished antigen-specific suppression, activated anti-idiotypic T-cells and inhibited arthritis. The extremely rapid appearance of anti-idiotype and antigen-specific suppressors so soon after immunization with the 65 kDa heat-shock protein again strongly suggests a pre-existing network linked to epitopes on this antigen as envisaged in the 'immunological homunculus' concept (cf. p. 208). If malfunctioning of the network produces autoimmune disease, vaccination with T-cell receptor epitopes would represent a logical attempt to re-establish natural control.

Manipulation by antigen

The object is to present the offending antigen in sufficient concentration and in the form which will turn off an ongoing autoimmune response. Since T-cells have been accorded such a pivotal role, it is natural to devise the strategy in terms of T-cell epitopes rather than whole antigen, obviously a far more practical proposition because this reduces the problem to dealing with relatively short peptides. One strategy is to design high affinity peptide analogs that will bind obstinately to the appropriate MHC molecule and antagonize the response to autoantigen (figure 20.22 (4)). Since we express several different MHC molecules, this should not impair microbial defenses unduly. However, we are now talking of patients not mice and this could involve repeated very high doses of peptide, although, much in their favor, peptides are well defined chemically and *relatively* cheap to produce. Antigen-specific suppression of T-cells (figure 20.22 (3)) would be advantageous in this respect, and giving the peptide under an umbrella of anti-CD4 or using partial agonists (cf. figure 9.8) could be feasible. Injection of an MBP peptide, particularly as a palmitoylated derivative inserted in liposomes, can block EAE and an hsp60 peptide can prevent the onset of diabetes in the NOD mouse (cf. p. 434). Awareness of the therapeutic benefit of injected insulin in the NOD model has fostered a large-scale trial in the human disease and considerable clinical improvement has been achieved in patients with exacerbating–remitting MS given Cop1, a random copolymer of alanine, glutamic acid, lysine and tyrosine meant to simulate MBP. Many thousands of patients have been injected with Cop1 subcutaneously every day, thereby reducing the risk of relapse from 1.5 per year at onset to less than 1 in every 5 years without an increase in neurological disability. The copolymer competes with MBP and other brain antigens for binding to the MHC and to the cognate T-cell receptors and induces T-suppressors which, it may be said, are also generated when the antigen is fed.

We have already noted that, because the mucosal surface of the gut is exposed to a horde of powerfully immunogenic microorganisms, and since enterocytes are especially vulnerable to damage by IFNγ and TNF, it has been important for the immune defenses of the gut to evolve mechanisms which deter Th1-type responses. This objective is attained by the stimulation of cells which release cytokines such as TGFβ, IL-4 and IL-10 and suppress the unwanted responses. Thus feeding antigens should tolerize Th1 cells and this has proved to be a successful strategy for blocking EAE, the collagen II arthritis model and the development of diabetes in NOD mice. Accordingly, MS patients are now being fed MBP and RA patients type II chicken collagen.

The tolerogen can also be delivered by inhalation of peptide aerosols (figure 20.23), and this could be a very attractive way of generating antigen-specific T-cell suppression in many hypersensitivity states. Induction of anergy or active suppression may contribute to different extents. Intranasal peptides have been used successfully to block collagen-induced arthritis, EAE, spontaneous diabetes (NOD) and a mouse model of allergy to the house dust mite antigen Der P1. Significantly, treatment can be effective even *after* induction of disease (figure 20.23), although in established human disease this may be more difficult to achieve and might require supplementary therapy, such as anti-CD4, and preliminary reduction of primed T-cells with cyclosporin or steroids. There is no shortage of strings to pull.

Now this is really important. A single internal epitope of MBP can inhibit disease induced by the *mixture* of epitopes or antigens contained within whole myelin. In other words, a single epitope can induce

Figure 20.23. Influence of peptide inhalation on experimental autoimmune encephalomyelitis (EAE) induced with pig spinal cord in complete Freund's adjuvant. Aerosols of the peptides were inhaled (a) 8 days before and (b) 8 days after injection of the encephalitogen. A single dose can give long-lived protection which is extended indefinitely if the mice are thymectomized. Regulation is IL-10 dependent and both Th1 and Th2 can be tolerized. Administration of a single peptide T-cell epitope can in-duce tolerance to other autoantigenic epitopes on the same protein (linked suppression) and to epitopes on different antigens within the nervous tissue used for immunization (bystander tolerance). PBS, phosphate-buffered saline; the peptide was an acetylated N-terminal 11-mer from myelin basic protein with lysine at position 4 substituted by alanine. (Data from Metzler B. & Wraith D.C. (1996) *Annals of the New York Academy of Science* **778**, 228, with permission of the publishers.)

Figure 20.24. Organ-related bystander tolerance induced by feeding or inhaling an organ-related autoantigen. Induced regulatory or anergic tolerogen-specific T-cells (Tr1/A) enter the organ and inhibit pathogenic T-cells (Tpath) on the same antigen-presenting cell which processes both the tolerogen and the other organ-derived antigen recognized by the pathogenic cell. Regulators act by production of IL-10 and possibly TGFβ, which downregulate the Th1 cells either directly or through an intermediate effect on the antigen-presenting cell.

suppression of the pathogenic T-cells specific for other epitopes on the same or other molecules provided that they are generated within the same organ or locality. We have referred to this already as **organ-related bystander tolerance**, a phenomenon best understood in terms of interactions on the same antigen-presenting cell between the regulatory cell, be it Th2 or anergic, recognizing the suppressor epitope and the patho-genic Th1 cell recognizing a **separate epitope** processed from the same or another molecule in the same organ (figure 20.24).

Another potentially valuable approach for the future involves 'switching off' primed B-cells by presenting hapten linked to a thymus-independent carrier like the copolymer of D-glutamic acid and D-lysine (D-GL) or IgG of the same species, particularly when given with high cortisone doses. This has certainly worked well in NZB×W hybrid mice where anti-DNA levels have been reduced using nucleosides as the haptens: we shall have to see whether human and mouse really are that different.

Another way to manipulate antigen is to remove it. For nucleosomal DNA this can be accomplished by injection of DNase. Sure enough, treatment with DNase I suppressed the manifestations of lupus nephritis in the NZB×W model. And last, back to the Holy Grail business, several groups are trying to evolve a strategy based upon the 'magic bullet', the essence of which is to fashion different types of cytotoxic weaponry by coupling bacterial toxins or lots of radioactivity to the antigen which selectively homes on to the lymphocytes bearing specific surface receptors. Something good has got to come out of all this!

Plasmapheresis

Plasma exchange to lower the rate of immune complex deposition in SLE provides only temporary benefit, although it may be of value in life-threatening cases of arteritis. Successful results have been obtained in Goodpasture's syndrome when the treatment has been applied in combination with antimitotic drugs (figure 20.25), the rationale being an increased tendency for antigen-reactive cells to divide as the negative feedback effect of IgG is lowered following removal of plasma proteins.

Figure 20.25. Treatment of a patient with antiglomerular basement membrane (anti-g.b.m.)-induced nephritis with plasma exchange, steroids and immunosuppressive drugs. Kidney function is here monitored by the serum creatinine level. The treatment leads to loss of autoantibody (the dashed line represents the amount of g.b.m. antigen bound in the assay by normal serum) and restoration of kidney function. (Courtesy of Dr C.M. Lockwood.)

SUMMARY

Pathogenic effects of humoral autoantibody

• Direct pathogenic effects of human autoantibodies to blood, surface receptors and several other tissues are listed in table 20.2.

• Passive transfer of disease is seen in 'experiments of nature' in which transplacental passage of maternal IgG autoantibody produces a comparable but transient disorder in the fetus and neonate.

• Disease can also be mimicked in experimental animals by passive transfer of monoclonal autoantibodies.

Pathogenic effects of complexes with autoantigens

• Immune complexes, usually with bound complement, appear in the kidneys, skin and joints of patients with SLE, associated with lesions in the corresponding organs.

• The formation of high affinity, mutated IgG anti-

bodies to anatomically clustered antigens (e.g. nucleosome components) attests to T-cell control and antigen selection of the antibody response. These antigen clusters can appear as blebs on the surface of apoptotic cells.

• Spontaneous lupus has been observed in certain pure-bred animal strains and the importance of autoimmunity for pathogenesis is shown by the amelioration of symptoms whenever the immune response is suppressed.

• The IgG in RA shows defective galactosylation of the Fc sugars.

• Most patients with RA produce autoantibodies to IgG (rheumatoid factors) as a result of immunological hyperreactivity in the deeper layers of the synovium. The IgG rheumatoid factors self-associate to form complexes.

(continued)

Table 20.2. Direct pathogenic effects of humoral antibodies.

DISEASE	AUTOANTIGEN	LESION
Autoimmune hemolytic anemia	Red cell	Erythrocyte destruction
Lymphopenia (some cases)	Lymphocyte	Lymphocyte destruction
Idiopathic thrombocytopenic purpura	Platelet	Platelet destruction
Anti-phospholipid syndrome	Cardiolipin/β2–glycoprotein 1 complex	Recurrent thromboembotic phenomena
Male infertility (some cases)	Sperm	Agglutination of spermatozoa
Pernicious anemia	H^+/K^+-ATPase, gastrin receptor	Block acid production
Hashimoto's disease	Thyroid peroxidase surface antigen	Cytotoxic effect on thyroid cells in culture
Primary myxedema	TSH receptor	Blocking of thyroid cell
Graves' disease	TSH receptor	Stimulation of thyroid cell
Goodpasture's syndrome	Glomerular basement membrane	Complement-mediated damage to basement membrane
Myasthenia gravis	Acetylcholine receptor	Blocking and destruction of receptors
Lambert-Eaton syndrome	Presynaptic Ca channel	Neuromuscular defect
Acanthosis nigricans (type B) and ataxia telangiectasia with insulin resistance	Insulin receptor	Blocking of receptors
Atopic allergy (some cases)	β-Adrenergic receptors	Blocking of receptors
Congenital heart block	Ro/SS-A	Distort fetal cardiac membrane action potential
Celiac disease	Endomysium	Small intestinal inflammation

• These give rise to acute inflammation in the joint space and stimulate the synovial lining cells to grow as a malign **pannus** which **produces erosions in the underlying cartilage and bone** through the release of IL-1, IL-6, TNF, prostaglandin E_2, collagenase, neutral proteinase and reactive oxygen intermediates.

T-cell-mediated hypersensitivity as a pathogenic factor

• Suppression of disease by cyclosporin or anti-CD4 treatment is strong evidence for T-cell involvement. So is an HLA-linked risk factor.

• There is a prevailing view that organ-specific inflammatory lesions are caused by autoreactive pathogenic Th1 cells.

• Activated T-cells are abundant in the rheumatoid synovium and their production of TNF and GM-CSF complements the immune complex stimulus for pannus formation.

• RA patients have poor corticosteroid responses to triggering of the pituitary–adrenal feedback loop and treatment with low, virtually maintenance doses of steroids is beneficial.

• Thyrocytes expressing MHC class II in autoimmune thyroid disease are direct targets for locally activated Th1 cells specific for thyroid peroxidase.

• That autoimmunity can cause thyroiditis is further shown by the deliberate induction of disease in rodents through immunization with thyroid antigens in complete Freund's adjuvant.

• The onset of IDDM is delayed by cyclosporin, HLA-DQ risk factors are prominent, and T-cell proliferative responses to β-islet cell antigens reflect prognosis of disease.

• Th1 cells from diseased NOD mice, which mimic the human disorder in histopathology and autoimmunity, can produce typical pancreatic lesions in young mice of the same strain. Introduction of a transgene encoding changes at residues 56 or 57 in the H-2 β chain dramatically ameliorates disease.

• Similarity to experimental allergic encephalomyelitis, a demyelinating disease induced by immunization with myelin in complete Freund's adjuvant, has made autoimmunity the front-running hypothesis in MS. Approximately one-third of the IL-2 or -4 activatable T-cells in the CSF of MS patients are specific for myelin and the DR2 phenotype is a strong risk factor.

(continued p. 448)

Some systemic disorders with a vascular component of unknown pathogenesis
• Immunologically mediated vascular lesions are of central importance in Wegener's granulomatosis, temporal arteritis, scleroderma and atherosclerosis.

Diagnostic value of autoantibody tests
• A wide range of serum autoantibodies now provide valuable diagnostic markers.
• Routine immunofluorescent screening is carried out on composite sections of human thyroid and stomach and rat kidney and liver, supplemented by agglutination tests for rheumatoid factors, thyroid and red cell antibodies, and by radioimmunoassays for intrinsic factor and acetylcholine receptor antibodies.
• Solid-phase ELISA tests are used for antibodies to DNA and other nuclear antigens and will increasingly displace fluorescence as purified autoantigens become available.

Treatment of autoimmune disorders
• Therapy conventionally involves metabolic control and the use of anti-inflammatory and immunosuppressive drugs.
• A whole variety of potential immunological control therapies are under intensive investigation. These include antibody and T-cell idiotype manipulations and attempts to induce antigen-specific unresponsiveness particularly to T-cells using peptides administered parenterally, orally or nasally.
• Organ-related bystander tolerance means that single epitopes can induce suppression of pathogenic cells within an organ reacting to other epitopes on the same or other antigens.
• Plasma exchange may be of value especially in combination with antimitotic drugs.
• The accompanying comparison of organ-specific and nonorgan-specific autoimmune disorders (table 20.3) gives an overall view of many of the points raised in the last two chapters.

See the accompanying website (**www.roitt.com**) for multiple choice questions.

Table 20.3. Comparison of organ-specific and nonorgan-specific diseases.

ORGAN-SPECIFIC (e.g. THYROIDITIS, GASTRITIS, ADRENALITIS)	NONORGAN-SPECIFIC (e.g. SYSTEMIC LUPUS ERYTHEMATOSUS)
DIFFERENCES	
Antigens only available to lymphoid system in low concentration	Antigens accessible at higher concentrations
Antibodies and lesions organ-specific	Antibodies and lesions nonorgan-specific
Clinical and serologic overlap – thyroiditis, gastritis and adrenalitis	Overlap SLE, rheumatoid arthritis, and other connective tissue disorders
Familial tendency to organ-specific autoimmunity	Familial connective tissue disease
Lymphoid invasion, parenchymal destruction by Th1 cell-mediated hypersensitivity and/or antibodies	Lesions largely due to deposition of antigen–antibody complexes but may also have Th1 component as in RA
Therapy aimed at controlling metabolic deficit or tolerizing T-cells	Therapy aimed at inhibiting inflammation and antibody synthesis
Tendency to cancer in organ	Tendency to lymphoreticular neoplasia
Antigens evoke organ-specific antibodies in normal animals with complete Freund's adjuvant	No antibodies produced in animals with comparable stimulation
Experimental lesions produced with antigen in Freund's adjuvant but also have spontaneous disease models	Diseases and autoantibodies arise spontaneously in certain animals (e.g. NZB mice and hybrids)
SIMILARITIES	
Circulating autoantibodies react with normal body constituents Patients often have increased immunoglobulins in serum Antibodies may appear in each of the main immunoglobulin classes particularly IgG and are usually high affinity and mutated Greater incidence in women Disease process not always progressive; exacerbations and remissions Association with HLA Spontaneous diseases in animals genetically programed Autoantibody tests of diagnostic value	

FURTHER READING

Anderton S.M. & Wraith D.C. (1998) Hierarchy in the ability of T-cell epitopes to induce peripheral tolerance to antigens from myelin. *European Journal of Immunology* **28**, 1251.

Austen K.F., Burakoff S.J., Rosen F.S. & Strom T.B. (eds) (1996) *Therapeutic Immunology*. Blackwell Science, Oxford.

Baum H. & Staines N.A. (1997) MHC-derived peptides and the CD4+ T-cell repertoire: implications for autoimmune disease. *Cytokines in Cellular and Molecular Therapy* **3**, 115.

Brostoff J., Scadding G.K., Male D. & Roitt I.M. (1991) *Clinical Immunology*. Gower Medical Publishing, London.

Celis E. (1993) T-helper cells and autoantibodies in autoimmune disease. *The Immunologist* **1**, 126.

Chapel M., Haeney M., Misbah S. & Snowden N. (1999) *Essentials of Clinical Immunology*, 4th edn. Blackwell Science, Oxford.

Datta S.K. (2000) Positive selection for autoimmunity. *Nature Medicine* **6**, 259.

Flavell R.A. & Hafler D.A. (eds) (1999) Autoimmunity. *Current Opinion in Immunology* **11**, 635. (Several critical essays in each annual volume.)

Gelfand E.W. (ed.) (1996) Intravenous immune globulin: mechanisms of action and model disease states. *Clinical and Experimental Immunology* **104** (Suppl. 1), 1.

Hanahan D. (1998) Peripheral antigen-expressing cells in thymic medulla: factors in self-tolerance and autoimmunity. *Current Opinion in Immunology* **10**, 656.

Lokki M-J. & Colten H.R. (1995) Genetic deficiencies of complement. *Annals of Medicine* **27**, 451.

Maini R.N., Breedveld F.C., Kalden J.R., Smolen J.S., Davis D., Macfarlane J.D., Antoni C., Leeb B., Elliott M.J., Woody J.N., Schaible T.F. & Feldmann M. (1998) Therapeutic efficacy of multiple intravenous infusions of anti-tumor necrosis factor α monoclonal antibody combined with low-dose weekly methotrexate in rheumatoid arthritis. *Arthritis and Rheumatism* **41**, 1552.

Peter J.B. & Schoenfeld Y. (eds) (1996) *Autoantibodies*. Elsevier, Amsterdam.

Rademacher T., Williams P. & Dwek R.A. (1994) Agalactosyl glycoforms of IgG autoantibodies are pathogenic. *Proceedings of the National Academy of Sciences of the United States of America* **91**, 6123.

Ramiya V.K., Maraist M., Arfors K.E., Schatz D.A., Cornelius J.G. & Peck A.B. (2000) Reversal of insulin-dependent diabetes using islets generated *in vitro* from pancreatic stem cells. *Nature Medicine* **6**, 278.

Schoenfeld Y. (ed.) (1999) Abstracts of 2nd International Congress on Autoimmunity, Tel Aviv, Israel. *Journal of Autoimmunity* (Supplement).

Schoenfeld Y. & Isenberg D. (1989) *The Mosaic of Autoimmunity (the Factors Associated with Autoimmune Disease)*. Elsevier, Amsterdam. (An excellent account.)

Schoenfeld Y. & Isenberg D.A. (eds) (1993) *Natural Autoantibodies. Their Physiological Role and Regulatory Significance*. CRC Press, Boca Raton, FL.

Sieper J. & Kingsley G. (1996) Recent advances in the pathogenesis of reactive arthritis. *Immunology Today* **17**, 160.

Song Y-H., Li Y. & Maclaren N.K. (1996) The nature of autoantigens targeted in autoimmune endocrine diseases. *Immunology Today* **17**, 232.

Tan E.M. (1999) Autoantibodies in diagnosis and in identifying autoantigens. *The Immunologist* **7**, 85.

Weetman A.P. (ed.) (1991) *Autoimmune Endocrine Disease*. Cambridge University Press, Cambridge.

Weiner H.L. & Mayer L.F. (1996) Oral tolerance: mechanisms and applications. *Annals of the New York Academy of Science* **778**, 1.

Wicker L. & Wekerle H. (eds) (1995) Autoimmunity. *Current Opinion in Immunology* **6**, 783. (Several critical essays in each annual volume.)

CD markers

CD (Cluster of differentiation) markers on hematopoietic cells.

CD	Identity	Function	Cellular distribution	Ligands
CD1a	Non-MHC, class I-like molecule	Presentation of lipid & glycolipid antigens	Thymocyte, DC, LC, B(sub)	Lipid & glycolipid antigens, αβ TCR
CD1b	Non-MHC, class I-like molecule	Presentation of lipid & glycolipid antigens	Thymocyte, DC, LC, B(sub)	Lipid & glycolipid antigens, αβ TCR
CD1c	Non-MHC, class I-like molecule	Presentation of lipid & glycolipid antigens	Thymocyte, DC, LC, B(sub)	Lipid & glycolipid antigens, αβ TCR
CD1d	Non-MHC, class I-like molecule	Presentation of lipid & glycolipid antigens	Leukocytes, epithelium	Lipid & glycolipid antigens, αβ TCR
CD1e	Non-MHC, class I-like molecule	Presentation of lipid & glycolipid antigens	Unknown	Lipid & glycolipid antigens, αβ TCR
CD2	LFA-2, T11	T cell adhesion to target cells or APC. T cell activation. Regulation of cytolysis	Thymocyte, T, NK	CD58 (LFA-3), CD59, CD48, CD15
CD3δ	TCR-associated molecule	T cell activation	Thymocyte, T	—
CD3ε	TCR-associated molecule	T cell activation	Thymocyte, T	—
CD3γ	TCR-associated molecule	T cell activation	Thymocyte, T	—
CD4	T4, L3T4	Co-receptor for MHC class II-restricted antigen-induced T cell activation	Thymocyte (sub), T(sub), Mo, Mφ	MHC class II, HIV gp120
CD5	Leu-1, Ly-1	Modulates signaling through TCR & BCR	Thymocyte, T, B(sub)	CD72
CD6	T12	T cell activation & thymocyte-stromal cell interaction	Thymocyte, T, B(sub)	CD166 (ALCAM)
CD7	Tp41	Regulation of cytokine production & sensitivity to LPS-induced shock syndromes	SC, Thymocyte, T, NK	Unknown
CD8α	T8, Lyt2/3	Co-receptor for MHC class I-restricted antigen-induced T cell activation	Thymocyte (sub), T(sub)	MHC class I
CD8β	T8, Lyt2/3	Co-receptor for MHC class I-restricted antigen-induced T cell activation	Thymocyte (sub), T(sub)	MHC class I
CD9	DRAP27	Platelet activation & aggregation	Pre-B, Plt, *B, *T, eosinophils, basophils, endothelium, epithelium	Pregnancy-specific glycoprotein-17 (PSG17)
CD10	CALLA, NEP	Neutral endopeptidase	BM	Unknown

(Continued on p. 452)

CD markers (*continued*)

CD	Identity	Function	Cellular distribution	Ligands
CD11a	LFA-1 α chain, α_L integrin chain	Leukocyte–leukocyte/leukocyte–endothelium interactions. Co-stimulation	All leukocytes	CD54 (ICAM-1), CD102 (ICAM-2), CD50 (ICAM-3), CD242 (ICAM-4)
CD11b	Mac-1 α chain, α_M integrin chain, CR3	Adhesion to vascular endothelium. Complement receptor	NK, Gr, Mo, T(sub), B(sub)	CD54 (ICAM-1), CD102 (ICAM-2), CD242 (ICAM-4), iC3b, C3dg, C3d, fibrinogen
CD11c	α_x integrin chain, CR4	Adhesion to vascular endothelium. Complement receptor	NK, Gr, Mo, Mφ	iC3b, C3dg, fibrinogen
CDw12	Phosphoprotein p90–120	Unknown	Mo, Gr, NK	Unknown
CD13	Aminopeptidase N	Trims peptides bound to MHC class II	Mo, Gr, Endothelium	Unknown
CD14	LPS receptor	Binds LPS, particularly in the presence of LPS-binding protein (LBP). Cellular activation	Mo, Mφ, Gr	LPS (endotoxin)
CD15	Lewis^X, 3-FAL, SSEA-1	Adhesion	Neutrophils, Mo, Plt	CD2
CD15s	Sialyl Lewis^X	Adhesion	Neutrophils, Mo, Plt	CD62E, CD62L, CD62P
CD15u	Sulfated CD15	Adhesion	Neutrophils, Mo, Plt	CD62P
CD16a	FcγRIIIA	Phagocytosis & ADCC	Gr, NK, Mφ, DC, B	Fcγ
CD16b	FcγRIIIB	Phagocytosis & ADCC	Neutrophils	Fcγ
CDw17	Lactosylceramide	Unknown	Mo, Gr, basophils, Plt, B(sub)	Unknown
CD18	β-chain for CD11, β_2 integrin chain	Adhesion & signaling	All leukocytes	see CD11a,b,c
CD19	B4	Component of CD19/CD21/CD81/CD225 signal transduction complex. B cell activation & proliferation	B, FDC	Heparin/heparan sulphate, IgM
CD20	B1, Bp35	B cell activation & proliferation	B	Unknown
CD21	CR2, EBV-R, C3dR	Complement receptor. Component of CD19/CD21/CD81/CD225 signal transduction complex. B cell activation & proliferation	B, FDC	iC3b, C3d, C3dg, CD23, EBV
CD22	BL-CAM	B cell adhesion & signaling	B(mat)	Sialyl proteins, CD45
CD23	FcεRII, low affinity IgE receptor	Regulation of IgE production. Adhesion and signaling	B, Mo, FDC	Fcε, CD21
CD24	HSA, BA-1	Apoptotic signaling	B, Gr(mat)	CD62P
CD25	IL-2R α-chain	Cytokine receptor	*T, *B, *Mo, *Mφ	IL-2
CD26	DPPIV	Endopeptidase. Costimulation for T cell activation	*T, B, Mφ, NK, thymocytes	Adenosine deaminase
CD27	S152, T14	Costimulation signal for T & B cell activation	Thymocytes, T, B(sub), NK	CD70
CD28	T44	Costimulatory molecule	Thymocytes, T, *B	CD80, CD86
CD29	VLA β-chain	Adhesion	Leukocytes, Plt, erythrocytes	See CD49a–f & CD51. CD171 (in mouse)
CD30	Ber-H2	Costimulatory for T cells	*T, *B, *NK, Mo	CD153

(Continued)

CD markers (*continued*)

CD	Identity	Function	Cellular distribution	Ligands
CD31	PECAM-1	Transendothelial migration of leukocytes	Mo, Plt, neutrophils, NK, endothelium, T(sub)	CD31 (homophilic), CD51/CD61 ($\alpha_v\beta_3$ integrin), CD38
CD32	FcγRII	Phagocytosis & ADCC	B, Mφ, Gr, Mo, FDC, NK	Fcγ
CD33	gp67	Adhesion	Mo, Mφ, mast cells	Sialic acid on sialo-glycoconjugates
CD34	gp105–120	Adhesion	SC, early lymphohematopoietic progenitor cells, endothelium	CD62L
CD35	CR1, C3b/C4bR	Complement receptor. Accelerates decay of C3 & C5 convertases. Facilitates phagocytosis	Erythrocytes, neutrophils, Mo, B, T(sub), eosinophils, FDC	C3b, C4b, iC3b
CD36	GPIIIb, MFGM, PAS IV	Adhesion. Scavenger receptor. Phagocytosis of apoptotic cells	Endothelium, Plt, Mo, Mφ, erythrocytes	Thrombospondin, collagen, oxidized LDL, long chain fatty acids, anionic phospholipids
CD37	gp52–40	Signal transduction	B, T, neutrophils, Mo	Unknown
CD38	T10	Like CD157, has ADP-ribosyl cyclase/cyclic ADP-ribose hydrolase activity. Modulates cell activation. Adhesion	Most leukocytes	CD31, hyaluronic acid
CD39	gp80	Adhesion	B(sub), *NK(sub), *T(sub)	CD39 (homophilic)
CD40	Bp50	B cell activation, proliferation & differentiation	B, Mφ, DC, FDC, endothelium	CD154
CD41	αIIb integrin chain	Platelet aggregation	Plt, megakaryocytes	VWF, fibrinogen, fibronectin
CD42a	GP IX	Plt adherence & aggregation at sites of vascular damage	Plt, megakaryocytes	—
CD42b	GP Ibα	Plt adherence & aggregation at sites of vascular damage	Plt, megakaryocytes	VWF, thrombin
CD42c	GP Ibβ	Plt adherence & aggregation at sites of vascular damage	Plt, megakaryocytes	—
CD42d	GP V	Plt adherence & aggregation at sites of vascular damage	Plt, megakaryocytes	—
CD43	Leucosialin, gp115	Anti-adhesion & pro-adhesion. Cellular activation	Most leukocytes	Sialoadhesin (Siglec-1)
CD44	HERMES, Pgp-1, H-CAM	Leukocyte attachment & rolling on endothelium. Homing to peripheral lymphoid organs & sites of inflammation. T cell activation	Widespread	Hyaluronan, osteopontin, ankyrin, fibronectin
CD44R	Variant isoform of CD44	Leukocyte attachment & rolling on endothelium. Homing to peripheral lymphoid organs & sites of inflammation	Mo, *T, *B, epithelium	Hyaluronan, osteopontin, ankyrin, fibronectin
CD45	Leukocyte common antigen (LCA), B220	Lymphocyte signaling	All leukocytes	Galectin-1, CD22
CD45RA	Restricted LCA	Lymphocyte signaling	Thymocytes, T(sub), B, Gr(sub), Mo, NK	Galectin-1, CD22

(*Continued on p. 454*)

CD markers (*continued*)

CD	Identity	Function	Cellular distribution	Ligands
CD45RB	Restricted LCA	Lymphocyte signaling	Thymocytes, T(sub), B, Gr, Mo, NK	Galectin-1, CD22
CD45RC	Restricted LCA	Lymphocyte signaling	Thymocytes, NK, T(sub), B	Galectin-1, CD22
CD45RO	Restricted LCA	Lymphocyte signaling	Thymocytes, T(sub), Gr, Mo, DC	Galectin-1, CD22
CD46	Membrane cofactor protein (MCP)	Limits formation & function of C3 convertases	Widespread	Serum factor I protease, C3b, C4b, measles virus
CD47	Integrin-associated protein (IAP)	Adhesion. Thrombospondin receptor	Widespread	Thrombospondin, CD172a
CD47R	MEM133, CDw149	Adhesion. Thrombospondin receptor	T, B, Mo	Thrombospondin
CD48	Blast-1, OX-45, BCM1	T cell adhesion to target cells & APC	Leukocytes (except neutrophils)	CD2
CD49a	VLA-1 α chain, α_1 integrin chain	Receptor for laminin & collagen	Fibroblasts, capillary endothelium, NK, *T	Laminin, collagen I & IV
CD49b	VLA-2 α chain, α_2 integrin chain	Regulates expression of MMP-1 & collagen type I	Fibroblasts, endothelium, Plt, B, T, keratinocytes	Collagen I–IV, laminin
CD49c	VLA-3 α chain, α_3 integrin chain	Adhesion	Fibroblasts, keratinocytes, epithelium, B	Fibronectin, collagen
CD49d	VLA-4 α chain, α_4 integrin chain	Leukocyte rolling, adhesion & migration	Widespread	CD106 (VCAM-1), fibronectin
CD49e	VLA-5 α chain, α_5 integrin chain	Cell adhesion, migration & matrix assembly	Fibroblasts, epithelium, endothelium, muscle, Plt	Fibronectin, CD171 (in mouse)
CD49f	VLA-6 α chain, α_6 integrin chain	Cell adhesion, spreading & migration	Widespread	Laminin
CD50	ICAM-3	Costimulatory molecule	Leukocytes, LC, endothelium	$\alpha_d\beta_2$ integrin, CD11a/CD18 (LFA-1), CD209
CD51	α_v chain of vitronectin receptor	Recruitment, distribution & retention of cells via extracellular matrix	Endothelium, Mo, Plt, osteoclasts, B(sub), T	CD31, CD171, laminin, fibrinogen, fibronectin
CD52	Campath-1	Unknown	Thymocytes, T, B, Mo, Mϕ	Unknown
CD53	MEM-53	Activation	Leukocytes	Unknown
CD54	ICAM-1	Leukocyte adhesion to endothelium in inflammation	Endothelium, *T, *B, epithelium, Mo	CD11a/CD18 (LFA-1), CD11b/CD18 (Mac-1), CD227, rhinovirus, *Plasmodium falciparum*-infected erythrocytes
CD55	Decay accelerating factor (DAF)	Limits formation & half life of C3 convertases	Widespread	C3 convertases, CD97
CD56	NCAM, D2-CAM, Leu-19, NKH1	Adhesion	NK, T(sub), brain	CD56 (homophilic), heparan sulfate
CD57	HNK-1, Leu-7	Non-MHC restricted cytotoxicity after activation	NK, T(sub), B(sub), Mo	Unknown
CD58	LFA-3	T cell adhesion to target cells & APC	Widespread	CD2

(*Continued*)

CD markers (*continued*)

CD	Identity	Function	Cellular distribution	Ligands
CD59	HRF20, MIRL	Inhibits formation of membrane atttack complex. T cell adhesion to target cells & APC	Widespread	C8, C9, CD2
CD60a	GD3	Costimulation of T cells	T(sub), Plt	Sialic acid on sialo-glycoconjugates
CD60b	9-O-acetyl-GD3	Costimulation of T cells	T(sub), Plt	Sialic acid on sialo-glycoconjugates
CD60c	7-O-acetyl-GD3	Costimulation of T cells	T(sub), Plt	Sialic acid on sialo-glycoconjugates
CD61	Vitronectin receptor β chain, β_3 integrin chain	Adhesion	Plt, megakaryocytes, Mo, Mϕ, endothelium	CD31, CD171
CD62E	E-selectin, ELAM-1	Tethering & rolling of leukocytes on cytokine-activated endothelium	Endothelium	ESL-1, CD15s (sialyl Lewis^X), sialyl Lewis^a, CLA, CD66a, CD66c, CD162, CD227
CD62L	L-selectin, Leu-8	Tethering & rolling of lymphocytes on LN HEV & leukocytes on endothelium	T, B, Mo, Gr, NK. Downregulated on activation by endoproteolysis (shedding)	CD34, MAdCAM, GlyCAM-1, CD15s (sialyl Lewis^X), sialyl Lewis^a
CD62P	P-selectin, GMP-140, PADGEM	Adhesion of Plt & leukocytes to endothelium	Thrombin/histamine activated Plt & endothelium. Stored in granules prior to activation	CD162, CD24, CD15s (sialyl Lewis^X), sialyl Lewis^a
CD63	LIMP, ME491	Unknown	*Plt, *Endothelium	Unknown
CD64	FcγRI	Phagocytosis & ADCC	Mo, Mϕ, DC	Fcγ
CD65	VIM-8, VIM-11, asialylated ceramide dodecasaccharide 4c	Unknown	Gr	Unknown
CD65s	VIM-2, sialylated ceramide dodecasaccharide 4c	Unknown	Mo, Gr	Unknown
CD66a	NCA-160, BGP (biliary glycoprotein)	Adhesion, neutrophil activation	Gr, Epithelium	CD62E, CD66a (homophilic), c, e
CD66b	NCA-95, CD67	Adhesion, neutrophil activation	Gr	CD66c
CD66c	NCA-50/90	Adhesion, neutrophil activation	Gr, Epithelium	CD62E, CD66a, b, c (homophilic), e
CD66d	CGM1	Neutrophil activation	Gr	Unknown
CD66e	Carcinoembryonic antigen (CEA)	Adhesion	Epithelium	CD66a, c, e (homophilic)
CD66f	SP1, Pregnancy-specific glycoprotein (PSG)	Maintenance of pregnancy?	Placental syncytiotrophoblasts	Unknown
CD68	Microsialin	Unknown	Mo, Mϕ, DC, neutrophils, basophils, mast cells, *T, B(sub)	Oxidized LDL
CD69	AIM, Leu-23	Activation, signal transduction	*T, *B, *NK, *neutrophils, *eosinophils	Unknown
CD70	Ki-24	Costimulation	*T(sub), *B(sub)	CD27
CD71	Transferrin receptor	Iron uptake	*T, *B, *NK, *Mo, Mϕ, SC	Transferrin
CD72	Lyb-2	B cell activation & proliferation	B	CD5, CD100
CD73	Ecto-5′-nucleotidase	Unknown	T(sub), B(sub), FDC, endothelium, epithelium	Adenosine monophosphate

(*Continued on p. 456*)

CD markers (*continued*)

CD	Identity	Function	Cellular distribution	Ligands
CD74	Invariant chain	Intracellular sorting of MHC class II molecules	B, Mφ, *T, *endothelium, *epithelium	MHC class II
CD75	Non-sialylated/masked lactosamine epitopes	Unknown	B, T(sub), erythrocytes	Unknown
CD75s	α-2,6-sialylated lactosamines, CDw76	Unknown	B(sub), T(sub), endothelium, epithelium, erythrocytes	Unknown
CD77	BLA, globotriaosylceramide	Unknown	Germinal center B	Shiga toxin, verotoxin-1
CD79a	Igα, mb1	Signal transduction as part of B cell receptor	B	—
CD79b	Igβ, B29	Signal transduction as part of B cell receptor	B	—
CD80	B7.1, BB1	Regulates T cell activation	*B, *T, Mφ, DC	CD28, CD152
CD81	TAPA-1	Component of CD19/CD21/CD81/CD225 signal transduction complex	Leukocytes (except neutrophils), endothelium, epithelium	—
CD82	R2, IA4	Signal transduction	Leukocytes	Unknown
CD83	HB15	Unknown	DC, LC	Unknown
CD84	2G7	Costimulation	Mo, Mφ, Plt, B, T(sub), thymocytes	CD84 (homophilic)
CD85	ILT/LIR family	Inhibition/activation of cytotoxicity	B, T(sub), NK(sub), Mo, Mφ, DC, Gr	HLA-G, some HLA-A & -B alleles
CD86	B7.2	Regulates T cell activation	B, Mo, DC, LC	CD28, CD152
CD87	Urokinase plasminogen activator (uPA) receptor	Inflammatory cell invasion	Mo, Mφ, *T, endothelium, NK, neutrophils	Vitronectin, uPA
CD88	C5a receptor	Complement receptor	Gr, Mo, DC	C5a
CD89	FcαR	Induces phagocytosis, degranulation & respiratory burst	Gr, Mo, Mφ, *eosinophils	IgA1, IgA2
CD90	Thy-1	T cell activation	Thymocytes, T (mouse), SC, HEV	Unknown
CD91	α₂-macroglobulin receptor, LDLR-related protein	Receptor	Mo, Mφ	α₂-macroglobulin
CD92	VIM15	Unknown	Gr, Mo	Unknown
CD93	p120	C1q receptor	Mo, Gr, endothelium	C1q
CD94	kp43	Inhibition/activation of cytotoxicity	T(sub), NK	Some HLA class I molecules
CD95	Fas, APO-1	Transduces an apoptotic signal	Widespread	CD178 (Fas-L)
CD96	Tactile	Adhesion?	*T, *NK	Unknown
CD97	BL-KDD/F12	Unknown	Gr, Mo, Mφ, DC, *T, *B	CD55
CD98	4F2	Cellular activation	Widespread	Unknown
CD99	E2, MIC2	Apoptotic signaling	Thymocytes, T, B, erythrocytes	Unknown
CD100	SEMA4D	Lymphocyte proliferation	All leukocytes	CD72
CD101	p126	Costimulation	Gr, Mo, Mφ, DC, *T	Unknown
CD102	ICAM-2	Lymphocyte recirculation & trafficking. Costimulation	Endothelium, neutrophils, lymphocytes, Mo, Plt	CD11a/CD18 (LFA-1)

(*Continued*)

CD markers (*continued*)

CD	Identity	Function	Cellular distribution	Ligands
CD103	α_E-integrin chain, HML-1	Adhesion of mucosal lymphocytes to epithelium	Most intraepithelial T & 50% of lamina propria lymphocytes. Absent from PBLs	E-cadherin
CD104	β_4-integrin chain	Adhesion molecule with α_6 integrin chain	Epithelium	Laminin, epiligrin
CD105	Endoglin	Regulatory component of TGFβ receptor	*Mo, Mφ, endothelium	TGFβ
CD106	VCAM-1	Leukocyte migration & recruitment to sites of inflammation	Mφ, DC, FDC, BM stromal cells, endothelium	CD49d/CD29 (VLA4), $\alpha_4\beta_7$ integrin
CD107a	LAMP-1	Unknown	*Plt, *T, *endothelium, *neutrophils	Unknown
CD107b	LAMP-2	Unknown	*Plt, *endothelium, *neutrophils	Unknown
CD108	JMH blood group antigen	Adhesion	T, B, erythrocytes	Unknown
CD109	Sialomucin	Unknown	Endothelium, stromal cells, Plt, *T	Unknown
CD110	MPL	Thrombopoietin receptor	Plt, megakaryocytes	Thrombopoietin
CD111	PRR1/Nectin1	Adhesion	Widespread	Herpes simplex virus, CD111 (homophilic)
CD112	PRR2/Nectin2	Adhesion	Widespread	Herpes simplex virus, CD112 (homophilic)
CD114	G-CSF receptor	Growth factor receptor	Gr, Mo, Plt, endothelium	G-CSF
CD115	CSF-1 receptor	Growth factor receptor	Mo, Mφ	M-CSF
CD116	GM-CSF receptor α-chain	Growth factor receptor	Mo, Mφ, neutrophils, eosinophils, DC	GM-CSF
CD117	Stem cell factor (SCF) receptor, c-*kit*	Growth factor receptor	SC, hematopoietic progenitors, mast cells	SCF
CDw119	IFNγ receptor	Cytokine receptor	Mo, Gr	IFNγ
CD120a	TNF receptor type I, p55	Cytokine receptor	Widespread	TNF (TNFα), lymphotoxin (TNFβ)
CD120b	TNF receptor type II, p75	Cytokine receptor	Widespread	TNF (TNFα), lymphotoxin (TNFβ)
CD121a	IL-1 RI	Cytokine receptor	Thymocytes, T, fibroblasts, endothelium	IL-1α,β,ra
CD121b	IL-1 RII	Cytokine receptor	B, T, Mo, Mφ	IL-1α,β,ra
CD122	IL-2 & IL-15 receptor β-chain	Cytokine receptor	T, B, Mo, Mφ, NK	IL-2, IL-15
CD123	IL-3 receptor α-chain	Cytokine receptor	Hematopoietic precursors	IL-3
CD124	IL-4 & IL-13 receptor α-chain	Cytokine receptor	T, B, hematopoietic precursors, fibroblasts	IL-4, IL-13
CDw125	IL-5 receptor α-chain	Cytokine receptor	Eosinophils, basophils, *B	IL-5
CD126	IL-6 receptor α-chain	Cytokine receptor	*B, plasma cells, T, Mo, epithelium, fibroblasts, neural cells	IL-6

(*Continued on p. 458*)

CD markers (*continued*)

CD	Identity	Function	Cellular distribution	Ligands
CD127	IL-7 receptor α-chain	Cytokine receptor	Immature thymocytes, hepatocytes, pre-B, T(mat)	IL-7
CDw128a	IL-8 receptor α-chain, CXCR1	Chemokine receptor	Gr, T(sub), Mo, endothelium	CXCL8 (IL-8), CXCL6 (GCP-2)
CDw128b	IL-8 receptor β-chain, CXCR2	Chemokine receptor	Gr, T(sub), Mo, endothelium	CXCL8 (IL-8), CXCL1 (GROα), CXCL2 (GROβ), CXCL3 (GROγ), CXCL5 (ENA-78), CXCL6 (GCP-2), CXCL7 (NAP-2)
CD130	gp130 component of IL-6, IL-11, LIF, OSM, CNTF & CT-1 receptors	Signal transduction	Widespread	Oncostatin M (OSM) is the only direct ligand
CDw131	Common β-chain of IL-3, IL-5 & GM-CSF receptors	Signal transduction	Mo, Gr, B	Not involved in cytokine binding
CD132	Common γ-chain of IL-2, 4, 7, 9 & 15 receptors	Cytokine binding & signaling	T, B, NK, Mo, Mφ, neutrophils, fibroblasts	IL-2, 4, 7, 9 & 15
CD133	AC133	Unknown	SC	Unknown
CD134	OX40	Adhesion of *T to vascular endothelium	*T	OX40 ligand, gp34
CD135	Flt3/Flk2	Receptor, tyrosine kinase	Myelomonocytic & B progenitors	Flt3/Flk2 ligand
CD136	MSP receptor, RON	Receptor, tyrosine kinase	Epithelium, some hematopoietic cells	Macrophage stimulating protein, HGF1
CDw137	4-1BB	Costimulatory molecule for T cell proliferation	T	4-1BB ligand
CD138	Syndecan-1	Heparan sulfate proteoglycan	B(sub)	Collagen type 1
CD139	—	Unknown	B, Mo, Gr	Unknown
CD140a	PDGF receptor α	Tyrosine kinase	Endothelium, stromal cells, mesangial cells	PDGF A
CD140b	PDGF receptor β	Tyrosine kinase	Endothelium, stromal cells, mesangial cells	PDGF B
CD141	Thrombomodulin	Downregulates coagulation	Megakaryocytes, Plt, Mo, neutrophils, endothelium, smooth muscle	Thrombin
CD142	Tissue factor, thromboplastin	Induces coagulation	Mo, endothelium, epithelium, keratinocytes	Factor VIIa
CD143	ACE, peptidyl-dipeptidase A	Metabolism of angiotensin & bradykinin	Endothelium, epithelium, Mφ	Angiotensin, bradykinin
CD144	VE-cadherin	Adhesion	Endothelium	Unknown
CDw145	—	Unknown	Endothelium	Unknown
CD146	MUC18, S-endo	Adhesion?	Endothelium, T	Unknown
CD147	Neurothelin, basigen, EMMPRIN, OX-47	Adhesion?	Leukocytes, endothelium, erythrocytes	Unknown
CD148	HPTP-eta, DEP-1	Tyrosine phosphatase RPTPase type III	Widespread	Tyrosine phosphorylated proteins

(*Continued*)

CD markers (*continued*)

CD	Identity	Function	Cellular distribution	Ligands
CD150	SLAM	Signaling	T(sub), B, thymocytes, DC, endothelium	CD150 (homophilic), measles virus
CD151	PETA3	Unknown	Megakaryocytes, Plt, Gr, endothelium, smooth muscle, epithelium	Unknown
CD152	CTLA-4	Negative regulator of T cell costimulation	*T	CD80, CD86
CD153	CD30L	Costimulatory for T cells	*T, Gr, B, Mφ	CD30
CD154	CD40L, TRAP	Costimulatory	*T, *B, NK, mast cells	CD40
CD155	Poliovirus receptor	Adhesion?	Mo, Mφ, thymocytes, CNS neurons	Vitronectin, poliovirus
CD156a	ADAM8	Extravasation of leukocytes?	Neutrophils, Mo	Unknown
CD156b	TACE (TNFα converting enzyme), ADAM17	Protease which releases soluble forms of TNF from cells	Widespread	Unknown
CD157	Bst-1	Like CD38, has ADP-ribosyl cyclase/cyclic ADP-ribose hydrolase activity	Mo, Mφ, neutrophils, endothelium, T(sub), B(sub)	NAD, cyclic ADP-ribose
CD158	KIR family	Inhibition/activation of cytoxicity	NK, T(sub)	Various MHC class I molecules
CD159a	NKG2A	Inhibition of cytoxicity	NK, T(sub)	HLA class I signal sequence derived peptides presented by HLA-E
CD160	BY55, NK1	Costimulation	NK, CD8$^+$ T	HLA-G
CD161	NKRP1A	Activation?	NK, T(sub)	Ganglioside GM2
CD162	BY55, PSGL-1 (P-selectin glycoprotein ligand-1)	Adhesion	Mo, Gr, T, B(sub)	CD62E, CD62P
CD162R	PEN5, PSGL-1 (P-selectin glycoprotein ligand-1)	Adhesion	NK, *T	CD62P
CD163	M130	Hemoglobin scavenger receptor	Mo, some Mφ	Haptoglobin–hemoglobin complexes
CD164	MGC-24	Adhesion of hematopoietic progenitor cells to stromal cells	Myeloid cells, T, epithelium, BM stromal cells, hematopoietic progenitor cells	Unknown
CD165	AD2, gp37	Adhesion of thymocytes to thymic epithelium	Plt, thymocytes, lymphocytes (sub), thymic epithelium, Mo, CNS neurons	Unknown
CD166	ALCAM, BEN	Adhesion	T, *Mo, epithelium, fibroblasts, neurons	CD6
CD167a	DDR1 (Discoid domain receptor 1)	Receptor tyrosine kinase	Epithelial cells	Collagen
CD168	RHAMM	Cell migration	Fibroblasts	Hyaluronan
CD169	Sialoadhesin, SIGLEC-1	Cell adhesion	Mφ	Sialic acid on sialo-glycoconjugates
CD170	SIGLEC-5	Cell adhesion	Neutrophils	Sialic acid
CD171	L1 (NCAM-L1)	Cell adhesion, costimulation	CD4$^+$ T, B(sub), Mo, DC, FDC, fibroblasts, neurons	Laminin, Neurocan, Phosphocan, CD51/CD61 ($\alpha_V\beta_3$ integrin) (and CD49e/CD29 $\alpha_5\beta_1$ integrin in mouse)

(*Continued on p. 460*)

CD markers (*continued*)

CD	Identity	Function	Cellular distribution	Ligands
CD172a	PTPNS1, SHPS1, SIRPα	Adhesion	Mo, Mφ, DC	CD47
CD173	Blood group H type 2	Glycocalyx component	Widespread	Unknown
CD174	Lewis^y	Adhesion	Widespread	Unknown
CD175	Tn	Mucin-type carbohydrate	Epithelium. Elevated expression in some tumors	Unknown
CD175s	Sialyl-Tn	Mucin-type carbohydrate	Epithelium. Elevated expression in some tumors	Unknown
CD176	TF (Thomsen–Friedenreich antigen)	Mucin-type carbohydrate	Epithelium, Mφ (sub). Elevated expression in some tumors	Unknown
CD177	NB1, HNA-2a	Receptor?	Gr	Unknown
CD178	Fas ligand	Induction of apoptosis	*T	CD95 (Fas)
CD179a	Vpre-B, surrogate light chain	B cell differentiation	Pro-B, early pre-B	Unknown
CD179b	λ5, surrogate light chain	B cell differentiation	Pro-B, early pre-B	Unknown
CD180	RP105, Bgp95	Controls B cell recognition of, & signaling by, LPS	B, Mo, DC	Unknown
CD183	CXCR3	Chemokine receptor, signaling	Effector/memory T, B(sub), NK(sub), DC(sub), eosinophils	CXCL9 (Mig), CXCL10 (IP-10), CXCL11 (I-TAC)
CD184	CXCR4	Chemokine receptor, signaling	T, B, DC, Mo	CXCL12 (SDF-1α/β)
CD195	CCR5	Chemokine receptor, signaling	T, NK, DC, Mo	CCL3 (MIP-1α), CCL4 (MIP-1β), CCL5 (RANTES)
CDw197	CCR7	Chemokine receptor, signaling	B, T, DC	CCL19 (MIP-3β), CCL21 (6Ckine)
CD200	OX2	Downregulates Mφ activation	Widespread	OX2R
CD201	EPCR	Protein C receptor	Endothelial cells	Protein C
CD202b	TEK, Tie2	Receptor tyrosine kinase	Endothelial cells	Angiopoietin-1
CD203c	E-NPP3, PDNP3	Enzyme involved in hydrolysis of extracellular nucleotides	Basophils, mast cells	Nucleoside di- and tri-phosphates
CD204	Macrophage scavenger receptor-1	Antigen uptake	Mφ	Negatively charged macromolecules
CD205	DEC205	Antigen uptake	DC, B, thymic epithelium	Unknown
CD206	Macrophage mannose receptor	Antigen uptake	Mφ, liver endothelial cells	Oligomannose-containing carbohydrates
CD207	Langerin	Antigen uptake	LC, DC	Mannose
CD208	DC-LAMP (Dendritic cell lysosome-associated membrane protein)	Regulation of MHC class II antigen processing compartments	DC	Unknown
CD209	DC-SIGN (DC-specific ICAM-3- grabbing nonintegrin)	Adhesion	DC	CD50 (ICAM-3)
CDw210	IL-10 receptor	Cytokine receptor	T, B, NK, Mo, Mφ	IL-10
CD212	IL-12 receptor	Cytokine receptor	*T, *NK	IL-12
CD213a1	IL-13 receptor α1	Cytokine receptor	B, Mo, fibroblasts, endothelial cells	IL-13

(Continued)

CD markers (*continued*)

CD	Identity	Function	Cellular distribution	Ligands
CD213a2	IL-13 receptor α2	Cytokine receptor	B, Mo, fibroblasts, endothelial cells	IL-13
CDw217	IL-17 receptor	Cytokine receptor	Widespread	IL-17
CD220	Insulin receptor	Hormone receptor	Muscle, adipose tissue, hepatocytes	Insulin
CD221	Insulin-like growth factor 1 (IGF-1) receptor	Cell survival	Bone, cartilage, muscle, adipose tissue	IGF-1
CD222	Mannose 6-phosphate receptor, insulin-like growth factor II receptor	Lysosomal sorting & internalization	Widespread	Molecules bearing mannose 6-phosphate
CD223	Lymphocyte activation gene 3 (LAG-3)	Lymphocyte activation	*T, *NK	MHC class II
CD224	γ-glutamyl transpeptidase (GGT)	Involved in uptake of extracellular glutathione	T, B, liver, kidney	Glutathione
CD225	Leu13	Component of CD19/CD21/CD81/CD225 signal transduction complex	Widespread	—
CD226	DNAM-1, PTA1	Adhesion, activation	NK, Plt, Mo, T(sub), B(sub)	Unknown
CD227	MUC1	Modulation of adhesion, signaling	T, DC, Mo, B, FDC, glandular and ductal epithelium	CD54, CD62E, Grb2
CD228	Melanotransferrin	Iron transport	Melanoma cells	Iron
CD229	Ly9	Adhesion	T, B	Unknown
CD230	PrP (prion protein)	Signal transduction?	Widespread	Unknown (plasminogen binds to the misfolded form of PrP)
CD231	TALLA-1, A15	Unknown	T cell ALL	Unknown
CD232	Plexin C1	Receptor for VESP	B	Virally-encoded semaphorin (VESP)
CD233	Band 3	Anion exchange	Erythrocytes	Chloride and bicarbonate
CD234	Duffy antigen receptor for chemokines (DARC)	Chemokine receptor	Erythrocytes, endothelium, epithelium, neurons	CXCL8 (IL-8), CCL5 (RANTES), CCL2 (MCP-1), *Plasmodium vivax*
CD235a	Glycophorin A	Mechanical stability & elastic properties of erythrocytes	Erythrocytes, endothelium, epithelium	*Plasmodium falciparum*
CD235b	Glycophorin B	Mechanical stability & elastic properties of erythrocytes	Erythrocytes, endothelium, epithelium	*Plasmodium falciparum*
CD235ab	Glycophorin A/B	Mechanical stability & elastic properties of erythrocytes	Erythrocytes, endothelium, epithelium	*Plasmodium falciparum*
CD236	Glycophorin C/D	Mechanical stability & elastic properties of erythrocytes	Erythrocytes, endothelium	—
CD236R	Glycophorin C	Mechanical stability & elastic properties of erythrocytes	Erythrocytes, endothelium	—
CD238	Kell blood group	Endopeptidase cleaves the endothelin-3 precursor (big ET3) to produce the multifunctional bioactive peptide ET3	Erythrocytes, myeloid progenitors	Big endothelin-3

(*Continued on p. 462*)

CD markers (*continued*)

CD	Identity	Function	Cellular distribution	Ligands
CD239	B-CAM (B-cell adhesion molecule), Lutheran blood group	Adhesion, signaling?	Widespread	Laminin
CD240CE	Rh blood group CcEe alleles	Transporter?	Erythrocytes	Unknown
CD240D	Rh blood group D antigen	Transporter?	Erythrocytes	Unknown
CD240 DCE	Rh blood group DCcEe alleles	Transporter?	Erythrocytes	Unknown
CD241	RHAG (Rh blood group associated glycoprotein)	Ammonium transport	Erythrocytes	Ammonium
CD242	ICAM-4	Adhesion	Erythrocytes	CD11a/CD18 (LFA-1), CD11b/CD18 (Mac-1)
CD243	MDR1	P-glycoprotein drug efflux pump	SC	—
CD244	2B4	Involved in non-MHC restricted cytotoxicity	NK, T(sub)	CD48
CD245	p220/240	Unknown	T	Unknown
CD246	ALK (Anaplastic lymphoma protein kinase)	Signaling	T	Unknown
CD247	ζ chain	TCR & FcγRIIIA signaling	T, Mφ, NK	None

Abbreviations: APC, antigen-presenting cell; BM, bone marrow; T, T-cell; B, B-cell; NK, natural killer cell; Mo, monocyte; Mφ, macrophage; Gr, granulocytes (neutrophils, basophils, eosinophils); Plt, platelet; LC, Langerhans' cell; DC, interdigitating dendritic cell; FDC, follicular dendritic cell; SC, stem cell; *, activated; (mat), mature; (sub), subset; EBV, Epstein–Barr virus; ECM, extracellular matrix; VWF, von Willebrand factor. Further information on each CD antigen can be freely accessed through Protein Reviews on the Web (PROW: Shaw S., Turni L.A. and Katz K.S. [editors], http://www.ncbi.nlm.nih.gov/prow). Another excellent reference source is *The Leucocyte Antigen Facts* book (Barclay A.N., Brown M.H., Law S.K.A., McKnight A.J., Tomlinson M.G. and van der Merwe P.A. 2nd edn, 1997, Academic Press, London).

Glossary

acquired immune response: Immunity mediated by lymphocytes and characterized by antigen-specificity and memory.

acute phase proteins: Serum proteins, mostly produced in the liver, which rapidly change in concentration (some increase, some decrease) during the initiation of an inflammatory response.

adjuvant: Any substance which nonspecifically enhances the immune response to antigen.

affinity (intrinsic affinity): The strength of binding (affinity constant) between a receptor (e.g. one antigen-binding site on an antibody) and a ligand (e.g. epitope on an antigen).

allele: Variants of a polymorphic gene at a given genetic locus.

allelic exclusion: The phenomenon whereby, following successful rearrangement of one allele of an antigen receptor gene, rearrangement of the other parental allele is suppressed, thereby ensuring each lymphocyte expresses only a single specificity of antigen receptor (although this does not occur for α chains in T-cells).

allergen: An antigen which causes allergy.

allergy: IgE-mediated hypersensitivity, e.g. asthma, eczema, hayfever and food allergy.

allogeneic: Refers to the genetic differences between individuals of the same species.

allograft: Tissue or organ graft between allogeneic individuals.

allotype: An allelic variant of an antigen which, because it is not present in all individuals, may be immunogenic in members of the same species which have a different version of the allele.

alternative pathway (of complement activation): Activation pathway involving complement components C3, Factor B, Factor D, and Properdin which, in the presence of a stabilizing activator surface such as microbial polysaccharide, generates the alternative pathway C3 convertase $\overline{C3bBb}$.

anaphylatoxin: A substance (e.g. C3a, C4a or C5a) capable of directly triggering mast cell degranulation.

anaphylaxis: An often fatal hypersensitivity reaction, triggered by IgE or anaphylatoxin-mediated mast cell degranulation, leading to anaphylactic shock due to vasodilatation and smooth muscle contraction.

anergy: Potentially reversible specific immunological tolerance in which the lymphocyte becomes functionally nonresponsive.

antibody-dependent cellular cytotoxicity (ADCC): A cytotoxic reaction in which an antibody-coated target cell is directly killed by an Fc receptor-bearing leukocyte, e.g. NK cell, macrophage or neutrophil.

antigen: Any molecule capable of being recognized by an antibody or T-cell receptor.

antigen-presenting cell (APC): A term most commonly used when referring to cells that present processed antigenic peptide and MHC class II molecules to the T-cell receptor on CD4$^+$ T-cells, e.g. macrophages, dendritic cells, B-cells. Note, however, that most types of cell are able to present antigenic peptides with MHC class I to CD8$^+$ T-cells, e.g. as occurs with virally infected cells.

antigenic determinant: A cluster of epitopes (*see* epitope).

apoptosis: A form of programmed cell death, characterized by endonuclease digestion of DNA.

atopic allergy: IgE-mediated hypersensitivity, i.e. asthma, eczema, hayfever and food allergy.

autologous: From the same individual.

avidity (functional affinity): The binding strength between two molecules (e.g. antibody and antigen) taking into account the valency of the interaction. Thus the avidity will always be equal to or greater than the intrinsic affinity (*see* affinity).

β_2-microglobulin: A 12 kDa protein, not itself encoded within the MHC, but forming part of the structure of MHC class I-encoded molecules.

B-1/B-2 cells: The two major subpopulations of B lymphocytes. B-1 cells bear high levels of surface IgM, lower levels of surface IgD, are CD43$^+$, CD23$^-$ and most express the cell surface antigen CD5; they are self-renewing, and frequently secrete high levels of antibody which binds to a range of antigens ('polyspecificity') with a relatively low affinity. The majority of B cells, however, are B-2 which express low levels of surface IgM, higher levels of surface IgD, do not express CD5, and are CD43⁻, CD23⁺; they are directly generated from precursors in the bone marrow, and secrete highly specific antibody.

basophil: A type of granulocyte found in the blood and resembling the tissue mast cell.

BCG (bacille Calmette–Guérin): Attenuated *Mycobacterium tuberculosis* used both as a specific vaccine for tuberculosis and as an adjuvant.

biolistics: The use of small particles, e.g. colloidal gold, as a vehicle for carrying agents (drugs, nucleic acid, etc.) into a cell. Following coating with the desired agent(s), the particles are fired into the dermis of the recipient using a helium-powered gun.

bispecific antibody: An artificially produced hybrid antibody in which each of the two antigen-binding arms is specific for a different antigenic epitope. Such antibodies, which can be produced either by chemical cross-linkage or by recombinant DNA techniques, can be used to link together two different antigens or cells, e.g. a cytotoxic T-cell and a tumor cell.

bursa of Fabricius: A primary lymphoid organ in avian species, located at the cloacal-hind gut junction; it is the site of B-cell maturation.

capping: An active process whereby cross-linking of cell surface molecules (e.g. by antibody) leads to aggregation and subsequent migration of the molecules to one pole of the cell.

carrier: Any molecule which when conjugated to a non-immunogenic molecule (e.g. a hapten) makes the latter immunogenic by providing epitopes for helper T-cells which the hapten lacks.

CD antigen: Cluster of differentiation designation assigned to leukocyte cell surface molecules which are identified by a given group of monoclonal antibodies.

CD3: A trimeric complex of γ, δ and ε chains which together with a $\zeta\zeta$ homodimer or $\zeta\eta$ heterodimer acts as a signal transducing unit for the T-cell receptor.

CD4: Cell surface glycoprotein, usually on helper T-cells, that recognizes MHC class II molecules on antigen-presenting cells.

CD8: Cell surface glycoprotein, usually on cytotoxic T-cells, that recognizes MHC class I molecules on target cells.

cell-mediated immunity (CMI): Refers to T-cell mediated immune responses.

chemokines: A family of structurally-related cytokines which selectively induce chemotaxis and activation of leukocytes. They also play important roles in lymphoid organ development, cell compart-

mentalization within lymphoid tissues, Th1/Th2 development, angiogenesis and wound healing.

chemotaxis: Movement of cells up a concentration gradient of chemotactic factors.

chimeric: Composite of genetically distinct individuals, e.g. following an allogeneic bone marrow graft.

class switching: The process by which a B-cell changes the class but not specificity of a given antibody it produces, e.g. switching from an IgM to an IgG antibody.

classical pathway (of complement activation): Activation pathway involving complement components C1, C2 and C4 which, following fixation of C1q, e.g. by antigen–antibody complexes, produces the classical pathway C3 convertase $C\overline{4b2a}$.

clonal deletion: A process by which contact with antigen (e.g. self antigen) at an early stage of lymphocyte differentiation leads to cell death by apoptosis.

clonal selection: The selection and activation by antigen of a lymphocyte bearing a complementary receptor, which then proliferates to form an expanded clone.

clone: Identical cells derived from a single progenitor.

colony stimulating factors (CSF): Factors that permit the proliferation and differentiation of hematopoietic cells.

complement: A group of serum proteins, some of which act in an enzymatic cascade, producing effector molecules involved in inflammation (C3a, C5a), phagocytosis (C3b), and cell lysis (C5b-9).

complementarity determining regions (CDR): The hypervariable amino acid sequences within antibody and T-cell receptor variable regions which interact with complementary amino acids on the antigen or peptide–MHC complex.

ConA (concanavalin A): A T-cell mitogen.

congenic: Animals which only differ at a single genetic locus.

conjugate: Covalently-linked complex of two or more molecules (e.g. fluorescein conjugated to antibody).

Coombs' test: Diagnostic test using anti-immunoglobulin to agglutinate antibody-coated erythrocytes.

cortex: Outer (peripheral) layer of an organ.

C-reactive protein: An acute phase protein which is able to bind to the surface of microorganisms where it functions as a stimulator of the classical pathway of complement activation, and as an opsonin for phagocytosis.

cyclophosphamide: Cytotoxic drug used as an immunosuppressive.

cyclosporin A: A T-cell specific immunosuppressive drug used to prevent graft rejection.

cytokines: Low molecular weight proteins that stimulate or inhibit the differentiation, proliferation or function of immune cells.

cytophilic: Binds to cells.

cytotoxic: Kills cells.

cytotoxic T lymphocyte (Tc): T-cells (usually CD8$^+$) which kill target cells following recognition of foreign peptide–MHC molecules on the target cell membrane.

delayed-type hypersensitivity (DTH): A hypersensitivity reaction occurring within 48–72 hours and mediated by cytokine release from sensitized T-cells.

differentiation antigen: A cell surface molecule expressed at a particular stage of development or on cells of a given lineage.

DiGeorge syndrome: Immunodeficiency caused by a congenital failure in thymic development resulting in a lack of mature functional T-cells.

diversity (D) gene segments: Found in the immunoglobulin heavy chain gene and T-cell receptor β and δ gene loci between the V and J gene segments. Encode part of the third hypervariable region in these antigen receptor chains.

edema: Swelling caused by accumulation of fluid in the tissues.

effector cells: Cells which carry out an immune function, e.g. cytokine release, cytotoxicity.

ELISA (enzyme-linked immunosorbent assay): Assay for detection or quantitation of an antibody or antigen using a ligand (e.g. an anti-immunoglobulin) conjugated to an enzyme which changes the color of a substrate.

endocytosis: Cellular ingestion of macromolecules by invagination of plasma membrane to produce an intracellular vesicle which encloses the ingested material.

endogenous: From within.

endosomes: Intracellular smooth surfaced vesicles in which endocytosed material passes on its way to the lysosomes.

endotoxin: Pathogenic cell wall-associated lipopolysaccharides of Gram-negative bacteria.

eosinophil: A class of granulocyte, the granules of which contain toxic cationic proteins.

epitope: That part of an antigen recognized by an antigen receptor (see antigenic determinant).

Epstein–Barr virus (EBV): The virus responsible for infectious mononucleosis and Burkitt's lymphoma. Used to immortalize human B-cells in vitro.

equivalence: The ratio of antibody to antigen at which immunoprecipitation of the reactants is virtually complete.

erythema: The redness produced during inflammation due to erythrocytes entering tissue spaces.

erythropoiesis: Erythrocyte production.

exotoxin: Pathogenic protein secreted by bacteria.

exudate: The extravascular fluid (containing proteins and cellular debris) which accumulates during inflammation.

Fab: Monovalent antigen-binding fragment obtained following papain digestion of immunoglobulin. Consists of an intact light chain and the N-terminal V_H and C_H1 domains of the heavy chain.

F(ab')$_2$: Bivalent antigen-binding fragment obtained following pepsin digestion of immunoglobulin. Consists of both light chains and the N-terminal part of both heavy chains linked by disulfide bonds.

Fas: A member of the TNF receptor gene family. Engagement of Fas (CD95) on the surface of the cell by the Fas ligand (CD178) present on cytotoxic cells, can trigger apoptosis in the Fas-bearing target cell.

Fc: Crystallizable, non-antigen binding fragment of an immunoglobulin molecule obtained following papain digestion. Consists of the C-terminal portion of both heavy chains which is responsible for binding to Fc receptors and C1q.

Fc receptors: Cell surface receptors which bind the Fc portion of particular immunoglobulin classes.

fibroblast: Connective tissue cell which produces collagen and plays an important part in wound healing.

fluorescein isothiocyanate (FITC): Green fluorescent dye used to 'tag' antibodies for use in immunofluorescence.

fluorescent antibody: An antibody conjugated to a fluorescent dye such as FITC.

follicular dendritic cell: MHC class II-negative Fc receptor-positive dendritic cells which bear immune complexes on their surface and are probably involved in the generation of antibody-secreting cells and maintenance of B-cell memory in germinal centres. (N.B. a different cell type to interdigitating dendritic cells).

framework regions: The relatively conserved amino acid sequences which flank the hypervariable regions in immunoglobulin and T-cell receptor variable regions and maintain a common overall structure for all V-region domains.

Freund's adjuvant: Complete Freund's adjuvant is an emulsion of aqueous antigen in mineral oil that contains heat-killed Mycobacteria. Incomplete Freund's adjuvant lacks the Mycobacteria.

gammaglobulin: The serum proteins, mostly immunoglobulins, which have the greatest mobility towards the cathode during electrophoresis.

germ line: The arrangement of the genetic material as transmitted through the gametes.

germinal center: Discrete areas within lymph node and spleen where B-cell maturation and memory development occur.

giant cell: Large multinucleate cell derived from fused macrophages and often present in granulomas.

glomerulonephritis: Inflammation of renal glomerular capillary loops, often resulting from immune complex deposition.

graft versus host (g.v.h.) reaction: Reaction occurring when T lymphocytes present in a graft recognize and attack host cells.

granulocyte: Myeloid cells containing cytoplasmic granules (i.e. neutrophils, eosinophils and basophils).

granuloma: A tissue nodule containing proliferating lymphocytes, fibroblasts, and giant cells and epithelioid cells (both derived from activated macrophages), which forms due to inflammation in response to chronic infection or persistence of antigen in the tissues.

granzymes: Serine esterases present in the granules of cytotoxic T lymphocytes and NK cells. They induce apoptosis in the target cell which they enter through perforin channels inserted into the target cell membrane by the cytotoxic lymphocyte.

gut-associated lymphoid tissue (GALT): Includes Peyer's patches, appendix, and solitary lymphoid nodules in the submucosa.

H-2: The mouse major histocompatibility complex (MHC).

haplotype: The set of allelic variants present at a given genetic region.

hapten: A low molecular weight molecule that is recognized by preformed antibody but is not itself immunogenic unless conjugated to a 'carrier' molecule which provides epitopes recognized by helper T-cells.

helper T lymphocyte (Th): A subclass of T-cells which provide help (in the form of cytokines and/or cognate interactions) necessary for the expression of effector function by other cells in the immune system.

hemagglutinin: Any molecule which agglutinates erythrocytes.

hematopoiesis: The production of erythrocytes and leukocytes.

high endothelial venule (HEV): Capillary venule composed of specialized endothelial cells allowing migration of lymphocytes into lymphoid organs.

hinge region: Amino acids between the Fab and Fc regions of immunoglobulin which permit flexibility of the molecule.

histamine: Vasoactive amine present in basophil and mast cell granules which, following degranulation, causes increased vascular permeability and smooth muscle contraction.

HLA (*h***uman ***l***eukocyte ***a***ntigen):** The human major histocompatibility complex (MHC).

humanized antibody: A genetically engineered monoclonal antibody of non-human origin in which all but the antigen-binding CDR sequences have been replaced with sequences derived from human antibodies. This procedure is carried out to minimize the immunogenicity of therapeutic monoclonal antibodies.

humoral: Pertaining to extracellular fluid such as plasma and lymph. The term humoral immunity is used to denote antibody-mediated immune responses.

hybridoma: Hybrid cell line obtained by fusing a lymphoid tumor cell with a lymphocyte which then has both the immortality of the tumor cell and the effector function (e.g. monoclonal antibody secretion) of the lymphocyte.

hypersensitivity: Excessive immune response which leads to undesirable consequences, e.g. tissue or organ damage.

hypervariable regions: Those amino acid sequences within the immunoglobulin and T-cell receptor variable regions which show the greatest variability and contribute most to the antigen or peptide–MHC binding site.

idiotope: An epitope made up of amino acids within the variable region of an antibody or T-cell receptor which reacts with an anti-idiotope.

idiotype: The complete set of idiotopes in the variable region of an antibody or T-cell receptor which react with an anti-idiotypic serum.

idiotype network: A regulatory network based on interactions of idiotypes and anti-idiotypes present on antibodies and T-cell receptors.

immune complex: Complex of antibody bound to antigen which may also contain complement components.

immunoadsorption: Method for removal of antibody or antigen by allowing it to bind to solid phase antigen or antibody.

immunofluorescence: Technique for detection of cell or tissue-associated antigens by the use of a fluorescently-tagged ligand (e.g. an anti-immunoglobulin conjugated to fluorescein isothiocyanate).

immunogen: Any substance which elicits an immune response. Whilst all immunogens are antigens, not all antigens are immunogens (*see* hapten).

immunoglobulin superfamily: Large family of proteins characterized by possession of 'immunoglobulin-type' domains of approximately 110 amino acids folded into two β-pleated sheets. Members include immunoglobulins, T-cell receptors and MHC molecules.

immunological synapse: A contact point between the T-cell and antigen-presenting cell which is generated by reorganization and clustering of cell surface molecules in lipid rafts. The synapse facilitates interactions between TCR and MHC and between adhesion molecules, thereby potentiating the TCR-mediated activation signal.

inflammation: The tissue response to trauma, characterized by increased blood flow and entry of leukocytes into the tissues, resulting in swelling, redness, elevated temperature and pain.

innate immunity: Immunity which is not intrinsically affected by prior contact with antigen, i.e. all aspects of immunity not directly mediated by lymphocytes.

interdigitating dendritic cell: MHC class II-positive, Fc receptor-negative, antigen-presenting dendritic cell found in T-cell areas of lymph nodes and spleen. (N.B. a different cell type to follicular dendritic cells).

interferons (IFN): IFNα is derived from various leukocytes, IFNβ from fibroblasts and IFNγ from T lymphocytes. All three types induce an anti-viral state in cells and IFNγ acts as a cytokine in the regulation of immune responses.

interleukins (IL): Designation for some of the cytokines secreted by leukocytes.

internal image: An epitope on an anti-idiotype which binds in a way that structurally and functionally mimics the antigen.

invariant chain: A polypeptide which binds MHC class II molecules in the endoplasmic reticulum, directs them to the late endosomal compartment and prevents premature association with self peptides.

Ir (*immune response*) **genes:** The genes, including those within the MHC, that together determine the overall level of immune response to a given antigen.

isotype: An antibody constant region structure present in all normal individuals, i.e. antibody class or subclass.

ITAM: *Immunoreceptor Tyrosine-based Activation Motifs* are consensus sequences for src-family tyrosine kinases. These motifs are found in the cytoplasmic domains of several signaling molecules including the signal transduction units of lymphocyte antigen receptors and of Fc receptors.

ITIM: *Immunoreceptor Tyrosine-based Inhibitory Motifs* present in the cytoplasmic domains of certain cell surface molecules, e.g. Fcγ RIIB, inhibitory NK cell receptors, and which mediate inhibitory signals.

J chain: A molecule which forms part of the structure of pentameric IgM and dimeric IgA.

joining (J) gene segments: Found in the immunoglobulin and T-cell receptor gene loci and, upon gene rearrangement, encode part of the third hypervariable region of the antigen receptors.

K (killer) cell: Large granular lymphocyte which mediates antibody-dependent cellular cytotoxicity (ADCC), is Fc receptor positive, but does not rearrange or express either immunoglobulin or T-cell receptor genes.

kinins: A family of polypeptides released during inflammatory responses and which increase vascular permeability and smooth muscle contraction.

KIRs: *Killer* cell *Immunoglobulin-like Receptors* found on NK cells, some $\gamma\delta$ and some $\alpha\beta$ T-cells. KIRs recognize MHC class I molecules and, like the C-type lectin receptors also found on these cells, can either inhibit or activate the killer cells. If ITIM sequences are present in their cytoplasmic domain they are inhibitory. KIRs lacking ITIMs can associate with ITAM-containing adaptor molecules, in which case they can activate the killer cell.

knockout: The use of homologous genetic recombination in embryonal stem cells to replace a functional gene with a defective copy of the gene. The animals that are produced by this technique can be bred to homozygosity, thus allowing the generation of a null phenotype for that gene product.

Kupffer cells: Fixed tissue macrophages lining the blood sinuses in the liver.

Langerhans' cell: Fc receptor and MHC class II-positive antigen-presenting dendritic cell found in the skin.

large granular lymphocyte (LGL): Large lymphocytes which contain cytoplasmic granules and function as natural killer (NK) and killer (K) cells. Activated CD8$^+$ cytotoxic T lymphocytes (Tc) also assume an LGL morphology.

lectins: A family of proteins, mostly of plant origin, which bind specific sugars on glycoproteins and glycolipids. Some lectins are mitogenic (e.g. PHA, ConA).

leukotrienes: Metabolic products of arachidonic acid which promote inflammatory processes (e.g. chemotaxis, increased vascular permeability) and are produced by a variety of cell types including mast cells, basophils and macrophages.

ligand: General term for a molecule recognized by a binding structure such as a receptor.

linkage disequilibrium: The occurrence of two alleles being inherited together at a greater frequency than that expected from the product of their individual frequencies.

lipid raft: Cholesterol- and glycosphingolipid-rich

membrane subdomain in which molecules involved in cellular activation become concentrated.

lipopolysaccharide (LPS): Endotoxin derived from Gram-negative bacterial cell walls which has inflammatory and mitogenic actions.

lymph: The tissue fluid which drains into and through the lymphatic system.

lymphadenopathy: Enlarged lymph nodes.

lymphokine: Cytokine produced by lymphocytes.

lymphokine-activated killer cells (LAK): Killer (K) and natural killer (NK) cells activated *in vitro* by IL-2 to give enhanced killing of target cells.

Lymphotoxin (also called TNFβ): A T-cell derived cytokine which is cytotoxic for certain tumor cells and also has immunoregulatory functions.

lysosomes: Cytoplasmic granules containing hydrolytic enzymes involved in the digestion of phagocytosed material.

lysozyme: Anti-bacterial enzyme present in phagocytic cell granules, tears and saliva, which digests peptidoglycans in bacterial cell walls.

macrophage: Large phagocytic cell, derived from the blood monocyte, which also functions as an antigen-presenting cell and can mediate ADCC.

mannose binding protein: A member of the collectin family of calcium-dependent lectins, and an acute phase protein. It functions as a stimulator of the classical pathway of complement activation, and as an opsonin for phagocytosis by binding to mannose, a sugar residue usually found in an exposed form only on the surface of microorganisms.

marginal zone: The outer area of the splenic periarteriolar lymphoid sheath (PALS) which is rich in B cells, particularly those responding to thymus-independent antigens.

margination: Leukocyte adhesion to the endothelium of blood vessels in the early phase of an acute inflammatory reaction.

mast cell: A tissue cell with abundant granules which resembles the blood basophil. Both these cell types bear Fc receptors for IgE, which when crosslinked by IgE and antigen cause degranulation and the release of a number of mediators including histamine and leukotrienes.

medulla: Inner (central) region of an organ.

megakaryocyte: A bone marrow precursor of platelets.

membrane attack complex (MAC): Complex of complement components C5b–C9 which inserts as a pore into the membrane of target cells leading to cell lysis.

memory (immunological): A characteristic of the acquired immune response of lymphocytes whereby a second encounter with a given antigen produces a secondary immune response; faster, greater and longer lasting than the primary immune response.

memory cells: Clonally expanded T- and B-cells produced during a primary immune response and which are 'primed' to mediate a secondary immune response to the original antigen.

MHC (*m*ajor *h*istocompatibility *c*omplex): A genetic region encoding molecules involved in antigen presentation to T-cells. Class I MHC molecules are present on virtually all nucleated cells and are encoded mainly by the H-2K, D, and L loci in mice and by HLA-A, B, and C in man, whilst class II MHC molecules are expressed on antigen-presenting cells (primarily macrophages, B-cells and interdigitating dendritic cells) and are encoded by H-2A and E in mice and HLA-DR, DQ, and DP in man. Allelic differences can be associated with the most intense graft rejection within a species.

MHC restriction: The necessity that T-cells recognize processed antigen only when presented by MHC molecules of the original haplotype associated with T-cell priming.

minor histocompatibility antigens: Non-MHC-encoded cell surface processed peptides which, in association with MHC-encoded molecules, contribute to graft rejection, albeit not usually as severe as that due to MHC mismatch.

mitogen: A substance which non-specifically induces lymphocyte proliferation.

mixed lymphocyte reaction (MLR): A T-cell proliferative response induced by cells expressing allogeneic MHC.

monoclonal antibody: Homogeneous antibody derived from a single B-cell clone and therefore all bearing identical antigen-binding sites and isotype.

monocyte: Mononuclear phagocyte found in blood and which is the precursor of the tissue macrophage.

mononuclear phagocyte system: A system comprising blood monocytes and tissue macrophages.

mucosal-associated lymphoid tissue (MALT): Lymphoid tissue present in the surface mucosa of the respiratory, gastrointestinal and genitourinary tracts.

multiple myeloma: Plasma cell malignancy resulting in high levels of monoclonal immunoglobulin in serum and of free light chains (Bence–Jones protein) in urine.

murine: Pertaining to mice.

myeloma protein: Monoclonal antibody secreted by myeloma cells.

negative selection: Deletion by apoptosis in the thymus of T-cells which recognize self peptides presented by self MHC molecules, thus preventing the development of autoimmune T-cells. Negative selection of developing B-cells is also thought to occur if they encounter high levels of self antigen in the bone marrow.

neutrophil: The major circulating phagocytic polymorphonuclear granulocyte. Enters tissues early in an inflammatory response and is also able to mediate antibody-dependent cellular cytotoxicity (ADCC).

NK (natural killer) cell: Large granular lymphocyte which does not rearrange nor express either immunoglobulin or T-cell receptor genes but is able to recognize and destroy certain tumor and virally-infected cells in an MHC and antibody-independent manner.

NK-T cell: NK1.1$^+$ lymphoid cells with a morphology and granule content intermediate between T-cells and NK cells. They are potent producers of IL-4, may be CD4$^-$8$^-$ or CD4$^+$8$^-$, and express low levels of $\alpha\beta$ TCR with an invariant α chain and very restricted β chain specificity. Many of these TCR recognize antigens presented by the non-classical MHC-like molecule CD1. Their lectin-like NK1.1 receptor may recognize microbial carbohydrates.

nude mouse: Mouse which is T-cell deficient due to a homozygous gene defect (*nu/nu*) resulting in the absence of a thymus (and also lack of body hair).

oncofetal antigen: Antigen whose expression is normally restricted to the fetus but which may be expressed during malignancy in adults.

opsonin: Substance, e.g. antibody or C3b, which enhances phagocytosis by promoting adhesion of the antigen to the phagocyte.

opsonization: Coating of antigen with opsonin to enhance phagocytosis.

PAF (platelet activating factor): An alkyl phospholipid released by a variety of cell types including mast cells and basophils, which has immunoregulatory effects on lymphocytes and monocytes/macrophages as well as causing platelet aggregation and degranulation.

paracortex: The part of an organ (e.g. lymph node) which lies between the cortex and the medulla.

pathogen-associated molecular pattern (PAMP): Molecules such as lipopolysaccharide, peptidoglycan, lipoteichoic acids and mannans, which are widely expressed by microbial pathogens as repetitive motifs but are not present on host tissues. They are therefore utilized by the pattern recognition receptors (PRRs) of the immune system to distinguish pathogens from self antigens.

pattern recognition receptor (PRR): Receptors on professional antigen-presenting cells and phagocytes which enable them to recognize pathogen-associated molecular patterns (PAMPs). Amongst the large number of different PRRs are the mannose receptor (CD206) and the macrophage scavenger receptor (CD204).

perforin: Molecule produced by cytotoxic T-cells and NK cells which, like complement component C9, polymerizes to form a pore in the membrane of the target cell leading to cell death.

periarteriolar lymphoid sheath (PALS): The lymphoid tissue which forms the white pulp of the spleen.

Peyer's patches: Part of the gut associated lymphoid tissue (GALT) and found as distinct lymphoid nodules mainly in the small intestine.

PHA (phytohemagglutinin): A plant lectin which acts as a T-cell mitogen.

phage antibody library: A collection of cloned antibody variable region gene sequences which can be expressed as Fab or scFv fusion proteins with bacteriophage coat proteins. These can be displayed on the surface of the phages. The gene encoding a monoclonal recombinant antibody is enclosed in the phage particle and can be selected from the library by binding of the phage to specific antigen.

phagocyte: Cells, including monocytes/macrophages and neutrophils, which are specialized for the engulfment of cellular and particulate matter.

phagolysosome: Intracellular vacuole where killing and digestion of phagocytosed material occurs following the fusion of a phagosome with a lysosome.

phagosome: Intracellular vacuole produced following invagination of the cell membrane around phagocytosed material.

phorbol myristate acetate (PMA): A mitogenic phorbol ester which directly stimulates protein kinase C and acts as a tumor promoter.

plaque forming cell (PFC): Antibody-secreting plasma cell detected *in vitro* by its ability to produce a 'plaque' of lysed antigen-sensitized erythrocytes in the presence of complement.

plasma cell: Terminally differentiated B lymphocyte which actively secretes large amounts of antibody.

pokeweed mitogen (PWM): A plant lectin which is a T-cell dependent B-cell mitogen.

polyclonal: Many different clones, or the product of many different clones, e.g. polyclonal antiserum.

poly-Ig receptor: A receptor molecule which specifically binds J-chain containing polymeric Ig, i.e. dimeric secretory IgA and pentameric IgM, and transports it across mucosal epithelium.

positive selection: The selection of those developing T-cells in the thymus which are able to recognize self

MHC molecules. This occurs by preventing apoptosis in these cells.

precipitin: Precipitate of antibody and multivalent antigen due to the formation of high molecular weight complexes.

primary immune response: The relatively weak immune response which occurs upon the first encounter of naive lymphocytes with a given antigen.

primary lymphoid organs: The sites at which immunocompetent lymphocytes develop, i.e. bone marrow and thymus in mammals.

prime: The process of giving an initial sensitization to antigen.

prostaglandins: Acidic lipids derived from arachidonic acid which are able to increase vascular permeability, mediate fever, and can both stimulate and inhibit immunological responses.

proteasome: Cytoplasmic proteolytic enzyme complex involved in antigen processing for association with MHC.

protein A: *Staphylococcus aureus* cell wall protein which binds to the Fc region of IgG.

protein tyrosine kinases: Enzymes which are able to phosphorylate proteins on tyrosines, and often act in a cascade-like fashion in the signal transduction systems of cells.

prozone effect: The loss of immune precipitation or agglutination which occurs when antibody concentration is increased to an extent that the antibody is in such excess that it is no longer able to effectively cross-link the antigen. A similar phenomenon may occur in antigen excess.

Qa antigens: 'Non-classical' MHC class I molecules of mice.

recombination signal sequence (RSS): Conserved heptamer (7-nucleotide)-nonamer (9-nucleotide) sequences, separated by a 12 or 23 base spacer, which occur 3' of variable gene segments, 5' and 3' of diversity gene segments, and 5' of joining gene segments, in both immunoglobulin and T cell receptor genes. They function as recognition sequences for the recombinase enzymes that mediate the gene rearrangement process involved in the generation of lymphocyte antigen receptor diversity.

respiratory burst: The increased oxidative metabolism which occurs in phagocytic cells following activation.

reticuloendothelial system (RES): A rather old term for the network of phagocytes and endothelial cells throughout the body.

rheumatoid factor: IgM, IgG and IgA autoantibodies to IgG, particularly the Fc region.

rosette: Particles or cells bound to the surface of a lymphocyte (e.g. sheep erythrocytes around a human T-cell).

scFv: A single chain molecule composed of the variable regions of an antibody heavy and light chain joined together by a flexible linker.

SCID (*severe combined immunodeficiency*)**:** Immunodeficiency affecting both T and B lymphocytes.

secondary immune response: The qualitatively and quantitatively improved immune response which occurs upon the second encounter of primed lymphocytes with a given antigen.

secretory component: Proteolytic cleavage product of the poly-Ig receptor which remains associated with dimeric IgA in sero-mucus secretions.

secretory IgA: Dimeric IgA found in sero-mucus secretions.

somatic hypermutation: The enhanced rate of point mutation in the immunoglobulin variable region genes which occurs following antigenic stimulation and acts as a mechanism for increasing antibody diversity and affinity.

stem cell: Multipotential cell from which differentiated cells derive.

superantigen: An antigen which reacts with all the T-cells belonging to a particular T-cell receptor V region family, and which therefore stimulates (or deletes) a much larger number of cells than does conventional antigen.

surface plasmon resonance: A technique based upon changes in the angle of reflected light which occur upon ligand binding to an immobilized target molecule on a biosensor chip. This permits the observation of protein–protein interactions (such as antibody binding to an antigen) in 'real-time', i.e. by continuous monitoring of the association and dissociation of the reversible reaction.

switch sequences: Highly conserved repetitive sequences which mediate class switching in the immunoglobulin heavy chain gene locus.

syngeneic: Genetically identical, e.g. a fully inbred strain of mice.

TAP: The *T*ransporters associated with *A*ntigen *P*rocessing (TAP-1 and TAP-2) are molecules which carry antigenic peptides from the cytoplasm into the lumen of the endoplasmic reticulum for incorporation into MHC class I molecules.

T-cell receptor (TCR): The heterodimeric antigen receptor of the T lymphocyte exists in two alternative forms, consisting of α and β chains, or γ and δ chains. The αβ TCR recognizes peptide fragments of protein antigens presented by MHC molecules on cell surfaces. The function of the γδ TCR is less clearly defined but it can recognize native proteins on the cell surface.

T-dependent antigen: An antigen which requires helper T-cells in order to elicit an antibody response.

T-independent antigen: An antigen which is able to elicit an antibody response in the absence of T-cells.

thymocyte: Developing T-cell in the thymus.

titer: Measure of the relative 'strength' (a combination of amount and avidity) of an antibody or antiserum, usually given as the highest dilution which is still operationally detectable in, for example, an ELISA.

tolerance: Specific immunological unresponsiveness.

tolerogen: An antigen used to induce tolerance. Often depends more on the circumstances of administration (e.g. route and concentration) than on any inherent property of the molecule.

toxoid: Chemically or physically modified toxin that is no longer harmful but retains immunogenicity.

tumor necrosis factor (TNF, also called TNFα): Together with the related cytokine lymphotoxin (TNFβ), was originally named for its cytotoxic effect on certain tumor cells, but also has immunoregulatory functions.

variable (V) gene segments: Genes that rearrange together with D (diversity) and J (joining) gene segments in order to encode the variable region amino acid sequences of immunoglobulins and T-cell receptors.

vasoactive amines: Substances including histamine and 5-hydroxytryptamine which increase vascular permeability and smooth muscle contraction.

xenogeneic: Genetic differences between species.

xenograft: A tissue or organ graft between individuals of different species.

Index